Textbook of Pharmaceutics

Textbook of Pharmaceutics

Edited by **Reginald Thornburg**

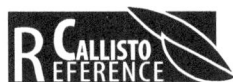

R CALLISTO REFERENCE

New York

Published by Callisto Reference,
106 Park Avenue, Suite 200,
New York, NY 10016, USA
www.callistoreference.com

Textbook of Pharmaceutics
Edited by Reginald Thornburg

International Standard Book Number: 978-1-63239-757-7 (Hardback)

Printed in the United States of America.

Contents

Preface

This book was inspired by the evolution of our times; to answer the curiosity of inquisitive minds. Many developments have occurred across the globe in the recent past which has transformed the progress in the field.

Pharmaceutics is the science of designing drug dosages. It has three subfields namely formulation science, biopharmaceutics and pharmacokinetics. After the formulation and production of an important drug, it is very essential to find the required proportion in which a drug is required. This discipline tries to study the interaction of various quantities of dosages of the formulated drug with the human body, its effects and optimum concentration. This book is a valuable compilation of topics, ranging from the basic to the most complex advancements in this field. For someone with an interest and eye for detail, this book covers the most significant topics in the field of pharmaceutics. It will serve as a valuable source of reference for pharmacologists, researchers and students.

This book was developed from a mere concept to drafts to chapters and finally compiled together as a complete text to benefit the readers across all nations. To ensure the quality of the content we instilled two significant steps in our procedure. The first was to appoint an editorial team that would verify the data and statistics provided in the book and also select the most appropriate and valuable contributions from the plentiful contributions we received from authors worldwide. The next step was to appoint an expert of the topic as the Editor-in-Chief, who would head the project and finally make the necessary amendments and modifications to make the text reader-friendly. I was then commissioned to examine all the material to present the topics in the most comprehensible and productive format.

I would like to take this opportunity to thank all the contributing authors who were supportive enough to contribute their time and knowledge to this project. I also wish to convey my regards to my family who have been extremely supportive during the entire project.

Editor

Spirulina platensis Lacks Antitumor Effect against Solid Ehrlich Carcinoma in Female Mice

Waleed Barakat,[1,2] Shimaa M. Elshazly,[1] and Amr A. A. Mahmoud[1]

[1]Department of Pharmacology, Faculty of Pharmacy, Zagazig University, Zagazig 44519, Egypt
[2]Department of Pharmacology, Faculty of Pharmacy, Tabuk University, Tabuk 71491, Saudi Arabia

Correspondence should be addressed to Amr A. A. Mahmoud; aamahmoud@pharmacy.zu.edu.eg

Academic Editor: Antonio Ferrer-Montiel

Spirulina is a blue-green alga used as a dietary supplement. It has been shown to possess anti-inflammatory, antioxidant, and hepatoprotective properties. This study was designed to evaluate the antitumor effect of spirulina (200 and 800 mg/kg) against a murine model of solid Ehrlich carcinoma compared to a standard chemotherapeutic drug, 5-fluorouracil (20 mg/kg). Untreated mice developed a palpable solid tumor after 13 days. Unlike fluorouracil, spirulina at the investigated two dose levels failed to exert any protective effect. In addition, spirulina did not potentiate the antitumor effect of fluorouracil when they were administered concurrently. Interestingly, their combined administration resulted in a dose-dependent increase in mortality. The present study demonstrates that spirulina lacks antitumor effect against this model of solid Ehrlich carcinoma and increased mortality when combined with fluorouracil. However, the implicated mechanism is still elusive.

1. Introduction

Cancer is considered one of the leading causes of death worldwide, accounting for approximately 8.2 million deaths in 2012. Success of cancer chemotherapy is limited by drug-induced adverse effects and multidrug resistance [1, 2]. Therefore, there is a growing interest in identifying antitumor agents of natural sources, which are effective and produce fewer side effects than the conventional chemotherapeutic drugs. Actually, many of the currently used anticancer agents originate from natural sources, such as marine organisms and plants [3, 4].

Spirulina (*Arthrospira platensis*) is a blue-green alga used as a dietary supplement. It is rich in proteins, carotenoids, polyunsaturated fatty acids, vitamin B complex, vitamin E, and minerals. Additionally, it possesses other potent antioxidants such as spirulans, C-phycocyanin, and allophycocyanin [5, 6].

Spirulina phycocyanin has been shown to possess anti-inflammatory, antioxidant, and hepatoprotective properties [7–9]. In addition, different studies demonstrated the potential anticancer activity of spirulina in different experimental models [10–12].

Ehrlich ascites carcinoma (EAC) is an undifferentiated carcinoma, which is characterized by rapid proliferation, high transplantable capability, and short life span [13]. EAC bears resemblance to human tumors; therefore, the solid and the ascetic forms of this tumor are frequently utilized to evaluate the antitumor activity of different products [14, 15].

Relying on the aforementioned, the present study was conducted to evaluate the effect of spirulina against Ehrlich solid tumor induced experimentally in mice. To our knowledge, this is the first report that describes the antitumor effect of spirulina in this experimental model of EAC solid tumor. In our attempt, we compared the effects of spirulina to a reference chemotherapeutic drug, fluorouracil, and examined the effect of their combined administration as well.

2. Materials and Methods

2.1. Animals. Adult female Swiss albino mice (23 ± 2 g) were used in the current study. Mice were acclimatized for one week before starting experiments. They were housed in stainless steel cages (5 mice/cage) and kept at controlled temperature (23 ± 2°C), humidity (60 ± 10%), and light/dark (12/12 hr) cycle. Animals had free access to food and water.

2.1.1. Ethical Statement. Experimental design and animal handling procedures were approved by the local authorities at the Faculty of Pharmacy, Zagazig University, Zagazig, Egypt—ECAHZU (Ethical Committee for Animal Handling at Zagazig University). Every effort was made to reduce the number of animals and their suffering.

2.2. Drugs. Spirulina tablets, containing 100% *Spirulina platensis* microalgae powder, were obtained from Allcura Naturheilmittel (Wertheim, Germany). 5-Fluorouracil (50 mg/mL ampoules) was obtained from Pharco Pharmaceuticals (Egypt). All other chemicals were of analytical grade. Spirulina tablets were manually crushed, ground, and then suspended in 1% gum acacia in distilled water just before administration.

2.3. Induction of Ehrlich Solid Tumor. On the day of induction (day 0), EAC cells were collected from the ascitic fluid of a female Swiss albino mouse bearing 8–10-day-old ascitic tumor obtained from the National Cancer Institute (Cairo, Egypt). The ascitic fluid was diluted with normal saline (1 : 10). Solid tumors were induced by intramuscular inoculation of 0.2 mL of ascitic fluid, containing approximately 2.5×10^6 EAC cells, in the right thigh of the hind limb of each mouse [16].

2.4. Experimental Design. On the following day (day 1), EAC-bearing mice were randomly divided into six groups ($n = 10$ each) as follows.

Group 1 (EAC). Mice were inoculated with EAC cells and received vehicle (1% gum acacia) by oral gavage daily from day 1 to 9.

Group 2 (FU). Mice were inoculated with EAC cells and received 5-fluorouracil (20 mg/kg, i.p.) daily from day 1 to 9.

Group 3 (SP200). Mice were inoculated with EAC cells and received spirulina (200 mg/kg) suspended in 1% gum acacia in distilled water by oral gavage daily from day 1 to 9.

Group 4 (SP800). Mice were inoculated with EAC cells and received spirulina (800 mg/kg) suspended in 1% gum acacia in distilled water by oral gavage daily from day 1 to 9.

Group 5 (FU/SP200). Mice were inoculated with EAC cells and received 5-fluorouracil (20 mg/kg, i.p.) plus spirulina (200 mg/kg) suspended in 1% gum acacia in distilled water by oral gavage daily from day 1 to 9.

Group 6 (FU/SP800). Mice were inoculated with EAC cells and received 5-fluorouracil (20 mg/kg, i.p.) plus spirulina (800 mg/kg) suspended in 1% gum acacia in distilled water by oral gavage daily from day 1 to 9.
     Doses of spirulina and 5-fluorouracil were chosen based on previous studies [17, 18].

2.5. Blood Sampling, Assessment of Hematological Parameters, and Serum Preparation. On day 13, mice were anaesthetized with intraperitoneal injection of urethane (2 g/kg), and blood samples were collected from the orbital sinus using heparinized microcapillary tubes as previously described [19]. Aliquot of blood was collected from each mouse into ethylenediamine tetra-acetic acid- (EDTA-) coated tubes for the analysis of hematological parameters using an automated analyzer Swelab Alfa (Boule Medical AB, Sweden). For serum preparation, another portion of blood was collected into microcentrifuge tube and then centrifuged at 3500 rpm for 15 min. Serum was stored at −20°C and thawed just before use.

2.6. Determination of Tumor Weight and Volume. After blood collection, tumor-bearing thigh of each mouse was shaved; tumors were dissected, weighed, and photographed on a graph paper. Digital images were processed using ImageJ software (National Institutes of Health, USA) in order to determine the length (mm) of the major and minor axes of the tumor. Tumor volume was calculated using the following formula [16]:

$$\text{Tumor volume } \left(\text{mm}^3 \right)$$
$$= 0.52 \times \left(\text{minor axis} \right) \times \left(\text{major axis} \right)^2 . \tag{1}$$

2.7. Determination of Alanine Transaminase Activity. Serum alanine transaminase (ALT) activity was determined colorimetrically using an ALT-kit supplied by Diamond Diagnostics (Egypt), following the manufacturer's instructions. Absorbance of the final product was read using Jenway Genova spectrophotometer supplied by Bibby Scientific (Staffordshire, UK).

2.8. Histopathological Analysis. Specimens of tumors from different groups were excised and fixed in 10% phosphate-buffered formalin solution at room temperature. Specimens were dehydrated in graded ethanol (70–100%), cleared in xylene, and embedded in paraffin. Paraffin-embedded tissue sections (5 μm thick) were prepared, mounted on slides, and kept at room temperature. Thereafter, slides were dewaxed in xylene, hydrated using graded ethanol, and stained by hematoxylin and eosin (HE) dyes. The sections were examined under light microscope and photographed with a digital camera (Canon, Japan).

2.9. Statistical Analysis. All data were expressed as mean ± standard error of mean (SEM). Statistical analysis was performed using GraphPad Prism software v.5 (GraphPad Software, Inc., La Jolla, CA, USA). The intergroup variation was measured by one-way analysis of variance (ANOVA) followed by Dunnett's posttest. A significant difference was assumed for values of $P < 0.05$.

3. Results

3.1. Effect on Mortality Rate. As represented in Table 1, there was no difference in mortality rate between untreated EAC tumor-bearing mice and 5-fluorouracil-treated mice. Only one mouse died from each group. On the other hand, treatment of tumor-bearing mice with spirulina (200 and

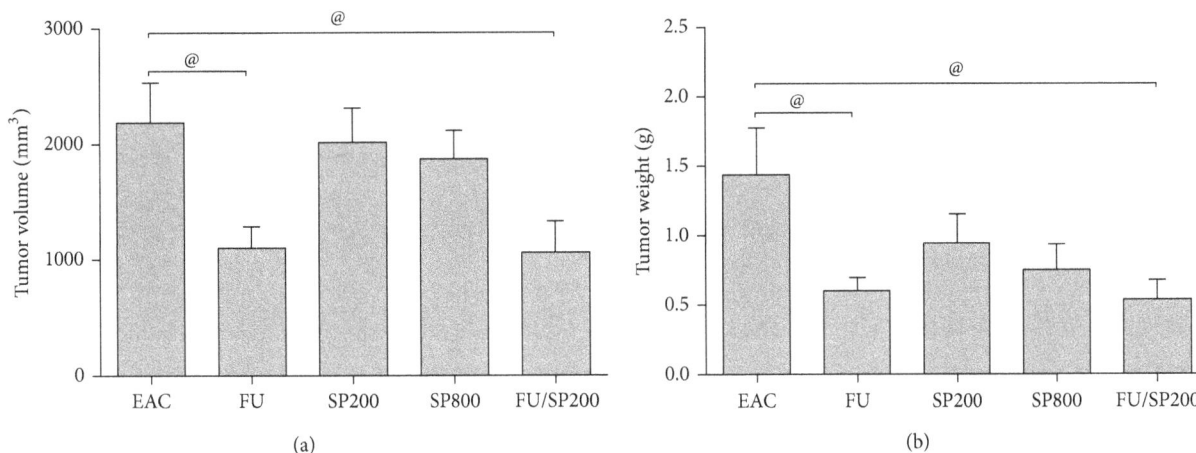

FIGURE 1: Effect of 5-fluorouracil (20 mg/kg), spirulina (200 or 800 mg/kg), and their combination on tumor volume (a) and tumor weight (b) of EAC tumor-bearing mice ($n = 5$–9). EAC: Ehrlich ascites carcinoma tumor-bearing mice; FU: Ehrlich ascites carcinoma tumor-bearing mice treated with 5-fluorouracil (20 mg/kg); SP200: Ehrlich ascites carcinoma tumor-bearing mice treated with spirulina (200 mg/kg); SP800: Ehrlich ascites carcinoma tumor-bearing mice treated with spirulina (800 mg/kg); FU/SP200: Ehrlich ascites carcinoma tumor-bearing mice treated with 5-fluorouracil (20 mg/kg) plus spirulina (200 mg/kg). Data are expressed as mean ± SEM. Statistical analysis using one-way ANOVA, followed by Dunnett's posttest. $^{@}P < 0.05$ versus EAC group.

TABLE 1: Effects of 5-fluorouracil (20 mg/kg), spirulina (200 or 800 mg/kg), and their combination on the survival of EAC tumor-bearing mice.

Group	Number tested	Survivors/total mice	% Mortality
EAC[a]	10	9/10	10%
FU[b]	10	9/10	10%
SP200[c]	10	5/10	50%
SP800[d]	10	7/10	30%
FU/SP200[e]	10	5/10	50%
FU/SP800[f]	10	1/10	90%

[a]EAC: Ehrlich ascites carcinoma tumor-bearing mice; [b]FU: Ehrlich ascites carcinoma tumor-bearing mice treated with 5-fluorouracil (20 mg/kg); [c]SP200: Ehrlich ascites carcinoma tumor-bearing mice treated with spirulina (200 mg/kg); [d]SP800: Ehrlich ascites carcinoma tumor-bearing mice treated with spirulina (800 mg/kg); [e]FU/SP200: Ehrlich ascites carcinoma tumor-bearing mice treated with 5-fluorouracil (20 mg/kg) plus spirulina (200 mg/kg); [f]FU/SP800: Ehrlich ascites carcinoma tumor-bearing mice treated with 5-fluorouracil (20 mg/kg) plus spirulina (800 mg/kg).

800 mg/kg) resulted in increased mortality rate reaching 50% and 30%, respectively. Similarly, combined administration of 5-fluorouracil plus spirulina (200 or 800 mg/kg) caused a noticeable dose-dependent increase in mortality rate in tumor-bearing mice reaching 50% and 90%, respectively. Therefore, further assessment of other parameters was not possible from mice that received fluorouracil plus spirulina (800 mg/kg) due to the high mortality rate (90%).

3.2. Effect on Tumor Weight and Volume. As depicted in Figure 1, administration of 5-fluorouracil significantly reduced tumor volume (−49.7%) and weight (−58.3%) compared to untreated EAC tumor-bearing mice ($P < 0.05$). On the other hand, treatment of tumor-bearing mice with spirulina (200 or 800 mg/kg) did not significantly reduce

either the tumor volume or tumor weight. Combined administration of 5-fluorouracil plus spirulina (200 mg/kg) diminished tumor growth as indicated by the significant reduction of tumor volume (−51.5%) and tumor weight (−62.7%) compared to untreated EAC tumor-bearing mice ($P < 0.05$). There was no significant difference between mice treated with 5-fluorouracil alone or 5-fluorouracil plus spirulina (200 mg/kg) regarding tumor volume or weight.

3.3. Effect on Hematological Parameters. Different treatment regimens used in the present study resulted in significant alterations of some hematological parameters compared to untreated tumor-bearing mice, while other parameters were not significantly altered. Hematocrit (HCT) level was significantly reduced by the administration of 5-fluorouracil (−19.7%), spirulina 200 mg/kg (−22.7%), spirulina 800 mg/kg (−19.3%), or 5-fluorouracil plus spirulina 200 mg/kg (−27.7%) compared to untreated EAC tumor-bearing mice. No significant differences were observed between group 2, treated with 5-fluorouracil alone, and group 5, treated with 5-fluorouracil plus spirulina (200 mg/kg). Similarly, mean corpuscular volume (MCV) of red blood cells (RBCs) was significantly reduced by the administration of 5-fluorouracil (−10%), spirulina 200 mg/kg (−16.2%), spirulina 800 mg/kg (−19.7%), or 5-fluorouracil plus spirulina 200 mg/kg (−22.3%) compared to untreated EAC tumor-bearing mice. Mice received 5-fluorouracil plus spirulina (200 mg/kg) showed a further significant reduction in MCV level when compared to mice treated with 5-fluorouracil alone. From all treatment regimens, only combined administration of 5-fluorouracil plus spirulina (200 mg/kg) resulted in significant elevation of both platelet count (PT) and plateletcrit (PCT) levels when compared to either untreated EAC tumor-bearing mice or fluorouracil-treated mice (Table 2).

TABLE 2: Effects of 5-fluorouracil (20 mg/kg), spirulina (200 or 800 mg/kg), and their combination on hematological parameters of EAC tumor-bearing mice.

	EAC	FU	SP200	SP800	FU/SP200
RBC (10^{12}/L)	7.6 ± 0.27	6.8 ± 0.27	6.9 ± 0.77	7.7 ± 0.48	7.1 ± 0.36
HGB (g/L)	11.4 ± 0.37	9.8 ± 0.41	10.1 ± 1.1	10.8 ± 0.65	10.3 ± 0.45
HCT (%)	46.8 ± 1.3	37.6 ± 1.5[a]	36.1 ± 4.1[a]	37.8 ± 2.3[a]	33.8 ± 1.5[a]
MCV (fL)	61.5 ± 0.9	55.3 ± 2.3[a]	51.6 ± 0.6[a]	49.4 ± 1.5[a]	47.8 ± 1.5[ab]
PT (10^9/L)	737 ± 64	959 ± 102	947 ± 39	806 ± 80	1403 ± 160[ab]
PCT (%)	0.47 ± 0.05	0.69 ± 0.08	0.59 ± 0.04	0.54 ± 0.07	1.0 ± 0.12[ab]
WBC (10^9/L)	8.1 ± 0.81	6.2 ± 1.4	10.2 ± 2.1	10.7 ± 2.0	8.9 ± 3.3
LYM (10^9/L)	7.3 ± 0.75	4.9 ± 0.97	7.8 ± 1.6	7.3 ± 1.3	6.9 ± 2.3
GRA (10^9/L)	0.28 ± 0.08	0.41 ± 0.17	0.48 ± 0.19	0.55 ± 0.19	0.53 ± 0.27

Values are expressed as mean ± SEM (n = 5–9). EAC: Ehrlich ascites carcinoma tumor-bearing mice; FU: Ehrlich ascites carcinoma tumor-bearing mice with 5-fluorouracil (20 mg/kg); SP200: Ehrlich ascites carcinoma tumor-bearing mice treated with spirulina (200 mg/kg); SP800: Ehrlich ascites carcinoma tumor-bearing mice treated with spirulina (800 mg/kg); FU/SP200: Ehrlich ascites carcinoma tumor-bearing mice treated with 5-fluorouracil (20 mg/kg) plus spirulina (200 mg/kg). RBC: red blood cell count; HGB: hemoglobin; HCT: hematocrit; MCV: mean corpuscular volume; PT: platelet count; PCT: plateletcrit; WBC: white blood cell count; LYM: lymphocyte count; GRA: granulocyte count. Statistical analysis using one-way ANOVA, followed by Dunnett's posttest. [a]P < 0.05 versus EAC and [b]P < 0.05 versus FU.

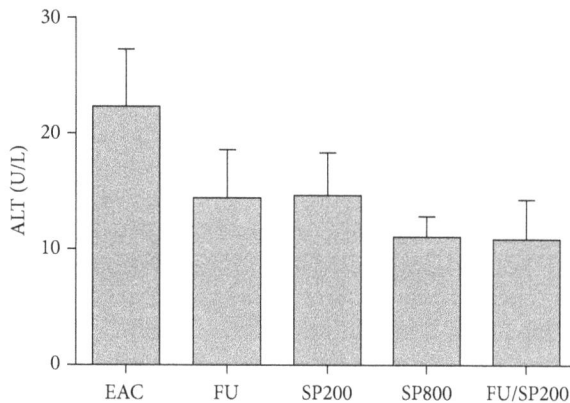

FIGURE 2: Effect of 5-fluorouracil (20 mg/kg), spirulina (200 or 800 mg/kg), and their combination on ALT level of EAC tumor-bearing mice (n = 4). ALT: alanine transaminase; EAC: Ehrlich ascites carcinoma tumor-bearing mice; FU: Ehrlich ascites carcinoma tumor-bearing mice treated with 5-fluorouracil (20 mg/kg); SP200: Ehrlich ascites carcinoma tumor-bearing mice treated with spirulina (200 mg/kg); SP800: Ehrlich ascites carcinoma tumor-bearing mice treated with spirulina (800 mg/kg); FU/SP200: Ehrlich ascites carcinoma tumor-bearing mice treated with 5-fluorouracil (20 mg/kg) plus spirulina (200 mg/kg). Data are expressed as mean ± SEM. Statistical analysis using one-way ANOVA, followed by Dunnett's posttest.

3.4. Effect on ALT. In our attempt to identify the cause of the increased mortality associated with the combined administration of fluorouracil and spirulina, we measured the changes in ALT levels. As shown in Figure 2, administration of different drugs resulted in reduction of ALT level when compared to untreated tumor-bearing mice. Nevertheless, this difference does not reach statistical significance. In addition, we did not notice any significant differences in ALT level between mice treated with fluorouracil alone and mice treated with spirulina alone (200 or 800 mg/kg) or fluorouracil plus spirulina (200 mg/kg).

3.5. Histopathological Examination. Examination of untreated tumor-bearing mice showed that EAC cells infiltrated and mostly replaced the subcutaneous tissue with necrosis of the remaining skeletal muscles. Numerous newly formed blood capillaries (neovascularization) were seen in the surrounding tissue with mild or no inflammatory response. Such tumor showed tissue architectural disarray, as well as marked degree of cellular anaplasia, pleomorphism, and anisocytosis, with nuclear vesicularity, atypicality, hyperchromasia, and mitoses. Some tumor cells were differentiated into gland-like structures surrounding a lumen containing eosinophilic material. Minimum necrotic areas with pyknosis and karyolysis, which appeared markedly in the central regions of the tumors, were noticed as well as few round-cell infiltrations and hemorrhage (Figures 3(a) and 3(b)).

On the other hand, mice treated with 5-flurourocil revealed minimal tumor cell infiltrations, extensive necrosis, and apoptosis at the margin of the tumor with destructed blood vessels and hemorrhage. Huge numbers of round cells of mostly lymphocytes and macrophages invaded the necrotic areas. Areas of the subcutaneous muscles were normal and others showed fibrous connective tissue proliferation infiltrated with leukocytes (Figures 3(c) and 3(d)).

Mice treated with spirulina alone (200 or 800 mg/kg) showed similar degree of infiltration as described with untreated tumor-bearing mice. Minimum necrosis and high vascularity of newly formed blood capillaries were also noticed. The inflammatory cell responses and necrosis in comparison with EAC were slightly increased, particularly with the higher dose of 800 mg/kg (Figures 3(e)–3(h)).

The tumor mass in mice treated with 5-flurouracil plus spirulina (200 mg/kg) was mostly necrotic (60–70%). In some parts, this was accompanied by a marked proliferation of fibrotic tissues as regeneration attempts of the subcutaneous tissue. Intense leukocyte aggregations, edema, and hemorrhage were visualized (Figures 3(i) and 3(j)). A scoring of histopathological findings is summarized in Table 3.

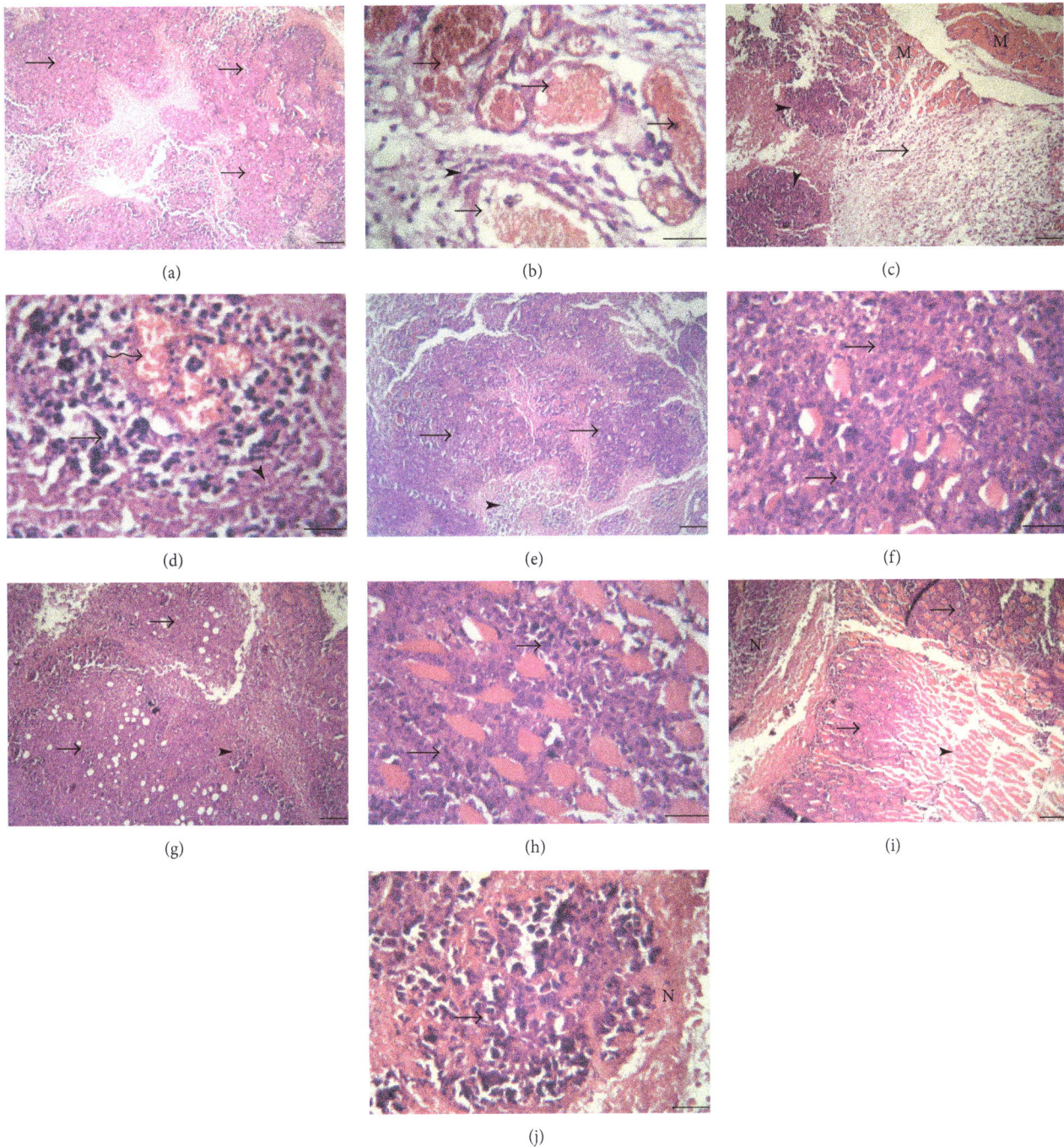

FIGURE 3: Histopathological examination of Ehrlich ascites carcinoma (EAC) solid tumor. Representative sections were obtained from (a) untreated EAC-bearing mice (arrows: infiltration of subcutaneous tissue with tumor cells), (b) untreated EAC-bearing mice (arrows: newly formed blood capillaries; arrowheads: leukocyte infiltration), (c) EAC tumor-bearing mice treated with 5-fluorouracil 20 mg/kg (arrowheads: extensive necrosis; arrow: fibrosis; M: skeletal muscles), (d) EAC tumor-bearing mice treated with 5-fluorouracil 20 mg/kg (irregular arrow: destructed blood vessels and hemorrhage), (e) EAC tumor-bearing mice treated with spirulina 200 mg/kg (arrows: extensive infiltration of the subcutaneous tissue with tumor cells), (f) EAC tumor-bearing mice treated with spirulina 200 mg/kg (arrows: tumor cells with cellular anaplasia and anisocytosis), (g) EAC tumor-bearing mice treated with spirulina 800 mg/kg (arrows: moderate infiltration of the tumor cells; arrowhead: numerous leukocyte infiltration), (h) EAC tumor-bearing mice treated with spirulina 800 mg/kg (arrows: huge numbers of tumor cells infiltrating the skeletal muscles), (i) EAC tumor-bearing mice treated with 5-fluorouracil 20 mg/kg plus spirulina 200 mg/kg (arrows: less infiltration with tumor cells; N: extensive necrosis and fibrosis), and (j) EAC tumor-bearing mice treated with 5-fluorouracil 20 mg/kg plus spirulina 200 mg/kg (arrows: islets of viable tumor cells; N: extensive necrosis). Sections were stained with HE dyes (scale bar = 50 μM).

TABLE 3: Histopathology scoring of tumor-bearing mice treated with 5-fluorouracil (20 mg/kg), spirulina (200 or 800 mg/kg), and their combination.

	Necrosis	Neovascularization	Leukocytes	Fibrosis
EAC[a]	8–12%	+++	+	−
FU[b]	50–60%	+	+++	++
SP200[c]	10–15%	+++	++	−
SP800[d]	10–15%	+++	++	−
FU/SP200[e]	60–70%	+	+++	+++

[a]EAC: Ehrlich ascites carcinoma tumor-bearing mice; [b]FU: Ehrlich ascites carcinoma tumor-bearing mice treated with 5-fluorouracil (20 mg/kg); [c]SP200: Ehrlich ascites carcinoma tumor-bearing mice treated with spirulina (200 mg/kg); [d]SP800: Ehrlich ascites carcinoma tumor-bearing mice treated with spirulina (800 mg/kg); [e]FU/SP200: Ehrlich ascites carcinoma tumor-bearing mice treated with 5-fluorouracil (20 mg/kg) plus spirulina (200 mg/kg). (−) none; (+) mild; (++) moderate; (+++) severe; (++++) more severe.

4. Discussion

Adjuvant and neoadjuvant chemotherapy represent important approaches in the management of cancer in order to reduce the recurrence following surgery or to reduce the tumor size enough to allow successful surgical removal [20, 21]. Considering various side effects caused by chemotherapeutic agents, development of new effective anticancer drugs is needed [22]. Increased attention is directed towards natural products as promising sources of anticancer therapeutic agents [23].

Spirulina is a plankton alga or cyanobacterium, which has been used as a food supplement for a long time [6, 24]. Spirulina exerts a wide array of pharmacological effects including anti-inflammatory, antioxidant, anticancer, and hepatoprotective properties [25, 26]. Therefore, in this study, we examined the effect of spirulina against Ehrlich solid tumor induced experimentally in mice.

Untreated mice inoculated with EAC cells intramuscularly in the right thigh of the hind limb developed a palpable solid tumor in 13 days following inoculation. This is consistent with other previous studies that used the same model [18, 27]. Administration of 5-fluorouracil (20 mg/kg) for 9 consecutive days starting from day 1 following EAC cells inoculation significantly reduced both tumor volume and tumor weight compared to untreated EAC tumor-bearing mice. On the other hand, administration of spirulina alone (200 or 800 mg/kg) did not significantly alter the tumor size compared to untreated EAC tumor-bearing mice. Although spirulina showed a dose-dependent tendency towards reducing the tumor volume, however, such change was not significant. These results reveal that spirulina alone lacks antitumor effect in this experimental model. We assume that this lack of activity is not attributed to the use of small doses of spirulina because even at a dose of 800 mg/kg no effect was observed. In addition, we rule out poor oral absorption of spirulina as a possible cause of the lack of the antitumor effect based on previous reports showing good bioavailability of different constituents of spirulina including carotenoids [28–30], iron [31], and proteins [32]. This lack of effect can be viewed also

at the histopathological level. Tumor specimen from mice treated with spirulina alone (200 or 800 mg/kg) showed EAC cells that infiltrated and mostly replaced the subcutaneous tissue. The observed degree of infiltration was similar to that found in specimens from untreated tumor-bearing mice. In addition, minimum necrosis was noticed in EAC tumor-bearing mice treated with spirulina alone at both dose levels (10–15%), which is very close to untreated mice (8–12%).

The lack of the antitumor effect of spirulina in our model does not conform to some other reports that described a potential anticancer activity of spirulina in other experimental models. Yogianti et al. [33] showed that spirulina exerts antitumor effects against UVB-induced skin tumor development in mice. In addition, it has been reported that spirulina exerts a chemopreventive effect against 7,12-dimethylbenz[a]anthracene-induced breast carcinogenesis [34] and against dibutyl nitrosamine-induced liver cytotoxicity and carcinogenesis [12] in rat. The discrepancy between these data and our results might be attributed to differences in the experimental conditions, the model of the solid tumor used, or the limited ability of spirulina to penetrate through Ehrlich solid tumor tissue and to reach all of the tumor cells in a potentially lethal concentration. The latter has been recognized as an important cause of anticancer drug resistance [35].

On the other hand, mice treated with 5-flurourocil alone showed minimal tumor cell infiltrations and extensive necrosis (50–60%). To test whether spirulina can at least potentiate the antitumor effect of fluorouracil, we examined the effect of their combined administration. Fluorouracil plus spirulina (200 mg/kg) significantly reduced both tumor volume and weight compared to untreated tumor-bearing mice; however, there were no significant differences in tumor volume or weight compared to mice treated with fluorouracil alone. In addition, histopathological examination revealed that the tumor mass in mice treated with both 5-flurouracil and spirulina (200 mg/kg) was mostly necrotic (60–70%) comparable to fluorouracil alone.

Interestingly, we observed a substantial, dose-dependent increase in mortality rate in mice treated with fluorouracil plus spirulina at a dose of 200 mg/kg (5 out of 10) and fluorouracil plus spirulina at a dose of 800 mg/kg (9 out of 10). We assume that this toxic effect is not attributed to EAC-tumor development *per se* or fluorouracil administration *per se* because only one animal died from group 1 (EAC-bearing mice) and group 2 (fluorouracil-treated mice). Therefore, it seems that the combined administration of fluorouracil and spirulina concurrently is responsible for such toxic effect.

We tried further to explain the mechanism implicated in the increased mortality by examining the effect on some hematological parameters and ALT level to see if this combination can cause acute hemotoxicity or fulminant hepatic damage. No significant alterations in complete blood count (CBC) were observed except for reduction in mean corpuscular volume (MCV) and increase in platelet count (PT) and plateletcrit (PCT) in mice treated with fluorouracil plus spirulina (200 mg/kg) when compared to mice treated with fluorouracil alone. In addition, there was no significant difference in ALT level between both groups. These results rule out hemotoxicity or hepatotoxicity as possible causes of increased mortality.

Depending on the present available results, the underlying mechanism of increased mortality is yet elusive; however, some postulations are worth mentioning. Different reports described a hypotensive effect associated with the administration of either 5-fluorouracil [36–38] or spirulina [39]. It is likely that combined administration of fluorouracil and spirulina, particularly at high dose level of 800 mg/kg, could enhance the reduction of blood pressure and might result in cardiovascular collapse. On the other hand, spirulina may have increased fluorouracil toxicity because of possible inhibition of the activity of dihydropyrimidine dehydrogenase, the enzyme that catalyzes the first rate-limiting step of fluorouracil degradation [40]. This assumption is based on a previous study reporting that spirulina resulted in inhibition of activities of some hepatic cytochrome P450 enzymes [41]. Although we could not find any report in the literature describing a direct relation between spirulina and dihydropyrimidine dehydrogenase, a possible effect could still be expected. Certainly, these assumptions need to be thoroughly investigated.

In conclusion, the present study describes the lack of antitumor activity of spirulina in EAC tumor-bearing mice model. In addition, spirulina administered simultaneously with fluorouracil did not enhance the antitumor activity of the later but rather resulted in increased dose-dependent mortality. In light of the present results, the mechanism of spirulina-induced mortality is not well understood. Although spirulina has been shown to possess anticancer effects in other models, the present study shows that it might not be a suitable therapeutic alternative for conventional chemotherapeutic agents in all settings such as EAC tumor-bearing mice model. In addition, spirulina might be not very safe, particularly when administered with other drugs such as fluorouracil. Therefore, we recommend that spirulina, or even other natural products, should be used cautiously and that possible interactions with other coadministered drugs should be monitored carefully.

Conflict of Interests

The authors declare that there is no conflict of interests.

Acknowledgment

The authors acknowledge Dr. Mohamed Hamed Mohamed, Professor of Pathology, Faculty of Veterinary Medicine, Zagazig University, for the histopathological examination.

References

[1] A. A. Stavrovskaya, "Cellular mechanisms of multidrug resistance of tumor cells," *Biochemistry*, vol. 65, no. 1, pp. 95–106, 2000.

[2] C. Moorthi, R. Manavalan, and K. Kathiresan, "Nanotherapeutics to overcome conventional cancer chemotherapy limitations," *Journal of Pharmacy and Pharmaceutical Sciences*, vol. 14, no. 1, pp. 67–77, 2011.

[3] G. M. Cragg and D. J. Newman, "Plants as a source of anticancer agents," *Journal of Ethnopharmacology*, vol. 100, no. 1-2, pp. 72–79, 2005.

[4] D. J. Newman, G. M. Cragg, and K. M. Snader, "Natural products as sources of new drugs over the period 1981–2002," *Journal of Natural Products*, vol. 66, no. 7, pp. 1022–1037, 2003.

[5] G. Chamorro, M. Salazar, L. Favila, and H. Bourges, "Pharmacology and toxicology of Spirulina alga," *Revista de Investigación Clínica*, vol. 48, no. 5, pp. 389–399, 1996.

[6] J. E. Piero Estrada, P. Bermejo Bescós, and A. M. Villar del Fresno, "Antioxidant activity of different fractions of *Spirulina platensis* protean extract," *Farmaco*, vol. 56, no. 5–7, pp. 497–500, 2001.

[7] C. Romay, J. Armesto, D. Remirez, R. González, N. Ledon, and I. García, "Antioxidant and anti-inflammatory properties of C-phycocyanin from blue-green algae," *Inflammation Research*, vol. 47, no. 1, pp. 36–41, 1998.

[8] B. B. Vadiraja, N. W. Gaikwad, and K. M. Madyastha, "Hepatoprotective effect of C-phycocyanin: protection for carbon tetrachloride and R-(+)-pulegone-mediated hepatotoxicty in rats," *Biochemical and Biophysical Research Communications*, vol. 249, no. 2, pp. 428–431, 1998.

[9] K. R. Roy, K. M. Arunasree, N. P. Reddy, B. Dheeraj, G. V. Reddy, and P. Reddanna, "Alteration of mitochondrial membrane potential by *Spirulina platensis* C-phycocyanin induces apoptosis in the doxorubicinresistant human hepatocellular-carcinoma cell line HepG2," *Biotechnology and Applied Biochemistry*, vol. 47, no. 3, pp. 159–167, 2007.

[10] T. Mishima, J. Murata, M. Toyoshima et al., "Inhibition of tumor invasion and metastasis by calcium spirulan (Ca–SP), a novel sulfated polysaccharide derived from a blue-green alga, *Spirulina platensis*," *Clinical and Experimental Metastasis*, vol. 16, no. 6, pp. 541–550, 1998.

[11] J. Schwartz and G. Shklar, "Regression of experimental hamster cancer by beta carotene and algae extracts," *Journal of Oral and Maxillofacial Surgery*, vol. 45, no. 6, pp. 510–515, 1987.

[12] M. F. Ismail, D. A. Ali, A. Fernando et al., "Chemoprevention of rat liver toxicity and carcinogenesis by Spirulina," *International Journal of Biological Sciences*, vol. 5, no. 4, pp. 377–387, 2009.

[13] M. Ozaslan, I. D. Karagoz, I. H. Kilic, and M. E. Guldur, "Ehrlich ascites carcinoma," *African Journal of Biotechnology*, vol. 10, no. 13, pp. 2375–2378, 2011.

[14] S. L. Da Silva, J. D. S. Chaar, and T. Yano, "Chemotherapeutic potential of two gallic acid derivative compounds from leaves of *Casearia sylvestris* Sw (Flacourtiaceae)," *European Journal of Pharmacology*, vol. 608, no. 1–3, pp. 76–83, 2009.

[15] A. M. Kabel, M. N. Abdel-Rahman, A. E.-D. E. El-Sisi, M. S. Haleem, N. M. Ezzat, and M. A. El Rashidy, "Effect of atorvastatin and methotrexate on solid Ehrlich tumor," *European Journal of Pharmacology*, vol. 713, no. 1–3, pp. 47–53, 2013.

[16] E. Noaman, N. K. Badr El-Din, M. A. Bibars, A. A. Abou Mossallam, and M. Ghoneum, "Antioxidant potential by arabinoxylan rice bran, MGN-3/biobran, represents a mechanism for its oncostatic effect against murine solid Ehrlich carcinoma," *Cancer Letters*, vol. 268, no. 2, pp. 348–359, 2008.

[17] G. Chamorro-Cevallos, L. Garduño-Siciliano, B. L. Barrón, E. Madrigal-Bujaidar, D. E. Cruz-Vega, and N. Pages, "Chemoprotective effect of *Spirulina* (*Arthrospira*) against cyclophosphamide-induced mutagenicity in mice," *Food and Chemical Toxicology*, vol. 46, no. 2, pp. 567–574, 2008.

[18] M. Mandal, S. K. Jaganathan, D. Mondhe, Z. A. Wani, and H. C. Pal, "Effect of honey and eugenol on ehrlich ascites and solid

carcinoma," *Journal of Biomedicine and Biotechnology*, vol. 2010, Article ID 989163, 5 pages, 2010.

[19] D. A. Sorg and B. Buckner, "A simple method of obtaining venous blood from small laboratory animals," *Proceedings of the Society for Experimental Biology and Medicine*, vol. 115, pp. 1131–1132, 1964.

[20] B. Fisher, J. Bryant, N. Wolmark et al., "Effect of preoperative chemotherapy on the outcome of women with operable breast cancer," *Journal of Clinical Oncology*, vol. 16, no. 8, pp. 2672–2685, 1998.

[21] D. Mauri, N. Pavlidis, and J. P. A. Ioannidis, "Neoadjuvant versus adjuvant systemic treatment in breast cancer: a meta-analysis," *Journal of the National Cancer Institute*, vol. 97, no. 3, pp. 188–194, 2005.

[22] S. Coseri, "Natural products and their analogues as efficient anticancer drugs," *Mini-Reviews in Medicinal Chemistry*, vol. 9, no. 5, pp. 560–571, 2009.

[23] D. J. Newman, "Natural products as leads to potential drugs: an old process or the new hope for drug discovery?" *Journal of Medicinal Chemistry*, vol. 51, no. 9, pp. 2589–2599, 2008.

[24] J. C. Dillon, A. P. Phuc, and J. P. Dubacq, "Nutritional value of the alga Spirulina," *World Review of Nutrition and Dietetics*, vol. 77, pp. 32–46, 1995.

[25] V. B. Bhat and K. M. Madyastha, "C-Phycocyanin: a potent peroxyl radical scavenger in vivo and in vitro," *Biochemical and Biophysical Research Communications*, vol. 275, no. 1, pp. 20–25, 2000.

[26] J. Subhashini, S. V. K. Mahipal, M. C. Reddy, M. M. Reddy, A. Rachamallu, and P. Reddanna, "Molecular mechanisms in C-Phycocyanin induced apoptosis in human chronic myeloid leukemia cell line-K562," *Biochemical Pharmacology*, vol. 68, no. 3, pp. 453–462, 2004.

[27] A. El-Moneim Mahmoud Osman, M. M. Sayed Ahmed, M. T. El-Din Khayyal, and M. M. El-Merzabani, "Hyperthermic potentiation of cisplatin cytotoxicity on solid Ehrlich carcinoma," *Tumori*, vol. 79, no. 4, pp. 268–272, 1993.

[28] R. Kapoor and U. Mehta, "Utilization of β-carotene from *Spirulina platensis* by rats," *Plant Foods for Human Nutrition*, vol. 43, no. 1, pp. 1–7, 1993.

[29] G. V. Mitchell, E. Grundel, M. Jenkins, and S. R. Blakely, "Effects of graded dietary levels of spirulina maxima on vitamins A and E in male rats," *Journal of Nutrition*, vol. 120, no. 10, pp. 1235–1240, 1990.

[30] V. Annapurna, N. Shah, P. Bhaskaram, M. S. Bamji, and V. Reddy, "Bioavailability of spirulina carotenes in preschool children," *Journal of Clinical Biochemistry and Nutrition*, vol. 10, no. 2, pp. 145–151, 1991.

[31] P. E. Johnson and L. E. Shubert, "Availability of iron to rats from spirulina, a blue-green alga," *Nutrition Research*, vol. 6, no. 1, pp. 85–94, 1986.

[32] C. Santillan, "Cultivation of the Spirulina for human consumption and for animal feed," in *Proceedings of the International Congress of Food Science and Technology*, Madrid, Spain, September 1974.

[33] F. Yogianti, M. Kunisada, E. Nakano et al., "Inhibitory effects of dietary *Spirulina platensis* on UVB-induced skin inflammatory responses and carcinogenesis," *Journal of Investigative Dermatology*, vol. 134, pp. 2610–2619, 2014.

[34] A. Ouhtit, M. F. Ismail, A. Othman et al., "Chemoprevention of rat mammary carcinogenesis by spirulina," *The American Journal of Pathology*, vol. 184, no. 1, pp. 296–303, 2014.

[35] O. Trédan, C. M. Galmarini, K. Patel, and I. F. Tannock, "Drug resistance and the solid tumor microenvironment," *Journal of the National Cancer Institute*, vol. 99, no. 19, pp. 1441–1454, 2007.

[36] A. Polk, M. Vaage-Nilsen, K. Vistisen, and D. L. Nielsen, "Cardiotoxicity in cancer patients treated with 5-fluorouracil or capecitabine: a systematic review of incidence, manifestations and predisposing factors," *Cancer Treatment Reviews*, vol. 39, no. 8, pp. 974–984, 2013.

[37] W. J. Gradishar and E. E. Vokes, "5-fluorouracil cardiotoxicity: a critical review," *Annals of Oncology*, vol. 1, no. 6, pp. 409–414, 1990.

[38] A. A. Jakubowski and N. Kemeny, "Hypotension as a manifestation of cardiotoxicity in three patients receiving cisplatin and 5-fluorouracil," *Cancer*, vol. 62, no. 2, pp. 266–269, 1988.

[39] G. Hsiao, P. O.-H. Chou, M.-Y. Shen, D.-S. Chou, C.-H. Lin, and J.-R. Sheu, "C-phycocyanin, a very potent and novel platelet aggregation inhibitor from *Spirulina platensis*," *Journal of Agricultural and Food Chemistry*, vol. 53, no. 20, pp. 7734–7740, 2005.

[40] R. B. Diasio and B. E. Harris, "Clinical pharmacology of 5-fluorouracil," *Clinical Pharmacokinetics*, vol. 16, no. 4, pp. 215–237, 1989.

[41] S. Savranoglu and T. B. Tumer, "Inhibitory effects of spirulina platensis on carcinogen-activating cytochrome P450 isozymes and potential for drug interactions," *International Journal of Toxicology*, vol. 32, no. 5, pp. 376–384, 2013.

2

Can Chronic Nitric Oxide Inhibition Improve Liver and Renal Dysfunction in Bile Duct Ligated Rats?

Mona Fouad Mahmoud, Sara Zakaria, and Ahmed Fahmy

Department of Pharmacology and Toxicology, Faculty of Pharmacy, University of Zagazig, Zagazig 44519, Egypt

Correspondence should be addressed to Mona Fouad Mahmoud; mona_pharmacology@yahoo.com

Academic Editor: Ismail Laher

The aims of the present work were to study the effects of chronic NO inhibition on liver cirrhosis and to analyze its relationship with liver and kidney damage markers. Two inhibitors of NO synthesis (inducible NO synthase (iNOS) inhibitor, aminoguanidine (AG), and nonselective NOS inhibitor, L-nitroarginine methyl ester (L-NAME)) were administered for 6 weeks to bile duct ligated (BDL) rats 3 days after surgery. The present study showed that BDL was associated with liver injury and renal impairment. BDL increased liver NO content and myeloperoxidase (MPO) activity. This was corroborated by increased oxidative stress, TNF-α, TGF-1β, and MMP-13 genes overexpression. Although both drugs reduced NO synthesis and TNF-α gene overexpression, only AG improved renal dysfunction and liver damage and reduced liver oxidative stress. However, L-NAME exacerbated liver and renal dysfunction. Both drugs failed to modulate TGF-1β and MMP-13 genes overexpression. In conclusion, inhibition of NO production by constitutive nitric oxide synthase (cNOS) plays a crucial role in liver injury and renal dysfunction while inhibition of iNOS by AG has beneficial effect. TNF-α is not the main cytokine responsible for liver injury in BDL model. Nitric oxide inhibition did not stop the progression of cholestatic liver damage.

1. Introduction

Increased nitric oxide (NO) is well recognized in patients with cholestatic liver diseases. Actually high levels of circulating bile salts during cholestasis disrupt intestinal mucosal barrier resulting in translocation of enteric bacteria to the mesenteric lymph nodes and the liver [1] and resulting endotoxemia is responsible for augmented nitric oxide (NO) synthesis by inducible NO synthase (iNOS) [2]. Excessive generation of NO has been observed both in experimental cholestasis and in primary biliary cirrhosis patients. The increase in hepatic and plasma circulating levels of NO and cytokines is the determinant for the hepatocellular injury and the rapid progression of hepatic dysfunction in cholestatic settings [3].

NO has a dual role. Beneficial role is mediated by its circulatory effects and its free radical scavenger properties. Under normal conditions NO has beneficial effect on vascular control including modulation of vascular tone and inflammation. The induction of NO synthesis in abnormal situations allows a more efficient defense not only because of local vascular effects but also because NO is thought to be involved in the macrophage-dependent killing of parasites and possibly cancer cells.

Negative role is mediated through its local toxic effects. NO has a multitude of potentially toxic effects, although many of these are probably mediated by oxidation products rather than by NO itself [4].

Strong inhibition of NO synthesis maintained for long periods by L-NAME may lead to adverse effects through different mechanisms [5]. Previous studies showed that inhibition of NO production in BDL rats may decrease liver blood flow promoting clot formation [6]. It also favors the production of oxyradicals [7]. Selective inhibition of iNOS by chronic administration of aminoguanidine (AG) could reduce systemic NO levels as it suppresses iNOS expression and activity in aorta of BDL rats. It also improves liver function possibly because of its ability to increase hepatic cNOS activity and to correct the systemic hemodynamic disorders by decreasing vascular NO production [8].

The role of NO produced by iNOS in bile duct ligation model was previously investigated. Some studies showed that iNOS gene transfer could inhibit hepatocytes apoptosis [9]. Furthermore, Dirlik et al. [10] reported that BDL caused a significant increase in iNOS staining on the 3rd day following surgery and decreased on the 5th day after BDL and reduction of iNOS expression was associated with increased hepatocytes apoptosis. However, the changes in NO production after longer periods following BDL have not been yet investigated.

From this point of view, the aim of the present work was to study the role of complete and partial inhibition of nitric oxide synthase enzymes in liver fibrosis and renal dysfunction induced by bile duct ligation in rats after 6 weeks of BDL. In addition the correlation between NO inhibition and matrix formation, and growth factors and the inflammatory process mediating liver fibrosis was also investigated.

2. Materials and Methods

2.1. Animals. Adult male Wistar rats weighing 180 ± 220 g were used in the present investigation. The animals were obtained from National Research Center, Cairo, Egypt. They were kept under constant environmental and nutritional conditions throughout the period of study. They were housed as six rats per cage in plastic cages with wood shave bedding and fed normal standard diet. They had free access to water and food. The protocol of the present study was approved by the Animal Care and Use Committee of the Pharmacology Department, Faculty of Pharmacy, Zagazig University, Egypt. Every effort was done to minimize the number of animals and their suffering.

2.2. Materials. Aminoguanidine (AG) and L-NAME were supplied from Sigma Co., USA. The required dose of AG was dissolved in normal saline but the required dose of L-NAME was dissolved in drinking water. All drugs and vehicle were given to rats by oral gavage.

2.3. Experimental Design. The animals were randomly divided into 5 groups of 20 rats/per each group. Group (1) received normal saline (2 mL/kg, orally) for 6 weeks and represents normal control group. Group (2) underwent a midline incision and manipulation of the bile duct without ligation and received saline (2 mL/kg, orally) and served as sham group. Group (3) was bile duct ligated and received saline (2 mL/kg, orally) and served as BDL group. Group (4) was bile duct ligated and received aminoguanidine (50 mg/kg, orally). Group (5) was bile duct ligated and received L-NAME (2 mg/kg, orally).

All treatments were given starting from 3rd day after surgery and for 6 weeks as single daily dose.

2.4. Induction of Fibrosis. Fibrosis was induced in rats by the ligation of the common bile duct. Bile duct ligation was performed under general anesthesia with a mixture of ketamine hydrochloride (50 mg/kg) and diazepam (3 mg/kg) [11]. The common bile duct was manipulated and then doubly ligated with 4-0 silk threads and excised between the ligatures to prevent regeneration. In sham operated group, the bile duct was identified, manipulated, and left *in situ* without ligation.

Meloxicam in a dose of 1 mg/kg [12] IM was given for 3 days after surgery to reduce pain. Meloxicam has a good record for effectiveness and safety for both short-term and long-term use in animals. Rats were also injected with Penicillin G (aqua-pen vial) by deep IM injection [13] for 3 days after surgery for prophylaxis against infection.

2.5. Blood Sampling and Serum Preparation. At the end of the experiment, blood was collected from the orbital sinus of rats [14] in clean dry centrifuge tubes. For the preparation of serum, blood was collected into tubes without anticoagulant. The tubes were left to clot for 15 minutes at room temperature. Serum was separated after centrifugation at 3500 r.p.m. (10,000 ×g) for 15 minutes using Heraeus Sepatech centrifuge (Labofuge 200, DJB Labcare Company). Serum was divided into two aliquots and all were frozen. The first aliquot was used for the determination of alanine aminotransferase (ALT), aspartate aminotransferase (AST), lactate dehydrogenase (LDH), and total bilirubin. The second aliquot was used for determination of creatinine and urea.

2.6. Tissue Sampling. Animals were anaesthetized by ether and livers were perfused with phosphate buffered solution (PBS) containing 0.16 mg/mL heparin. Livers were isolated and dissected into 3 parts. All parts were immersed immediately in liquid nitrogen and kept at −80°C. These parts were used to measure tumor necrosis factor alpha (TNF-α), transforming growth factor one beta (TGF-1β), matrix metalloproteinase-13 (MMP-13), myeloperoxidase (MPO), malondialdehyde (MDA), reduced glutathione content (GSH), and nitric oxide (NO).

2.7. Biochemical Analysis

2.7.1. Liver Function Tests. Serum ALT and AST activities were determined by a colorimetric method according to the principle of Reitman and Frankel [15].

2.7.2. Liver Cell Death. Serum lactate dehydrogenase activity as indicator of cytolytic cell death was determined using a kinetic method according to the method of Fasce Jr. and Rej [16].

2.7.3. Serum Total Bilirubin. It was measured colorimetrically as described by Gellis et al. [17].

2.7.4. Kidney Function Tests. Serum urea was measured colorimetrically as described by Fawcett and Scott [18] and also creatinine level was measured colorimetrically as described by Bowers and Wong [19].

2.7.5. Liver TNF-α, TGF-1β, and MMP-13. Detection of TNF-α, TGF-1β, and MMP-13 gene expression was performed by semiquantitative reverse transcriptase-polymerase chain reaction (RT-PCR).

Briefly, total RNA was extracted from liver tissue using E.Z.N.A. RNA extraction kit. The extracted RNA was

TABLE 1: Effect of different treatments on liver and renal functions of bile duct ligated rats.

Treatment	Control	Sham	BDL	Aminoguanidine	L-NAME
ALT	24.3 ± 1.8	56.1* ± 2.1	1012# ± 6.4	290.2$ ± 3.5	1517$ ± 8.3
AST	126.3 ± 5.9	310.4* ± 5.7	1379# ± 11.0	1102$ ± 5.3	1801$ ± 6.4
LDH	929.7 ± 6.9	1637* ± 14.7	2607# ± 10.1	2050$ ± 18.8	2428$ ± 16.1
T. bilirubin	0.02 ± 0.002	0.08 ± 0.003	4.06# ± 0.1	3.51$ ± 0.04	6.07$ ± 0.07
Urea	11.8 ± 0.4	31.5* ± 0.8	327.7# ± 3.8	172.4$ ± 2.7	516.4$ ± 5.8
Creatinine	0.24 ± 0.02	0.72* ± 0.05	2.72# ± 0.06	1.95$ ± 0.06	2.78 ± 0.02

Data are presented as mean ± S.E., $n = 6$. *Significantly different from control at $P < 0.05$*, #significantly different from sham at $P < 0.05$, and $significantly different from BDL at $P < 0.05$, using one-way ANOVA and Tukey's *post hoc* test.

reverse transcribed into cDNA using RT-PCR kit (Stratagene, USA). The cDNA was amplified using the following primers:

TNF alpha, Forward: 5′-ATTGGCAAATGGGAA-AATGA-3′

Reverse: 5′-TTATGACCTCCTTTTGGTCTGA-3′,

TGF beta, Forward: 5′-TTGAGTGTCAGCCCA-CAGAG-3′

Reverse: 5′-TCCGACAGCCACACTTCTTC-3′,

MMP-13, Forward: 5′-GCTGGTCAGTCGCCCTTT-T-3′

Reverse: 5′-GCTAAGGAAAGCAGAGAGGGATT-3′.

Gene expression of β-actin was used as a house keeping gene.

The primer sequence of β-actin was Forward: 5′-TCA CCC TGA AGT ACC CCA TGG AG-3′ and Reverse: 5′-TTG GCC TTG GGG TTC AGG GGG-3′. At the end of the amplification process, the DNA product was detected using agarose gel electrophoresis. Semiquantitation was performed using the gel documentation system (BioDO, Analyser) supplied by Biometra. Relative expression of each studied gene (R) was calculated following the formula: R = Densitometrical Units of each studied gene/Densitometrical Units of β-actin.

2.7.6. Liver MPO. Liver MPO activity was determined by a colorimetric method using myeloperoxidase chlorination activity determination kit as described by Kettle and Winterbourn [20].

2.7.7. Liver GSH and Membrane Lipid Peroxidation. The reduced form of glutathione (GSH) was determined in the liver homogenate by colorimetric method according to Beutler et al. [21]. Malondialdehyde (MDA) content as indicator of lipid peroxidation was determined in the liver homogenate, by a colorimetric method according to Ohkawa et al. [22].

2.7.8. Liver Nitric Oxide. Liver content of nitric oxide was quantitatively measured indirectly as nitrite and nitrate by a colorimetric method as described by Montgomery and Dymock [23] using a diagnostic kit supplied by Tocris Bioscience, Boston Biochem join R&D systems (Minneapolis, USA).

2.8. Statistical Analysis. Results were expressed as mean ± S.E.M. Graph Pad Prism software version 5 was used to perform statistical analysis. Comparison between different groups was carried out using one-way analysis of variance (ANOVA) followed by Tukey's *post hoc* test. The statistical associations between functional parameters were assayed using Spearman nonparametric correlation analysis. P values less than 0.05 were considered significant.

3. Results

3.1. General Observations. The animals started to have the signs of cholestasis such as jaundice, dark urine, and steatorrhea at the 4th day from the bile duct ligation operation with higher mortality rate during the first 2 weeks after the operation; then mortality rate decreased during the 3rd and 4th weeks and then increased at last two weeks. Untreated BDL group had the highest mortality rate.

3.2. Effect on Liver Enzymes and Total Bilirubin. Table 1 showed that BDL significantly increased serum activities of ALT, AST, and serum total bilirubin level as compared to sham group ($P < 0.05$). Aminoguanidine caused significant ($P < 0.05$) reduction of ALT, AST serum activities and serum total bilirubin levels. However, L-NAME caused significant ($P < 0.05$) increase in the activities of serum ALT, AST, and total bilirubin level.

3.3. Effect on Liver Cell Death. Bile duct ligation significantly increased serum activity of LDH, an indicator of necrotic cell death as compared to sham group ($P < 0.05$). Aminoguanidine reduced LDH activity as compared to BDL group (Table 1). On the other hand, L-NAME did not affect LDH activity when compared to BDL group ($P > 0.05$).

3.4. Effect on Kidney Function. Bile duct ligation significantly increased serum levels of urea and creatinine as compared to sham ($P < 0.05$). Aminoguanidine caused significant ($P < 0.05$) reduction of urea and creatinine as compared to BDL group. L-NAME caused significant ($P < 0.05$) increase in serum urea levels and had no effect on serum creatinine levels as compared to BDL group.

3.5. Effect on Oxidative Stress and Nitric Oxide Levels. Bile duct ligation significantly increased liver MDA, a lipid peroxidation product ($P < 0.05$), and significantly decreased

TABLE 2: Effect of different treatments on nitrosative and oxidative stress in bile duct ligated rats.

Treatment	Control	Sham	BDL	Aminoguanidine	L-NAME
MPO	1.8 ± 0.1	$2.9^* \pm 0.2$	$4.6^\# \pm 0.2$	4.2 ± 0.3	4.5 ± 0.3
GSH	2.7 ± 0.2	$1.6^* \pm 0.1$	$0.4^\# \pm 0.1$	$0.9^\$ \pm 0.1$	0.6 ± 0.1
MDA	24.6 ± 0.1	$41.1^* \pm 1.3$	$62.7^\# \pm 2.3$	$52.7^\$ \pm 2.6$	58.2 ± 2.5
NO	0.21 ± 0.02	$0.33^* \pm 0.03$	$0.94^\# \pm 0.02$	$0.19^\$ \pm 0.02$	$0.08^\$ \pm 0.004$

Data are presented as mean $\pm$ S.E., $n = 6$. *Significantly different from control at $P < 0.05$, $^\#$significantly different from sham at $P < 0.05$, and $^\$$significantly different from BDL at $P < 0.05$, using one-way ANOVA and Tukey's *post hoc* test.

liver GSH as compared to sham ($P < 0.05$). Aminoguanidine caused significant ($P < 0.05$) decrease in liver MDA and significant ($P < 0.05$) increase in liver GSH as compared to BDL group (Table 2). L-NAME had no significant effect on liver contents of both MDA and GSH as compared to BDL group (Table 2). Both aminoguanidine and L-NAME caused a significant ($P < 0.05$) reduction of liver NO compared to BDL group (Table 2).

3.6. Effect on Inflammation Markers. Myeloperoxidase is an enzyme released by infiltrating inflammatory cells during inflammation and was increased significantly in BDL rats as compared to sham rats ($P < 0.05$). Aminoguanidine and L-NAME did not affect liver MPO activity (Table 2). TNF-α gene expression was upregulated in the liver cells of BDL when compared to sham group ($P < 0.05$). Both aminoguanidine and L-NAME produced significant reduction of TNF-α gene expression ($P < 0.05$) as shown in Figure 1.

3.7. Effect on Growth Factors and Matrix Formation. Bile duct ligation induced a significant increase in liver expression of both TGF-1β and MMP-13 as compared to sham rats. Aminoguanidine and L-NAME had no significant effect on both TGF-1β and MMP-13 gene expression as compared to BDL group (Figures 2 and 3).

3.8. Correlation Analysis between Liver Content of Nitrite and Different Studied Parameters. There was positive correlation between liver nitrite and serum activity of LDH ($r = 0.4$ at $P < 0.05$), serum creatinine level ($r = 0.3$ at $P < 0.05$), and liver TGF-1β, MMP-13, TNF-α, MDA, and GSH ($r = 0.4$ for all at $P < 0.05$). However, serum activities of ALT, AST, and total bilirubin level were not correlated to liver nitrite ($r = 0.2, 0.1,$ and 0.1, resp., at $P > 0.05$). Serum urea level and liver MPO activity were not correlated to liver nitrite ($r = 0.1$ and 0.3, resp., at $P > 0.05$).

4. Discussion

Although some previous studies investigated the effect of aminoguanidine on cholestatic liver damage, the present study was the first up to our knowledge which compares chronic partial or complete inhibition of NO by aminoguanidine or L-NAME, respectively, on liver and renal dysfunction in bile duct ligated rat model. It is one of the longest treatment periods in the literature using these inhibitors. We found that bile duct ligation for six weeks caused a significant increase in serum activities of ALT, AST and in serum level of total bilirubin compared to sham group indicating liver injury due

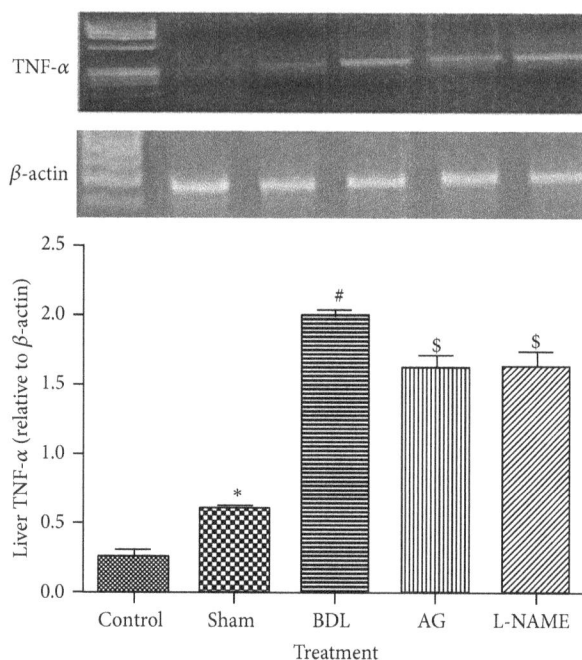

FIGURE 1: Effect of aminoguanidine (AG) and L-NAME on liver TNF-α gene expression relative to β-actin in bile duct ligated (BDL) rats and an agarose gel electrophoresis show PCR products of TNF alpha. Lane M: DNA marker with 100 bp; Lane 1: PCR products of TNF alpha in control group; Lane 2: PCR products of TNF alpha in sham group; Lane 3: PCR products of TNF alpha in BDL group; Lane 4: PCR products of TNF alpha in aminoguanidine group; Lane 5: PCR products of TNF alpha in L-NAME group.

to cholestasis. The mortality rate in the untreated bile duct rats was the highest rate among the experimental groups. This may be attributed to the great elevation of bilirubin in the blood of untreated animals during the first two weeks after surgery and due to complications of hepatic damage at the last two weeks of the experiment. It also increased serum levels of urea and creatinine as markers for kidney function compared to sham group. Lactate dehydrogenase, a marker of cytolytic cell death, was also elevated. Liver genes expression of TGF-1β, TNF-α, and MMP-13, MPO activity, MDA, and nitric oxide levels were significantly increased but the liver content of GSH was decreased compared to sham group.

One of the proposed mechanisms by which BDL induces liver injury was investigated in the present study, the role of NO in liver injury. Some studies suggested that NO has a dual role in cholestatic liver disease; one is beneficial, mediated by its circulatory effects, and the second is negative, through its

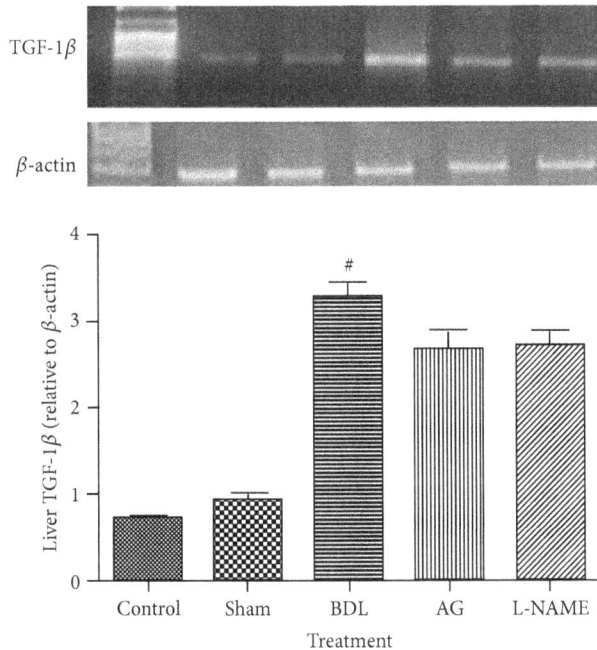

FIGURE 2: Effect of aminoguanidine (AG) and L-NAME on liver TGF-1β gene expression relative to β-actin in bile duct ligated (BDL) rats and an agarose gel electrophoresis show PCR products of TGF beta in different studied groups. Lane M: DNA marker with 100 bp; Lane 1: PCR products of TGF beta in control group; Lane 2: PCR products of TGF beta in sham group; Lane 3: PCR products of TGF beta in BDL group; Lane 4: PCR products of TGF beta in aminoguanidine group; Lane 5: PCR products of TGF beta in L-NAME group.

FIGURE 3: Effect of aminoguanidine (AG) and L-NAME on liver MMP-13 gene expression relative to β-actin in bile duct ligated (BDL) rats and an agarose gel electrophoresis show PCR products of MMP-13 in different studied groups. Lane M: DNA marker with 100 bp; Lane 1: PCR products of MMP-13 in control group; Lane 2: PCR products of MMP-13 in sham group; Lane 3: PCR products of MMP-13 in BDL group; Lane 4: PCR products of MMP-13 in aminoguanidine group; Lane 5: PCR products of MMP-13 in L-NAME group.

local toxic effects [24]. Increased NO level and NO synthase activity in patients with liver cirrhosis have adverse effects on the functions of renal tubules and glomeruli [25]. Inhibition of NO synthase prevented the development of renal failure in an animal model of hepatorenal syndrome [26].

Based on the previous studies that indicate that nitric oxide (NO) plays an important role in the systemic and renal alterations of liver cirrhosis, in this study, we used aminoguanidine (AG), a preferential inhibitor of inducible nitric oxide synthase (iNOS), to evaluate the role of this NOS isoform in the pathogenesis of liver cirrhosis and its subsequent alteration in renal function. AG was orally administered in a dose 50 mg/kg as it totally inhibits iNOS with no effect on constitutive NOS but the 100 mg/kg dose also inhibits some constitutive NOS isoform [27].

Oral administration of AG (50 mg/kg) for bile duct ligated rats three days after surgery for six weeks produced a significant decrease in the serum activities of ALT, AST, LDH, and serum total bilirubin level compared to BDL group. It also decreased liver content of TNF-α compared to BDL group. Previous studies showed that AG may be useful in the preservation of liver injury in cholestasis as it reduces cytokine induced liver damage and ductular proliferation [28]. Inhibition of iNOS is thought to control the injury of liver. The present study showed that AG decreased liver NO production compared to BDL group. It was reported

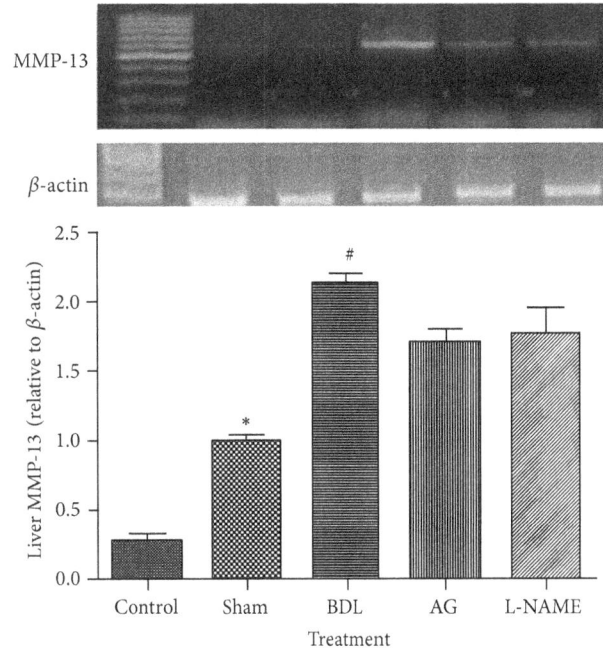

previously that iNOS was expressed in liver tissue from control rats but its expression was increased in BDL animals [24]. On the other hand, cNOS was expressed to a similar extent in normal and BDL animals which make the iNOS responsible for liver injury.

AG improved renal dysfunction as revealed by reduction of both urea and creatinine levels. Previous studies showed that iNOS is involved in the renal alterations observed in BDL animals [29]. NO plays an important role as a mediator of the systemic and renal alterations of liver cirrhosis. NO inhibition in experimental animals resulted in a reduction of the hyperdynamic circulation [30] and produces the beneficial effects on renal excretory function [31].

The present study showed that aminoguanidine has antioxidant effects. It decreased liver MDA and increased liver GSH compared to BDL group. During cholestasis, there is a high oxidative stress and more free radicals are produced. Interactions between reactive oxygen species and reactive nitrogen species, mainly NO, could mediate some of the pathological effects associated with chronic inflammation [32]. AG may attenuate liver and kidney damage during cholestasis through its inhibition of iNOS and its antioxidant effect.

Although aminoguanidine improved liver and renal dysfunction, it failed to modulate the fibrotic process in liver. The present study showed that AG did not modulate TGF-1β or

MMP-13 genes expression. In spite of reducing liver TNF-α gene expression, AG had no significant effect on MPO activity indicating that it could not modulate leukocyte infiltration. It seems that TNF-α is not the only player in the fibrotic process in liver. Other cytokines may have a more important role in fibrosis induced by BDL. A previous study of Bautista-García et al. [33] showed that the inhibition of iNOS by 0.1% AG reduced TGF-1β over expression in 5/6 nephrectomized rats. Another study of Kelly et al. [34] revealed that AG (1 g/L) reduces TGF-1β in diabetic nephropathy due to inhibition of advanced glycation end products (AGEs) formation but not due to NO inhibition. These variations in results may be related to the difference in experimental model and AG dose.

In contrast to the present findings, AG increased the expression of MMP-13 in diabetic mice kidney [35] via blocking AGEs formation. It was also reported that both AG and L-NAME upregulated MMP-13 mRNA expression in rat thioacetamide-induced fibrosis model [36]. The AG effects were more pronounced and it also inhibits TGF-1β. Both NOS inhibitors developed a clear profibrotic effect in the liver. Aminoguanidine was more fibrotic than L-NAME. Again in these studies, AG was administered in a dose of 100 mg/kg for three months, which may inhibit both constitutive and inducible NOS.

In this study, we also used L-NAME, a potent nonselective NOS inhibitor to determine the effects of nonselective NO inhibition during cholestatic liver disease. Oral administration of L-NAME (2 mg/kg) for BDL rats three days after surgery for six weeks produced a significant increase in the activities of serum enzymes of ALT, AST and serum level of total bilirubin with no effect on serum LDH compared to BDL group, indicating an aggravation of liver dysfunction and damage. It had no effect on liver contents of TGF-1β, MMP-13, and MPO but it decreased the liver content of NO compared with BDL group. Previous studies showed similar effects on liver [24]. We showed for the first time that L-NAME administration has detrimental effect on the renal function as manifested by elevation of urea level when compared by untreated BDL rats.

The deleterious effect of L-NAME may be attributed to inhibition of NO production by cNOS which may decrease liver blood flow, promoting clot formation and ROS generation [7].

5. Conclusion

Both aminoguanidine and L-NAME did not modulate the fibrotic process in liver of BDL rats in spite of reducing liver TNF-α gene expression. AG only decreased liver and kidney dysfunction due to its partial inhibition of nitric oxide synthase and antioxidant effects. L-NAME increased liver injury and deteriorates renal function due to its complete inhibition of nitric oxide synthase.

Abbreviations

AG: Aminoguanidine
BDL: Bile duct ligation/bile duct ligated

L-NAME: L-Nitroarginine methyl ester
MMP-13: Matrix metalloproteinase-13
TNF-α: Tumour necrosis factor alpha
TGF-1β: Transforming growth factor 1β
MPO: Myeloperoxidase
cNOS: Constitutive nitric oxide synthase
iNOS: Inducible nitric oxide synthase.

Conflict of Interests

The authors declared no conflict of interests.

Acknowledgment

The authors would like to thank Professor Dr. Laila Rashed, Professor of Biochemistry, Faculty of Medicine, Cairo University, for her help in PCR technique.

References

[1] S. F. Assimakopoulos, C. D. Scopa, A. Charonis et al., "Experimental obstructive jaundice disrupts intestinal mucosal barrier by altering occludin expression: beneficial effect of bombesin and neurotensin," *Journal of the American College of Surgeons*, vol. 198, no. 5, pp. 748–757, 2004.

[2] A. Hokari, M. Zeniya, H. Esumi, T. Kawabe, M. E. Gershwin, and G. Toda, "Detection of serum nitrite and nitrate in primary biliary cirrhosis: possible role of nitric oxide in bile duct injury," *Journal of Gastroenterology and Hepatology*, vol. 17, no. 3, pp. 308–315, 2002.

[3] I. Grattagliano, P. Portincasa, V. O. Palmieri, and G. Palasciano, "Mutual changes of thioredoxin and nitrosothiols during biliary cirrhosis: results from humans and cholestatic rats," *Hepatology*, vol. 45, no. 2, pp. 331–339, 2007.

[4] J. S. Beckman and W. H. Koppenol, "Nitric oxide, superoxide, and peroxynitrite: the good, the bad, and ugly," *American Journal of Physiology—Cell Physiology*, vol. 271, no. 5, part 1, pp. C1424–C1437, 1996.

[5] A. K. Nussler, M. Di Silvio, Z.-Z. Liu et al., "Further characterization and comparison of inducible nitric oxide synthase in mouse, rat, and human hepatocytes," *Hepatology*, vol. 21, no. 6, pp. 1552–1560, 1995.

[6] B. G. Harbrecht, T. R. Billiar, J. Stadler et al., "Inhibition of nitric oxide synthesis during endotoxemia promotes intrahepatic thrombosis and an oxygen radical-mediated hepatic injury," *Journal of Leukocyte Biology*, vol. 52, no. 4, pp. 390–394, 1992.

[7] V. Darley-Usmar, H. Wiseman, and B. Halliwell, "Nitric oxide and oxygen radicals: a question of balance," *FEBS Letters*, vol. 369, no. 2-3, pp. 131–135, 1995.

[8] C.-L. Wei, W.-M. Hon, K.-H. Lee, and H.-E. Khoo, "Chronic administration of aminoguanidine reduces vascular nitric oxide production and attenuates liver damage in bile duct-ligated rats," *Liver International*, vol. 25, no. 3, pp. 647–656, 2005.

[9] E. Tzeng, T. R. Billiar, D. L. Williams et al., "Adenovirus-mediated inducible nitric oxide synthase gene transfer inhibits hepatocyte apoptosis," *Surgery*, vol. 124, no. 2, pp. 278–283, 1998.

[10] M. Dirlik, H. Canbaz, D. Düşmez Apa et al., "The monitoring of progress in apoptosis of liver cells in bile duct-ligated rats," *Turkish Journal of Gastroenterology*, vol. 20, no. 4, pp. 247–256, 2009.

[11] G. A. Volger, "Anesthesia and analgesia," in *The Laboratory Rat*, M. A. Suckow, S. H. Weisbroth, and C. L. Franklin, Eds., pp. 627–664, Academic Press, 2nd edition, 2006.

[12] A. R. Blickman and L. J. Brossia, "Anesthesia and Analgesia for research animals," in *Animal Models of Acute Neurological Injuries*, J. Chen and J. H. Zhang, Eds., pp. 11–18, Springer, 1st edition, 2008.

[13] Z.-X. Xi and E. A. Stein, "Opiate self-adminstration," in *Opioid Research: Methods and Protocols*, Z. Z. Pan, Ed., pp. 251–264, Humana Press, 1st edition, 2003.

[14] D. A. Sorg and B. Buckner, "A simple method of obtaining venous blood from small laboratory animals," *Proceedings of the Society for Experimental Biology and Medicine*, vol. 115, pp. 1131–1132, 1964.

[15] S. Reitman and S. Frankel, "A colorimetric method for the determination of serum glutamic oxalacetic and glutamic pyruvic transaminases," *American Journal of Clinical Pathology*, vol. 28, no. 1, pp. 56–63, 1957.

[16] C. F. Fasce Jr. and R. Rej, "An automated system for kinetic multiple-point determinations exemplified by serum lactic dehydrogenase determination," *Clinical Chemistry*, vol. 16, no. 12, pp. 972–979, 1970.

[17] S. S. Gellis, R. M. Gofstein, D. Y. Hsia, H. H. Hsia, and A. Winter, "Determination of concentration of bilirubin in serum. I. Rapid micro-method employing photoelectric colorimeter. II. Rapid micro-method employing color standards," *Pediatrics*, vol. 18, no. 3, pp. 433–437, 1956.

[18] J. K. Fawcett and J. E. Scott, "A rapid and precise method for the determination of urea," *Journal of Clinical Pathology*, vol. 13, pp. 156–159, 1960.

[19] L. D. Bowers and E. T. Wong, "Kinetic serum creatinine assays. II. A critical evaluation and review," *Clinical Chemistry*, vol. 26, no. 5, pp. 555–561, 1980.

[20] A. J. Kettle and C. C. Winterbourn, "Assays for the chlorination activity of myeloperoxidase," *Methods in Enzymology*, vol. 233, pp. 502–512, 1994.

[21] E. Beutler, O. Duron, and B. M. Kelly, "Improved method for the determination of blood glutathione," *The Journal of Laboratory and Clinical Medicine*, vol. 61, pp. 882–888, 1963.

[22] H. Ohkawa, N. Ohishi, and K. Yagi, "Assay for lipid peroxides in animal tissues by thiobarbituric acid reaction," *Analytical Biochemistry*, vol. 95, no. 2, pp. 351–358, 1979.

[23] H. A. C. Montgomery and J. F. Dymock, "The rapid determination of nitrate in fresh and saline waters," *The Analyst*, vol. 87, no. 1034, pp. 374–378, 1962.

[24] P. Mayoral, M. Criado, F. Hidalgo et al., "Effects of chronic nitric oxide activation or inhibition on early hepatic fibrosis in rats with bile duct ligation," *Clinical Science*, vol. 96, no. 3, pp. 297–305, 1999.

[25] C. Türkay, Ö. Yönem, O. Arikan, and E. Baskin, "Nitric oxide and renal functions in liver cirrhosis," *The Turkish Journal of Gastroenterology*, vol. 15, no. 2, pp. 73–76, 2004.

[26] M. Saracyn, P. Wesołowski, Z. Nowak, J. Patera, W. Kozłowski, and Z. Wańkowicz, "Role of nitric oxide system in pathogenesis of experimental model of hepatorenal syndrome," *Polski Merkuriusz Lekarski: Organ Polskiego Towarzystwa Lekarskiego*, vol. 24, no. 142, pp. 293–297, 2008.

[27] M. C. Ortíz, L. A. Fortepiani, C. Martínez, N. M. Atucha, and J. García-Estañ, "Renal and pressor effects of aminoguanidine in cirrhotic rats with ascites," *Journal of the American Society of Nephrology*, vol. 7, no. 12, pp. 2694–2699, 1996.

[28] M. Yilmaz, C. Ara, B. Isik et al., "The effect of aminoguanidine against cholestatic liver injury in rats," *Cell Biochemistry and Function*, vol. 25, no. 6, pp. 625–632, 2007.

[29] M. Criado, O. Flores, M. C. Ortíz et al., "Elevated glomerular and blood mononuclear lymphocyte nitric oxide production in rats with chronic bile duct ligation: role of inducible nitric oxide synthase activation," *Hepatology*, vol. 26, no. 2, pp. 268–276, 1997.

[30] M. Niederberger, P.-Y. Martin, P. Ginès et al., "Normalization of nitric oxide production corrects arterial vasodilation and hyperdynamic circulation in cirrhotic rats," *Gastroenterology*, vol. 109, no. 5, pp. 1624–1630, 1995.

[31] N. M. Atucha, J. Garcia-Estan, A. Ramirez, M. D. C. Perez, T. Quesada, and J. C. Romero, "Renal effects of nitric oxide synthesis inhibition in cirrhotic rats," *The American Journal of Physiology—Regulatory Integrative and Comparative Physiology*, vol. 267, no. 6, pp. R1454–R1460, 1994.

[32] M. Galicia-Moreno, L. Favari, and P. Muriel, "Antifibrotic and antioxidant effects of N-acetylcysteine in an experimental cholestatic model," *European Journal of Gastroenterology and Hepatology*, vol. 24, no. 2, pp. 179–185, 2012.

[33] P. Bautista-García, L. G. Sánchez-Lozada, M. Cristóbal-García et al., "Chronic inhibition of NOS-2 ameliorates renal injury, as well as COX-2 and TGF-β1 overexpression in 5/6 nephrectomized rats," *Nephrology Dialysis Transplantation*, vol. 21, no. 11, pp. 3074–3081, 2006.

[34] D. J. Kelly, R. E. Gilbert, A. J. Cox, T. Soulis, G. Jerums, and M. E. Cooper, "Aminoguanidine ameliorates overexpression of prosclerotic growth factors and collagen deposition in experimental diabetic nephropathy," *Journal of the American Society of Nephrology*, vol. 12, no. 10, pp. 2098–2107, 2001.

[35] R. Tamarat, J.-S. Silvestre, M. Huijberts et al., "Blockade of advanced glycation end-product formation restores ischemia-induced angiogenesis in diabetic mice," *Proceedings of the National Academy of Sciences of the United States of America*, vol. 100, no. 14, pp. 8555–8560, 2003.

[36] O. Lukivskaya, E. Patsenker, R. Lis, and V. U. Buko, "Inhibition of inducible nitric oxide synthase activity prevents liver recovery in rat thioacetamide-induced fibrosis reversal," *European Journal of Clinical Investigation*, vol. 38, no. 5, pp. 317–325, 2008.

3

Anti-Inflammatory Effects of Heparin and Its Derivatives: A Systematic Review

Sarah Mousavi,[1] Mandana Moradi,[2] Tina Khorshidahmad,[3] and Maryam Motamedi[3]

[1]Department of Clinical Pharmacy and Pharmacy Practice, Faculty of Pharmacy and Pharmaceutical Sciences,
 Isfahan University of Medical Sciences, Isfahan, Iran
[2]Faculty of Pharmacy, Zabol University of Medical Sciences, Zabol, Iran
[3]Faculty of Pharmacy, Tehran University of Medical Sciences, Tehran, Iran

Correspondence should be addressed to Sarah Mousavi; s.mousavi@pharm.mui.ac.ir

Academic Editor: Berend Olivier

Background. Heparin, used clinically as an anticoagulant, also has anti-inflammatory properties. The purpose of this systematic review was to provide a comprehensive review regarding the efficacy and safety of heparin and its derivatives as anti-inflammatory agents. *Methods.* We searched the following databases up to March 2012: Pub Med, Scopus, Web of Science, Ovid, Elsevier, and Google Scholar using combination of Mesh terms. Randomized Clinical Trials (RCTs) and trials with quasi-experimental design in clinical setting published in English were included. Quality assessments of RCTs were performed using Jadad score and Consolidated Standards of Reporting Trials (CONSORT) checklist. *Results.* A total of 280 relevant studies were reviewed and 57 studies met the inclusion criteria. Among them 48 studies were RCTs. About 65% of articles had score of 3 and higher according to Jadad score. Twelve studies had a quality score > 40% according to CONSORT items. Asthma ($n = 7$), inflammatory bowel disease ($n = 5$), cardiopulmonary bypass ($n = 8$), and cataract surgery ($n = 6$) were the most studied disease condition. Forty studies use unfractionated heparin (UFH) for intervention; the remaining studies use low molecular weight heparin (LMWH). *Conclusion.* Despite the conflicting results, heparin seems to be a safe and effective anti-inflammatory agent; although it is shown that heparin can decrease the level of inflammatory biomarkers and improves patient conditions, still more data from larger rigorously designed studies are needed to support use of heparin as an anti-inflammatory agent in clinical setting. However, because of the association between inflammation, atherogenesis, thrombogenesis, and cell proliferation, heparin and related compounds with pleiotropic effects may have greater therapeutic efficacy than compounds acting against a single target.

1. Introduction

Heparin is a highly sulfated glycosaminoglycan (GAG) that is found in the mast cells of most mammals. The endogenous GAGs are highly acidic and actively charged. Heparin is the most sulfated, and acidic GAGs enable it to bind to different component such as coagulating and fibrinolysing proteins, many growth factors, and immune response proteins such as cytokines and chemokines [1, 2]. Heparin is mostly known for its anticoagulant properties, so commercially form of heparin including unfractionated heparin (UFH) and low molecular weight heparin (LMWH) used currently in treatment and prevention of thrombotic events like deep vein thrombosis, pulmonary emboli, acute coronary syndromes, and ischemic cerebrovascular events as well as prevention of thrombosis in extracorporeal circuits and hemodialysis [3, 4]. Apart from its anticoagulant effects, there are several studies which have shown that heparin possesses various anti-inflammatory and immunomodulatory properties and the mechanisms of anti-inflammatory actions of heparin have been discussed recently [5, 6]. But the exact benefit and safety of heparin and its derivatives as anti-inflammatory agents in clinical setting have not definitely proved yet. Our objective was to systematically review and summarize the literature supporting anti-inflammatory role of heparin to provide evidence about the clinical effectiveness and safety of heparin in inflammatory conditions.

2. Methods

2.1. Search Strategy. A comprehensive literature search was conducted in PubMed, Scopus, Web of Science, Ovid, Elsevier, and Google Scholar from inception to March 2012 using the following Mesh keywords: (1) heparin, (2) UFH, (3) anticoagulants, (4) dalteparin, (5) enoxaparin, (6) nadroparin, (7) tinzaparin, (8) heparinoids, (9) inflammation, (10) inflammatory process, (11) anti-inflammation, (12) inflammation mediators, (13) inflammatory bowel disease, and (14) anti-inflammatory agents. All keywords from 1 to 8 were separately combined with each keyword from 9 to 14 in all databases. Articles were initially scanned based on titles and abstracts by two reviewers (Sarah Mousavi and Mandana Moradi) and related articles were retrieved in full and assessed for eligibility by two reviewers (Sarah Mousavi and Mandana Moradi). The reference list of each eligible study was checked to identify additional studies.

2.2. Inclusion Criteria. All Randomized Clinical Trials (RCTs) and studies with quasi-experimental design which evaluated efficacy, using inflammatory biomarkers levels, and safety (significant hemorrhage or thrombocytopenia) of anti-inflammatory effects of heparin and heparin-related derivatives (LMWH or other heparinoids) with an English abstract regardless of rout of administration (intravenous, subcutaneous, topical, or inhaler), age, gender, race, and ethnic origin of participants were included.

2.3. Exclusion Criteria. The following were excluded: studies based on animal models; preclinical and biological studies, letters, and editorials; report published as meeting abstract only; where insufficient data were reported to allow inclusion.

2.4. Data Extraction and Quality Assessment. Data from each eligible study were extracted individually and compared by two authors (Sarah Mousavi and Mandana Moradi) using standard form that included study design, setting, sample size, duration and follow up, dosing regimen, intervention type, and outcomes. Disagreements were resolved through discussion; if necessary they consulted a third person. A narrative synthesis was conducted.

Quality assessment of clinical trials included in the analysis were performed utilizing the Jadad score, a previously validated instrument that assesses trials based on appropriate randomization, blinding, and description of study withdrawals or dropouts [7]. The description of this score is as follows: (1) whether it is randomized (yes = 1 point, no = 0); (2) whether randomization was described appropriately (yes = 1 point, no = 0); (3) whether it is double-blind (yes = 1 point, no = 0); (4) whether the double-blinding was described appropriately (yes = 1 point, no = 0); (5) whether withdrawals and dropouts were described (yes = 1 point, no = 0). The quality score ranges from 0 to 5 points; a low-quality report score is ≤2; and a high-quality report score is at least 3.

The Consolidated Standards of Reporting Trials (CONSORT) checklist was also used for randomized trials as it is

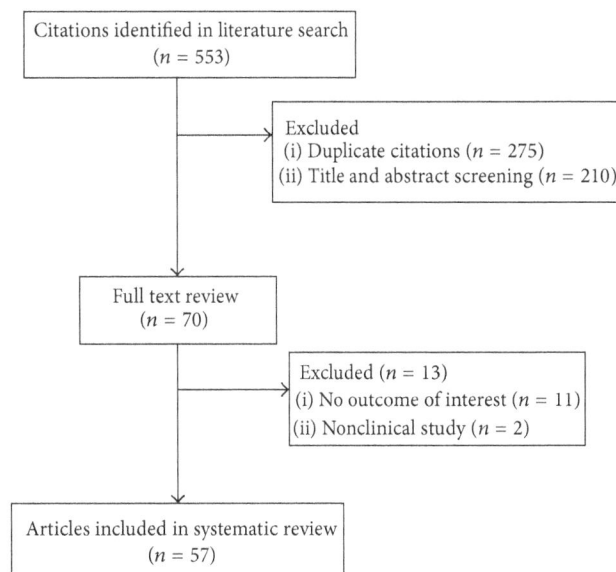

FIGURE 1: Flow diagram of literature search process.

strongly endorsed by prominent journals and leading editorial organizations [8]. Total possible score for CONSORT checklist was considered as 74: two points for adequate description, one point for inadequate description, and zero for no description.

2.5. Statistical Methods. To summarize and extract data, the database was designed by Microsoft office Access 2007 (Microsoft Corporation, Redmond, WA). A narrative synthesis was conducted and data were extracted into tables and summarized.

3. Results

Following Initial screening of mentioned databases total of 553 citations (275 duplicates) were extracted but only 70 of them were potentially eligible for investigation of our objectives (according to our proposed inclusion criteria) based on titles and abstracts. The full text screening excluded other 13 citations and the remaining 57 papers were considered relevant for data extraction and following analysis. The flow chart of studies' selection processes is as shown in Figure 1.

3.1. Study and Patient Characteristic. Sample sizes ranged from 8 to 555 patients in 57 studies that met the criteria to be included. Research designs mostly were randomized controlled trial ($n = 48$) and the remaining ($n = 9$) had quasi-experimental designs using pre-post studies ($n = 6$).

Tables 1 and 2 [9–62] list the characteristics of the included studies. The most studied clinical conditions was cardiopulmonary bypass ($n = 12$), followed by Asthma ($n = 8$), inflammatory bowel disease (IBD) ($n = 5$), acute coronary syndrome (ACS) ($n = 8$), and ophthalmological disease ($n = 8$). Other less common studied conditions were as follows: burn, cystic fibrosis, allergic rhinitis, superficial

TABLE 1: Summary and findings of common studied diseases.

Clinical setting	Heparin preparation	Mode of administration	Comparator	Number of patients	Clinical outcome	Laboratory outcome	Study design
Exercise-induced Asthma [9]	UFH	Inhaler	Cromolyn sodium or placebo	12	Significantly reduction of exercise-induced asthma	Heparin had no effect on histamine-induced bronchoconstriction	Single-blind, randomized, crossover clinical trial
Asthma [10]	UFH	Inhaler	Placebo	8	Significant reduction of late asthmatic response after allergen administration (P: 0.005)	—	Randomized, double-blind, crossover clinical trial
Atopic asthma [11]	Heparin (IVX-0142)	Nebulizer	Placebo	19	No significant decrease in early (P: 0.06) and late (P: 0.24) asthmatic response	—	Randomized single-blind, placebo-controlled, crossover trial
Asthma [12]	LMWH	Nebulizer	—	24	Effective as an add-on therapy to standard treatment	Reduction in eosinophil (P: 0.0006) and lymphocyte (P: 0.049) in bronchoalveolar lavage. No changes in IL-5 or ECP concentrations in serum	Quasi-experimental (pretest-posttest design)
Allergic asthma [13]	UFH	Inhaler	Placebo	25	Heparin inhalation significantly reduced bronchial hyperreactivity ($P < 0.05$)	—	Randomized, double-blind, placebo-controlled, crossover trial
Asthma [14]	UFH	Inhaler	—	12	Transient (time-dependent) inhibitory role in allergic reactions	Increased the methacholine PC20 value (P: 0.05) but did not prevent an increase in Raw and/or a decrease in SGAW	Randomized, double-blind, placebo-controlled, crossover trial
Asthma (children) [15]	UFH	Inhaler	Placebo	14	Single dose of heparin significantly (P: 0.005) reduced bronchial hyperreactivity	Provocation test used leukotriene D4	Randomized, double-blind, placebo-controlled, crossover trial
Asthma [16]	UFH	Inhaler	Placebo	23	Significant reduction of bronchial hyperreactivity to histamine and leukotriene	—	Randomized, double-blind, placebo controlled, crossover trial
IBD [17]	UFH	IV/SC	Hydrocortisone + prednisolone	20 (12 in control group)	Clinical activity index, stool frequency, and endoscopic and histopathological grading were similar in both treatment groups	CRP and $\alpha 1$ acid glycoprotein did not change	Open label randomized, crossover clinical trial

TABLE 1: Continued.

Clinical setting	Heparin preparation	Mode of administration	Comparator	Number of patients	Clinical outcome	Laboratory outcome	Study design
IBD [18]	UFH	SC	—	17	Histology improved significantly in ulcerative colitis patients (UFH is effective in ulcerative colitis but not Crohn disease)	CRP (P: 0.0119) and ESR (P: 0.0096) significantly reduced in ulcerative colitis but not Crohn disease	Quasi-experimental (pretest-posttest design)
IBD [19]	UFH	IV	Methyl prednisolone	25 (13 in control group)	No effect of heparin, also increased bleeding	No change in CRP	Randomized, double-blind, parallel-group trial
IBD [20]	Enoxaparin + standard treatment	SC	Aminosalicylate + corticosteroid	34 (18 in control group)	Significant improvement in disease severity in both groups (P: 0.001)	No difference ESR, CRP and fibrinogen and coagulation	Randomized controlled trial
IBD [21]	Nadroparin	SC	—	25	Endoscopic and histological sign of inflammation significantly improved	—	Quasi-experimental (Non-randomized clinical trial)
Cataract surgery [22]	UFH	Intraocular lens (IOL)	Polymethylmethacrylate	524	—	Heparin surface modification reduced the cellular deposit compared to control group	Randomized, double-blind, parallel group clinical trial
Cataract surgery [23]	UFH	Intraocular lens (IOL)	Polymethylmethacrylate	58 (31 in control group)	Postoperative inflammation decreased significantly in heparin group (P: 0.02)	Giant cell and cell deposit decreased significantly ($P < 0.05$)	Randomized, double-blind, clinical trial
Cataract surgery (pediatric) [24]	UFH	Irrigation	Balanced salt solution	33 (19 in control group)	Heparin irrigation reduced number of postoperative inflammatory related complication	Anterior chamber reaction including fibrin formation was lower in heparin group	Randomized prospective double-blind trial
Cataract surgery (pediatrics) [25]	Enoxaparin	Irrigation	No treatment	40 (20 in each group)	Increase of flare and cell deposit after surgery (1 and 3 months) (P: 0.99)	Increase in large cell deposits	Randomized, double-blind, controlled trial
Cataract surgery [26]	UFH	Irrigation	Regular irrigation solution	72	Significant reduction of inflammation in the early (days 1–3) postoperative period ($P < 0.01$)	—	Randomized controlled trial
Cardiopulmonary bypass (pediatric) [27]	Heparin-coated circuit ($n = 11$)	—	Non-heparin-coated circuit ($n = 10$)	21	Decrease of systemic inflammatory response with the use of heparin-bonded oxygenators	Significantly decreased levels of IL-6, IL-8, terminal complement complex, neutrophils, and elastase in heparin coated circuit	Randomized controlled trial
Cardiopulmonary bypass [28]	Heparin-coated circuit ± aprotinin	—	Uncoated circuit ± aprotinin	200 (4 groups)	Aprotinin and heparin had no effect on cytokine release	TNF-α, IL-6, IL-8 and myeloperoxidase did not change	Randomized, double-blind, clinical trial

TABLE 1: Continued.

Clinical setting	Heparin preparation	Mode of administration	Comparator	Number of patients	Clinical outcome	Laboratory outcome	Study design
Cardiopulmonary bypass [29]	UFH	—	Uncoated circuit	51 (26 in each group)	Decreased pulmonary vascular resistance index and pulmonary shunt fraction, and increased PaO2/FIO2 ratio	Lower levels of phospholipase A2 and complement activation (P: 0.001)	Randomized, double-blind, clinical trial
Cardiopulmonary bypass [30]	Heparin-coated circuit	—	Non-heparin-coated circuit	16 (9 in control group)	—	No significant difference between groups regarding: granulocyte elastase IL-6, IL-8	Quasi-experimental (pretest-posttest design)
Cardiopulmonary bypass [31]	Heparin concentration-based system	—	Activated clotting time-based management	200 (100 in control group)	No effect on postoperative blood loss	Significant reduction of neutrophil activation and fibrinolysis and thrombin generation ($P < 0.05$)	Randomized controlled trial
Cardiopulmonary bypass (pediatric) [32]	Heparin-coated circuit	—	Non-heparin-coated circuit	19 (10 in control group)	Improvement of the biocompatibility of CPB during heart surgery	Levels of complement factor C3a ($P < 0.001$) and IL-6 (P: 0.005) significantly reduced in heparin-coated circuit	Randomized controlled trial
Cardiopulmonary bypass (pediatric) [33]	Heparin-coated circuit	—	Non-heparin-coated circuit	34 (12 in control group)	No differences in duration of intubation, intensive care unit or hospital stay, or postoperative blood loss	IL-6, IL-8, and TNF-α were significantly lower in heparin group ($P < 0.01$, $P < 0.01$, and $P < 0.05$, resp.)	Randomized controlled trial
Cardiopulmonary bypass [34]	Heparin-coated circuit (heparin + aprotinin)	—	Non-heparin-coated circuit (heparin + aprotinin)	30 (15 in each group)	No significant differences between the two groups in terms of bleeding and transfusional requirements, the time spent on a ventilator, or in duration of stay in the intensive care unit (ICU)	Levels of IL-6, CRP, and neutrophil count did not change by heparin-coated circuit. Monocyte count increased in heparin-coated circuit	Randomized controlled trial
Coronary artery bypass grafting (CABG) [35]	Heparin-coated circuit	—	Non-heparin-coated circuit	18 (9 in each group)	—	Reduction of levels of IL-8 and TNF-α and increase of neutrophil elastase	Randomized controlled trial

CRP: C-Reactive Protein, CPB: Cardio Pulmonary Bypass, ECP: Eosinophil Cationic Protein, ESR: Erythrocyte Sedimentation, ICU: Intensive Care Unit, IL: interleukin, IV: intravenous, SC: subcutaneous, SGAW: Specific Airway Conductance, TNF: Tumor Necrosis Factor, and UFH: unfractionated heparin.

TABLE 2: Summary and findings of other studied diseases.

Clinical setting	Heparin preparation	Mode of administration	Comparator	Number of patients	Clinical outcome	Laboratory outcome	Study design
Pancreatitis after ERCP [36]	UFH	SC	Saline solution	105 (54 in control group)	Rate of postoperative pancreatitis was not significant between both groups	—	Randomized placebo-controlled clinical trial
Acute coronary syndrome (ACS) [37]	UFH	SC	Enoxaparin	201	—	No significant difference between CD4 ligand and PAI-1 in both groups	Open label, randomized, clinical trial
Skin or pulmonary allergy [38]	UFH	IV/nebulizer	Normal saline/placebo	25	Significant inhibition of mast cell-mediated allergic inflammation (P: 0.04)	—	Double-blind, placebo-controlled, crossover clinical trial
COPD [39]	UFH	IV	—	37 (18 in control group)	Significant improvement in bronchospasm and bronchial secretions (58% response rate)	—	Randomized placebo-controlled clinical trial
COPD [40]	Nadroparin	SC	Conventional treatment	66 (33 in each group)	Decrease of duration of mechanical ventilation and length of hospital and ICU stay ($P < 0.01$)	Significant decrease in levels of CRP, IL-6, and fibrinogen	Randomized controlled trial
Ischemic stroke [41]	UFH	IV	Aspirin	167 (97 in control group)	Early onset initiation of heparin might improve recovery after stroke	Rise of sVCAM-1 at 48 h was significantly lower in patients treated with UFH ($P < 0.01$)	Quasi-experimental (controlled observational study)
Ligneous conjunctivitis [42]	UFH	Topical	Alpha chymotrypsin or steroid	17 (12 in control group)	Intensive and early use of topical heparin may improve therapy results in disease	—	Quasi-experimental (nonrandomized Clinical trial)
Endotoxemia (induced by lipopolysaccharide in healthy subjects) [43]	UFH	IV	LMWH or placebo	30 (10 in each group)	—	No effect on TNF-α, IL-6 and 8, CRP, and E-selectin	Randomized, double-blinded, placebo-controlled parallel group trial
Mechanical ventilation [44]	UFH	Nebulizer	Normal saline (placebo)	50 (25 in each group)	Fewer days on mechanical ventilation, better Pao2/Fio2 ratio	—	Double-blind, randomized, placebo-controlled trial
Percutaneous coronary intervention [45]	Bivalirudin	IV	UFH + eptifibatide	63 (29 in control group)	—	Increase in IL-6 and CRP after 1 day. Decrease in CRP in bivalirudin group after 30 days (P: 0.002)	Randomized controlled trial
Cystic fibrosis (adults) [46]	UFH	Inhaler	—	12 (6 in control group)	Spirometry parameters did not change	IL-6 reduced after treatment	Quasi-experimental (pretest-posttest design)

TABLE 2: Continued.

Clinical setting	Heparin preparation	Mode of administration	Comparator	Number of patients	Clinical outcome	Laboratory outcome	Study design
Cystic fibrosis (adults) [47]	UFH	Inhaler	Placebo	14	No effect on FEV1	No effect on sputum inflammatory markers	Randomized, double-blind, placebo-controlled crossover trial
Hemodialysis patients [48]	UFH	IV/SC	LMWH and no drug	33	LMWH decreased oxidative stress and inflammation whereas heparin increased them	CRP, TNF-α, superoxide dismutase, MDA increased in heparin group but comparable to LMWH group	Quasi-experimental (pretest-posttest design)
Stable angina [49]	Heparin + Aspirin ($n = 15$)	—	Argatroban + Aspirin ($n = 12$)	27	No difference in inflammatory response after angioplasty	Fibrinogen decreased significantly in argatroban group. No difference in von Willbrand factor between both groups. PAI-1 increased in argatroban group	Randomized controlled trial
Phacoemulsification [50]	Heparin	Coated lenses	Polymethylmethacrylate lenses	367	Heparin coated lenses reduced significantly inflammation early postoperation (P: 0.05)	—	Randomized, double-blind, multicenter, parallel group trial
Allergic rhinitis [51]	UFH	Intranasal	—	10	—	Reduction of eosinophil cationic protein in the nasal wash	Quasi-experimental (pretest-posttest design)
Phacomorphic glaucoma [52]	Dalteparin	Irrigation	Balanced salt solution	46 (23 in each group)	Significant decrease of postoperative inflammation in dalteparin group	—	Randomized, double-blind, clinical trial
Burn [53]	Dalteparin	SC	No treatment	24	—	Decrease of nitric oxide synthetase activity significantly	Quasi-experimental (nonrandomized clinical trial)
Unstable coronary artery disease [54]	Enoxaparin ($n = 46$) Dalteparin ($n = 48$)	SC	UFH ($n = 47$)	68	Von Willberand factor may have prognostic value, but other biological variables did not predict outcome	CRP, fibrinogen, Von Willberand factor increased over first 2 days despite medical treatment. Enoxaparin (13%) and dalteparin (19%) reduced release of Von Willberand factor	Open label, randomized, clinical trial
ST-Elevated Myocardial Infarction (STEMI) [55]	Enoxaparin	SC	UFH	34 (17 in each group)	Both heparin and enoxaparin show anti-inflammatory effects in STEMI patients	Serum Amyloid A (P: 0.02), CRP (P: 0.02), and ferritin (P: 0.01) reduced in heparin group. IL-6 (P: 0.002), SAA (P: 0.009), CRP (P: 0.01) were significantly decreased in enoxaparin group. The overall difference between groups was not significant	Open label, randomized, clinical trial

23

TABLE 2: Continued.

Clinical setting	Heparin preparation	Mode of administration	Comparator	Number of patients	Clinical outcome	Laboratory outcome	Study design
Coronary artery disease [56]	Dalteparin	SC	Placebo	555 (285 in control group)	Dalteparin reduced coagulation and so Myocardial Infarction but has not inflammatory activity	No effects on IL-6, C-reactive protein and fibrinogen	Randomized, double-blind, parallel-group, multicentre trial
Stable coronary artery disease [57]	Enoxaparin	SC	Sodium chloride	62 (31 in each group)	By mobilizing vessel bound MPO, enoxaparin improves endothelial function	Significant increase of MPO levels	Randomized, double-blind, placebo-controlled trial
Acute coronary syndrome and PCI [58]	Tirofiban (high dose) + enoxaparin	SC	Tirofiban (high dose) + UFH	60 (30 in each group)	The combination of tirofiban (high dose) + enoxaparin reduced inflammation after PCI	Von willberand, CRP, D-dimer, and prothrombin fragment were significantly lower in enoxaparin group than UFH	Open label randomized controlled trial
Superficial venous thrombophlebitis [59]	Dalteparin	SC	Ibuprofen	72 (37 in dalteparin group)	Significant reduction of pain form baseline to day 14 of follow-up. No difference on thrombosis progression after 3 months	—	Randomized, double-blind, controlled trial
Superficial venous thrombosis [60]	Nadroparin	SC	Naproxen	117 (39 in control group)	Nadroparin reduced symptom and signs of thrombosed superficial vein better than naproxen (P: 0.007)	—	Randomized, open label clinical trial
Superficial venous thrombosis [61]	Nadroparin	SC	Nadroparin + acemetacin	50	Significant symptom improvement in both groups (P: 0.001). The combination group was better	—	Randomized controlled trial
Peritoneal dialysis patients [62]	Tinzaparin	Intraperitoneal	Isotonic saline	21	Reduction of local and systemic inflammation in peritoneal dialysis patients	Reduced levels of CRP (P: 0.032) and fibrinogen (P: 0.042) and IL-6 (P: 0.007) in dialysate.	Randomized, double-blind, placebo-controlled crossover trial

COPD: Chronic Obstructive Pulmonary Disease, CRP: C-Reactive Protein, CPB: Cardio Pulmonary Bypass, ECP: Eosinophil Cationic Protein, ERCP: Endoscopic Retrograde Cholangiopancreatography, ESR: Erythrocyte Sedimentation, ICU: Intensive Care Unit, IL: interleukin, IV: intravenous, LMWH: low molecular weight heparin, MDA: malondialdehyde, PAI: Plasminogen Activator Inhibitor, SC: subcutaneous, sVCAM: Soluble Vascular Cell Adhesion Molecule, TNF: Tumor Necrosis Factor, and UFH: unfractionated heparin.

TABLE 3: Summary of numbers and percentages of adequately reported items in each trial according to CONSORT checklist and Jadad score.

Trials	Jadad score	Adequately reported items (n/N)	Percentage (%)
Abdollahi et al. [52]	4	29/74	39.2%
Ahmed et al. [9]	3	20/74	27%
Ang et al. [17]	2	24/74	32.4%
Ashraf et al. [27]	2	22/74	29.7%
Becker et al. [37]	3	28/74	37.8%
de Vroege et al. [29]	3	26/74	35.1%
Defraigne et al. [28]	4	28/74	37.8%
Derhaschnig et al. [43]	3	32/74	43.2%
Dixon et al. [44]	4	50/74	67.5%
Duong et al. [11]	3	30/74	40.5%
Gu et al. [71]	2	16/74	21.6%
Jerzynska et al. [13]	3	20/74	27%
Keating et al. [45]	2	21/74	28.4%
Koster et al. [31]	2	26/74	35.1%
Montalescot et al. [54]	3	35/74	47.3%
Nasiripour et al. [55]	2	34/74	46%
Oldgren et al. [56]	3	27/74	36.5%
Olsson et al. [32]	2	25/74	33.8%
van Ophoven et al. [79]	2	27/74	36.5%
Ozawa et al. [33]	2	27/74	36.5%
Özkurt et al. [24]	3	18/74	24.3%
Paparella et al. [72]	2	22/74	29.7%
Polosa et al. [67]	3	23/74	31.1%
Rathbun et al. [59]	5	44/74	59.5%
Rudolph et al. [57]	3	31/74	41.2%
Serisier et al. [47]	5	45/74	60.8%
Stelmach et al. [16]	3	31/74	41.2%
Suzuki et al. [49]	2	23/74	31%
Vancheri et al. [51]	4	22/74	29.7%
Vasavada et al. [25]	5	52/74	70.2%
Walters et al. [58]	3	32/74	43.2%
Zezos et al. [20]	3	37/74	50%

thrombophlebitis, and hemodialysis. Unfractionated heparin (UFH) was used in forty studies as subcutaneous, intravenous, inhaler, or heparin-coated circuits while others used enoxaparin ($n = 3$), dalteparin ($n = 4$), nadroparin ($n = 4$), and tinzaparin ($n = 1$).

Table 3 provides information on the adequately reported items according to Jadad score and CONSORT items. Among these 32 papers, 11 (35.4%) scored 2 and the remaining studies scored 3 or higher according to Jadad score and just three studies fulfill the criteria of Jadad score. Calculated quality scores according to CONSORT checklist range from 21% to 70% in our object studies with twelve studies scoring greater than 40%. The following characteristics were not exactly reported in more than half of the trials: identification as

a randomized trial in the title, information about the setting and location of studies, determination of sample size, allocation and implementation of randomization, participant flow, recruitment and follow-up, subgroup analysis, limitations of study, harms, registration number, access to full trial protocol, and funding source.

4. Discussion

We discuss evidence from clinical studies supporting an anti-inflammatory role for heparin and heparin-related derivatives.

4.1. Asthma. Asthma is a chronic inflammatory disorder of airways characterized by bronchial hyperresponsiveness resulting in episodic bronchospasm. Several studies in 1960s described subjective improvement of symptoms in asthmatic patients using intravenous heparin for the first time [39, 63]. Inhaled heparin or its derivatives have been shown to possess antiasthmatic properties in various clinical models: allergen induced [38, 64], exercise [9], adenosine [6], and distilled water challenge models [65]. Seven randomized controlled crossover trials studied anti-inflammatory effects of heparin in exercise-induced or allergen-induced asthma having sample size range from 8 to 25 in 5 trials.

Heparin inhalation reduced bronchial hyperreactivity in a single-blind randomized crossover trial ($n = 12$) by Ahmed et al. [9]. Heparin inhalation (1000 μ/kg) prevents exercise-induced asthma ($P < 0.05$) without prevention of histamine-induced bronchoconstriction. Stelmach et al. [66] provoke challenge tests with histamine or leukotriene D4 before and after inhalation of heparin; showed that heparin (5000 Iu) decreases histamine and leukotriene-induced bronchial hyperreactivity compared to placebo significantly (P: 0.043 and 0.005) but changes in Forced Expiratory Volume (FEV 1) were not significant (P: 0.064). The inhibitory effects of inhaled heparin in the airways in the absence of bronchodilation might be related to suppressive action on mast cell degranulation. A randomized, double-blind study in 10 subjects with asthma showed that heparin inhalation attenuates airway response to adenosine $5'$-monophosphate (AMP) but not to methacholine ($P < 0.01$) suggesting the theory that heparin acts more likely in association to modulation of mediator release compared to a direct effect on smooth muscle [67].

Our results showed that inhaled enoxaparin was used just in a pre-post study of 24 asthmatic patients, measuring inflammatory biomarkers, and showed a reduction in eosinophil (P: 0.006) and lymphocytes of bronchoalveolar lavage without any significant change in IL-5 or Eosinophil Cationic Protein (ECP) concentrations [12]. Therefore, it seems that enoxaparin could be a valuable add on treatment in asthma like UFH. Duong et al. [11] evaluated IVX-0142 nebulizer, a heparin-derived hypersulfated disaccharide, in asthma and showed nonsignificant decrease in early and late asthmatic response.

Performed studies did not show any adverse events or harms with heparin or related compounds except increase in the plasma partial thromboplastin time reported by Ahmed et al. [9].

All in one, considering the results of these studies, we can conclude that heparin and its derivatives could have anti-inflammatory effects and could be considered along with other treatments in asthma.

4.2. Cardiopulmonary Bypass. Contact and interaction of blood with foreign surfaces during cardiopulmonary bypass (CPB) cause systemic inflammatory response syndrome (SIRS) through activation of several humoral cascades including cytokines such as IL-6, IL-8, and Tumor Necrosis Factor-α (TNF-α) [68]. The inflammatory response can be attenuated by promoting the biocompatibility of the CPB circuit. Use of heparin-treated surfaces in CPB circuits has been shown to decrease activation of leukocytes and the complement cascades [5]. As a result, need to inotropic support, postoperative time of mechanical ventilation, and rate of acute lung injury decrease and patients duration of hospital stay shortens, which reflects the positive effect of heparin in CPB circuits [69, 70]. Twelve studies whose endpoints were the effects of heparin-bonded circuits on inflammatory markers were included in our analysis and in the majority of these trials [27, 29, 32–35, 71]; heparin-coated circuit significantly decreased the level of cytokines such as IL-6, IL-8, TNF-α, complement complex, neutrophils, and elastase compared to non-heparin-coated circuit.

Defraigne et al. [28] randomized 200 patients in 4 groups; heparin-coated circuit with or without aprotinin administration and uncoated circuit with or without aprotinin administration. They measured IL-6, IL-8, TNF-α, myeloperoxidase (MPO), and elastase level and concluded that cytokine release and neutrophil activation were not attenuated by heparin-coated circuit or by the administration of aprotinin. Misawa et al. [30] evaluated cytokines level under normothermic CPB, in a small observational controlled study ($n = 19$, 9 in control group). Levels of IL-6, IL-8, and ICAM-1 (indicator of endothelial damage) were not different between study and control group. However, as mentioned before, most studies indicate the favorable effect of heparin-coated circuit on inflammatory responses in CPB.

Paparella et al. [72] compared two doses of heparin and 300 Iu/kg and 600 Iu/kg in 40 patients undergoing CPB in an RCT and showed that IL-6 and TNF-α plasma levels were in association to heparin dose. It seems that lower heparin dose had small influence on proinflammatory cytokines release; however, higher doses make a better regulatory effect on coagulation system.

The side effects of heparin-coated circuits were not reported. In these studies, just a number of included studies reported a decrease in platelet levels in both groups (coated and noncoated circuit). No major events including hemorrhage were reported.

4.3. Inflammatory Bowel Diseases (IBD). Hypercoagulable state may be an important contributing factor in the pathogenesis of IBD, especially ulcerative colitis (UC) [73]. A number of studies evaluate the effects of heparin administration on UC but the results obtained are controversial [17, 19].

Bloom et al. [74] did not find any favorable effect of LMWH, tinzaparin, over placebo in the treatment of active UC in a double-blind randomized, placebo controlled, multicenter trial ($n = 100$) evaluating mean change in colitis activity as the primary endpoint. Ang et al. [17] compared heparin to hydrocortisone plus prednisolone in 20 patients (UC, $n = 17$, Crohn's colitis, $n = 3$) in open-label randomized crossover trial which measured endpoints; clinical disease activity, stool frequency and α_1 acid glycoprotein, and endoscopic and histopathological grading indicate the efficacy and safety of heparin compared to corticosteroids ($P > 0.05$); in contrast the study by Panes et al. [19] did not show the efficacy of heparin in UC compared to methylprednisolone.

Zezos et al. [20] compared enoxaparin with standard treatment (aminosalicylate + corticosteroids) in 34 patients with active UC. The inflammatory biomarkers including C-Reactive Protein (CRP), Erythrocyte Sedimentation Rate (ESR), and fibrinogen did not show any difference in study group compared to control and both groups showed similar rate of disease improvement ($P > 0.05$); furthermore, coagulation factors did not change from one to another. Authors concluded that enoxaparin is a safe adjuvant but has no additive benefit over standard treatment of UC.

Generally the studies show conflicting results. The heparin and LMWHs showed efficacy in regard of disease activity and also well tolerated but inflammatory markers did not change significantly. Therefore the improvement in disease activity might be the result of heparin's anticoagulant effects.

4.4. Acute Coronary Syndrome (ACS). Inflammation has a key role in the pathogenesis of coronary artery plaque destabilization and rupture leading to acute coronary syndromes (ACS) [75]. Leukocyte activation, monocyte, and neutrophil infiltration result in local and systemic inflammatory responses [76]. Heparin and LMWHs are commonly used in ACS to prevent clot formation; they also seem to have desirable effects on inflammatory markers level based on sparse data.

We found 8 studies about heparin and LMWHs in CADs evaluating anti-inflammatory effects as their endpoints. Oldgren et al. [56] found that dalteparin administration in patients with unstable CAD ($n = 555$) did not affect IL-6, C-Reactive Protein (CRP), and fibrinogen levels, although it reduced coagulation activity and mortality rate in long term, so it is concluded that these effects are not related to its anti-inflammatory properties. Walters et al. [58] compared high dose of tirofiban/enoxaparin ($n = 30$) with tirofiban/heparin ($n = 30$) in an open-label randomized controlled trial in high risk percutaneous intervention. They found that combination of high dose of tirofiban with enoxaparin significantly attenuate inflammatory process (decreased levels of CRP, and von Willebrand factor) compared to tirofiban and heparin.

The ARMADA study [54] evaluated anti-inflammatory effects of heparin and enoxaparin in Non-ST-Elevated Myocardial Infarction (Non-STEMI) and reported that inflammatory markers (CRP and von Willebrand factor) are affected more by LMWH compared to UFH. However because of the small sample size of the study ($n = 68$)

it did not acquire sufficient statistical power to prove any effects on defined outcomes. Nasiripour et al. [55] found that both enoxaparin and heparin reduce inflammatory markers in STEMI patients at the same level; however, this study had the same limitations of sample size ($n = 34$) and power too.

In summary considering heparins as the main stay treatment of ACS, its effects are more pronounced as anticoagulating than as an anti-inflammatory agent in this pathological condition.

4.5. Cataract Surgery. Postoperative inflammation is observed in cataract surgery especially in children. Newer techniques as lensectomy and phacoemulsification cause less complication but still pose potential risks [77, 78]. It has been suggested that a heparin surface-modified intraocular lens (IOL) or augmenting the irrigating solution with heparin during cataract surgery may reduce the incidence of postoperative inflammation. Borgioli et al. [22] confirm this hypothesis that heparin surface-modified IOL will reduce the inflammatory response compared to conventional IOL at least in short term period (3 months) in a large (524 patients) double-blind, multicenter trial. A similar study by Colin et al. [23] ($n = 58$) confirms their results; however, the power of Borgioli et al. study was higher. Heparinized lenses showed also more anti-inflammatory effects during long term follow-up (1 year). Heparinized irrigating solution was used during cataract surgery in two different studies and inflammation decrease observed in the early postoperative period of both studies (Kohnen et al. [26] and Özkurt et al. [24]). Therefore, it seems that heparin in both forms have anti-inflammatory effects in cataract surgery.

Vasavada et al. [25] used enoxaparin irrigation solution in 20 children undergoing bilateral cataract surgery but they did not find any beneficial effect in early postoperative inflammation. This study acquired the highest quality in the study quality assessment process, based on Jadad score and CONSORT items (52/74, 70.2%). It is worth noticing that the majority of items mentioned in the CONSORT checklist were adequately reported and covered in this paper.

Potential mechanisms of anti-inflammatory effects of heparin have been discussed completely in a review by Young [6]. Binding of heparin to different mediators involved in the immune system response (cytokines and chemokines), acute phase proteins, and complement complex proteins may contribute to the anti-inflammatory activity of heparin. Neutralizing of cytokines at the inflammation site is another possible mechanism. In most of the studies level of cytokines such as IL-6, IL-8, TNF-α, and CRP was decreased after heparin administration, which can confirm this mechanism; also heparin and LMWHs inhibit adhesion of leukocytes and neutrophils to endothelial cells by binding to p-selectin, and consequently prevent release of oxygen radicals and proteolytic enzymes. Other possible mechanisms are as follows: inhibition of nuclear factor κB (NF-κB) and induction of apoptosis by modulation of activity of TNF-α and NF-κB. In a double-blind placebo-controlled trial ($n = 62$) in patients with stable coronary artery disease, following administration of 1 mg/kg subcutaneous enoxaparin, plasma levels of myeloperoxidase (MPO) increased significantly ($P < 0.001$) and subsequently endothelial function improved ($r = 0.67$, $P < 0.001$) through MPO binding to endothelium and depleting vascular nitric oxide [57]. This study confirms another possible mechanism of heparins anti-inflammatory effects.

5. Conclusion

As we discussed heparins potential effects as anti-inflammatory agents, supported by several clinical trials in various setting. Heparin and its related derivatives have been shown to benefit patients with asthma and patients undergoing cardiopulmonary bypass and cataract surgery. In other inflammatory diseases, such as IBD (ulcerative colitis), the studies are heterogeneous and incongruent. Most studies did not report any unwanted event with heparins when they used them as anti-inflammatory agents whether through systemic or through local (as inhaler or irrigation or heparin-coated circuit) administration. However, because the majority of these trials did not pose optimal quality scores, we cannot draw a definite conclusion on the efficacy of heparin and its derivatives as anti-inflammatory agents.

The present review included studies which measured inflammatory markers as their endpoints and in most of them these markers were decreased though not significantly. To come to a definite conclusion further double-blind, randomized, placebo-controlled clinical trials with a larger sample size are needed. However, because the inflammation, atherogenesis, thrombogenesis, and cell proliferation are associated with each other, the pleiotropic effects of heparin and related compounds may have greater therapeutic effect than compounds that are directed against a single target.

Conflict of Interests

The authors declare that there is no conflict of interests regarding the publication of this paper.

References

[1] B. Casu, "Heparin structure," *Pathophysiology of Haemostasis and Thrombosis*, vol. 20, supplement 1, pp. 62–73, 1990.

[2] J. Hirsh, R. Raschke, T. E. Warkentin, J. E. Dalen, D. Deykin, and L. Poller, "Heparin: mechanism of action, pharmacokinetics, dosing considerations, monitoring, efficacy, and safety," *Chest*, vol. 108, no. 4, supplement, pp. 258S–275S, 1995.

[3] J. Fareed, D. A. Hoppensteadt, and R. L. Bick, "An update on heparins at the beginning of the new millennium," *Seminars in Thrombosis and Hemostasis*, vol. 26, no. 3, pp. 5–21, 2000.

[4] J. Hirsh, "Drug therapy: heparin," *The New England Journal of Medicine*, vol. 324, no. 22, pp. 1565–1574, 1991.

[5] R. J. Ludwig, "Therapeutic use of heparin beyond anticoagulation," *Current Drug Discovery Technologies*, vol. 6, no. 4, pp. 281–289, 2009.

[6] E. Young, "The anti-inflammatory effects of heparin and related compounds," *Thrombosis Research*, vol. 122, no. 6, pp. 743–752, 2008.

[7] A. R. Jadad, R. A. Moore, D. Carroll et al., "Assessing the quality of reports of randomized clinical trials: is blinding necessary?" *Controlled Clinical Trials*, vol. 17, no. 1, pp. 1–12, 1996.

[8] K. F. Schulz, D. G. Altman, and D. Moher, "CONSORT 2010 statement: updated guidelines for reporting parallel group randomised trials," *International Journal of Surgery*, vol. 9, no. 8, pp. 672–677, 2011.

[9] T. Ahmed, J. Garrigo, and I. Danta, "Preventing bronchoconstriction in exercise-induced asthma with inhaled heparin," *The New England Journal of Medicine*, vol. 329, no. 2, pp. 90–95, 1993.

[10] Z. Diamant, M. C. Timmers, H. Van Der Veen, C. P. Page, F. J. Van Der Meer, and P. J. Sterk, "Effect of inhaled heparin on allergen-induced early and late asthmatic responses in patients with atopic asthma," *American Journal of Respiratory and Critical Care Medicine*, vol. 153, no. 6, pp. 1790–1795, 1996.

[11] M. Duong, D. Cockcroft, L.-P. Boulet et al., "The effect of IVX-0142, a heparin-derived hypersulfated disaccharide, on the allergic airway responses in asthma," *Allergy*, vol. 63, no. 9, pp. 1195–1201, 2008.

[12] A. M. Fal, M. Kraus-Filarska, J. Miecielica, and J. Malolepszy, "Mechanisms of action of nebulized low-molecular-weight heparin in patients with bronchial asthma," *The Journal of Allergy and Clinical Immunology*, vol. 113, no. 2, supplement, p. S36, 2004.

[13] J. Jerzynska, I. Stelmach, P. Majak, and P. Kuna, "The effect of inhaled heparin on airway responsiveness to histamine and metacholine in asthmatic children," *Journal of Allergy and Clinical Immunology*, vol. 109, no. 1, supplement 1, p. S39, 2002.

[14] A. F. Kalpaklioğlu, Y. S. Demirel, S. Saryal, and Z. Misirligil, "Effect of pretreatment with heparin on pulmonary and cutaneous response," *Journal of Asthma*, vol. 34, no. 4, pp. 337–343, 1997.

[15] I. Stelmach, J. Jerzynska, A. Brzozowska, and P. Kuna, "The effect of inhaled heparin on postleukotriene bronchoconstriction in children with asthma," *Journal of Allergy and Clinical Immunology*, vol. 109, no. 1, supplement 1, p. S39, 2002.

[16] I. Stelmach, J. Jerzynska, W. Stelmach et al., "The effect of inhaled heparin on airway responsiveness to histamine and leukotriene D4," *Allergy and Asthma Proceedings*, vol. 24, no. 1, pp. 59–65, 2003.

[17] Y. S. Ang, N. Mahmud, B. White et al., "Randomized comparison of unfractionated heparin with corticosteroids in severe active inflammatory bowel disease," *Alimentary Pharmacology and Therapeutics*, vol. 14, no. 8, pp. 1015–1022, 2000.

[18] C. Folwaczny, B. Wiebecke, and K. Loeschke, "Unfractioned heparin in the therapy of patients with highly active inflammatory bowel disease," *The American Journal of Gastroenterology*, vol. 94, no. 6, pp. 1551–1555, 1999.

[19] J. Panes, M. Esteve, E. Cabre et al., "Comparison of heparin and steroids in the treatment of moderate and severe ulcerative colitis," *Gastroenterology*, vol. 119, no. 4, pp. 903–908, 2000.

[20] P. Zezos, G. Papaioannou, N. Nikolaidis et al., "Low-molecular-weight heparin (enoxaparin) as adjuvant therapy in the treatment of active ulcerative colitis: a randomized, controlled, comparative study," *Alimentary Pharmacology and Therapeutics*, vol. 23, no. 10, pp. 1443–1453, 2006.

[21] A. A. Vrij, J. M. Jansen, E. J. Schoon, H. C. Hemker, and R. W. Stockbrügger, "Low molecular weight heparin treatment in steroid refractory ulcerative colitis: clinical outcome and influence on mucosal capillary thrombi," *Scandinavian Journal of Gastroenterology, Supplement*, vol. 36, no. 234, pp. 41–47, 2001.

[22] D. M. Borgioli, D. J. Coster, R. F. T. Fan et al., "Effect of heparin surface modification of polymethylmethacrylate intraocular lenses on signs of postoperative inflammation after extracapsular cataract extraction: one-year results of a double-masked multicenter study," *Ophthalmology*, vol. 99, no. 8, pp. 1248–1255, 1992.

[23] J. Colin, S. Roncin, and M. Wenzel, "Efficacy of heparin surface-modified IOLs in reducing postoperative inflammatory reactions in patients with exfoliation syndrome—a double-blind comparative study," *European Journal of Implant and Refractive Surgery*, vol. 7, no. 5, pp. 266–270, 1995.

[24] Y. B. Özkurt, A. Taşkiran, N. Erdogan, B. Kandemir, and Ö. K. Doğan, "Effect of heparin in the intraocular irrigating solution on postoperative inflammation in the pediatric cataract surgery," *Clinical Ophthalmology*, vol. 3, no. 1, pp. 363–365, 2009.

[25] V. A. Vasavada, M. R. Praveen, S. K. Shah, R. H. Trivedi, and A. R. Vasavada, "Anti-inflammatory effect of low-molecular-weight heparin in pediatric cataract surgery: a randomized clinical trial," *The American Journal of Ophthalmology*, vol. 154, no. 2, pp. 252–258, 2012.

[26] T. Kohnen, B. Dick, V. Hessemer, D. D. Koch, and K. W. Jacobi, "Effect of heparin in irrigating solution on inflammation following small incision cataract surgery," *Journal of Cataract & Refractive Surgery*, vol. 24, no. 2, pp. 237–243, 1998.

[27] S. Ashraf, Y. Tian, D. Cowan, A. Entress, P. G. Martin, and K. G. Watterson, "Release of proinflammatory cytokines during pediatric cardiopulmonary bypass: heparin-bonded versus nonbonded oxygenators," *Annals of Thoracic Surgery*, vol. 64, no. 6, pp. 1790–1794, 1997.

[28] J.-O. Defraigne, J. Pincemail, R. Larbuisson, F. Blaffart, and R. Limet, "Cytokine release and neutrophil activation are not prevented by heparin- coated circuits and aprotinin administration," *Annals of Thoracic Surgery*, vol. 69, no. 4, pp. 1084–1091, 2000.

[29] R. de Vroege, W. van Oeveren, J. van Klarenbosch et al., "The impact of heparin-coated cardiopulmonary bypass circuits on pulmonary function and the release of inflammatory mediators," *Anesthesia and Analgesia*, vol. 98, no. 6, pp. 1586–1594, 2004.

[30] Y. Misawa, K. Kawahito, H. Konishi, and K. Fuse, "Cytokine mediated endothelial activation during and after normothermic cardiopulmonary bypass: Heparin-bonded versus non heparin-bonded circuits," *ASAIO Journal*, vol. 46, no. 6, pp. 740–743, 2000.

[31] A. Koster, T. Fischer, M. Praus et al., "Hemostatic activation and inflammatory response during cardiopulmonary bypass: impact of heparin management," *Anesthesiology*, vol. 97, no. 4, pp. 837–841, 2002.

[32] C. Olsson, A. Siegbahn, A. Henze et al., "Heparin-coated cardiopulmonary bypass circuits reduce circulating complement factors and interleukin-6 in paediatric heart surgery," *Scandinavian Cardiovascular Journal*, vol. 34, no. 1, pp. 33–40, 2000.

[33] T. Ozawa, K. Yoshihara, N. Koyama, Y. Watanabe, N. Shiono, and Y. Takanashi, "Clinical efficacy of heparin-bonded bypass circuits related to cytokine responses in children," *The Annals of Thoracic Surgery*, vol. 69, no. 2, pp. 584–590, 2000.

[34] A. Parolari, F. Alamanni, T. Gherli et al., "'High dose' aprotinin and heparin-coated circuits: Clinical efficacy and inflammatory response," *Cardiovascular Surgery*, vol. 7, no. 1, pp. 117–127, 1999.

[35] H. Yamada, I. Kudoh, Y. Hirose, M. Toyoshima, H. Abe, and K. Kurahashi, "Heparin-coated circuits reduce the formation of

TNFα during cardiopulmonary bypass," *Acta Anaesthesiologica Scandinavica*, vol. 40, no. 3, pp. 311–317, 1996.

[36] O. Barkay, E. Niv, E. Santo, R. Bruck, A. Hallak, and F. M. Konikoff, "Low-dose heparin for the prevention of post-ERCP pancreatitis: a randomized placebo-controlled trial," *Surgical Endoscopy and Other Interventional Techniques*, vol. 22, no. 9, pp. 1971–1976, 2008.

[37] R. C. Becker, K. W. Mahaffey, H. Yang et al., "Heparin-associated anti-Xa activity and platelet-derived prothrombotic and proinflammatory biomarkers in moderate to high-risk patients with acute coronary syndrome," *Journal of Thrombosis and Thrombolysis*, vol. 31, no. 2, pp. 146–153, 2011.

[38] S. D. Bowler, S. M. Smith, and P. S. Lavercombe, "Heparin inhibits the immediate response to antigen in the skin and lungs of allergic subjects," *American Review of Respiratory Disease*, vol. 147, no. 1, pp. 160–163, 1993.

[39] J. P. Boyle, R. H. Smart, and J. K. Shirey, "Heparin in the treatment of chronic obstructive bronchopulmonary disease," *The American Journal of Cardiology*, vol. 14, no. 1, pp. 25–28, 1964.

[40] Y. Qian, H. Xie, R. Tian, K. Yu, and R. Wang, "Efficacy of low molecular weight heparin in patients with acute exacerbation of chronic obstructive pulmonary disease receiving ventilatory support," *COPD: Journal of Chronic Obstructive Pulmonary Disease*, vol. 11, no. 2, pp. 171–176, 2014.

[41] Á. Chamorro, Á. Cervera, J. Castillo, A. Dávalos, J. J. Aponte, and A. M. Planas, "Unfractionated heparin is associated with a lower rise of serum vascular cell adhesion molecule-1 in acute ischemic stroke patients," *Neuroscience Letters*, vol. 328, no. 3, pp. 229–232, 2002.

[42] R. de Cock, L. A. Ficker, J. G. Dart, A. Garner, and P. Wright, "Topical heparin in the treatment of ligneous conjunctivitis," *Ophthalmology*, vol. 102, no. 11, pp. 1654–1659, 1995.

[43] U. Derhaschnig, T. Pernerstorfer, M. Knechtelsdorfer, U. Hollenstein, S. Panzer, and B. Jilma, "Evaluation of antiinflammatory and antiadhesive effects of heparins in human endotoxemia," *Critical Care Medicine*, vol. 31, no. 4, pp. 1108–1112, 2003.

[44] B. Dixon, M. J. Schultz, R. Smith, J. B. Fink, J. D. Santamaria, and D. J. Campbell, "Nebulized heparin is associated with fewer days of mechanical ventilation in critically ill patients: a randomized controlled trial," *Critical Care*, vol. 14, no. 5, article R180, 2010.

[45] F. K. Keating, H. L. Dauerman, D. A. Whitaker, B. E. Sobel, and D. J. Schneider, "The effects of bivalirudin compared with those of unfractionated heparin plus eptifibatide on inflammation and thrombin generation and activity during coronary intervention," *Coronary Artery Disease*, vol. 16, no. 6, pp. 401–405, 2005.

[46] M. Ledson, M. Gallagher, C. A. Hart, and M. Walshaw, "Nebulized heparin in *Burkholderia cepacia* colonized adult cystic fibrosis patients," *European Respiratory Journal*, vol. 17, no. 1, pp. 36–38, 2001.

[47] D. J. Serisier, J. K. Shute, P. M. Hockey, B. Higgins, J. Conway, and M. P. Carroll, "Inhaled heparin in cystic fibrosis," *European Respiratory Journal*, vol. 27, no. 2, pp. 354–358, 2006.

[48] O. K. Poyrazoglu, A. Dogukan, M. Yalniz, D. Seckin, and A. L. Gunal, "Acute effect of standard heparin versus low molecular weight heparin on oxidative stress and inflammation in hemodialysis patients," *Renal Failure*, vol. 28, no. 8, pp. 723–727, 2006.

[49] S. Suzuki, T. Matsuo, H. Kobayashi et al., "Antithrombotic treatment (argatroban vs. heparin) in coronary angioplasty in angina pectoris: effects on inflammatory, hemostatic, and

endothelium-derived parameters," *Thrombosis Research*, vol. 98, no. 4, pp. 269–279, 2000.

[50] S. D. Trocme and H.-I. Li, "Effect of heparin-surface-modified intraocular lenses on postoperative inflammation after phacoemulsification: a randomized trial in a United States patient population," *Ophthalmology*, vol. 107, no. 6, pp. 1031–1037, 2000.

[51] C. Vancheri, C. Mastruzzo, F. Armato et al., "Intranasal heparin reduces eosinophil recruitment after nasal allergen challenge in patients with allergic rhinitis," *Journal of Allergy and Clinical Immunology*, vol. 108, no. 5, pp. 703–708, 2001.

[52] A. Abdollahi, M.-T. Naini, H. Shams, and R. Zarei, "Effect of low-molecular-weight heparin on postoperative inflammation in phacomorphic glaucoma," *Archives of Iranian Medicine*, vol. 5, no. 4, pp. 225–229, 2002.

[53] R. T. S. Lakshmi, T. Priyanka, J. Meenakshi, K. R. Mathangi, V. Jeyaraman, and M. Babu, "Low molecular weight heparin mediated regulation of nitric oxide synthase during burn wound healing," *Annals of Burns and Fire Disasters*, vol. 24, no. 1, pp. 24–29, 2011.

[54] G. Montalescot, C. Bal-dit-Sollier, D. Chibedi et al., "Comparison of effects on markers of blood cell activation of enoxaparin, dalteparin, and unfractionated heparin in patients with unstable angina pectoris or non-ST-segment elevation acute myocardial infarction (the ARMADA study)," *The American Journal of Cardiology*, vol. 91, no. 8, pp. 925–930, 2003.

[55] S. Nasiripour, K. Gholami, S. Mousavi et al., "Comparison of the effects of enoxaparin and heparin on inflammatory biomarkers in patients with ST-segment elevated myocardial infarction: a prospective open label pilot clinical trial," *Iranian Journal of Pharmaceutical Research*, vol. 13, no. 2, pp. 583–590, 2014.

[56] J. Oldgren, C. Fellenius, K. Boman et al., "Influence of prolonged dalteparin treatment on coagulation, fibrinolysis and inflammation in unstable coronary artery disease," *Journal of Internal Medicine*, vol. 258, no. 5, pp. 420–427, 2005.

[57] T. K. Rudolph, V. Rudolph, A. Witte et al., "Liberation of vessel adherent myeloperoxidase by enoxaparin improves endothelial function," *International Journal of Cardiology*, vol. 140, no. 1, pp. 42–47, 2010.

[58] D. L. Walters, M. J. Ray, P. Wood, E. J. Perrin, J. H. N. Bett, and C. N. Aroney, "High-dose tirofiban with enoxaparin and inflammatory markers in high-risk percutaneous intervention," *European Journal of Clinical Investigation*, vol. 40, no. 2, pp. 139–147, 2010.

[59] S. W. Rathbun, C. E. Aston, and T. L. Whitsett, "A randomized trial of dalteparin compared with ibuprofen for the treatment of superficial thrombophlebitis," *Journal of Thrombosis and Haemostasis*, vol. 10, no. 5, pp. 833–839, 2012.

[60] J. P. Titon, D. Auger, P. Grange et al., "Therapeutic management of superficial venous thrombosis with calcium nadroparin. Dosage testing and comparison with a non-steroidal anti-inflammatory agent," *Annales de Cardiologie et d Angéiologie*, vol. 43, no. 3, pp. 160–166, 1994.

[61] H. Uncu, "A comparison of low-molecular-weight heparin and combined therapy of low-molecular-weight heparin with an anti-inflammatory agent in the treatment of superficial vein thrombosis," *Phlebology*, vol. 24, no. 2, pp. 56–60, 2009.

[62] J. A. Sjøland, R. S. Pedersen, J. Jespersen, and J. Gram, "Intraperitoneal heparin ameliorates the systemic inflammatory response in PD patients," *Nephron—Clinical Practice*, vol. 100, no. 4, pp. c105–c110, 2005.

[63] N. L. Fine, C. Shim, and M. H. Williams Jr., "Objective evaluation of heparin in the treatment of asthma," *American Review of Respiratory Disease*, vol. 98, no. 5, pp. 886–887, 1968.

[64] Z. Diamant, M. C. Timmers, H. van der Veen, C. P. Page, F. J. van der Meer, and P. J. Sterk, "Effect of inhaled heparin on allergen-induced early and late asthmatic responses in patients with atopic asthma," *American Journal of Respiratory and Critical Care Medicine*, vol. 153, no. 6 I, pp. 1790–1795, 1996.

[65] C. M. E. Tranfa, A. Vatrella, R. Parrella, G. Pelaia, F. Bariffi, and S. A. Marsico, "Effect of inhaled heparin on water-induced bronchoconstriction in allergic asthmatics," *European Journal of Clinical Pharmacology*, vol. 57, no. 1, pp. 5–9, 2001.

[66] I. Stelmach, J. Jerzyńska, A. Brzozowska, and P. Kuna, "The effect of inhaled heparin on postleukotriene bronchoconstriction in children with asthma," *Polski Merkuriusz Lekarski*, vol. 12, no. 68, pp. 95–98, 2002.

[67] R. Polosa, S. Magrì, C. Vancheri et al., "Time course of changes in adenosine $5'$-monophosphate airway responsiveness with inhaled heparin in allergic asthma," *Journal of Allergy and Clinical Immunology*, vol. 99, no. 3, pp. 338–342, 1997.

[68] J. Butler, G. M. Rocker, and S. Westaby, "Inflammatory response to cardiopulmonary bypass," *The Annals of Thoracic Surgery*, vol. 55, no. 2, pp. 552–559, 1993.

[69] J. M. Redmond, A. M. Gillinov, R. S. Stuart et al., "Heparin-coated bypass circuits reduce pulmonary injury," *The Annals of Thoracic Surgery*, vol. 56, no. 3, pp. 474–479, 1993.

[70] S. Svenmarker, E. Sandström, T. Karlsson et al., "Clinical effects of the heparin coated surface in cardiopulmonary bypass," *European Journal of Cardio-Thoracic Surgery*, vol. 11, no. 5, pp. 957–964, 1997.

[71] Y. J. Gu, W. van Oeveren, C. Akkerman, P. W. Boonstra, R. J. Huyzen, and C. R. H. Wildevuur, "Heparin-coated circuits reduce the inflammatory response to cardiopulmonary bypass," *The Annals of Thoracic Surgery*, vol. 55, no. 4, pp. 917–922, 1993.

[72] D. Paparella, O. O. Al Radi, Q. H. Meng, T. Venner, K. Teoh, and E. Young, "The effects of high-dose heparin on inflammatory and coagulation parameters following cardiopulmonary bypass," *Blood Coagulation and Fibrinolysis*, vol. 16, no. 5, pp. 323–328, 2005.

[73] S. Danese, A. Papa, S. Saibeni, A. Repici, A. Malesci, and M. Vecchi, "Inflammation and coagulation in inflammatory bowel disease: the clot thickens," *The American Journal of Gastroenterology*, vol. 102, no. 1, pp. 174–186, 2007.

[74] S. Bloom, S. Kiilerich, M. R. Lassen et al., "Low molecular weight heparin (tinzaparin) vs. placebo in the treatment of mild to moderately active ulcerative colitis," *Alimentary Pharmacology & Therapeutics*, vol. 19, no. 8, pp. 871–878, 2004.

[75] P. Libby, "Coronary artery injury and the biology of atherosclerosis: inflammation, thrombosis, and stabilization," *American Journal of Cardiology*, vol. 86, no. 8, 2000.

[76] N. T. Mulvihill and J. B. Foley, "Inflammation in acute coronary syndromes," *Heart*, vol. 87, no. 3, pp. 201–204, 2002.

[77] N. A. Jameson, W. V. Good, and C. S. Hoyt, "Inflammation after cataract surgery in children," *Ophthalmic Surgery*, vol. 23, no. 2, pp. 99–102, 1992.

[78] R. M. Sinskey, P. A. Amin, and R. Lingua, "Cataract extraction and intraocular lens implantation in an infant with a monocular congenital cataract," *Journal of Cataract & Refractive Surgery*, vol. 20, no. 6, pp. 647–651, 1994.

[79] A. van Ophoven, A. Heinecke, and L. Hertle, "Safety and efficacy of concurrent application of oral pentosan polysulfate and subcutaneous low-dose heparin for patients with interstitial cystitis," *Urology*, vol. 66, no. 4, pp. 707–711, 2005.

4

Evaluation of Antidiarrheal Activity of Methanolic Extract of *Maranta arundinacea* Linn. Leaves

Md. Khalilur Rahman,[1] Md. Ashraf Uddin Chowdhury,[2] Mohammed Taufiqual Islam,[2] Md. Anisuzzaman Chowdhury,[3] Muhammad Erfan Uddin,[4] and Chandra Datta Sumi[5]

[1]*Department of Pharmacology, Dongguk University, Gyeongju 780-714, Republic of Korea*
[2]*Department of Systems Immunology, Kangwon National University, Chuncheon 200-701, Republic of Korea*
[3]*Department of Pharmacy, Chosun University, Gwangju 61452, Republic of Korea*
[4]*Department of Pharmacy, International Islamic University Chittagong, Chittagong 4203, Bangladesh*
[5]*Department of Systems Biotechnology, Chung-Ang University, Anseong 456-756, Republic of Korea*

Correspondence should be addressed to Chandra Datta Sumi; sumi.datta.chandra@gmail.com

Academic Editor: Antonio Ferrer-Montiel

Diarrhea is one of the most common causes for thousands of deaths every year. Therefore, identification of new source of antidiarrheal drugs becomes one of the most prominent focuses in modern research. Our aim was to investigate the antidiarrheal and cytotoxic activities of methanolic extract of *Maranta arundinacea* linn. (MEMA) leaves in rats and brine shrimp, respectively. Antidiarrheal effect was evaluated by using castor oil-induced diarrhea, enteropooling, and gastrointestinal motility tests at 200 mg/kg and 400 mg/kg body weight in rats where the cytotoxic activity was justified using brine shrimp lethality bioassay at different concentrations of MEMA. The extract showed considerable antidiarrheal effect by inhibiting 42.67% and 57.75% of diarrheal episode at the doses of 200 and 400 mg/kg, respectively. MEMA also significantly ($p < 0.01$) reduced the castor oil-induced intestinal volume (2.14 ± 0.16 to 1.61 ± 0.12 mL) in enteropooling test as well as intestinal transit (33.00 to 43.36%) in GI motility test, compared to their respective control. These observed effects are comparable to that of standard drug loperamide (5 mg/kg). On the other hand, in brine shrimp lethality test after 24 h, surviving brine shrimp larvae were counted and LD_{50} was assessed. Result showed that MEMA was potent against brine shrimp with LD_{50} value of 420 μg/mL. So the highest dose of 400 μg/mL of MEMA was not toxic to mice. So these results indicate that bioactive compounds are present in methanolic extract of *Maranta arundinacea* leaves including significant antidiarrheal activity and could be accounted for pharmacological effects.

1. Introduction

Due to unhygienic livelihood condition, peoples of the third world counties are very prone to several common diseases including diarrhea. According to the World Health Organization (WHO), diarrhea is the second leading reason of death of children less than five years of age [1]. During diarrhea, the normal bowel movement becomes changed, which results in an increase in water content, volume, or frequency of the stools [2]. The common reason for causing diarrhea is gastrointestinal infection by various types of bacteria, virus, and parasites. This infection can be spread out through food, drinking water, and unhygienic environment. Besides other pathological conditions, usually four major mechanisms are responsible for pathophysiology in electrolyte and water transportation, such as increasing of luminal osmolarity and electrolyte secretion, decreasing of electrolyte absorption, and acceleration of intestinal motility ultimately decreasing of transition time [3].

Despite the efforts of international organizations to control this disease, still the incidence of diarrhea is very high [4]. Some antibiotics are used as antidiarrheal drug, but these drugs sometimes show some adverse effects and microorganisms are tend to develop resistance towards them [5]. Therefore the search for safe and more effective agents from plant origin has continued to be an important area of active research. However, plants have long been a very important source of new drugs. Many plant species have been screened for substances with therapeutic activity. For the treatment of diarrhea, medicinal plants are a potential source of antidiarrheal drugs [6]. Moreover, many international organizations including WHO have encouraged studies pertaining to the treatment and prevention of diarrheal diseases using traditional medical practices [7–9]. At present, around 25% of drugs are isolated from plants and there are numerous evidences available about the use of medicinal plants including their pharmacological and biochemical properties [10].

Maranta arundinacea Linn. is a tropical and perennial tuberous plant belonging to the family Marantaceae. Locally, this plant is called arrowroot which contains more than 20% of starch in its tubers. It increases digestion and used as nourishing diet for convalescents, mainly in bowel illness. Arrowroot is also popular in traditional medicine for its demulcent properties [11, 12]. However, there are no available medicinal claims about antidiarrheal activity and cytotoxicity of this plant. That is why we are interested in examining the antidiarrheal and cytotoxic activities of methanolic extract of *Maranta arundinacea* L. leaves.

2. Materials and Methods

2.1. Plant Materials and Extract Preparation. *Maranta arundinacea* L. leaves were collected from Saint Martin Island, Bangladesh, and authenticated by the expert of Bangladesh Forest Research Institute, Chittagong, Bangladesh (Voucher number 5646). The leaves of *Maranta arundinacea* L. were air dried at room temperature and ground into fine powder by pulverization in electric grinder. The powder was successively extracted in methanol (55–60°C) with occasional agitation and then filtered through a cotton plug followed by Whitman Filter Paper number 1. The solvent was evaporated under vacuum at room temperature to yield semisolid extract. Then, the methanolic extract of *Maranta arundinacea* L. (MEMA) leaves was collected in Eppendorf tube and preserved in a refrigerator at 4°C for further use.

2.2. Drugs and Chemicals. Castor oil (WELL's Heath Care, Spain), 0.9% sodium chloride solution (normal saline) (Orion Infusions Ltd., Bangladesh), charcoal meal (10% activated charcoal in 5% gum acacia), and loperamide (Square Pharmaceuticals Ltd., Bangladesh) were used for antidiarrheal activity test, and dimethyl sulfoxide (DMSO) (Sigma-Aldrich, USA) and sodium chloride (Sigma) were used for cytotoxic activity test.

2.3. Experimental Animals. Long-Evans rats (95–100 g) were collected from International Centre for Diarrheal Disease and Research, Bangladesh (ICDDR, B), which were used as the experimental model for investigation of the antidiarrheal activity. All the animals housed under standard laboratory condition at 25.0 ± 2.0°C and 12 h light: dark cycle, acclimatized for 10 days before experiment. Standard diet and water were provided constantly. All experiments on rat were conducted in accordance with the National Institute of Health

Guide for Care and Use of Laboratory Animal (Publication Number 85-23, revised 1985).

2.4. Castor Oil-Induced Diarrhea in Rats. Rats of both sexes (95–100 g) were fasted for 18 hours. The selected rats for castor oil-induced diarrheal test were divided into four groups (*n* = 5). Group I was given normal saline (2 mL/kg) orally as control group and Group II received loperamide (5 mg/kg) as standard group. Groups III-IV received MEMA (200 and 400 mg/kg b. wt. i.p., resp.). After 1 h, all groups received castor oil 1 mL each orally. Then they were placed in cages lined with adsorbent papers and observed for 4 h for the presence of characteristic diarrheal droppings. 100% was considered as the total number of feces of control group [13]. The activity was expressed as % inhibition of diarrhea. The percent (%) inhibition of defecation was measured using the following formula:

$$\text{Percent (\%) inhibition of defecation} = \left[\frac{(A - B)}{A} \right] \times 100, \tag{1}$$

where A is mean number of defecation time caused by castor oil and B is mean number of defecation time caused by drug or extract.

2.5. Castor Oil-Induced Enteropooling. Castor oil-induced enteropooling test helps to determine the prevention of fluid accumulation ability of extract. Here also rats of both sexes (95–100 g) were fasted for 18 hours. The selected rats for this test were divided into four groups (*n* = 5). Group I (controlled group) was given normal saline (2 mL/kg) orally while Group II (standard group) received loperamide (5 mg/kg). The rest of the groups (Groups III-IV) received MEMA (200 and 400 mg/kg b. wt. i.p. resp.). After 1 h, all groups received castor oil, 1 mL orally per animal. Two hours later, all rats were sacrificed and the small intestine from the pylorus to the caecum was isolated. The intestinal contents were collected by milking into a graduated tube and their volume was measured [14].

2.6. Gastrointestinal Motility Test. This test was done according to the method of Mascolo et al. and Rahman et al. For this test, selected rats were divided into four groups of five rats in each. At first, 1 mL castor oil was given orally in every rat of each group to produce diarrhea. After 1 h, Group I (control group) received saline (2 mL/kg) orally. Group II received standard drug (loperamide 5 mg/kg b. wt. i.p) and Groups III-IV (the rest of the two groups) received MEMA (200 and 400 mg/kg b. wt. i.p. resp.). After 1 h, all animals received 1 mL of charcoal meal (10% charcoal suspension in 5% gum acacia) orally. One hour after following the charcoal meal administration, all animals were sacrificed and the distance covered by the charcoal meal in the intestine, from the pylorus to the caecum, was measured and expressed as percentage of distance moved [15, 16].

2.7. Brine Shrimp Lethality Bioassay. Brine shrimp lethality bioassay was conducted for investigating the cytotoxicity of

TABLE 1: Effect of MEMA leaves on castor oil-induced diarrhea in rats.

Group	Treatment	Total number of feces	% Inhibition of defecation	Total number of diarrheal feces	% Inhibition of diarrhea
I	Castor oil + Saline (2 mL/kg p.o)	$18.18 \pm 1.91^{**}$	—	$11.05 \pm 1.08^{**}$	—
II	Castor oil + Loperamide (5 mg/kg i.p)	$7.76 \pm 0.66^{**}$	57.32	$5.00 \pm 0.33^{**}$	54.75
III	Castor oil + Leaves Extract (200 mg/kg i.p)	$10 \pm 0.81^{**}$	44.99	$6.33 \pm 0.93^{**}$	42.67
IV	Castor oil + Leaves Extract (400 mg/kg i.p)	$8 \pm 1.52^{**}$	55.99	$5.79 \pm 0.52^{**}$	57.75

Values were expressed as mean $\pm$ SEM. ($n = 5$). $^*p < 0.05$, $^{**}p < 0.01$ when compared with control group (ANOVA followed by Dunnett's t-test).

TABLE 2: Effect of MEMA leaves on castor oil induced enterpooling in rats.

Group	Treatment	Weight of intestinal content (g)	Volume of intestinal content (mL)	Inhibition (%)
I	Castor oil + Saline (2 mL/kg p.o)	$3.22 \pm 0.05^{**}$	$2.77 \pm 0.23^{**}$	—
II	Castor oil + Loperamide (5 mg/kg i.p)	$1.84 \pm 0.44^{**}$	$1.57 \pm 0.07^{**}$	42.58
III	Castor oil +Leaves extract (200 mg/kg i.p)	$2.46 \pm 0.08^{*}$	$2.14 \pm 0.016^{*}$	30.33
IV	Castor oil + Leaves extract (400 mg/kg i.p)	$1.92 \pm 0.03^{**}$	$1.61 \pm 0.12^{**}$	40.16

Values were expressed as mean $\pm$ SEM. ($n = 5$). $^*p < 0.05$, $^{**}p < 0.01$ when compared with control group (ANOVA followed by Dunnett's t-test).

MEMA. For this test, brine shrimps (*Artemia salina*) were hatched in a round shaped vessel (1 L), filled with sterile artificial seawater (prepared using sea salt of sodium chloride $38 \, g \, L^{-1}$ and adjusted to pH 8.5 using 1N NaOH) with continuous oxygen supply. After 48 h of hatching, the active nauplii were identified and collected from clear part of the vessel and used for the study. Twenty nauplii were withdrawn through a glass capillary and transferred to each test tube containing 4.5 mL of brine solution. Then 0.5 mL of the extract solution(s) was added to each test tube and kept them in room temperature for 24 h under light. After that time, surviving larvae were counted. This experiment was done along with control (vehicle treated), different concentrations (50–800 μg/mL) [17].

2.8. Statistical Analysis. The results are presented as mean $\pm$ standard error of mean (SEM). The one-way ANOVA test with Dunnett's post hoc test was used to analyze and compare the data using SPSS 11.5 software, while $p < 0.05$–0.001 were considered as statistically significant.

3. Results

3.1. Castor Oil-Induced Diarrhea. In case of castor oil-induced diarrheal test, the methanol extract of *Maranta arundinacea* L. showed a marked antidiarrheal effect in the rats (Table 1). In both doses, 200 mg/kg and 400 mg/kg, extract produced significant ($p < 0.01$) defecation. The leaves extract doses of 200 mg/kg and 400 mg/kg decrease the total amount of wet feces produced upon administration of castor oil (6.33 ± 0.93 and 5.79 ± 0.52 g) at doses 200 mg/kg and

400 mg/kg compared to the control group (5.00 ± 0.33 g) at the dose of 5 mg/kg.

3.2. Castor Oil-Induced Enteropooling. In this test, MEMA at both of the 200 and 400 mg/kg doses produced significant and dose dependent reduction in intestinal weight and volume (Table 2). The leaves extract decreased intestinal volume by 30.33% and 40.16% at doses 200 and 400 mg/kg, respectively. The standard drug loperamide (5 mg/kg) also significantly inhibited ($p < 0.01$) the intestinal fluid accumulation (42.58%).

3.3. Gastrointestinal Motility Test. The methanolic extract of *Maranta arundinacea* L. lessened gastrointestinal distance (101 ± 2.82 cm to 57.2 ± 1.41 cm) traveled by the charcoal meal in the rats noticeably compared with the control group. Loperamide (5 mg/kg) produced a marked (46.53%) decrease in the propulsion of charcoal meal through gastrointestinal tract (Table 3).

3.4. Brine Shrimp Lethality Bioassay. The cytotoxicity activity of methanolic extract of *M. arundinacea* leaves assayed by the brine shrimp lethality bioassay test. The effect of the extract was dose dependent. In this assay, at 50 μg/mL, MEMA showed the lowest 5% of mortality where, at 800 μg/mL, extract showed the highest 75% of mortality (Table 4). However, at 300 μg/mL concentration, % of mortality was only 20. Overall LD_{50} of MEMA was 420 μg/mL. So, potent bioactive compounds were present in the extract of *M. arundinacea* leaves.

TABLE 3: Effect of MEMA leaves on small intestinal transition in rats.

Group	Treatment	Total length of intestine (cm)	Distance traveled by marker (cm)	Inhibition (%)
I	Castor oil + Saline (2 mL/kg p.o)	107.8 ± 2.36	101 ± 2.82[***]	—
II	Castor oil + Loperamide (5 mg/kg i.p)	103.36 ± 1.66	44 ± 0.07[***]	46.53
III	Castor oil + leaves extract (200 mg/kg i.p)	101.03 ± 3.08[***]	67.6 ± 2.11[***]	33.00
IV	Castor oil + Leaves extract (400 mg/kg i.p)	93.7 ± 2.61[***]	57.2 ± 1.41[***]	43.36

Values were expressed as mean ± SEM. (n = 5). [*]$p < 0.05$, [**]$p < 0.01$ [***]$p < 0.001$ when compared with control group (ANOVA followed by Dunnett's t-test).

TABLE 4: Cytotoxic effect of MEMA leaves on shrimp nauplii. Cytotoxicity effect of MEMA at various concentrations on the viability of brine shrimp nauplii was examined after 24 hrs incubation.

Concentration (μg/mL)	% of mortality	LD$_{50}$ (μg/mL)
50	5	
100	15	
300	20	420
500	60	
800	75	

All values were the mean of three replicates.

4. Discussion

Traditionally, people use plant(s) or plant-derived preparations considering them to be efficacious against diarrheal disorders without any scientific basis [18]. These experimental models were therefore employed to validate antidiarrheal efficacy of methanolic extract of *M. arundinacea* leaves in the current study.

Diarrhea can be described as the abnormally frequent defecation of feces of low consistency which may be due to a disturbance in the transport of water and electrolytes in the intestines. Instead of the multiplicity of etiologies, (i) increased electrolytes secretion (secretory diarrhea), (ii) increased luminal osmolarity (osmotic diarrhea), (iii) deranged intestinal motility causing a decreased transit time, and (iv) decreased electrolytes absorption may be responsible for pathophysiology [19, 20]. Recent study claims that nitric oxide in castor oil is responsible for the diarrheal effect, although it is evidenced that ricinoleic acid produces diarrhea through a hypersecretory response which is the most active component of castor oil [21, 22]. There are several mechanisms proposed to explain the diarrheal effect of castor oil including inhibition of intestinal Na$^+$ K$^+$ ATPase activity, consequently reducing normal fluid absorption [23, 24], activation of adenylate cyclase or mucosal cAMP-mediated active secretion [25], and stimulation of prostaglandin formation and platelet activating factor [15]. Usually castor oil is metabolized into ricinoleic acid in the gut, which causes irritation and inflammation in the intestinal mucosa, resulting in the release of inflammatory mediators (e.g., prostaglandins and histamine). The released prostaglandins initiate vasodilatation, smooth muscle contraction, and mucus secretion in the small intestines. In experimental animals as well as in human beings, prostaglandins of the E series are considered to be good diarrheagenic agents.

Our study showed that the overall antidiarrheal study reveals the dose dependent activity. In our study, MEMA leaves showed significantly reduced amount of feces in castor oil-induced rat by 44.99% and 55.99% at the doses of 200 and 400 mg/kg, respectively, and % inhibition of diarrhea was 42.67 and 57.57 at 200 and 400 mg/kg, respectively. Moreover, our results directly demonstrate an inhibition of castor oil-induced enteropooling with reduction of the weight and volume of intraluminal contents by 30.33% and 40.16% at 200 and 400 mg/mL, respectively. These results suggest that leaves of *M. arundinacea* contain antidiarrheal components. Also, from these results, it can be predicted that reduction of water and electrolytes secretion into the small intestine may enhance electrolyte absorption from the intestinal lumen consistent with inhibition of hypersecretion [26]. Besides different pathophysiological conditions of diarrhea, hypermotility characterizes diarrhea where the secretory component is not the causative factor [27]. Castor oil produces ricinoleic acid leading to irritation, inflammation of intestinal mucosa, and ultimately diarrhea. At this condition, prostaglandins stimulate gastrointestinal motility and secrete water and electrolytes. It is also well established that loperamide inhibits diarrhea induced by castor oil and charcoal passage test is used to determine the effect of test substance on gut motility [10]. In gastrointestinal motility, MEMA suppressed the propulsive movement or transit of charcoal meal through the gastrointestinal tract which demonstrates that the leaves extract may be able to reduce the frequency of stool in diarrheal conditions.

Previous report on the phytochemical screening on *M. arundinacea* leaves has shown that alkaloids, tannin, cardiac glycosides, steroids, and saponins are absent but phenols and flavonoids are significantly present [28]. It was reported that flavonoids and polyphenols were responsible for the antidiarrheal activity properties [29]. However, previous studies also have shown that flavonoids have ability to inhibit intestinal motility and water and electrolytes secretion [30]. Moreover, in vivo and in vitro tests have also shown that flavonoids are able to inhibit prostaglandin E2 induced intestinal secretion and spasmogens induced contraction and also inhibit release of prostaglandins and autocoids [29]. Thereby, flavonoids as the inhibitors of prostaglandins biosynthesis are considered to delay castor oil-induced diarrhea [31]. Polyphenols also can show antidiarrheal property by interacting and inhibiting cytochrome P450 systems [32]. So, the antidiarrheal activity of the methanolic extract of the leaves of *M. arundinacea* could therefore be due to the presence of flavonoids and phenols.

The brine shrimp lethality test was considered as a convenient probe for primary assessment of toxicity, detection of fungal toxins, heavy metals, and pesticides, and cytotoxicity testing of dental materials. It can also be extrapolated for cell-line toxicity and antitumor activity [17, 32]. MEMA was also assessed for its cytotoxicity using a sensitive in vitro brine shrimp lethality bioassay (Table 4). LD_{50} value of the extract was 420 μg/mL. From this result, it can be well predicted that the *M. arundinacea* extracts do not have considerable cytotoxic activity.

5. Conclusion

The findings of the present study provide convincing evidence that methanolic extract of *M. arundinacea* (MEMA) leaves possesses remarkable antidiarrheal activity but has slight cytotoxic effect. Antidiarrheal effect is rapid, long lasting, and statistically significant at both 200 and 400 mg/kg doses. Determination of antidiarrheal effect in other models as well as the effect on gut motility may give a clear idea about the mechanism(s) of antidiarrheal activity. However, further chemical and pharmacological studies are required to isolate the bioactive compounds and elucidate the precise mechanisms responsible for the observed pharmacological activities of this plant.

Conflict of Interests

The authors declare that there is no conflict of interests.

Acknowledgments

The authors wish to thank Dr. Shaikh Bokhtear Uddin, Associate Professor, Department of Botany, University of Chittagong, for identification of the plant. The authors are also grateful to the authority of International Centre for Diarrhoeal Disease and Research, Bangladesh (ICDDR, B), for providing the experimental rats.

References

[1] WHO, *Diarrheal Disease: Fact Sheet*, 2009, http://www.who.int/mediacentre/factsheets/fs330/en/index.html.

[2] R. L. Guerrant, T. Van Gilder, T. S. Steiner et al., "Practice guidelines for the management of infectious diarrhea," *Clinical Infectious Diseases*, vol. 32, no. 3, pp. 331–351, 2001.

[3] G. D. Lutterodt, "Inhibition of microlax-induced experimental diarrhoea with narcotic-like extracts of *Psidium guajava* leaf in rats," *Journal of Ethnopharmacology*, vol. 37, no. 2, pp. 151–157, 1992.

[4] M. Kouitcheu, B. Penlap, J. Kouam, B. Ngadjui, Z. Fomum, and F. Etoa, "Evaluation of antidiarrheal activity of the stem bark of *Cylocodiscus ganbunensis* (Mimosaceae)," *African Journal of Biotechnology*, vol. 5, no. 11, pp. 1062–1066, 2006.

[5] H. Knecht, S. C. Neulinger, F. A. Heinsen et al., "Effects of β-lactam antibiotics and fluoroquinolones on human gut microbiota in relation to *Clostridium difficile* associated diarrhea," *PLoS ONE*, vol. 9, no. 2, Article ID e89417, 2014.

[6] R. Maïkere-Faniyo, L. Van Puyvelde, A. Mutwewingabo, and F. X. Habiyaremye, "Study of Rwandese medicinal plants used in the treatment of diarrhoea I," *Journal of Ethnopharmacology*, vol. 26, no. 2, pp. 101–109, 1989.

[7] J. D. Snyder and M. H. Merson, "The magnitude of the global problem of acute diarrhoeal disease: a review of active surveillance data," *Bulletin of the World Health Organization*, vol. 60, no. 4, pp. 605–613, 1982.

[8] G. D. Lutterodt, "Inhibition of gastrointestinal release of acetylchoune byquercetin as a possible mode of action of *Psidium guajava* leaf extracts in the treatment of acute diarrhoeal disease," *Journal of Ethnopharmacology*, vol. 25, no. 3, pp. 235–247, 1989.

[9] K. Park, *Park's Textbook of Preventive and Social Medicine*, M/S Banarsidas Bharat Publishers, Jabalpur, India, 2000.

[10] S. E. Bahekar and R. S. Kale, "Antidiarrheal activity of ethanolic extract of *Manihot esculenta* Crantz leaves in Wistar rats," *Journal of Ayurveda and Integrative Medicine*, vol. 6, no. 1, pp. 35–40, 2015.

[11] M. N. Madineni, S. Faiza, R. S. Surekha, R. Ravi, and M. Guha, "Morphological, structural, and functional properties of maranta (*Maranta arundinacea* L) starch," *Food Science and Biotechnology*, vol. 21, no. 3, pp. 747–752, 2012.

[12] Arrowroot, Pure, 2010, http://www.frontiercoop.com/products.php?ct=spicesaz&cn=Arrowroot%2C%20Pure.

[13] M. Abdullahi, G. Muhammad, and N. U. Abdulkadir, *Combretaceae. Medicinal and Economic Plants of Nupeland*, Jube Evans Books and Publications, Bida, Nigeria, 2003.

[14] J. M. Sini, I. A. Umar, K. M. Anigo, I. Stantcheva, E. N. Bage, and R. Mohammed, "Antidiarrhoeal activity of aqueous extract of *Combretum sericeum* roots in rats," *African Journal of Biotechnology*, vol. 7, no. 17, pp. 3134–3137, 2008.

[15] N. Mascolo, A. A. Izzo, G. Autore, F. Barbato, and F. Capasso, "Nitric oxide and castor oil induced diarrhea," *Journal of Pharmacology and Experimental Therapeutics*, vol. 268, no. 1, pp. 291–295, 1994.

[16] M. M. Rahman, A. M. T. Islam, M. A. U. Chowdhury, M. E. Uddin, and A. Jamil, "Antidiarrheal activity of leaves extract of *Microcos paniculata* Linn in mice," *International Journal of Pharmacy*, vol. 2, no. 1, pp. 21–25, 2012.

[17] B. N. Meyer, N. R. Ferrigni, J. E. Putnam, L. B. Jacobsen, D. E. Nichols, and J. L. Mclaughlin, "Brine shrimp: a convenient general bioassay for active plant constituents," *Planta Medica*, vol. 45, no. 5, pp. 31–34, 1982.

[18] A. H. Atta and S. M. Mouneir, "Evaluation of some medicinal plant extracts for antidiarrhoeal activity," *Phytotherapy Research*, vol. 19, no. 6, pp. 481–485, 2005.

[19] G. A. Agbor, T. Léopold, and N. Y. Jeanne, "The antidiarrheal activity of *Alchornea cordifolia* leaf extract," *Phytotherapy Research*, vol. 18, no. 11, pp. 873–876, 2004.

[20] S. Umer, A. Tekewe, and N. Kebede, "Antidiarrheal and antimicrobial activity of *Calpurnia aurea* leaf extract," *BMC Complementary and Alternative Medicine*, vol. 13, article 21, 5 pages, 2013.

[21] L. C. Racusen and H. J. Binder, "Ricinoleic acid stimulation of active anion secretion in colonic mucosa of the rat," *Journal of Clinical Investigation*, vol. 63, no. 4, pp. 743–749, 1979.

[22] C. Vieira, S. Evangelista, R. Cirillo, A. Lippi, C. A. Maggi, and S. Manzini, "Effect of ricinoleic acid in acute and subchronic experimental models of inflammation," *Mediators of Inflammation*, vol. 9, no. 5, pp. 223–228, 2000.

[23] F. Capasso, N. Mascolo, A. A. Izzo, and T. S. Gaginella, "Dissociation of castor oil-induced diarrhoea and intestinal mucosal injury in rat: effect of N(G)-nitro-L-arginine methyl ester," *British Journal of Pharmacology*, vol. 113, no. 4, pp. 1127–1130, 1994.

[24] M. Z. Imam, S. Sultana, and S. Akter, "Antinociceptive, antidiarrheal, and neuropharmacological activities of *Barringtonia acutangula*," *Pharmaceutical Biology*, vol. 50, no. 9, pp. 1078–1084, 2012.

[25] A. Pinto, G. Autore, N. Mascolo et al., "Time course of PAF formation by gastrointestinal tissue in rats after castor oil challenge," *Journal of Pharmacy and Pharmacology*, vol. 44, no. 3, pp. 224–226, 1992.

[26] S. Shah, "Evaluation of diarrhea: the challenge continues! Part-1," *Indian Journal of Medical Sciences*, vol. 58, no. 2, pp. 75–78, 2004.

[27] H. R. Chitme, R. Chandra, and S. Kaushik, "Studies on antidiarrhoeal activity of *Calotropis gigantea* R.Br. in experimental animals," *Journal of Pharmacy and Pharmaceutical Sciences*, vol. 7, no. 1, pp. 70–75, 2004.

[28] Y. Vaghasiya, R. Dave, and S. Chanda, "Phytochemical analysis of some medicinal plants from western region of India," *Research Journal of Medicinal Plant*, vol. 5, no. 5, pp. 567–576, 2011.

[29] K. Dosso, B. B. N'guessan, A. P. Bidie et al., "Antidiarrhoeal activity of an ethanol extract of the stem bark of *Piliostigma reticulatum* (Caesalpiniaceae) in rats," *African Journal of Traditional, Complementary and Alternative Medicines*, vol. 9, no. 2, pp. 242–249, 2011.

[30] G. Di Carlo, G. Autore, A. A. Izzo et al., "Inhibition of intestinal motility and secretion by flavonoids in mice and rats: structure-activity relationships," *Journal of Pharmacy and Pharmacology*, vol. 45, no. 12, pp. 1054–1059, 1993.

[31] S. Brijesh, P. Daswani, P. Tetali, N. Antia, and T. Birdi, "Studies on the antidiarrhoeal activity of *Aegle marmelos* unripe fruit: validating its traditional usage," *BMC Complementary and Alternative Medicine*, vol. 9, article 47, 12 pages, 2009.

[32] J. E. Anderson, C. M. Goetz, J. L. McLaughlin, and M. A. Suffness, "A blind comparison of simple bench-top bioassays and human tumour cell cytotoxicities as antitumor prescreens," *Phytochemical Analysis*, vol. 2, no. 3, pp. 107–111, 1991.

5

Integrating TRPV1 Receptor Function with Capsaicin Psychophysics

Gregory Smutzer and Roni K. Devassy

Department of Biology, Temple University, 1900 N. 12th Street, Philadelphia, PA 19122, USA

Correspondence should be addressed to Gregory Smutzer; smutzerg@temple.edu

Academic Editor: Antonio Ferrer-Montiel

Capsaicin is a naturally occurring vanilloid that causes a hot, pungent sensation in the human oral cavity. This trigeminal stimulus activates TRPV1 receptors and stimulates an influx of cations into sensory cells. TRPV1 receptors function as homotetramers that also respond to heat, proinflammatory substances, lipoxygenase products, resiniferatoxin, endocannabinoids, protons, and peptide toxins. Kinase-mediated phosphorylation of TRPV1 leads to increased sensitivity to both chemical and thermal stimuli. In contrast, desensitization occurs via a calcium-dependent mechanism that results in receptor dephosphorylation. Human psychophysical studies have shown that capsaicin is detected at nanomole amounts and causes desensitization in the oral cavity. Psychophysical studies further indicate that desensitization can be temporarily reversed in the oral cavity if stimulation with capsaicin is resumed at short interstimulus intervals. Pretreatment of lingual epithelium with capsaicin modulates the perception of several primary taste qualities. Also, sweet taste stimuli may decrease the intensity of capsaicin perception in the oral cavity. In addition, capsaicin perception and hedonic responses may be modified by diet. Psychophysical studies with capsaicin are consistent with recent findings that have identified TRPV1 channel modulation by phosphorylation and interactions with membrane inositol phospholipids. Future studies will further clarify the importance of capsaicin and its receptor in human health and nutrition.

1. Introduction

The chemosensory properties of capsaicin have been widely examined in the human oral cavity. This review describes how psychophysical studies with capsaicin complement molecular and physiological studies of the capsaicin receptor, Transient Receptor Potential Vanilloid type 1 (TRPV1).

Capsaicin (8-methyl-*N*-vanillyl-*trans*-6-nonenamide) is a hydrophobic compound that is produced by the plant genus *Capsicum* and gives chili peppers their spicy taste [1]. The chemical structure of capsaicin and the related compound dihydrocapsaicin are shown in Figure 1. These vanilloids act as deterrents against ingestion of the plant by mammals, and as a means to inhibit fungal infections caused by insects [2, 3]. Due to its pharmacological properties, capsaicin is widely used as a topical analgesic to decrease muscle and joint pain [4]. In the human oral cavity, capsaicin is an irritant that produces both thermal (hot) and nociceptive (burning or stinging) sensations [5] by activating neurons of the maxillary and mandibular branches of the trigeminal nerve (Cranial Nerve V) [6]. TRPV1 receptor cells in oral tissue project via the lingual branch of the trigeminal nerve to the trigeminal spinal nucleus, which is also known as the trigeminal nuclear complex of the brain stem [7].

In addition, capsaicin stimulates metabolic activity, promotes negative energy balance through an increase in energy exposure, plays a role in weight control, and increases the oxidation of fatty acids [8–11]. In humans, this vanilloid may also suppress orexigenic (appetite-stimulating) sensations [8]. This compound may also exhibit antitumorigenic properties [12] and may function as a vasodilator that facilitates heat dissipation [13]. Finally, morbidity studies suggest that the consumption of spicy foods that contain chili peppers may increase human longevity [14].

Transient Receptor Potential Vanilloid Type 1 in the Oral Cavity. The mandibular branch of the trigeminal nerve provides sensation to the lower third of the face, the anterior

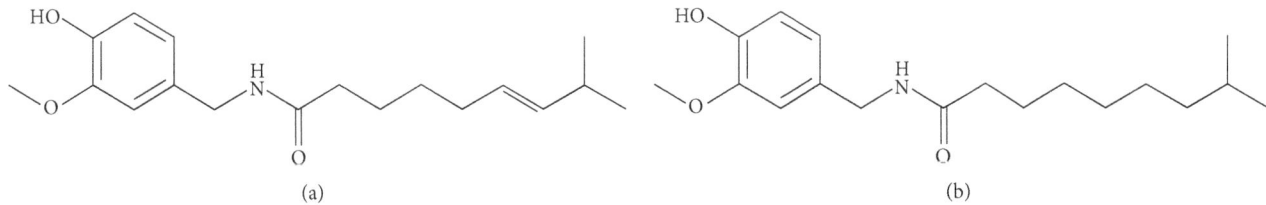

FIGURE 1: Chemical structure of (a) capsaicin and (b) dihydrocapsaicin (image 1b by Vyacheslav Nasretdinov via Wikimedia Commons).

two-thirds of the tongue, the oral mucosa, and the lower jaw [6]. Since capsaicin binds to receptors located within trigeminal neurons, sensitivity to this oral stimulant is usually restricted to the anterior two-thirds of the tongue [15].

Capsaicin is an agonist that binds to the TRPV1 receptor [16–19], a well characterized ion channel that localizes to peripheral terminals of primary afferent neurons that sense both pain and heat. TRPV1 is widely expressed in central nervous system (CNS) tissue and highly expressed in sensory neurons of the dorsal root ganglion [19]. This receptor also localizes to neurons that line the oral and nasal cavities [10], where it is found in a subpopulation of sensory afferent nociceptive nerve fibers [20]. The two major trigeminal fiber systems that express functional TRPV1 receptors are the myelinated A_{delta}-fibers and the unmyelinated C-fibers [10, 21, 22]. In addition to gustatory tissue, TRPV1 is also expressed in afferent fibers and in keratinocytes of the oral and nasal cavities [8, 17]. Keratinocytes are important in maintaining the integrity of the immune response in skin cells [23].

Within cells, TRPV1 receptors localize to both plasma membranes and internal membranes (such as ER membranes) where this channel mobilizes internal calcium (Ca^{2+}) stores [18]. This nonselective cation channel has a tenfold higher preference for Ca^{2+} where it functions as a biosensor of noxious heat and chemical agonists [19]. Activators for this receptor include proinflammatory substances such as 9-hydroxyoctadecadienoic acid, lipoxygenase products, resiniferatoxin from *Euphorbia resinifera* plants, endocannabinoids, capsaicin and its *cis* isomer zucapsaicin, dihydrocapsaicin, protons, and peptide toxins [16, 17, 19, 24, 25]. The alkaloid piperine from black pepper [26] and zingerone (vanillylacetone, commonly known as ginger) may also activate TRPV1 receptors in heterologous systems [27], and in trigeminal ganglia [28]. Gingerol also activates TRPV1 in cultured neurons [29]. In heterologous systems, sodium cyclamate, saccharin, aspartame, and acesulfame potassium may also function as TRPV1 agonists [30]. Finally, TRPV1 channels are also activated by increases in membrane voltage (>+60 mV), and at temperatures with thresholds near 43°C [19].

At the receptor level, capsaicin binds to the region that spans transmembrane domains 3 to 4 of the TRPV1 receptor [31] (see Figure 2(a)). Bound capsaicin orients in a "tail-up, head-down" configuration where the vanillyl and amide groups form specific interactions that anchor the ligand to the receptor [32]. Amino acids Y512 (helix S3), S513 (helix S3), E571 (S4-S5 linker), and T671 (helix S6) of murine TRPV1 bind the ring of capsaicin via hydrogen bonding while amino acid residue T551 (helix S4) binds the amide group of

capsaicin [32]. (Murine Y512 corresponds to Y511 of human TRPV1.) Since ligands bind to the cytosolic side of TRPV1 [18], these agonists must traverse the plasma membrane to access the intracellular ligand-binding site of TRPV1 [19, 33]. One exception is proton activation at pH of <6.0. Below this pH, protons bind to the extracellular outer-pore domain of TRPV1 [33] for activation of homotetrameric TRPV1 channels [34].

Several antagonists have been identified that block TRPV1 function. Ruthenium red (ammoniated ruthenium oxychloride) is a noncompetitive TRPV1 antagonist, and this dye functions as a pore blocker [35]. In addition, the capsaicin analogue capsazepine is a powerful antagonist for human TRPV1 channels [36].

TRPV1 is also an important heat sensor in peripheral sensory neurons [33]. This channel exhibits high sensitivity to heat, with Q10 values of approximately 25 [16, 33]. TRPV1 channel activation leads to the elevation of cytosolic Ca^{2+}, and the subsequent release of neuropeptides such as substance P and calcitonin-gene related peptide by exocytosis [37]. Substance P is found in nociceptive sensory fibers that express TRPV1, and in sensory fibers near taste buds of several mammalian species [38]. This neurotransmitter modulates signals for both heat and pain [39]. This undecapeptide is released from neurons following an increase in cytosolic Ca^{2+} levels, which may be mediated by TRPV1 channels. The release of substance P causes an increase in vasodilatation and vascular permeability, which may cause local edema [40]. Finally, this neuropeptide may stimulate mast cells to release inflammatory mediators such as histamine [41].

However, sustained activation of trigeminal neurons by capsaicin depletes presynaptic concentrations of substance P [42]. This depletion can interfere with a variety of sensory functions, including the response of animals to noxious heat stimuli [42].

2. Structure and Function of TRPV1 Receptor

The fully assembled TRPV1 receptor is a homotetramer that forms an outwardly rectifying cation channel that is permeable to both monovalent and divalent cations [33]. This channel exhibits single-channel conductance of 50–100 picosiemens [33]. Each TRPV1 subunit contains six transmembrane domains and a hydrophobic pore region between transmembrane domains 5 and 6 [19, 33]. The N and C termini of this receptor both localize to the cytoplasm [19, 33]. A schematic diagram of the structure and regulatory sites of TRPV1 is shown in Figure 2.

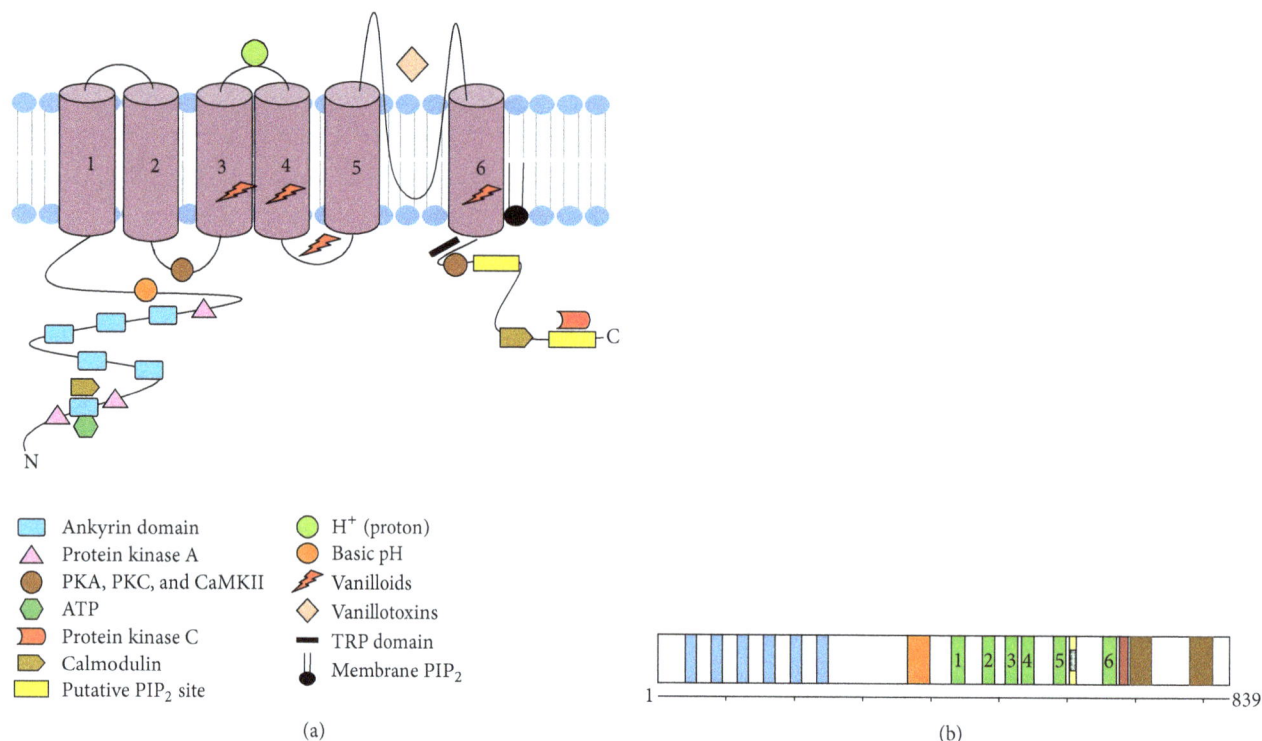

FIGURE 2: Schematic diagram that illustrates key structural features of TRPV1 control and regulation of channel activity and ion transport. (a) Each TRPV1 subunit is a 95 kDa protein that contains six transmembrane domains, a pore region between the fifth and sixth transmembrane domains, and extended intracellular N- and C-terminal tails. Modified from Bevan et al. [33]. Vanilloid binding site from Yang et al. [32]. (b) Protein domains of canonical TRPV1 receptor (human TRPV1 receptor contains 839 amino acid residues). Blue columns represent N-terminal ankyrin repeats, and orange column represents the cytosolic linker domain. The six numbered green columns represent transmembrane domain regions of the receptor, and light yellow column represents the alpha helical domain of the pore-forming region found between transmembrane domains 5 and 6. The red column represents the cytosolic TRP domain, and the two brown columns represent putative C-terminal PIP_2 binding domains. Horizontal line represents the linear sequence of amino acids from the N-terminus to the C-terminus. Modified from Liao et al. [43].

At the subunit level, six consecutive ankyrin repeats localize to the cytosolic N terminus, followed by a conserved linker region that connects the last N-terminal ankyrin repeat domain to the pre-S1 helix that contains α-helical and β-strand secondary structure [43]. This helix is followed by four transmembrane domains (S1–S4), and the S4-S5 linker region. Transmembrane domain 5 (S5) adjoins the hydrophobic pore region, a region that is required for proton activation, heat activation, or activation by chloroform and isoflurane [44]. Transmembrane domain six (S6) links the receptor to its C-terminal cytosolic region, which contains the 25-amino acid long TRP domain [TRP box] [45].

Ankyrin repeats at the cytoplasmic N-terminal domain bind calmodulin and ATP for modulating TRPV1 activation [45, 46]. The N-terminal domain also contains several putative phosphorylation sites that serve as binding sites for both calmodulin and ATP [47] (see Figure 2(a)).

The 150-amino acid residue C-terminus also interacts with cytosolic proteins and ligands. This terminus contains phosphoinositide and calmodulin binding domains, and protein kinase C (PKC) consensus sites [48–51]. This C-terminal

cytosolic region of TRPV1 also includes the conserved transient receptor potential (TRP) domain that interacts with the S4-S5 cytoplasmic linker for involvement in channel gating, and binding sites for phosphatidylinositol 4,5-bisphosphate (PIP_2) [18, 43]. The highly conserved TRP box also interacts with the pre-S1 helix of TRPV1. The TRP box is necessary for allosteric channel activation [52] and may also regulate the formation of functional tetrameric TRPV1 receptors [53].

Single particle electron cryomicroscopy (cryo-EM) permits the three-dimensional reconstruction of large protein complexes at high atomic resolution without the need to crystallize the protein [32, 43, 54]. The transmembrane topology and subunit organization of TRPV1 have recently been identified by cryo-EM structures at 4.2 to 4.5 Å resolution [43, 46]. These studies indicate that TRPV1 resembles voltage-gated potassium channels [32] where the symmetrical arrangement of four identical protein subunits forms a centrally located ion-conducting pore [19, 32, 33] (see Figure 3). This pore-forming loop of TRPV1 homotetramers contains an outer-pore turret, a pore helix, and a selectivity filter [55, 56], where each of the four subunits contributes to the ion-conducting

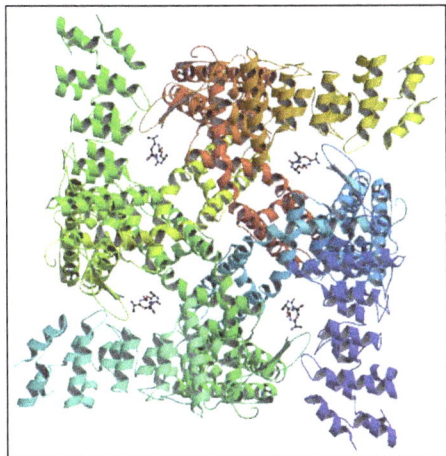

FIGURE 3: Reconstruction of homotetrameric rodent TRPV1 ion channel complexed with capsaicin that was obtained by single particle electron cryomicroscopy. Image from PDB ID 3J5R. Liao et al. [43] (http://www.rcsb.org/ [112]).

pore and selectivity filter [45]. Also, a second intervening pore loop is flanked by Segment 1–Segment 4 voltage-sensor-like domains [43]. See Figure 3.

2.1. Mutagenesis Studies of TRPV1. Mutagenesis studies have shown that M547 and T551 of human and rodent TRPV1 are required for sensitivity to capsaicin [57]. In addition, Glu600 and Glu648 (pK_a of side chain is 4.07) of TRPV1 receptors both face the extracellular surface. These two residues flank the pore-forming region of the receptor and regulate channel activation by extracellular protons [19]. At pH below 6.0, protons open the TRPV1 channel. Above this pH, protons lower the threshold for TRPV1 activation by agonists including capsaicin [19]. Finally, replacing a glutamate with the neutral amino acid glutamine (E600Q) causes a greater than tenfold leftward shift in the capsaicin dose-response curve [58], with EC_{50} values shifting from 520 nM to 40 nM. The physiological characteristics of these TRPV1 E600Q mutant receptors were thought to resemble wild-type channels operating under acidic conditions [58].

Several domains of the TRPV1 receptor are critical for heat sensitivity. In particular, several amino acid residues in the pore region and the C-terminal domains are critical for heat sensitivity [33]. Mutagenesis studies have further shown that I696A, W697A, and R701A in the C-terminal TRP box domain of this receptor resulted in complete loss or reduction of heat sensitivity, capsaicin sensitivity, or voltage activation [59]. In contrast, an F640L mutation in the pore-forming region of this receptor enhanced channel sensitivity to heat and capsaicin but abolished the potentiating effect of extracellular protons [60].

2.2. G-Protein-Coupled Receptors and TRPV1 Sensitization. Sensitization (activation) at the receptor level is consistent with psychophysical studies with capsaicin. Sensitization is thought to occur by phosphorylating this receptor, and

maximal stimulation (and mobilization to the plasma membrane) of TRPV1 may occur when the receptor is maximally phosphorylated [19]. TRPV1 channels contain multiple phosphorylation sites that stimulate sensitization [35, 51]. Sensitization may arise following phosphorylation of TRPV1 by either PKC (via IP_3 signaling) or protein kinase A (PKA) (via cyclic AMP signaling). These kinases are both activated by distinct G-protein-coupled receptors [20, 35, 61].

Agonists such as prostaglandin E_2 and serotonin bind to receptors that activate the stimulatory G-protein $G\alpha_s$. This G-protein subunit then triggers the synthesis of cyclic AMP by adenylate cyclase. The resulting increase in cytosolic cyclic AMP activates PKA, which in turn phosphorylates serine 116 and threonine 370 in the N-terminal region of TRPV1 (see Figure 2(a)). The phosphorylation of serine 116 likely inhibits dephosphorylation of TRPV1 after activation by capsaicin [35]. Finally, PKA activity reduces desensitization of TRPV1 by phosphorylating serine 116 [19], which allows increased sensitivity to the agonist anandamide [62].

TRPV1 also interacts with signal transduction pathways that activate G-protein-coupled receptors such as bradykinin B_2 and endothelin receptors [19, 63]. These receptors trigger the release of $G\alpha_q$ subunits from heterotrimeric G-proteins, which in turn activate the enzyme phospholipase C-beta (PLCβ). PLCβ then hydrolyzes PIP_2 to the second messengers inositol 1,4,5-trisphosphate (IP_3) and diacylglycerol (DAG) [64]. DAG activates PKCε, which in turn phosphorylates TRPV1 receptors at serine and threonine residues [51, 64, 65]. This phosphorylation sensitizes this receptor to heat, protons, or chemical agonists [19]. In general, inflammatory agents enhance TRPV1 activity by phosphorylation pathways that stimulate IP_3 turnover and enzymatic activation of PKCε [19, 20, 35].

Phosphorylation of serine/threonine residues at both N- and C-termini of TRPV1 receptors by PKCε increases the sensitivity of this channel to both capsaicin and heat by lowering thresholds for these two stimuli [66]. In addition, phosphorylation of serine 800 reverses the desensitization of TRPV1 that occurs from prolonged stimulation with capsaicin, and subsequently increases the sensitivity of this channel to agonists [19].

In addition to serine 800, PKC enhances TRPV1 function by phosphorylating serine 502 [51]. Phosphorylation by PKC at these residues is thought to modulate TRPV1-evoked currents [51], by possibly lowering temperature thresholds for opening TRPV1 channels [35, 51]. Sensitization (potentiation) of TRPV1 by PKC-mediated phosphorylation may also increase SNARE-dependent exocytosis of TRPV1-containing vesicles to the plasma membrane [67]. This mobilization of TRPV1 to the plasma membrane could then increase the overall channel activity of these receptors in sensory cells by increasing access to capsaicin.

In summary, TRPV1 may be most responsive to agonists if the channels are maximally phosphorylated prior to exposure to agonist. Increases in the intensity of capsaicin perception in the oral cavity may mirror greater numbers of phosphorylated TRPV1 receptors, or increased phosphorylation of individual TRPV1 receptors.

2.3. TRPV1 Desensitization and Calcium. The repeated exposure of TRPV1 to agonists such as capsaicin fails to activate this receptor or may only minimally activate this receptor. This process is known as desensitization and occurs by a Ca^{2+}-dependent mechanism that leads to dephosphorylation of TRPV1 receptors [19]. Since the activation of TRPV1 transiently increases cytosolic Ca^{2+} levels, even low concentrations of agonist can raise cytosolic Ca^{2+} concentrations and desensitize the receptor. This dephosphorylation occurs by enzymes such as calcineurin (protein phosphatase 3) [68], which can dephosphorylate serine and threonine residues that were previously phosphorylated by PKA [69]. This decrease in TRPV1 phosphorylation could then diminish capsaicin channel sensitivity [68] and cause a decrease in response to agonists such as capsaicin. In support of this hypothesis, receptor phosphorylation by PKC has been shown to diminish Ca^{2+}-induced desensitization of TRPV1 receptors [68, 69].

Conversely, TRPV1 may exhibit the lowest responses to agonist if the receptor is dephosphorylated prior to agonist (capsaicin) binding. TRPV1 phosphorylation by PKC may mobilize TRPV1 to the plasma membrane from internal (vesicular) membranes [67]. If true, then these results would imply that dephosphorylated receptors localize primarily to internal membranes where TRPV1 receptors might have less access to hydrophobic agonists such as capsaicin. If so, then this internal pool of dephosphorylated (and possibly nontetrameric) receptors might underlie capsaicin desensitization.

TRPV1 receptors are also stabilized by the cytoskeleton [70]. Tubulin dimers directly bind the C-terminus of TRPV1, and this interaction could decrease TRPV1 activity under depolymerizing conditions [71], possibly at high Ca^{2+} concentrations. Finally, capsaicin-sensitive channels can form heterotetramers with either TRPA1 or TRPV3 subunits in heterologous systems [72, 73]. These heterotetramers have channel properties that differ from TRPV1 homotetrameric channels.

2.4. Regulation of TRPV1 Channels by Membrane Lipids. TRPV1 is highly sensitive to its membrane environment. For example, this receptor requires membrane cholesterol for optimal channel activity in CHO cells [74]. In addition, TRPV1 channels are highly sensitive to their phospholipid environment [75]. One important modulator of TRPV1 activity is PIP_2, a membrane phospholipid that directly interacts with TRPV1 channels [74, 76, 77]. PIP_2 is a physiologically important phospholipid that is formed from phosphatidylinositol and localizes to the inner leaflet of native mammalian plasma membranes [78]. The C-terminal regions of TRPV1 channels between amino acids 777–820 as well as amino acids R701 and K710 near the TRP domain are thought to be responsible for directly interacting with PIP_2 [31, 76] (see Figure 2(a)).

Activation of the phosphatidylinositol signaling cascade by TRPV1 agonists such as bradykinin will decrease membrane PIP_2 concentrations (a substrate for $PLC\beta$) by hydrolyzing this lipid to IP_3 and DAG. This decrease in membrane PIP_2 could directly modulate TRPV1 activity in plasma membranes [39, 76]. This modulation may occur by

releasing TRPV1 from PIP_2-dependent inhibition [79], or by PKA-mediated recovery from inactivation [62].

Several lines of evidence suggest that PIP_2 is a positive modulator of TRPV1 activity [76]. For example, positively charged epsilon amino groups of polylysine sequester anionic membrane lipids by electrostatic interactions with negatively charged phosphoinositide headgroups [80]. The addition of polylysine to TRPV1-containing membranes inhibits capsaicin-activated currents [81].

Several excised inside-out patch clamp studies have shown that inositol phospholipids directly affect TRPV1 channel activity [76]. The application of PIP_2 to the intracellular leaflet of excised membrane patches, or application of this lipid to one side of a planar membrane containing reconstituted TRPV1 channels, activates TRPV1 channels [75, 77]. PIP_2-activated TRPV1 also shows a decrease in activity due to the gradual dephosphorylation of PIP_2 and its precursor phosphatidylinositol 4-phosphate (PI_4P) by phosphatases in membrane patches [76, 82]. The activity of TRPV1 channels at low capsaicin levels decreased by approximately 90% from initial activity after excision of the membrane patch into an ATP-free medium [75, 76]. TRPV1 channel activity was restored by directly adding Mg^{++}ATP to excised patches. This restoration was prevented by adding inhibitors of phosphatidylinositol 4-kinase, or inhibitors to a phosphatidylinositol-specific bacterial phospholipase C enzyme [75, 76]. These results indicate that PIP_2 sensitizes TRPV1 channels, and the depletion of this membrane lipid may lead to channel desensitization [76].

Membrane PIP_2 concentrations may be decreased by mechanisms that do not involve the generation of second messengers via PLC. For example, the immunosuppressive compound rapamycin from the bacterium *Streptomyces hygroscopicus* causes the translocation of $5'$-phosphatase to the plasma membrane where this enzyme dephosphorylates PIP_2 to PI_4P [77]. Studies with this inducible $5'$-phosphatase indicated that TRPV1 was not inhibited by rapamycin [77] at high concentrations of capsaicin. These results suggested an important role for PI_4P in modulating TRPV1 channel activity under these conditions [77]. Taken together, these studies suggest that endogenous inositol phosphates enhance TRPV1 channel activity in excised membrane patches [76, 77, 81, 83, 84] similar to their effect on K channels [85]. Finally, the combined depletion of both PIP_2 and PI_4P in native membranes inhibits capsaicin-induced TRPV1 channel activity in these membranes [86].

After initial activation of TRPV1 by capsaicin, high levels of this agonist reduce channel responsiveness in trigeminal neurons [87]. One interpretation is that maximal stimulation of TRPV1 receptors and subsequent Ca^{2+} influx depletes PIP_2 in membrane bilayers. This decrease in PIP_2 and its precursor PI_4P may be caused by hydrolysis of PIP_2 by Ca^{2+}-sensitive isoforms of phospholipase Cδ. If PIP_2 stimulates channel activity, then a decrease in PIP_2 would limit channel activity [88]. TRPV1 channel activity may then be inhibited and possibly undergo desensitization [89]. If true, then degradation of PIP_2 by PLC isoforms (which hydrolyze PIP_2 to IP_3 and DAG) would decrease membrane PIP_2 concentrations and subsequently limit channel activity during capsaicin-induced desensitization [76].

Alternatively, PIP_2 may inhibit TRPV1 function [48, 90]. Purified TRPV1 protein that was reconstituted into artificial lipid membranes devoid of phosphoinositides was fully active, which suggested no dependence of TRPV1 channel activity on phosphoinositides [90]. However, the response of purified TRPV1 to both capsaicin and heat decreased when phosphatidylinositol, PIP_2, or PI_4P was added to membranes. This finding suggested that membrane phosphoinositides inhibited TRPV1 in reconstituted systems [90]. In addition, recent studies suggest that purified TRPV1 channel activity is inhibited at its C-terminus by PIP_2 when this phospholipid localizes to both leaflets of the plasma membrane [86]. Finally, a TRPV1 mutant protein lacking a putative PIP_2 binding site in the C-terminal region suggested that PIP_2 binding caused an inhibitory effect on channel activity [48, 79].

The contradictory results concerning PIP_2 modulation of TRPV1 channel activity may be explained by phosphatidylinositol distribution in membranes. In native plasma membranes, PIP_2 localizes to the inner leaflet of the bilayer where this inositol lipid may positively regulate TRPV1 channel activity [76]. Recent data has suggested that PIP_2 localized to the inner (cytoplasmic) leaflet activates TRPV1 while PIP_2 localized to both the outer (extracellular) and inner (cytoplasmic) leaflets inhibited TRPV1 [91]. Patch clamp fluorometry studies with synthetic PIP_2 further indicated that PIP_2 must incorporate into the outer leaflet for inhibition to occur [91]. This observation could explain why PIP_2 inhibited TRPV1 activity in reconstituted membranes where this phospholipid is presumed to be distributed equally between both membrane leaflets [91].

However, PIP_2 is a lipid component of both plasma membranes and internal membranes. Some evidence suggests that membrane phospholipids are symmetrically distributed between the two leaflets of ER (microsomal) membranes [92]. If membrane asymmetry is required for PIP_2 to function as a positive regulator of TRPV1, then a symmetric distribution of PIP_2 in ER membranes could modulate TRPV1 differently from an asymmetric distribution of PIP_2 (and PI_4P) in plasma membranes. Nonetheless, these studies do indicate a dependence of TRPV1 channel activity on membrane phosphoinositides. The relative contributions of PIP_2 and PI_4P in plasma membranes and internal membranes, and partitioning of TRPV1 in membranes following agonist binding, remain to be determined [76].

2.5. Capsaicin Perception in the Human Oral Cavity. The consumption of chili peppers in the human diet dates back to 7000 BC [93]. This consumption resulted in the domestication of these plants approximately 1000 years later in Mexico or northern Central America from wild bird pepper plants [93, 94]. Hot-tasting foods from these plants were subsequently introduced to Europeans when these early explorers returned from the Caribbean [95].

Capsaicin and dihydrocapsaicin are the two major capsaicinoids synthesized by chili peppers, and these two vanilloids are responsible for approximately 90% of the total pungency of chili peppers [96]. Currently, chili peppers are some of the most widely consumed spices in the world [97]. The food industry is the largest consumer of chili peppers, which uses these compounds as flavoring agent in foods, noncarbonated drinks, and alcoholic beverages [98]. Chili peppers can also interact with other foods such as cheese sauces, chicken patties, pork patties, sucrose, sodium chloride, and citric acid [99–102]. Chili peppers may also increase the flavor of vegetables. This flavor enhancement would presumably enhance the ingestion of vegetables and decrease the consumption of fats and cholesterol-rich foods [103].

Due to its dietary importance, capsaicin perception in the oral cavity has been extensively examined in human psychophysical studies. As opposed to taste stimuli, capsaicin is a hydrophobic compound that is difficult to administer to the oral cavity in aqueous solution by "sip and spit" chemosensory assays. Since capsaicin exhibits low solubility in water (0.0013 g/100 mL), psychophysical testing of this stimulus at suprathreshold concentrations is often performed in ethanolic solutions [104], or with impregnated (dried) filter papers [105]. Other delivery methods include the use of rapidly dissolving edible films [106]. Edible film delivery of capsaicin can identify chemosensory properties of this vanilloid in the oral cavity and can demonstrate that a variety of oral stimuli modulate capsaicin chemosensation in the oral cavity [106].

3. Psychophysics of Capsaicin Perception

Capsaicin causes a burning sensation and affects the perception of temperature in the oral cavity [107]. Interestingly, the tip of the tongue is thought to be the most responsive region to capsaicin [108]. This burning sensation may alter preferences for this vanilloid in humans. Frequent consumers of chili peppers generally indicate that "hot-tasting" spices enhance the taste of food, while individuals who avoid spicy foods indicate that hot spices reduce or mask food flavors [109]. In some instances, development of preferences for capsaicin in the oral cavity can be associated with an affective (mood) shift from "dislike to like" for hot-tasting foods [110, 111].

In humans, capsaicin-rich foods may produce "gustatory sweating." This phenomenon causes flushing of the face and the appearance of perspiration on the face and scalp [113]. "Gustatory sweating" is thought to be caused by the effect of capsaicin on the control of thermoregulation [113].

Rats normally avoid diets that contain chili pepper and rarely develop preferences for oral irritants [114]. In 1960, Jancsó reported that systemic application of capsaicin could cause an extended loss in chemical irritant sensitivity in rodents [115], and rats became indifferent to these diets after systemic desensitization to this stimulus [114].

Human studies have demonstrated that topical application of high concentrations of capsaicin to the tongue for ten-minute periods caused a large drop in irritant sensitivity, and this loss of sensitivity did not recover for up to 48 hours [116, 117]. In addition, changes in taste perception from exposure to capsaicin did not occur. However, interactions were predicted to occur between taste receptors and TRP receptors [17, 118].

Exposure to gradually increasing amounts of chili in the human diet appears to be a sufficient condition for developing a preference for spicy foods [110]. Individuals that consume spicy foods begin to enjoy this burning sensation in the oral cavity. The basic change to "liking" for chili peppers is thought to correspond to an affective shift that represents a change in the evaluation of peripheral sensory input [110, 111]. Finally, this hedonic shift toward acceptance may result from an understanding that the burning sensation is harmless and may correspond to the enjoyment of constrained risks [110].

Few studies have examined the effect of temperature on capsaicin perception in the oral cavity [107]. In 1986, Green demonstrated that the perceived intensity of the burning sensation of 2 ppm capsaicin increased in a linear fashion when the solution temperature varied from 34 to 45 degrees Celsius [107]. Tongue surface temperature was not measured, and no conclusions could be drawn as to whether TRPV1 receptors were activated by heat (at a temperature $\geq 43°C$). However, capsaicin can affect sensitivity to pain. Heat stimulation with a Peltier thermode is a standard procedure for examining human sensitivity to pain. The surface temperature of the tongue can be transiently increased with a square Peltier thermode in order to induce oral pain. Capsaicin ($33 \mu M$) significantly enhanced pain ratings to heat stimuli in the temperature range of 47°C to 50°C for a period of at least 5 minutes after presentation of this irritant [119]. The authors concluded that capsaicin enhanced the thermal gating of TRPV1 in cells that mediated thermal pain sensation [119].

The effect of primary taste qualities on capsaicin perception in the oral cavity has been examined. Stevens and Lawless [120] reported that all four primary taste qualities (sweet, sour, salty, and bitter) attenuated the burning sensation of capsaicin in the oral cavity. The decline in the intensity of capsaicin perception following an oral rinse with a taste stimulus occurred most rapidly with citric acid (sour taste) and sucrose. Sodium chloride produced less of an attenuating effect on capsaicin, while the bitter taste stimulus quinine had the least effect on capsaicin perception [120]. Capsaicin underwent exponential decay in perceived intensity following oral rinses with primary taste stimuli [120].

Nasrawi and Pangborn [121] reported that room temperature rinses with 10% sucrose or whole milk at 5°C reduced the oral burn of 3 ppm capsaicin. Sizer and Harris [99] further noted that thresholds for capsaicin mouth-burn were suppressed by sucrose, but not by sodium chloride and/or citric acid.

Psychophysical studies have also identified the effect of capsaicin on the perception of primary taste stimuli. Lawless and Stevens [122] reported that oral rinses with capsicum oleoresin (chili extract containing capsaicin and related compounds) decreased perceived intensities of sour taste (citric acid), bitter taste (quinine), and sweet taste (at high concentrations of sucrose). In contrast, they reported no decrease in salty taste following a capsicum rinse. Their results suggested an inhibitory effect of oral chemical irritation on the perception of primary taste qualities, perhaps by recruiting gustatory nerves for carrying irritant information at the expense of gustatory signals [122].

Lawless and Stevens [108] also reported that capsaicin partially masked both taste and olfactory stimuli. These results suggested an inhibitory effect of oral chemical irritants on the perception of sweet, sour, and bitter taste [108, 120] and supported the earlier results of Sizer and Harris [99]. In contrast, Cowart [123] simultaneously presented capsaicin and individual primary taste stimuli and reported that the perceived intensity of primary taste qualities was generally unaffected by oral irritation with capsaicin. Finally, animal studies have shown that capsaicin at $100 \mu M$ concentrations reduced the strong preference for sucrose in $TRPV1^{-/-}$ null mice [118].

The ability of capsaicin to variably mask primary taste stimuli may suggest that capsaicin alone does not directly activate the human gustatory system [124]. However, capsaicin (and the trigeminal stimulus menthol) may stimulate taste responses in some individuals. For example, cotton swabs that contain 100 or $320 \mu M$ capsaicin elicit a bitter taste response in the human oral cavity, most notably when applied to circumvallate papillae [124]. In addition, a modified TRPV1 channel has been proposed as a candidate Na^+ taste receptor/channel [125–127].

Overall, these results suggest that primary taste stimuli can partially mask the burning sensation of capsaicin and that capsaicin rinses may also attenuate primary taste stimuli in the oral cavity. These findings suggest that interactions may occur between trigeminal neurons and taste receptor cells in the oral cavity, or that signal integration between trigeminal neurons and the gustatory system might occur in the CNS.

These results may imply that TRPV1 receptors and taste receptors are expressed in the same sensory cell or that trigeminal neurons directly communicate and interact with specific populations of taste receptor cells. However, the expression of TRPV1 in taste receptor cells remains controversial [17, 128]. If coexpression of taste receptors and TRPV1 receptors is conclusively shown to occur within a sensory cell [128], this finding could explain how capsaicin attenuates taste responses that stimulate cytosolic Ca^{2+} flux. For example, sweet or bitter taste stimuli could deplete TRPV1-containing cells of Ca^{2+}, a signal that is common to all three cellular transduction pathways. The amount of cytosolic Ca^{2+} could be rate limiting if sensory cells coexpressing TRPV1 and sweet or bitter taste receptors did not activate plasma membrane store-operated channels for subsequent influx of extracellular Ca^{2+}. If true, these findings would also argue against the labeled line model for information coding of chemosensory signals in the oral cavity.

3.1. Capsaicin Thresholds in the Oral Cavity. The threshold for an oral chemosensory stimulus is defined as the lowest concentration or amount at which a subject is able to detect that stimulus. A variety of oral thresholds have been reported for capsaicin in the human oral cavity. In an early study, Sizer and Harris [99] reported a mean threshold value of 5.9 nanomoles (in 10 mL volumes) for capsaicin. In addition, they reported that thresholds decreased (became more sensitive) as solution temperature increased. Finally, these authors demonstrated that sucrose increased thresholds for capsaicin when both stimuli were presented simultaneously [99].

When investigating concentrations between 0.06 and 4.00 parts per million (ppm) in 0.5 $\log_2$ unit steps, Rozin et al. [129] reported a threshold of approximately 0.310 ppm in aqueous solutions (5.1 nmol in 5 mL volume). Lawless et al. [130] compared capsaicin thresholds in aqueous solutions and oil-based delivery methods. The concentration of capsaicin in water varied from 0.03125 to 0.500 ppm. The mean threshold was also 0.310 ($\pm$0.03) ppm in aqueous solution, which is consistent with the results of Rozin et al. [129]. The findings of Rozin et al. [129] and Lawless et al. [130] generally agreed with the results of Sizer and Harris [99], who reported threshold values between 0.090 and 0.350 ppm (2.9 nmol to 11.5 nmol in 10 mL volumes). Karrer and Bartoshuk [131] reported that a concentration of 0.100 ppm did not induce a response in all test subjects. However, Green [132] used capsaicin-impregnated filter paper disks as the delivery method and identified mean thresholds near 0.09–0.10 ppm. Finally, Rentmeister-Bryant and Green [133] reported mean thresholds of 0.299 ppm for capsaicin on the tongue.

More recent studies have reported absolute thresholds of 0.050 ppm (1.6 nmol) for total capsaicinoids, where total capsaicinoid content was taken as the sum of capsaicin and dihydrocapsaicin in the test sample [134]. In these studies, detection thresholds for capsaicin and dihydrocapsaicin in aqueous solutions, or emulsified with polysorbate 80, were identified by a three-alternative forced-choice method. Mean thresholds were near 0.080 ppm (1.3 nmol). In this study, "users" and "nonusers" of chili did not differ significantly in their perception of capsaicin [134]. Finally, Smutzer et al. [106] reported mean recognition thresholds for capsaicin near 1 nmol when the stimulus was delivered by pullulan-based edible strips. A possible explanation for these variations in thresholds could be due to the placement of stimulus on different regions of the tongue surface. Variations in thresholds could also be explained by the different methods that were used for stimulus delivery. Finally, diet could affect capsaicin thresholds since diets rich in spicy foods could cause chronic desensitization in some individuals [132]. Nonetheless, these thresholds are considerably lower (more sensitive) than mean thresholds for bitter taste stimuli [135], including n-propylthiouracil (PROP) [136].

In humans, thresholds to oral chemosensory stimuli may be affected by anxiety levels [135]. Behavioral factors may also affect responses to trigeminal stimuli. In particular, personality factors may drive differences in the liking and consumption of spicy foods that contain capsaicin [137]. These affective responses may influence responses to the previously aversive burning sensation of capsaicin.

Finally, some evidence suggests that the pleasure obtained from the irritating qualities of capsaicin in the oral cavity can be learned following repeated exposure to this irritant [110, 138]. This increased pleasure may be caused by repeated exposure to a cuisine rich in spicy foods [139]. In addition to genetic and cultural factors, human personality traits may have an important role in determining hedonic responses to capsaicin-containing spicy foods [140].

3.2. *Capsaicin Sensitization.* Sensitization is caused by an increase in perceived intensity following the repeated exposure of that irritant at short stimulus intervals [132, 141–144].

Psychophysical studies have shown that sensitization has been observed following either oral or cutaneous application of capsaicin [132]. Also, test subjects show variation in sensitization patterns to capsaicin in the oral cavity [145]. However, not all chemosensory stimuli cause sensitization. For example, repeated stimulation with odors generally shows a reduction in stimulus intensity if the interstimulus interval is brief [146].

In psychophysical studies, low (3 ppm) concentrations of capsaicin that do not elicit oral pain produce an increase in perception (piquancy) during repeated stimulation with interstimulus intervals between 30 and 60 seconds [132, 145]. In the human oral cavity, repeated stimulation with capsaicin resulted in a monotonic increase in perceived intensity. This sensitization occurred after only a few applications of stimulus [132] and continued for up to 25 sequential exposures when no oral rinse was presented between exposures [132]. In this study, filter papers saturated with 3 ppm capsaicin were presented at one-minute intervals. This procedure caused more than a doubling in rating intensity for capsaicin following ten successive applications of irritant [132]. Capsaicin sensitization may have occurred from an increase in stimulus concentration at the site of application on the tongue surface, rather than from spatial summation from converging neurons [147]. However, the mobilization of TRPV1 receptor to the plasma membrane, formation of functional homotetrameric channels, interactions with inositol phospholipids, or receptor phosphorylation could also underlie sensitization.

Capsaicin sensitization in the human oral cavity may be independent of the delivery method since filter paper applications and whole mouth rinses composed of 0.6 or 3 ppm capsaicin in 5% ethanol yielded similar increases in perception of this irritant [145]. However, trigeminal irritants such as zingerone (which may also activate TRPV1 receptors [28]) and menthol (a TRPM8 agonist) show little or no sensitization in the human oral cavity [147–149]. Rather, zingerone induces a progressive decline in irritant intensity after repeated stimulation in the majority of test subjects [147, 148].

Secondly, cross-sensitization of TRP channels could contribute to an enhanced sensitivity to TRPV1 agonists [150]. The sensitization of TRPV1 may occur via activation of TRPA1 receptors in cells that express both cation channels [151]. Since 30% of TRPV1-expressing nociceptive neurons also express TRPA1 channels [152], TRPV1 sensitization could be modulated by TRPA1. In the oral cavity, sensitization of TRPV1 could also involve the activation of adenylyl cyclase, increased cyclic AMP levels, the subsequent translocation and activation of PKA, and phosphorylation of TRPV1 at PKA phosphorylation residues. A possible role for regulatory proteins such as Tmem100 in modulating TRPA1-TRPV1 interactions [153] in oral trigeminal neurons remains to be explored.

Thirdly, low sodium levels may lead to capsaicin sensitization [61]. The lowering of external sodium concentrations directly activates TRPV1 channels in heterologous expression systems [61]. The lowering of external cellular sodium levels could directly gate and sensitize human TRPV1 channels by allowing a greater influx of Ca^{2+}, a cation that could be rate limiting under physiological sodium concentrations [61].

Finally, sensitization may occur by mobilizing dimeric capsaicin receptors into functional homotetramers. Since TRPV1 dimers bind ligand before forming functional tetrameric receptors [53], sensitization may be associated with mobilization of functional tetrameric receptors in neuronal membranes.

3.3. Capsaicin Desensitization. Desensitization is defined as the diminished sensory response to an aversive stimulus after repeated (discontinuous) exposure to that stimulus. Capsaicin desensitization differs from sensory adaptation because a delay of several minutes is required for capsaicin desensitization to occur [154]. Desensitization may be the result of strong or repeated activation of nociceptors that in turn cause a loss in sensitivity to an irritant [150]. Two different types of desensitization have been associated with TRPV1 receptors. One type is classified as acute desensitization, which is a rapid loss of receptor activity during agonist binding. Acute desensitization of TRPV1 is caused by agonist-induced conformational changes, which close TRPV1 channel pores [31]. This pore closing is dependent on cytosolic Ca^{2+} levels [16]. The second type of desensitization is tachyphylaxis, which is identified as a gradually diminishing response of agonist following repeated administrations of that agonist [14, 31]. Capsaicin-induced tachyphylaxis has been widely examined in the human oral cavity [105]. In general, tachyphylaxis may involve the cycling of TRPV1 channels between resting and active states [28].

In the oral cavity, repeated exposure to capsaicin at identical concentrations causes an increase in perceived intensity. Following an interval of 15 minutes, the sensation produced by capsaicin is less than that of the initial application of capsaicin [141]. Thus, the initial burning sensation of capsaicin in the mouth is generally followed by an extended refractory period [82, 155]. Following an extended time period, the reapplication of capsaicin to the tongue produces a diminished intensity that is identified as self-desensitization [131]. Intervals as short as 5 to 15 minutes can decrease the intensity of subsequent capsaicin applications in the oral cavity. In humans, capsaicin induces desensitization [150, 156], and this property is thought to give capsaicin its anesthesia-like properties.

Under certain conditions, repeated exposure to capsaicin and spicy foods in the diet can cause chronic desensitization in humans [109, 131, 157]. Chronic desensitization may in part be responsible for variations in capsaicin perception in the oral cavity among test subjects in psychophysical studies that are described below [158].

Rozin and Schiller [110] identified capsaicin thresholds and salivation volumes and found a small desensitization effect from capsaicin in chili peppers that were consumed at moderate amounts by test subjects. They reported a modest increase in capsaicin thresholds in subjects who liked chili peppers. These authors also reported that liking of the orally irritating qualities of capsaicin could be learned with repeated exposure to this vanilloid in the human diet [110, 159].

In 1989, Green [132] reported that varying the amount of time between applications of capsaicin produced either sensitization or desensitization. Desensitization could occur with as few as five oral applications of stimulus, as long as a minimum delay of 2.5 to 5 minutes between applications was provided [131]. This capsaicin desensitization could last for several days [131].

Nasrawi and Pangborn [160] demonstrated that the intensity of mouth-burn from repeated stimulation with capsaicin did not increase in an additive fashion for all subjects. They further reported that "eaters and noneaters" of chili pepper showed no differences in their perception of capsaicin. However, capsaicin desensitization may be associated with diet where regular users of chili have reported desensitization to the perception of capsaicin-containing foods [132, 161]. Finally, chronic capsaicin desensitization in the oral cavity may be caused by personality differences that drive a wide range of hedonic responses and subsequent consumption of spicy foods [137].

Capsaicin also desensitizes bitter taste [104]. Desensitization with 100 ppm capsaicin decreased the perceived bitterness of several taste stimuli [131]. Pretreatment with capsaicin desensitized the lingual epithelium and reduced the perception of bitter stimuli that included quinine HCl, urea, and PROP [162].

3.4. Long-Lasting (Chronic) Desensitization to Capsaicin. An extended exposure to capsaicin may cause long-lasting desensitization to this stimulus [163]. For example, desensitization to capsaicin increases as exposure to this irritant occurs over a span of weeks [164]. The mechanism for long-term desensitization has been explained as an excessive influx of cations and anions across the plasma membrane of capsaicin-sensitive cells [163]. This ion influx is thought to cause a progressive fatigue-like process in sensory neurons of the oral cavity [154]. However, these conclusions do not agree with more recent studies where desensitization could be produced by rapid and repeated topical exposure to this stimulus, followed by an interval where exposure was stopped for several minutes and then resumed [154].

However, intensity responses to oral capsaicin do vary in humans [165]. This variation could be explained by the frequency of exposure to capsaicin in the diet. For example, intensity responses to capsaicin could decrease over time as dietary consumption of this vanilloid increases [109, 123] or becomes an integral component of the diet. This increased (or continued) consumption could in turn lead to long-lasting desensitization to oral capsaicin.

3.5. Desensitization at the Receptor Level. For TRPV1, desensitization may be mediated by Ca^{2+} influx, which leads to a loss of sensitivity to capsaicin [68, 166]. Calcium ions activate calmodulin, which then stimulates calcineurin-mediated dephosphorylation and desensitization of TRPV1 channels [49]. Calcineurin causes capsaicin-induced desensitization by dephosphorylating amino acids that were previously phosphorylated by PKA [55].

After exposure to high capsaicin concentrations, an increase in cytosolic Ca^{2+} levels may activate PLCδ [76], an enzyme that hydrolyzes PIP_2 to DAG and IP_3. This hydrolysis depletes PIP_2 (and PI_4P) levels in the inner leaflet of plasma membranes, which in turn likely decreases TRPV1 channel activity in native membranes [76, 89, 92]. This depletion could limit TRPV1 channel activity and lead to desensitization [77]. A possible role for disassembly of tetrameric TRPV1 channels into dimeric complexes as a model for channel desensitization has not been examined. Finally, desensitization of TRPV1 channels may be caused by a decrease in affinity for capsaicin since receptor responses can be recovered by raising capsaicin concentrations [167].

Following a protracted exposure to capsaicin, TRPV1 activity may decrease by desensitization (self-desensitization) [132, 168]. Desensitization of TRPV1 may produce the analgesic effect of capsaicin [49]. Extracellular Ca^{2+} ions are required for channel desensitization because Ca^{2+} influx and release of intracellular Ca^{2+} stores mediate this effect [169]. Calcium influx leads to a loss of sensitivity to capsaicin along with a reduction in heat sensitivity [166]. Also, desensitization of TRPV1 by capsaicin decreases the apparent affinity for this agonist since responses can be recovered by raising capsaicin concentrations [167].

At the molecular level, long-lasting desensitization to capsaicin could be caused by a decrease in functional TRPV1 receptors in sensory neurons, lack of mobilization of functional receptors to the plasma membrane, a decrease in kinase activity in these cells, or changes in membrane lipid interactions with this receptor. An explanation for long-term desensitization to capsaicin in the oral cavity, and the possible role of diet in this phenomenon, awaits further study.

3.6. Stimulus Induced Recovery following Desensitization. The repeated application of capsaicin to previously desensitized oral epithelium induces irritation that approaches the original perceived intensity of capsaicin [105, 154, 170]. These results indicate that desensitization can be temporarily reversed if oral stimulation with a trigeminal stimulant such as capsaicin is resumed. This response to desensitized tissue has been named stimulus induced recovery (SIR). SIR occurs when lingual application of capsaicin induces the activation of TRPV1 receptors, and this activation overcomes prior desensitization by this stimulus [105, 154, 170].

SIR is caused by rapid exposure to capsaicin in concentrations at least as high as the desensitizing stimulus, and at short interstimulus intervals [133]. This reapplication of stimulus may result in maximal intensities that were previously observed during sensitization with agonist [105, 154]. These findings suggest that capsaicin desensitization could be reversed by further application of this irritant and that desensitization and SIR were likely facilitated by opposing cellular (or TRPV1 receptor) processes.

At the receptor level, SIR may be the result of mobilization of low-affinity TRPV1 receptors that were not desensitized during initial applications of capsaicin [170]. Therefore, SIR may involve cellular mechanisms similar or identical to those that trigger capsaicin sensitization [170] (i.e., low-affinity receptors that failed to form homotetramers). Finally, some evidence suggests that PIP_2 synthesis from PI_4P by PI_4P

kinase is required for the recovery of TRPV1 channels from prior desensitization [171].

Interestingly, SIR is not unique to capsaicin. The trigeminal stimulant piperine (a component of black pepper) is a vanilloid that also induces SIR under conditions of self-sensitization, or by cross-desensitization with capsaicin [154]. Both capsaicin and piperine are TRPV1 agonists [172].

Zingerone (from ginger) is primarily a TRPA1 agonist [173] that does not exhibit SIR [154]. However, zingerone can activate TRPV1 channels in heterologous systems where inositol phospholipids may be uniformly distributed in both leaflets of the bilayer [27]. Menthol is also a trigeminal stimulus (counterirritant) and a TRPM8 agonist that does not induce SIR when capsaicin is the stimulus [149]. However, menthol does show transient desensitization (cross-desensitization) of capsaicin irritation in the oral cavity [174].

SIR may occur from interacting factors at the cellular level or may be the result of higher order neuronal processing. However, these results do suggest a functional role for TRPV1 receptors in SIR. As previously mentioned, PIP_2 enhances TRPV1 activity in native membranes. At the present time, a possible role for membrane PIP_2 levels (or receptor phosphorylation) in SIR has not been explored. However, activation of PKC reverses the capsaicin-induced desensitization of TRPV1 channels [65], which could explain the underlying mechanism of SIR.

4. Conclusions

In summary, capsaicin is a naturally occurring compound that causes a pungent sensation in the human oral cavity when this vanilloid binds to TRPV1 receptors. Functional TRPV1 receptors form homotetramers in biological membranes, are highly regulated in neuronal tissue, and are highly sensitive to their membrane lipid environment. Along with receptor phosphorylation, recent data have suggested that inositol lipids such as PIP_2 and PI_4P stimulate this receptor in native membranes. TRPV1 mobilization to the plasma membrane and the effects of receptor phosphorylation and TRPV1 interactions with inositol phospholipids on capsaicin perception in the oral cavity remain largely unexplored.

Human psychophysical studies have indicated that capsaicin may modulate the perception of primary taste stimuli and that some primary taste stimuli may in turn modulate capsaicin perception. Recent psychophysical studies have further indicated that capsaicin causes sensitization, desensitization, and SIR in the oral cavity. Further studies are required to determine possible interactions between TRPV1-expressing cells and taste receptor cells in the human oral cavity. Future studies are also needed to more fully integrate molecular studies with psychophysical studies and to clarify possible interactions involving signals from primary taste stimuli and trigeminal irritants in the CNS. Finally, the possible role of TRPV1 single nucleotide polymorphisms in modulating vanilloid perception in the oral cavity remains largely unexplored [175]. The results of these studies will serve to clarify the effects of capsaicin on the human diet, and its role as an analgesic for treating pain.

Conflict of Interests

The authors certify that they have no involvement in any organization or entity with any financial interests in the subject matter discussed in this paper.

Acknowledgments

This work was funded by an FSSMF grant from Temple University and from the Temple University Undergraduate Research Program. The authors thank Judith Stull and Harry Rappaport for their valuable assistance.

References

[1] G. K. Jones, "The chemistry and pharmacy of capsicum," *Manufacturing Chemist and Aerosol News*, vol. 17, no. 8, pp. 342–344, 1946.

[2] J. J. Tewksbury, K. M. Reagan, N. J. Machnicki et al., "Evolutionary ecology of pungency in wild chilies," *Proceedings of the National Academy of Sciences of the United States of America*, vol. 105, no. 33, pp. 11808–11811, 2008.

[3] D. C. Haak, L. A. McGinnis, D. J. Levey, and J. J. Tewksbury, "Why are not all chilies hot? A trade-off limits pungency," *Proceedings of the Royal Society B: Biological Sciences*, vol. 279, no. 1735, pp. 2012–2017, 2012.

[4] J. A. Rumsfield and D. P. West, "Topical capsaicin in dermatologic and peripheral pain disorders," *DICP: The Annals of Pharmacotherapy*, vol. 25, no. 4, pp. 381–387, 1991.

[5] S. Mandadi and B. D. Roufogalis, "ThermoTRP channels in nociceptors: taking a lead from capsaicin receptor TRPV1," *Current Neuropharmacology*, vol. 6, no. 1, pp. 21–38, 2008.

[6] R. D. Sanders, "The trigeminal (V) and facial (VII) cranial nerves: head and face sensation and movement," *Psychiatry*, vol. 7, no. 1, pp. 13–16, 2010.

[7] N. Amano, J. W. Hu, and B. J. Sessle, "Responses of neurons in feline trigeminal subnucleus caudalis (medullary dorsal horn) to cutaneous, intraoral, and muscle afferent stimuli," *Journal of Neurophysiology*, vol. 55, no. 2, pp. 227–243, 1986.

[8] M.-J. Ludy, G. E. Moore, and R. D. Mattes, "The effects of capsaicin and capsiate on energy balance: critical review and meta-analyses of studies in humans," *Chemical Senses*, vol. 37, no. 2, pp. 103–121, 2012.

[9] K. Lim, M. Yoshioka, S. Kikuzato et al., "Dietary red pepper ingestion increases carbohydrate oxidation at rest and during exercise in runners," *Medicine & Science in Sports & Exercise*, vol. 29, no. 3, pp. 355–361, 1997.

[10] M.-J. Ludy and R. D. Mattes, "The effects of hedonically acceptable red pepper doses on thermogenesis and appetite," *Physiology & Behavior*, vol. 102, no. 3-4, pp. 251–258, 2011.

[11] M. A. Eskander, S. Ruparel, D. P. Green et al., "Persistent nociception triggered by nerve growth factor (NGF) is mediated by TRPV1 and oxidative mechanisms," *Journal of Neuroscience*, vol. 35, no. 22, pp. 8593–8603, 2015.

[12] A. M. Sánchez, M. G. Sánchez, S. Malagarie-Cazenave, N. Olea, and I. Díaz-Laviada, "Induction of apoptosis in prostate tumor PC-3 cells and inhibition of xenograft prostate tumor growth by the vanilloid capsaicin," *Apoptosis*, vol. 11, no. 1, pp. 89–99, 2006.

[13] J. Donnerer and F. Lembeck, "Heat loss reaction to capsaicin through a peripheral site of action," *British Journal of Pharmacology*, vol. 79, no. 3, pp. 719–723, 1983.

[14] J. Lv, L. Qi, C. Yu et al., "Consumption of spicy foods and total and cause specific mortality: population based cohort study," *The BMJ*, vol. 351, article h3942, 2015.

[15] C. M. Mistretta, "Developmental neurobiology of the taste system," in *Smell and Taste in Health and Disease*, T. V. Getchell, R. L. Doty, L. M. Bartoshuk, and J. B. Snow, Eds., chapter 3, Raven Press, New York, NY, USA, 1991.

[16] M. J. Caterina, M. A. Schumacher, M. Tominaga, T. A. Rosen, J. D. Levine, and D. Julius, "The capsaicin receptor: a heat-activated ion channel in the pain pathway," *Nature*, vol. 389, no. 6653, pp. 816–824, 1997.

[17] S. D. Roper, "TRPs in taste and chemesthesis," *Handbook of Experimental Pharmacology*, vol. 223, pp. 827–871, 2014.

[18] Z. Olah, T. Szabo, L. Karai et al., "Ligand-induced dynamic membrane changes and cell deletion conferred by vanilloid receptor 1," *Journal of Biological Chemistry*, vol. 276, no. 14, pp. 11021–11030, 2001.

[19] K. W. Ho, N. J. Ward, and D. J. Calkins, "TRPV1: a stress response protein in the central nervous system," *American Journal of Neurodegenerative Disease*, vol. 1, no. 1, pp. 1–14, 2012.

[20] M. J. Caterina and D. Julius, "The vanilloid receptor: a molecular gateway to the pain pathway," *Annual Review of Neuroscience*, vol. 24, pp. 487–517, 2001.

[21] K. Kobayashi, T. Fukuoka, K. Obata et al., "Distinct expression of TRPM8, TRPA1, and TRPV1 mRNAs in rat primary afferent neurons with $A\delta$/C-fibers and colocalization with trk receptors," *Journal of Comparative Neurology*, vol. 493, no. 4, pp. 596–606, 2005.

[22] S. Benemei, R. Patacchini, M. Trevisani, and P. Geppetti, "TRP channels," *Current Opinion in Pharmacology*, vol. 22, pp. 18–23, 2015.

[23] A. Gröne, S. Fonfara, and W. Baumgärtner, "Cell type-dependent cytokine expression after canine distemper virus infection," *Viral Immunology*, vol. 15, no. 3, pp. 493–505, 2002.

[24] K. Sałat, A. Jakubowska, and K. Kulig, "Zucapsaicin for the treatment of neuropathic pain," *Expert Opinion on Investigational Drugs*, vol. 23, no. 10, pp. 1433–1440, 2014.

[25] M. Hakim, W. Jiang, L. Luo et al., "Scorpion toxin, BmP01, induces pain by targeting TRPV1 channel," *Toxins*, vol. 7, no. 9, pp. 3671–3687, 2015.

[26] F. N. McNamara, A. Randall, and M. J. Gunthorpe, "Effects of piperine, the pungent component of black pepper, at the human vanilloid receptor (TRPV1)," *British Journal of Pharmacology*, vol. 144, no. 6, pp. 781–790, 2005.

[27] Y. Iwasaki, A. Morita, T. Iwasawa et al., "A nonpungent component of steamed ginger—[10]-shogaol—increases adrenaline secretion via the activation of TRPV1," *Nutritional Neuroscience*, vol. 9, no. 3-4, pp. 169–178, 2006.

[28] L. Liu and S. A. Simon, "Similarities and differences in the currents activated by capsaicin, piperine, and zingerone in rat trigeminal ganglion cells," *Journal of Neurophysiology*, vol. 76, no. 3, pp. 1858–1869, 1996.

[29] V. N. Dedov, V. H. Tran, C. C. Duke et al., "Gingerols: a novel class of vanilloid receptor (VR1) agonists," *British Journal of Pharmacology*, vol. 137, no. 6, pp. 793–798, 2002.

[30] C. E. Riera, H. Vogel, S. A. Simon, and J. le Coutre, "Artificial sweeteners and salts producing a metallic taste sensation activate TRPV1 receptors," *American Journal of Physiology: Regulatory Integrative and Comparative Physiology*, vol. 293, no. 2, pp. R626–R634, 2007.

[31] A. Jara-Oseguera, S. A. Simon, and T. Rosenbaum, "TRPV1: on the road to pain relief," *Current Molecular Pharmacology*, vol. 1, no. 3, pp. 255–269, 2008.

[32] F. Yang, X. Xiao, W. Cheng et al., "Structural mechanism underlying capsaicin binding and activation of the TRPV1 ion channel," *Nature Chemical Biology*, vol. 11, no. 7, pp. 518–524, 2015.

[33] S. Bevan, T. Quallo, and D. A. Andersson, "TRPV1," *Handbook of Experimental Pharmacology*, vol. 222, pp. 207–245, 2014.

[34] A. Hazan, R. Kumar, H. Matzner, and A. Priel, "The pain receptor TRPV1 displays agonist-dependent activation stoichiometry," *Scientific Reports*, vol. 5, article 12278, 2015.

[35] J. Vriens, G. Appendino, and B. Nilius, "Pharmacology of vanilloid transient receptor potential cation channels," *Molecular Pharmacology*, vol. 75, no. 6, pp. 1262–1279, 2009.

[36] R. J. Docherty, J. C. Yeats, and A. S. Piper, "Capsazepine block of voltage-activated calcium channels in adult rat dorsal root ganglion neurones in culture," *British Journal of Pharmacology*, vol. 121, no. 7, pp. 1461–1467, 1997.

[37] I. Devesa, C. Ferrándiz-Huertas, S. Mathivanan et al., "αCGRP is essential for algesic exocytotic mobilization of TRPV1 channels in peptidergic nociceptors," *Proceedings of the National Academy of Sciences of the United States of America*, vol. 111, no. 51, pp. 18345–18350, 2014.

[38] J. Grant, "Tachykinins stimulate a subset of mouse taste cells," *PLoS ONE*, vol. 7, no. 2, Article ID e31697, 2012.

[39] K. Srinivasan, "Biological activities of red pepper (*Capsicum annuum*) and its pungent principle capsaicin: a review," *Critical Reviews in Food Science and Nutrition*, 2015.

[40] P. Holzer, "Neurogenic vasodilatation and plasma leakage in the skin," *General Pharmacology*, vol. 30, no. 1, pp. 5–11, 1998.

[41] M. L. Kowalski, M. Sliwinska-Kowalska, and M. A. Kaliner, "Neurogenic inflammation, vascular permeability, and mast cells: II. Additional evidence indicating that mast cells are not involved in neurogenic inflammation," *The Journal of Immunology*, vol. 145, no. 4, pp. 1214–1221, 1990.

[42] T. F. Burks, S. H. Buck, and M. S. Miller, "Mechanisms of depletion of substance P by capsaicin," *Federation Proceedings*, vol. 44, no. 9, pp. 2531–2534, 1985.

[43] M. Liao, E. Cao, D. Julius, and Y. Cheng, "Structure of the TRPV1 ion channel determined by electron cryo-microscopy," *Nature*, vol. 504, no. 7478, pp. 107–112, 2013.

[44] C. Kimball, J. Luo, S. Yin, H. Hu, and A. Dhaka, "The pore loop domain of TRPV1 is required for its activation by the volatile anesthetics chloroform and isoflurane," *Molecular Pharmacology*, vol. 88, no. 1, pp. 131–138, 2015.

[45] B. H. Lee and J. Zheng, "Proton block of proton-activated TRPV1 current," *The Journal of General Physiology*, vol. 146, no. 2, pp. 147–159, 2015.

[46] V. Y. Moiseenkova-Bell, L. A. Stanciu, I. I. Serysheva, B. J. Tobe, and T. G. Wensel, "Structure of TRPV1 channel revealed by electron cryomicroscopy," *Proceedings of the National Academy of Sciences of the United States of America*, vol. 105, no. 21, pp. 7451–7455, 2008.

[47] N. Kedei, T. Szabo, J. D. Lile et al., "Analysis of the native quaternary structure of vanilloid receptor 1," *Journal of Biological Chemistry*, vol. 276, no. 30, pp. 28613–28619, 2001.

[48] E. D. Prescott and D. Julius, "A modular PIP$_2$ binding site as a determinant of capsaicin receptor sensitivity," *Science*, vol. 300, no. 5623, pp. 1284–1288, 2003.

[49] M. Numazaki, T. Tominaga, K. Takeuchi, N. Murayama, H. Toyooka, and M. Tominaga, "Structural determinant of TRPV1 desensitization interacts with calmodulin," *Proceedings of the National Academy of Sciences of the United States of America*, vol. 100, no. 13, pp. 8002–8006, 2003.

[50] M. Numazaki, T. Tominaga, H. Toyooka, and M. Tominaga, "Direct phosphorylation of capsaicin receptor VR1 by protein kinase Cε and identification of two target serine residues," *Journal of Biological Chemistry*, vol. 277, no. 16, pp. 13375–13378, 2002.

[51] G. Bhave, H.-J. Hu, K. S. Glauner et al., "Protein kinase C phosphorylation sensitizes but does not activate the capsaicin receptor transient receptor potential vanilloid 1 (TRPV1)," *Proceedings of the National Academy of Sciences of the United States of America*, vol. 100, no. 21, pp. 12480–12485, 2003.

[52] L. Gregorio-Teruel, P. Valente, J. M. González-Ros, G. Fernández-Ballester, and A. Ferrer-Montiel, "Mutation of I696 and W697 in the TRP box of vanilloid receptor subtype I modulates allosteric channel activation," *Journal of General Physiology*, vol. 143, no. 3, pp. 361–375, 2014.

[53] N. García-Sanz, A. Fernández-Carvajal, C. Morenilla-Palao et al., "Identification of a tetramerization domain in the C terminus of the vanilloid receptor," *Journal of Neuroscience*, vol. 24, no. 23, pp. 5307–5314, 2004.

[54] X. Li, P. Mooney, S. Zheng et al., "Electron counting and beam-induced motion correction enable near-atomic-resolution single-particle cryo-EM," *Nature Methods*, vol. 10, no. 6, pp. 584–590, 2013.

[55] K. Venkatachalam and C. Montell, "TRP channels," *Annual Review of Biochemistry*, vol. 76, pp. 387–417, 2007.

[56] R. Latorre, C. Zaelzer, and S. Brauchi, "Structure-functional intimacies of transient receptor potential channels," *Quarterly Reviews of Biophysics*, vol. 42, no. 3, pp. 201–246, 2009.

[57] N. R. Gavva, L. Klionsky, Y. Qu et al., "Molecular determinants of vanilloid sensitivity in TRPV1," *Journal of Biological Chemistry*, vol. 279, no. 19, pp. 20283–20295, 2004.

[58] S.-E. Jordt, M. Tominaga, and D. Julius, "Acid potentiation of the capsaicin receptor determined by a key extracellular site," *Proceedings of the National Academy of Sciences of the United States of America*, vol. 97, no. 14, pp. 8134–8139, 2000.

[59] P. Valente, N. García-Sanz, A. Gomis et al., "Identification of molecular determinants of channel gating in the transient receptor potential box of vanilloid receptor I," *The FASEB Journal*, vol. 22, no. 9, pp. 3298–3309, 2008.

[60] B. R. Myers, C. J. Bohlen, and D. Julius, "A yeast genetic screen reveals a critical role for the pore helix domain in TRP channel gating," *Neuron*, vol. 58, no. 3, pp. 362–373, 2008.

[61] T. Ohta, T. Imagawa, and S. Ito, "Novel gating and sensitizing mechanism of capsaicin receptor (TRPV1): tonic inhibitory regulation of extracellular sodium through the external protonation sites on TRPV1," *Journal of Biological Chemistry*, vol. 283, no. 14, pp. 9377–9387, 2008.

[62] L. De Petrocellis, S. Harrison, T. Bisogno et al., "The vanilloid receptor (VR1)-mediated effects of anandamide are potently enhanced by the cAMP-dependent protein kinase," *Journal of Neurochemistry*, vol. 77, no. 6, pp. 1660–1663, 2001.

[63] S. Mistry, C. C. Paule, A. Varga et al., "Prolonged exposure to bradykinin and prostaglandin E2 increases TRPV1 mRNA but does not alter TRPV1 and TRPV1b protein expression in cultured rat primary sensory neurons," *Neuroscience Letters*, vol. 564, pp. 89–93, 2014.

[64] D. L. Gill, T. K. Ghosh, and J. M. Mullaney, "Calcium signalling mechanisms in endoplasmic reticulum activated by inositol 1,4,5-trisphosphate and GTP," *Cell Calcium*, vol. 10, no. 5, pp. 363–374, 1989.

[65] V. Vellani, S. Mapplebeck, A. Moriondo, J. B. Davis, and P. A. McNaughton, "Protein kinase C activation potentiates gating of the vanilloid receptor VR1 by capsaicin, protons, heat and anandamide," *Journal of Physiology*, vol. 534, no. 3, pp. 813–825, 2001.

[66] E. D. Por, R. Gomez, A. N. Akopian, and N. A. Jeske, "Phosphorylation regulates TRPV1 association with β-arrestin-2," *Biochemical Journal*, vol. 451, no. 1, pp. 101–109, 2013.

[67] C. Morenilla-Palao, R. Planells-Cases, N. García-Sanz, and A. Ferrer-Montiel, "Regulated exocytosis contributes to protein kinase C potentiation of vanilloid receptor activity," *Journal of Biological Chemistry*, vol. 279, no. 24, pp. 25665–25672, 2004.

[68] D. P. Mohapatra and C. Nau, "Regulation of Ca^{2+}-dependent desensitization in the vanilloid receptor TRPV1 by calcineurin and cAMP-dependent protein kinase," *Journal of Biological Chemistry*, vol. 280, no. 14, pp. 13424–13432, 2005.

[69] S. Mandadi, M. Numazaki, M. Tominaga, M. B. Bhat, P. J. Armati, and B. D. Roufogalis, "Activation of protein kinase C reverses capsaicin-induced calcium-dependent desensitization of TRPV1 ion channels," *Cell Calcium*, vol. 35, no. 5, pp. 471–478, 2004.

[70] B. Storti, R. Bizzarri, F. Cardarelli, and F. Beltram, "Intact microtubules preserve transient receptor potential vanilloid 1 (TRPV1) functionality through receptor binding," *Journal of Biological Chemistry*, vol. 287, no. 10, pp. 7803–7811, 2012.

[71] B. Storti, C. Di Rienzo, F. Cardarelli, R. Bizzarri, and F. Beltram, "Unveiling TRPV1 spatio-temporal organization in live cell membranes," *PLoS ONE*, vol. 10, no. 3, Article ID e0116900, 2015.

[72] L. R. Sadofsky, K. T. Sreekrishna, Y. Lin et al., "Unique responses are observed in transient receptor potential ankyrin 1 and vanilloid 1 (TRPA1 and TRPV1) co-expressing cells," *Cells*, vol. 3, no. 2, pp. 616–626, 2014.

[73] W. Cheng, F. Yang, C. L. Takanishi, and J. Zheng, "Thermosensitive TRPV channel subunits coassemble into heteromeric channels with intermediate conductance and gating properties," *Journal of General Physiology*, vol. 129, no. 3, pp. 191–207, 2007.

[74] G. Picazo-Juárez, S. Romero-Suárez, A. Nieto-Posadas et al., "Identification of a binding motif in the S5 helix that confers cholesterol sensitivity to the TRPV1 ion channel," *Journal of Biological Chemistry*, vol. 286, no. 28, pp. 24966–24976, 2011.

[75] V. Lukacs, J.-M. Rives, X. Sun, E. Zakharian, and T. Rohacs, "Promiscuous activation of Transient Receptor Potential Vanilloid 1 (TRPV1) channels by negatively charged intracellular lipids: the key role of endogenous phosphoinositides in maintaining channel activity," *Journal of Biological Chemistry*, vol. 288, no. 49, pp. 35003–35013, 2013.

[76] T. Rohacs, "Phosphoinositide regulation of TRPV1 revisited," *Pflügers Archiv—European Journal of Physiology*, vol. 467, no. 9, pp. 1851–1869, 2015.

[77] V. Lukacs, B. Thyagarajan, P. Varnai, A. Balla, T. Balla, and T. Rohacs, "Dual regulation of TRPV1 by phosphoinositides," *Journal of Neuroscience*, vol. 27, no. 26, pp. 7070–7080, 2007.

[78] P. J. Quinn, "Plasma membrane phospholipid asymmetry," *Subcellular Biochemistry*, vol. 36, pp. 39–60, 2002.

[79] H.-H. Chuang, E. D. Prescott, H. Kong et al., "Bradykinin and nerve growth factor release the capsaicin receptor from PtdIns(4,5)P2-mediated inhibition," *Nature*, vol. 411, no. 6840, pp. 957–962, 2001.

[80] M. Toner, G. Vaio, A. McLaughlin, and S. McLaughlin, "Adsorption of cations to phosphatidylinositol 4,5-bisphosphate," *Biochemistry*, vol. 27, no. 19, pp. 7435–7443, 1988.

[81] A. T. Stein, C. A. Ufret-Vincenty, L. Hua, L. F. Santana, and S. E. Gordon, "Phosphoinositide 3-kinase binds to TRPV1 and mediates NGF-stimulated TRPV1 trafficking to the plasma membrane," *Journal of General Physiology*, vol. 128, no. 5, pp. 509–522, 2006.

[82] L. Liu and S. A. Simon, "Capsaicin-induced currents with distinct desensitization and Ca2+ dependence in rat trigeminal ganglion cells," *Journal of Neurophysiology*, vol. 75, no. 4, pp. 1503–1514, 1996.

[83] D. Kim, E. J. Cavanaugh, and D. Simkin, "Inhibition of transient receptor potential A1 channel by phosphatidylinositol-4,5-bisphosphate," *The American Journal of Physiology—Cell Physiology*, vol. 295, no. 1, pp. C92–C99, 2008.

[84] C. A. Ufret-Vincenty, R. M. Klein, L. Hua, J. Angueyra, and S. E. Gordon, "Localization of the PIP2 sensor of TRPV1 ion channels," *Journal of Biological Chemistry*, vol. 286, no. 11, pp. 9688–9698, 2011.

[85] S. B. Hansen, X. Tao, and R. MacKinnon, "Structural basis of PIP_2 activation of the classical inward rectifier K^+ channel Kir2.2," *Nature*, vol. 477, no. 7365, pp. 495–498, 2011.

[86] G. R. V. Hammond, M. J. Fischer, K. E. Anderson et al., "PI4P and $PI(4,5)P_2$ are essential but independent lipid determinants of membrane identity," *Science*, vol. 337, no. 6095, pp. 727–730, 2012.

[87] H. Knotkova, M. Pappagallo, and A. Szallasi, "Capsaicin (TRPV1 agonist) therapy for pain relief: farewell or revival?" *Clinical Journal of Pain*, vol. 24, no. 2, pp. 142–154, 2008.

[88] V. Lukacs, Y. Yudin, G. R. Hammond, E. Sharma, K. Fukami, and T. Rohacs, "Distinctive changes in plasma membrane phosphoinositides underlie differential regulation of TRPV1 in nociceptive neurons," *The Journal of Neuroscience*, vol. 33, no. 28, pp. 11451–11463, 2013.

[89] T. Rohacs, B. Thyagarajan, and V. Lukacs, "Phospholipase C mediated modulation of TRPV1 channels," *Molecular Neurobiology*, vol. 37, no. 2-3, pp. 153–163, 2008.

[90] E. Cao, J. F. Cordero-Morales, B. Liu, F. Qin, and D. Julius, "TRPV1 channels are intrinsically heat sensitive and negatively regulated by phosphoinositide lipids," *Neuron*, vol. 77, no. 4, pp. 667–679, 2013.

[91] E. N. Senning, M. D. Collins, A. Stratiievska, C. A. Ufret-Vincenty, and S. E. Gordon, "Regulation of TRPV1 ion channel by phosphoinositide (4,5)-bisphosphate: the role of membrane asymmetry," *Journal of Biological Chemistry*, vol. 289, no. 16, pp. 10999–11006, 2014.

[92] G. Van Meer, D. R. Voelker, and G. W. Feigenson, "Membrane lipids: where they are and how they behave," *Nature Reviews Molecular Cell Biology*, vol. 9, no. 2, pp. 112–124, 2008.

[93] B. Pickersgill, "Domestication of plants in the Americas: insights from Mendelian and molecular genetics," *Annals of Botany*, vol. 100, no. 5, pp. 925–940, 2007.

[94] B. Pickersgill, "The domestication of chili peppers," in *The Domestication and Exploitation of Plants and Animals*, P. J. Ucko and G. W. Dimbleby, Eds., p. 443, Gerald Duckworth, London, UK, 1969.

[95] F. Lembeck, "Columbus, *Capsicum* and capsaicin: past, present and future," *Acta Physiologica Hungarica*, vol. 69, no. 3-4, pp. 265–273, 1987.

[96] G. F. Barbero, M. Palma, and C. G. Barroso, "Determination of capsaicinoids in peppers by microwave-assisted extraction-high-performance liquid chromatography with fluorescence detection," *Analytica Chimica Acta*, vol. 578, no. 2, pp. 227–233, 2006.

[97] L. Orellana-Escobedo, J. J. Ornelas-Paz, G. I. Olivas, J. A. Guerrero-Beltran, J. Jimenez-Castro, and D. R. Sepulveda, "Determination of absolute threshold and just noticeable difference in the sensory perception of pungency," *Journal of Food Science*, vol. 77, no. 3, pp. S135–S139, 2012.

[98] A. G. Mathew, Y. S. Lewis, R. Jagadishan, E. S. Nambudiri, and N. Krishnamurthy, "Oleoresin *Capsicum*," *Flavour Industry*, vol. 2, no. 1, pp. 23–26, 1971.

[99] F. Sizer and N. Harris, "The influence of common food additives and temperature on threshold perception of capsaicin," *Chemical Senses*, vol. 10, no. 3, pp. 279–286, 1985.

[100] L. A. Carden, M. P. Penfield, and A. M. Saxton, "Perception of heat in cheese sauces as affected by capsaicin concentration, fat level, fat mimetic and time," *Journal of Food Science*, vol. 64, no. 1, pp. 175–179, 1999.

[101] M. E. Emrick, M. P. Penfield, C. D. Bacon, R. V. L. Van Laack, and C. J. Brekke, "Heat intensity and warmed-over flavor in precooked chicken patties formulated at 3 fat levels and 3 pepper levels," *Journal of Food Science*, vol. 70, no. 9, pp. S600–S604, 2005.

[102] H. C. Reinbach, M. Toft, and P. Møller, "Relationship between oral burn and temperature in chili spiced pork patties evaluated by time-intensity," *Food Quality and Preference*, vol. 20, no. 1, pp. 42–49, 2009.

[103] H. Lawless, "Pepper potency and the forgotten flavor sense," *Food Technology*, vol. 11, pp. 52, 57–58, 1989.

[104] J. Lim and B. G. Green, "The psychophysical relationship between bitter taste and burning sensation: evidence of qualitative similarity," *Chemical Senses*, vol. 32, no. 1, pp. 31–39, 2007.

[105] B. G. Green and H. Rentmeister-Bryant, "Temporal characteristics of capsaicin desensitization and stimulus-induced recovery in the oral cavity," *Physiology & Behavior*, vol. 65, no. 1, pp. 141–149, 1998.

[106] G. S. Smutzer, J. C. Jacob, D. I. Shah, J. T. Tran, and J. C. Stull, "Modulation of chemosensory properties of capsaicin in the human oral cavity," in *Proceedings of the 35th Annual Meeting of the Association for Chemoreception Sciences*, Abstract #179, Association for Chemoreception Sciences, Bonita Springs, Fla, USA, 2014.

[107] B. G. Green, "Sensory interactions between capsaicin and temperature in the oral cavity," *Chemical Senses*, vol. 11, no. 3, pp. 371–382, 1986.

[108] H. T. Lawless and D. A. Stevens, "Responses by humans to oral chemical irritants as a function of locus of stimulation," *Perception and Psychophysics*, vol. 43, no. 1, pp. 72–78, 1988.

[109] H. Lawless, P. Rozin, and J. Shenker, "Effects of oral capsaicin on gustatory, olfactory and irritant sensations and flavor identification in humans who regularly or rarely consume chili pepper," *Chemical Senses*, vol. 10, no. 4, pp. 579–589, 1985.

[110] P. Rozin and D. Schiller, "The nature and acquisition of a preference for chili pepper by humans," *Motivation and Emotion*, vol. 4, no. 1, pp. 77–101, 1980.

[111] P. Rozin, L. Ebert, and J. Schull, "Some like it hot: a temporal analysis of hedonic responses to chili pepper," *Appetite*, vol. 3, no. 1, pp. 13–22, 1982.

[112] H. M. Berman, J. Westbrook, Z. Feng et al., "The protein data bank," *Nucleic Acids Research*, vol. 28, no. 1, pp. 235–242, 2000.

[113] T. S. Lee, "Physiological gustatory sweating in a warm climate," *The Journal of Physiology*, vol. 124, no. 3, pp. 528–542, 1954.

[114] P. Rozin, L. Gruss, and G. Berk, "Reversal of innate aversions: attempts to induce a preference for chili peppers in rats," *Journal of Comparative and Physiological Psychology*, vol. 93, no. 6, pp. 1001–1014, 1979.

[115] N. Jancsó, "Role of the nerve terminals in the mechanism of inflammatory reactions," *Bulletin of the Millard Fillmore Hospital*, vol. 7, pp. 53–77, 1960.

[116] N. Jancsó, "Desensitization with capsaicin and related acrylamides as a tool for studying the function of pain receptors," in *Pharmacology of Pain*, R. K. S. Lim, D. Armstrong, and E. G. Pardo, Eds., pp. 33–55, Pergamon Press, Oxford, UK, 1968.

[117] J. Szolcsanyi and A. Jancsó-Gábor, "Capsaicin and other pungent agents as pharmacological tools in studies on thermoregulation," in *The Pharmacology of Thermoregulation*, E. Schonbaum and P. Lomax, Eds., pp. 395–409, Karger Publishers, Basel, Switzerland, 1973.

[118] R. M. Costa, L. Liu, M. A. L. Nicolelis, and S. A. Simon, "Gustatory effects of capsaicin that are independent of TRPV1 receptors," *Chemical Senses*, vol. 30, supplement 1, pp. i198–i200, 2005.

[119] K. C. Albin, M. I. Carstens, and E. Carstens, "Modulation of oral heat and cold pain by irritant chemicals," *Chemical Senses*, vol. 33, no. 1, pp. 3–15, 2008.

[120] D. A. Stevens and H. T. Lawless, "Putting out the fire: effects of tastants on oral chemical irritation," *Perception & Psychophysics*, vol. 39, no. 5, pp. 346–350, 1986.

[121] C. W. Nasrawi and R. M. Pangborn, "Temporal effectiveness of mouth-rinsing on capsaicin mouth-burn," *Physiology & Behavior*, vol. 47, no. 4, pp. 617–623, 1990.

[122] H. Lawless and D. A. Stevens, "Effects of oral chemical irritation on taste," *Physiology & Behavior*, vol. 32, no. 6, pp. 995–998, 1984.

[123] B. J. Cowart, "Oral chemical irritation: does it reduce perceived taste intensity?" *Chemical Senses*, vol. 12, no. 3, pp. 467–479, 1987.

[124] B. G. Green and M. T. Schullery, "Stimulation of bitterness by capsaicin and menthol: differences between lingual areas innervated by the glossopharyngeal and chorda tympani nerves," *Chemical Senses*, vol. 28, no. 1, pp. 45–55, 2003.

[125] V. Lyall, G. L. Heck, A. K. Vinnikova, S. Ghosh, T.-H. T. Phan, and J. A. DeSimone, "A novel vanilloid receptor-1 (VR-1) variant mammalian salt taste receptor," *Chemical Senses*, vol. 30, supplement 1, pp. i42–i43, 2005.

[126] Y. Treesukosol, V. Lyall, G. L. Heck, J. A. DeSimone, and A. C. Spector, "A psychophysical and electrophysiological analysis of salt taste in *Trpv1* null mice," *American Journal of Physiology—Regulatory Integrative and Comparative Physiology*, vol. 292, no. 5, pp. R1799–R1809, 2007.

[127] C. Ruiz, S. Gutknecht, E. Delay, and S. Kinnamon, "Detection of NaCl and KCl in TRPV1 knockout mice," *Chemical Senses*, vol. 31, no. 9, pp. 813–820, 2006.

[128] Y. W. Moon, J.-H. Lee, S. B. Yoo, and J. W. Jahng, "Capsaicin receptors are colocalized with sweet/bitter receptors in the taste sensing cells of circumvallate papillae," *Genes & Nutrition*, vol. 5, no. 3, pp. 251–255, 2010.

[129] P. Rozin, M. Mark, and D. Schiller, "The role of desensitization to capsaicin in chili pepper ingestion and preference," *Chemical Senses*, vol. 6, no. 1, pp. 23–31, 1981.

[130] H. T. Lawless, C. Hartono, and S. Hernandez, "Thresholds and suprathreshold intensity functions for capsaicin in oil and aqueous based carriers," *Journal of Sensory Studies*, vol. 15, no. 4, pp. 437–447, 2000.

[131] T. Karrer and L. Bartoshuk, "Capsaicin desensitization and recovery on the human tongue," *Physiology & Behavior*, vol. 49, no. 4, pp. 757–764, 1991.

[132] B. G. Green, "Capsaicin sensitization and desensitization on the tongue produced by brief exposures to a low concentration," *Neuroscience Letters*, vol. 107, no. 1–3, pp. 173–178, 1989.

[133] H. Rentmeister-Bryant and B. G. Green, "Perceived irritation during ingestion of capsaicin or piperine: comparison of trigeminal and non-trigeminal areas," *Chemical Senses*, vol. 22, no. 3, pp. 257–266, 1997.

[134] D. J. Schneider, I. Seuss-Baum, and E. Schlich, "Comparison between chemical senses thresholds for capsaicin and dihydrocapsaicin in aqueous solutions and identification of the area of burning sensation," *Advance Journal of Food Science and Technology*, vol. 6, no. 1, pp. 36–41, 2014.

[135] T. P. Heath, J. K. Melichar, D. J. Nutt, and L. F. Donaldson, "Human taste thresholds are modulated by serotonin and noradrenaline," *The Journal of Neuroscience*, vol. 26, no. 49, pp. 12664–12671, 2006.

[136] H. Desai, G. Smutzer, S. E. Coldwell, and J. W. Griffith, "Validation of edible taste strips for identifying PROP taste recognition thresholds," *The Laryngoscope*, vol. 121, no. 6, pp. 1177–1183, 2011.

[137] N. K. Byrnes and J. E. Hayes, "Personality factors predict spicy food liking and intake," *Food Quality and Preference*, vol. 28, no. 1, pp. 213–221, 2013.

[138] P. Rozin, "Acquisition of food preferences and attitudes to food," *International Journal of Obesity*, vol. 4, no. 4, pp. 356–363, 1980.

[139] A. W. Logue and M. E. Smith, "Predictors of food preferences in adult humans," *Appetite*, vol. 7, no. 2, pp. 109–125, 1986.

[140] D. A. Stevens, "Individual differences in taste perception," *Food Chemistry*, vol. 56, no. 3, pp. 303–311, 1996.

[141] B. G. Green, "Temporal characteristics of capsaicin sensitization and desensitization on the tongue," *Physiology & Behavior*, vol. 49, no. 3, pp. 501–505, 1991.

[142] B. G. Green and G. S. Shaffer, "The sensory response to capsaicin during repeated topical exposures: differential effects on sensations of itching and pungency," *Pain*, vol. 53, no. 3, pp. 323–334, 1993.

[143] J.-M. Dessirier, M. O'Mahony, and E. Carstens, "Oral irritant effects of nicotine: psychophysical evidence for decreased sensation following repeated application and lack of cross-desensitization to capsaicin," *Chemical Senses*, vol. 22, no. 5, pp. 483–492, 1997.

[144] J.-M. Dessirier, N. Nguyen, J.-M. Sieffermann, E. Carstens, and M. O'Mahony, "Oral irritant properties of piperine and nicotine: psychophysical evidence for asymmetrical desensitization effects," *Chemical Senses*, vol. 24, no. 4, pp. 405–413, 1999.

[145] J. Prescott, "The generalizability of capsaicin sensitization and desensitization," *Physiology & Behavior*, vol. 66, no. 5, pp. 741–749, 1999.

[146] G. Brand and L. Jacquot, "Sensitization and desensitization to allyl isothiocyanate (mustard oil) in the nasal cavity," *Chemical Senses*, vol. 27, no. 7, pp. 593–598, 2002.

[147] J. Prescott and R. J. Stevenson, "Psychophysical responses to single and multiple presentations of the oral irritant zingerone: relationship to frequency of chili consumption," *Physiology & Behavior*, vol. 60, no. 2, pp. 617–624, 1996.

[148] J. Prescott and R. J. Stevenson, "Desensitization to oral zingerone irritation: effects of stimulus parameters," *Physiology & Behavior*, vol. 60, no. 6, pp. 1473–1480, 1996.

[149] M. A. Cliff and B. G. Green, "Sensory irritation and coolness produced by menthol: evidence for selective desensitization of irritation," *Physiology & Behavior*, vol. 56, no. 5, pp. 1021–1029, 1994.

[150] F. Touska, L. Marsakova, J. Teisinger, and V. Vlachova, "A 'cute' desensitization of TRPV1," *Current Pharmaceutical Biotechnology*, vol. 12, no. 1, pp. 122–129, 2011.

[151] V. Spahn, C. Stein, and C. Zöllner, "Modulation of transient receptor vanilloid 1 activity by transient receptor potential ankyrin 1," *Molecular Pharmacology*, vol. 85, no. 2, pp. 335–344, 2014.

[152] G. M. Story, A. M. Peier, A. J. Reeve et al., "ANKTM1, a TRP-like channel expressed in nociceptive neurons, is activated by cold temperatures," *Cell*, vol. 112, no. 6, pp. 819–829, 2003.

[153] H.-J. Weng, K. N. Patel, N. A. Jeske et al., "Tmem100 is a regulator of TRPA1-TRPV1 complex and contributes to persistent pain," *Neuron*, vol. 85, no. 4, pp. 833–846, 2015.

[154] B. G. Green, "Rapid recovery from capsaicin desensitization during recurrent stimulation," *Pain*, vol. 68, no. 2-3, pp. 245–253, 1996.

[155] X. L. Ma, F. X. Zhang, F. Dong, L. Bao, and X. Zhang, "Experimental evidence for alleviating nociceptive hypersensitivity by single application of capsaicin," *Molecular Pain*, vol. 11, no. 1, pp. 22–31, 2015.

[156] N. Jancsó, A. Jancsó-Gabor, and I. Takats, "Pain and inflammation induced by nicotine, acetylcholine and structurally related compounds and their prevention by desensitizing agents," *Acta Physiologica Hungarica*, vol. 19, pp. 113–132, 1961.

[157] R. J. Stevenson and J. Prescott, "The effects of prior experience with capsaicin on ratings of its burn," *Chemical Senses*, vol. 19, no. 6, pp. 651–656, 1994.

[158] P. Gazerani and L. Arendt-Nielsen, "The impact of ethnic differences in response to capsaicin-induced trigeminal sensitization," *Pain*, vol. 117, no. 1-2, pp. 223–229, 2005.

[159] P. Rozin, "Acquisition of stable food preferences," *Nutrition Reviews*, vol. 48, no. 2, pp. 106–113, 1990.

[160] C. W. Nasrawi and R. M. Pangborn, "Temporal gustatory and salivary responses to capsaicin upon repeated stimulation," *Physiology & Behavior*, vol. 47, no. 4, pp. 611–615, 1990.

[161] B. G. Green, "Capsaicin cross-desensitization on the tongue: psychophysical evidence that oral chemical irritation is mediated by more than one sensory pathway," *Chemical Senses*, vol. 16, no. 6, pp. 675–689, 1991.

[162] B. G. Green and J. E. Hayes, "Capsaicin as a probe of the relationship between bitter taste and chemesthesis," *Physiology & Behavior*, vol. 79, no. 4-5, pp. 811–821, 2003.

[163] P. Holzer, "Capsaicin: cellular targets, mechanisms of action, and selectivity for thin sensory neurons," *Pharmacological Reviews*, vol. 43, no. 2, pp. 143–201, 1991.

[164] R. B. Carter, "Topical capsaicin in the treatment of cutaneous disorders," *Drug Development Research*, vol. 22, no. 2, pp. 109–123, 1991.

[165] A. Astrup, M. Kristensen, N. T. Gregersen et al., "Can bioactive foods affect obesity?" *Annals of the New York Academy of Sciences*, vol. 1190, pp. 25–41, 2010.

[166] L. Vyklický, V. Vlachová, Z. Vitásková, I. Dittert, M. Kabát, and R. K. Orkand, "Temperature coefficient of membrane currents induced by noxious heat in sensory neurones in the rat," *Journal of Physiology*, vol. 517, no. 1, pp. 181–192, 1999.

[167] K. Novakova-Tousova, L. Vyklicky, K. Susankova et al., "Functional changes in the vanilloid receptor subtype 1 channel during and after acute desensitization," *Neuroscience*, vol. 149, no. 1, pp. 144–154, 2007.

[168] A. Szallasi and P. M. Blumberg, "Vanilloid (capsaicin) receptors and mechanisms," *Pharmacological Reviews*, vol. 51, no. 2, pp. 159–212, 1999.

[169] E. Iwaoka, S. Wang, N. Matsuyoshi et al., "Evodiamine suppresses capsaicin-induced thermal hyperalgesia through activation and subsequent desensitization of the transient receptor potential V1 channels," *Journal of Natural Medicines*, vol. 70, no. 1, pp. 1–7, 2016.

[170] J.-M. Dessirier, C. T. Simons, M. Sudo, S. Sudo, and E. Carstens, "Sensitization, desensitization and stimulus-induced recovery of trigeminal neuronal responses to oral capsaicin and nicotine," *Journal of Neurophysiology*, vol. 84, no. 4, pp. 1851–1862, 2000.

[171] B. Liu, C. Zhang, and F. Qin, "Functional recovery from desensitization of vanilloid receptor TRPV1 requires resynthesis of phosphatidylinositol 4,5-bisphosphate," *The Journal of Neuroscience*, vol. 25, no. 19, pp. 4835–4843, 2005.

[172] T. Gevaert, J. Vandepitte, G. Hutchings, J. Vriens, B. Nilius, and D. De Ridder, "TRPV1 is involved in stretch-evoked contractile changes in the rat autonomous bladder model: a study with piperine, a new TRPV1 agonist," *Neurourology and Urodynamics*, vol. 26, no. 3, pp. 440–450, 2007.

[173] H.-Y. Yue, C.-Y. Jiang, T. Fujita, and E. Kumamoto, "Zingerone enhances glutamatergic spontaneous excitatory transmission by activating TRPA1 but not TRPV1 channels in the adult rat substantia gelatinosa," *Journal of Neurophysiology*, vol. 110, no. 3, pp. 658–671, 2013.

[174] B. G. Green and B. L. McAuliffe, "Menthol desensitization of capsaicin irritation: evidence of a short-term anti-nociceptive effect," *Physiology & Behavior*, vol. 68, no. 5, pp. 631–639, 2000.

[175] O. Carreño, R. Corominas, J. Fernández-Morales et al., "SNP variants within the vanilloid *TRPV1* and *TRPV3* receptor genes are associated with migraine in the Spanish population," *American Journal of Medical Genetics, Part B: Neuropsychiatric Genetics*, vol. 159, no. 1, pp. 94–103, 2012.

6

Therapeutic Potential of Dietary Phenolic Acids

Venkata Saibabu,[1] **Zeeshan Fatima,**[1] **Luqman Ahmad Khan,**[2] **and Saif Hameed**[1]

[1]*Amity Institute of Biotechnology, Amity University Haryana, Gurgaon, Manesar 122413, India*
[2]*Department of Biosciences, Jamia Millia Islamia, New Delhi 110025, India*

Correspondence should be addressed to Saif Hameed; saifhameed@yahoo.co.in

Academic Editor: Robert Gogal

Although modern lifestyle has eased the quality of human life, this lifestyle's related patterns have imparted negative effects on health to acquire multiple diseases. Many synthetic drugs are invented during the last millennium but most if not all of them possess several side effects and proved to be costly. Convincing evidences have established the premise that the phytotherapeutic potential of natural compounds and need of search for novel drugs from natural sources are of high priority. Phenolic acids (PAs) are a class of secondary metabolites spread throughout the plant kingdom and generally involved in plethora of cellular processes involved in plant growth and reproduction and also produced as defense mechanism to sustain various environmental stresses. Extensive research on PAs strongly suggests that consumption of these compounds hold promise to offer protection against various ailments in humans. This paper focuses on the naturally derived PAs and summarizes the action mechanisms of these compounds during disease conditions. Based on the available information in the literature, it is suggested that use of PAs as drugs is very promising; however more research and clinical trials are necessary before these bioactive molecules can be made for treatment. Finally this review provides greater awareness of the promise that natural PAs hold for use in the disease prevention and therapy.

1. Introduction

Since ancient times, plants and their products have been used as folk medicine in different parts of the world. It is believed that over 400,000 tropical flowering plant species have healing properties [1]. Several studies on medicinal plants determined the variety of compounds contributing to treatment of life-threatening diseases such as diabetes, cancer, and infections. Numbers of methods have been introduced for qualitative and quantitative analysis of plant secondary metabolites such as polyphenols, alkaloids, saponins, glycosides, resins, oleoresins, sesquiterpene, and lactones. These secondary compounds are involved in plant growth, development, reproduction, and disease resistance. Phenolic acids (PAs) are among the most common bioactive compounds throughout plant kingdom which have role in growth, reproduction, and defense against environmental stress and microorganisms [2, 3]. The antioxidant activities of PAs are extensively implemented in food industry as preservatives since antiquity. They also have function in plethora of important biological activities such as antiageing, reducing the risk of life-threatening diseases such as HIV, diabetes, CVDs, and cancer. Bulk information available about potential health benefits regarding PAs has led to an increased interest in PAs and this review illustrates the role that PAs possess in important biological conditions (Figure 1). A comprehensive literature search was conducted in PubMed and Google Scholar by using the following mesh keywords: (1) phenolic acids, (2) antioxidants, (3) anticancer, (4) cardioprotective, (5) antiulcer, (6) anti-diabetic, (7) antimicrobial, and (8) hepatoprotective. Thus, the aim of the present paper is to systematically review and summarize the literature supporting the health benefits of PAs at a common platform.

2. Phenolic Acids: Classification, Occurrence, and Bioavailability

PAs are aromatic carboxylic acids naturally appearing in the plant kingdom. The term phenolic acid describes a phenol ring that possesses at least one carboxylic acid functionality.

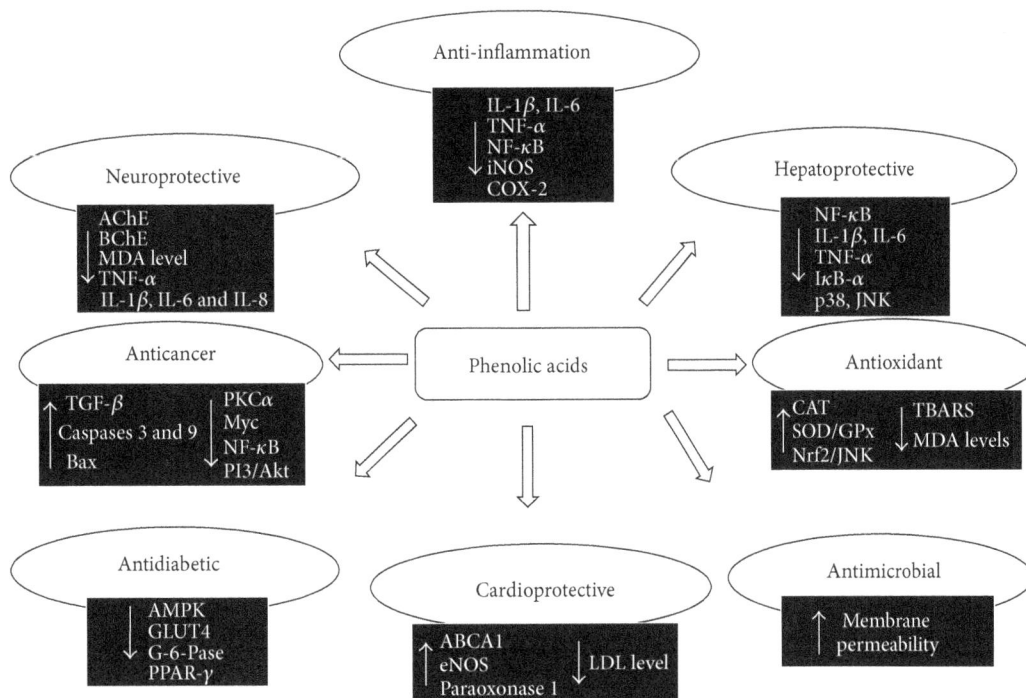

FIGURE 1: Key factors involved in health beneficial effects of natural PAs.

However, in case of plant metabolites, these refer to a distinct group of organic acids which contains two distinguishing carbon frameworks, hydroxybenzoic and hydroxycinnamic acid structures. PAs are usually subclassified into benzoic acids containing seven carbon atoms (C6-C1) and cinnamic acids with nine carbon atoms (C6-C3).

PAs are widely distributed in the plant kingdom and found in a wide variety of nuts and fruits, such as raspberries, grapes, strawberries, walnuts, cranberries, and black currants. These are secondary metabolites derived from pheny-lalanine and tyrosine via shikimate/chorismate pathway. However, these compounds exist predominantly as hydrox-ybenzoic acids which include gallic acid (GA), salicylic acid (SA), protocatechuic acid (PCA), ellagic acid (EA), and gentisic acid (GeA) and hydroxycinnamic acids which include p-coumaric acid (p-CA), caffeic acid (CA), ferulic acid (FA), chlorogenic acid (CGA), and sinapic acids (SA) or alternatively may occur as conjugated forms (Figure 2).

The chemical properties of PAs in terms of availability of the phenolic hydroxyl groups predict their activity *in vitro*. The effective *in vivo* potential of PAs depends on multiple factors such as quantity of the compound ingested, absorbed, and/or metabolized, plasma and/or tissue concentrations, type and amount of single PA, and synergistic effects. However, the chemical structure of phenolic compounds differently affects all the factors described above. For instance, sulfate derivatives of FA and CA showed lower activities when compared with the antioxidant activities of the parental phenolic acids indicating the importance of the phenolic acids and their metabolites [4].

3. Antioxidant Properties

Biological system generates reactive oxygen species (ROS) as the byproduct of various metabolic activities and mitochondria are said to be major site responsible for ROS production. These free radicals are highly unstable or reactive and can cause direct damage to cell components such as nucleic acids, lipids, and proteins [5]. ROS is the major contributor to many diseases which include CVDs, cancer, age-related decline in the immune system, and degenerative diseases such as Parkinson's and Alzheimer's disease. Human body possesses several stress response enzymes including superoxide dismutase (SOD) and catalase (CAT) to counteract radical-induced damage. PAs counteract both ROS and RNS-induced cell damage by their direct free radical scavenging activity as well as the upregulation of the HO/BVR system, superoxide dismutase (SOD), and catalase (CAT) whose final aim is to detoxify ROS and RNS.

Oxidative stress has been implicated in the pathogenesis of multiple cardiovascular complications. Antioxidant role of FA in cardioprotection is well studied [6]. In hypersensitive rats, treatment with FA for 4–12 weeks increased SOD and CAT activities. FA treatment also increased SOD and CAT levels in myocardium and pancreatic tissue of streptozotocin-induced diabetic rats in dose and time dependent manner [7].

Antioxidant activities of PCA along with known antioxidant Trolox were measured *in vitro* using various antioxidant assays including 1,1-diphenyl-2-picrylhydrazyl (DPPH$^{\bullet}$), 2,2'-azino-bis(3-ethylbenzthiazoline-6-sulfonic acid) (ABTS$^{+\bullet}$), superoxide anion radicals (O$_2^{-\bullet}$) and hydroxyl

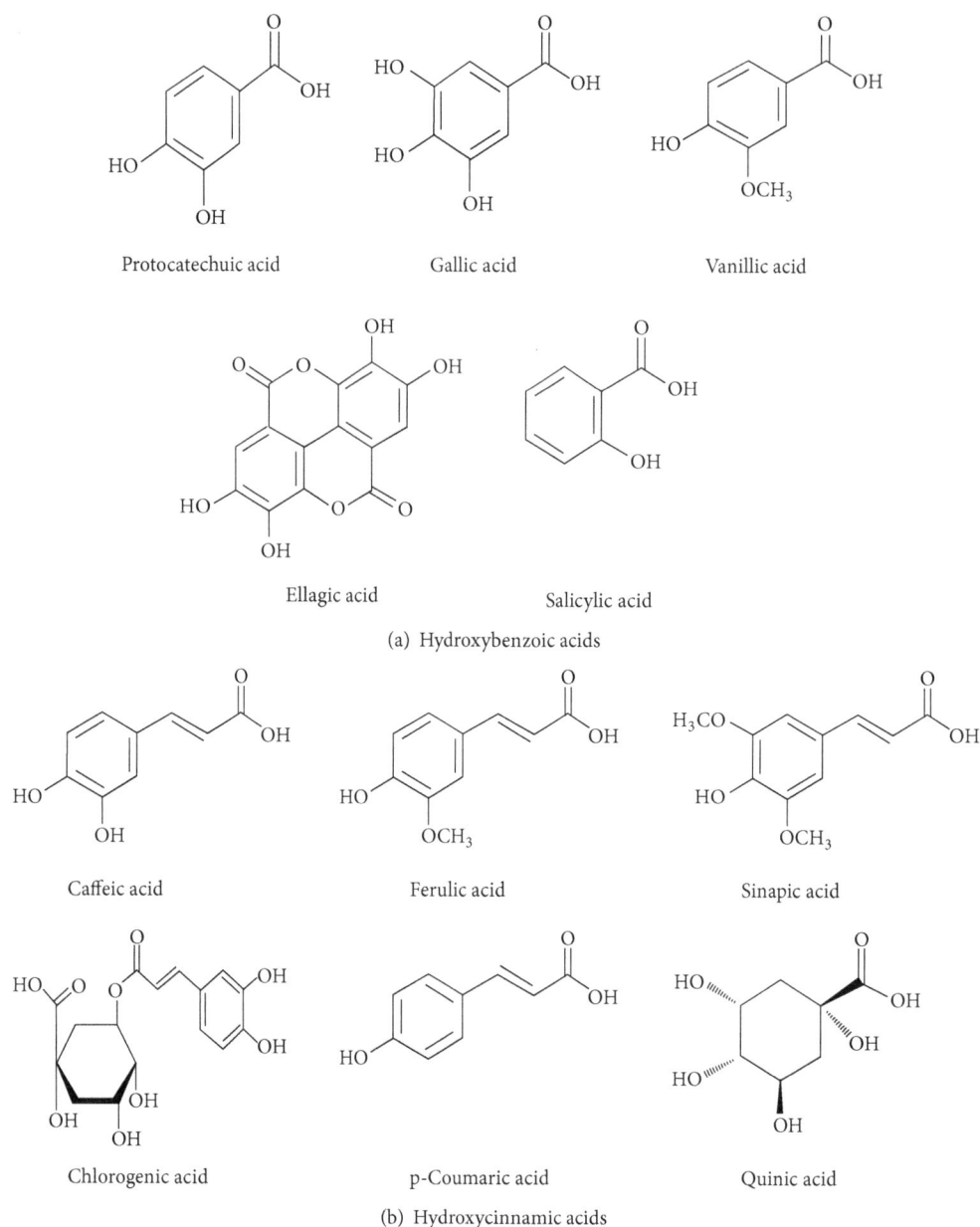

Protocatechuic acid

Gallic acid

Vanillic acid

Ellagic acid

Salicylic acid

(a) Hydroxybenzoic acids

Caffeic acid

Ferulic acid

Sinapic acid

Chlorogenic acid

p-Coumaric acid

Quinic acid

(b) Hydroxycinnamic acids

FIGURE 2: Structural classification of natural PAs discussed in the review.

radical (•OH) scavenging activity, ferric ions (Fe^{3+}) and cupric ions (Cu^{2+}) reducing power, ferrous ions (Fe^{2+}), and cupric ions (Cu^{2+}) chelating activity. The antioxidant activity of PCA could be attributed to both its transition metal ions chelation and by free radicals scavenging via donating hydrogen atom (H•) or electron [8].

Oral administration of vanillic acid (VA) at high doses (100 mg/kg) increased the antioxidant status by reducing lipid peroxidation and increased the SOD, CAT, and glutathione peroxidase (GPx) activities and reduced glutathione (GSH) levels in cisplatin induced nephrotoxicity in albino rats [9]. Similarly, GA consumption diminished this harmful effect via its antioxidant action by inhibiting the initiation and/or propagation of the lipid peroxidation [10]. In the later studies

same group investigated the antioxidant properties of GA derived from *Peltiphyllum peltatum* against sodium fluoride (NaF-) induced hepatotoxicity in rats [11]. Pretreatment of animals with GA could mitigate the NaF-induced hepatotoxicity through suppression of lipid peroxidation expressed in reduced Thiobarbituric Acid Reactive Substances (TBARS) levels, restoration of GPx levels, CAT, and SOD corroborating its antioxidative role.

Antioxidant properties of PAs depend on not only their direct activity as a scavenger but also their capacity to strengthen the endogenous antioxidant defenses. Nuclear factor erythroid 2- (NFE2-) related factor 2 (Nrf2) is a key transcription factor which strictly regulates the antioxidant/ detoxifying enzyme genes by antioxidant response elements, present in the promoter region of those genes [12]. PAs such as PCA have been demonstrated to induce the ARE-dependent antioxidant/detoxifying phase II enzymes such as GR and GPx by activating the transcription factor Nrf2 through JNK-mediated phosphorylation [13]. Similarly, PCA induces anti-apoptotic mechanism that likely related to the activation of the JNK-mediated survival signals that strengthen the cellular antioxidant defenses rather than antioxidant power of PCA. PAs induce phase II hepatic antioxidant enzyme and increase the antioxidant status of liver [14]. PAs including GEA, GA, p-CA, and FA selectively induce hepatic mRNA transcripts for CuZnSOD, GPx, and catalase likely through upregulation of gene transcription as well as the Nrf2 transcription factor indicating their potential antioxidant role in liver [15].

4. Antiulcer Activity

Gastric ulcer is a recurrent chronic illness caused by both endogenous and exogenous factors which include pepsin, stress, and noxious factors such as nonsteroidal anti-inflammatory drugs, *Helicobacter pylori* bacteria, smoking, and alcohol consumption [16]. Natural PAs have been investigated for their antiulcer activities which are apparent from wide ranges of studies in experimental animals. GA has been reported to be antiulcer in aspirin plus pylorus ligation model. GA exerts this effect by improving mucosal defensive with activation of antioxidant parameters and inhibition of some toxic oxidant parameters. Similarly, GA in combination with famotidine, an antiulcer drug, synergistically protected the experimentally induced peptic ulcer models [17]. Animals treated with low dose combinations like GA (50 mg/kg) + FM (10 mg/kg) along with high dose GA (100 mg/kg) + FM (10 mg/kg) showed significant ulcer protective effect induced by aspirin plus pylorus ligation.

Gastroprotective properties of another phenolic acid, EA, have also been reported. EA are well documented in acute and chronic ulcer rat models [18]. The gastroprotective properties of EA are partly due to increased endogenous production of nitric oxide which is an antioxidant effect by replenishing non-protein-sulfhydryls and attenuation of TNF-α, whereas in indomethacin ulcer, gastroprotective properties are partly due to attenuation of elevated levels of TNF-α, interferon-γ, and interleukins 4 and 6.

5. Antidiabetic Activity

Impairment in glucose metabolism leads to physiological imbalance with the onset of the hyperglycemia and subsequently diabetes mellitus which can be either type 1 or type 2. It is well known that several physiological parameters of the body get altered in the diabetic conditions. Long term effects of diabetes may cause development of specific complications such as retinopathy, nephropathy, neuropathy, foot ulcers, sexual dysfunctions, and cardiovascular complications.

Insulin stimulates glucose transport by inducing the translocation of glucose transporter 4 (GLUT4) to the plasma membrane which is mediated by two major pathways, an insulin independent AMPK pathway and an insulin dependent PI3K pathway. The antidiabetic effects of natural PAs

are well documented as evident from wide range of studies. CGA could enhance the glucose uptake in L6 myotubes via increasing expression of GLUT4 and PPAR-γ transcript [19]. Similarly, PCA also exerts its insulin-like activity in human omental adipocytes. PCA induces the glucose uptake associated with enhanced GLUT4 translocation and increased PPARg transcript [20]. GA derived from *sea buckthorn* leaf extract stimulated GLUT4 translocation and glucose transport in a concentration dependent manner with maximum stimulation at 10 μM concentration [21]. Further, the role of atypical protein kinase Cf/k is revealed in GA mediated GLUT4 translocation and glucose uptake.

Similarly, CGA stimulates glucose transport in both skeletal muscle isolated from mice and L6 skeletal muscle cells [22]. Furthermore, in L6 myotubes, CGA increased glucose transport via GLUT4 transporter and in skeletal muscle via the activation of AMPK. CGA lowered AUC glucose, inhibited hepatic glucose-6-phosphatase (G-6-Pase) expression, and improved skeletal muscle glucose uptake and lipid profiles, in Lepr$^{db/db}$ mice. Mechanistically, CGA activated AMPK leading to suppression of hepatic glucose production and fatty acid biosynthesis. Inhibition and knockdown of AMPK abrogating these metabolic alterations suggested that CGA can improve glucose and lipid metabolism via the activation of AMPK. Another phenolic acid p-CA modulated glucose and lipid metabolism via AMPK activation in L6 skeletal muscle cells [23]. p-CA also promoted fatty acid β-oxidation, decreased oleic acid-induced triglyceride accumulation, and enhanced glucose uptake proving its beneficial effects in improving or treating metabolic disorders.

6. Cardioprotective Activity

Cardiac disease is the major cause of morbidity and mortality among the noncommunicable diseases. Implication of cardiovascular complications including cardiomyopathy in diabetes can be attributed to hyperlipidemia, hyperglycemia, and oxidative stress which promote atherosclerosis [24–26]. Cardiovascular complications are higher in diabetic patients than nondiabetics [27]. Cardioprotective role of the two phenolic acids caffeic acid (CA) and ellagic acid (EA) has been reported in STZ-induced diabetic mice. Treatment with CA or EA markedly elevated the insulin secretion, which might attenuate the dyslipidemia, improved glycemic control, and diminished cardiac oxidative stress [28].

Atherosclerosis is a chronic inflammatory disease characterized by accumulation of leukocytes in the vascular wall. Platelets play essential role in formation of atherosclerotic plaques and thrombosis by coaggregating with leukocytes via P-selectin glycoprotein ligand-1 (PSGL-1) and P-selectin interactions [29, 30]. GA has been found to possess antiatherosclerotic activity by inhibiting platelet activation and its association with leukocytes, P-selectin expression stimulated by ADP which is likely to be through decreasing intracellular Ca^{2+} mobilization via regulating the signals of PKCα/p38MAPK and Akt/GSK3β [31]. Protocatechuic aldehyde (structurally similar to PCA) isolated from root of *Salvia miltiorrhiza* attenuated PDGF-induced proliferation and migration of VSMCs via (PI3K)/Akt and MAPK kinase pathways which regulate key enzymes associated with migration and proliferation of VSMCs [32]. It is reported that FA effectively reduced copper ion induced LDL oxidation and facilitated the uptake and degradation of cholesterol in the liver. p-CA is known to protect the LDL from ROS by scavenging ˙OH *in vivo* and thereby reduce lipid peroxidation and serum LDL cholesterol levels [33].

Cardioprotective activities of EA have also been investigated. EA effectively reduces oxidative stress, lowers the levels of plasma lipids, and inhibits lipid peroxidation. EA reduced the uptake of oxidized LDL in murine macrophages by downregulating membrane expression of SR-B1 [34]. SR-B1 is a membrane receptor on macrophages responsible for the internalization of oxidized LDL that promotes cellular accumulation of cholesterol [35]. Similarly, EA also promotes cholesterol efflux in lipid-loaded macrophages by inducing membrane receptor ABCA1 expression. ABCA1 is a membrane transporter abundant in macrophages and plays a crucial role in cholesterol homeostasis, thereby protecting against atherosclerosis [36]. Salicylic acid (SA) treatment has been reported to prevent complications of atherosclerotic cardiovascular disease such as myocardial infarction and occlusive stroke [37]. These effects of SA are attributed to its platelet-inhibitory function and stimulation of Paraoxonase 1, an enzyme that protects the serum lipids from oxidation and can reduce macrophage foam cell formation and attenuates atherosclerosis development [38].

Hypertension is the most common cardiovascular disorder mainly affected by lifestyle and dietary habits [39]. Nitric oxide (NO) plays a key role in the physiologic control of blood pressure and myocardial injury. Alterations in NO synthesis or bioavailability can cause vasoconstriction and might be involved in the pathogenesis of hypertension. VA has been proven to act against cardiovascular complications aroused due to hypertension [40]. VA normalized hypertension and left ventricular function in Nω-nitro-L-arginine methyl ester (L-NAME) induced hypertensive rat models. L-NAME is NO synthase inhibitor which causes reduction in its activity, leading to hypertension and arteriosclerosis [41–43]. Vanillic acid (VA) possessed cardioprotective effect, which is evident by lowered cardiac marker enzymes (CK, CK-MB, and LDH), left ventricular functions, improved tissue nitric oxide metabolite levels, and upregulated mRNA expression of eNOS in L-NAME induced hypertensive rat.

7. Anticancer Activity

Cancer is one of the leading causes of the deaths worldwide and chemotherapy is mainly used to treat cancer. However, occurrence of severe side effects of the drugs led to search for alternatives. Phytochemicals exert their anticancer activities by protecting critical cellular components (DNA, proteins, and lipids) from oxidative insult and interfere with proliferative activity and induction of apoptosis of cancer cells. Epidemiological and experimental studies confirmed that consumption of dietary products such as fruits and vegetables may have significant impact on the development of different types of cancers. EA is proven to be capable of decreasing oxidative stress, a hallmark of developing cancer.

EA downregulates the expression and activity of PKCα in lymphoma bearing mice via decreasing the oxidative stress as evident by reduced lipid peroxidation and protein carbonylation [44]. Similarly, EA downregulates the expression of oncogene Myc and upregulates tumor suppressor gene TGF-β in lymphoma bearing mice. EA also exerts apoptosis through targeting PI3K/Akt kinases that in turn resulted in attenuation of its downstream Bcl-2 family proteins in 1,2-dimethyl hydrazine- (DMH-) induced rat colon carcinogenesis [45]. EA could stimulate the apoptosis by decreasing NF-κB activity, thus activating the mitochondrial death pathway associated with caspase 3 activation and cytochrome C release [46]. Additionally EA also lowers the expression of cyclins against inflammation mediated cell proliferation by downregulation of NF-κB in EA-administered rats. Induction of apoptosis features were observed in prostate cancer using the transgenic rat for adenocarcinoma of prostate (TRAP) model and human prostate cancer cell line (LNCaP). These findings showed that EA inhibits the early stage of prostate carcinogenesis through induction of apoptosis via activation of caspase 3 [47]. Similarly inactivation of phosphatidyl inositol 3-kinase (PI3K)/Akt pathway, Bcl-2 downregulation and increased expression of Bax, caspase 3, and cytochrome c, increased annexin V apoptotic cells, and DNA fragmentation were observed in human adenocarcinoma cells [46]. Cytotoxic effects of EA have been reported in TSGH8301 [48]. Cells treated with EA resulted in arresting cell cycle at G0/G1, promoted ROS and Ca²⁺ production, activities of caspases 9 and 3, and decreased the level of ΔΨm. EA and Embelin isolated from *Ardisia japonica* at low concentrations synergistically increased the apoptosis thereby decreasing the proliferation *in vitro*. Similarly, EA alone or in combination with Embelin alone decreased tumor size and tumor cellularity in a subcutaneous xenograft mouse model of pancreatic cancer.

Angiogenesis is a critical process in tumor development and metastasis. PAs have been showed to inhibit the angiogenesis in various cancer cell lines and *in vivo*. Caffeic acid phenethyl ester (CAPE), a major medicinal component of propolis, showed dose dependent VEGF secretion in MDA-231 cells and formation of capillary-like tubes by endothelial cells, implicate on antiangiogenesis [49]. Antiangiogenic actions of p-CA have been studied in the ECV304 human endothelial cell line. p-CA reduced the mRNA levels of two important angiogenic factors VEGF and bFGF that stimulate permeability, proliferation, and tube formation of endothelial cells [50].

Tumor metastasis is a complex cascade that is accompanied by metalloproteinase (MMP) upregulation and extracellular matrix degradation. Metastasis allows cancer cells to proliferate and invade blood or lymphatic system, further enhancing cancer cell invasion and worsening prognosis. Pomegranate juice (*Punica granatum*) and its three constituents luteolin, ellagic acid, and punicic acid (L + EA + P) have been shown to interfere with multiple biological processes such as suppression of cell growth, increased cell adhesion, inhibition of cell migration, and inhibition of chemotaxis towards proteins (SDF1α) involved in breast cancer metastasis [51]. Similarly, L + EA + P exhibited beneficial effect on metastasis of prostate cancer in SCID mouse tumor model and $Pten^{-/-}$, $K\text{-}rasG^{12D}$ prostate tumors. Studies were conducted by injecting luciferase-expressing human PCa cells in the region of the prostate ectopically and monitored the tumor progression with bioluminescence imaging weekly. Results revealed that L + E + P inhibit PC-3M-luc primary tumor growth and suppress the CXCL12/CXCR4, implicated as therapeutic target for metastasis [52]. Further, L + E + P significantly inhibited the growth and metastasis *in vivo*. GA is known to inhibit metastasis and invasive growth of gastric cancer cells via increased expression of RhoB, downregulation of AKT/small GTPase signals, and inhibition of NF-κB activity [53].

8. Anti-Inflammatory Activity

Inflammation is the complex biological process of vascular tissues to harmful stimuli, such as pathogens, chemical irritants, and damaged cells or tissue. It is a protective attempt by the organism in which immune system plays a major role. Inflammatory response includes (1) migration of immune cells from blood vessels and release of mediators at the site of damage followed by (2) recruitment of inflammatory cells, (3) release of ROS, RNS, and proinflammatory cytokines to eliminate foreign pathogens, and (4) repairing injured tissues. Though acute inflammation is rapid and self-limiting, prolonged inflammation causes various chronic disorders [54]. The link between chronic inflammation and various diseases such as cancer, metabolic disorder, type II diabetes, arthritis, autoimmune diseases, neurological diseases, pulmonary diseases, and cardiovascular complications is well known. Among other natural bioactive compounds, PAs are widely recognized for their anti-inflammatory properties in wide range disease conditions.

Platelets are key mediators of inflammation that may trigger an inflammatory response in vessel wall early in the development of atherosclerosis and contribute to the destabilization of advanced atherosclerotic lesions [55]. CGA possesses antiplatelet activity by reducing release of atherosclerotic-related inflammatory mediators (sP-selectin, IL-1β, sCD40L, and CCL5) and inhibits *in vivo* thrombus formation [56]. In addition, antiplatelet and antithrombotic effects shown by CGA are associated with A$_{2A}$ receptor activation. Similarly, CGA induced an anti-inflammatory effect in lipopolysaccharide- (LPS-) inflamed murine RAW 264.7 macrophage cells through (1) suppression of proinflammatory cytokines such as IL-1β, TNF-α, and IL-6, as well as the chemokine CXCL1 through downregulation of NF-κB; (2) decreased NO production mediated by downregulation of iNOS; and (3) inhibition of an important adhesion molecule Ninjurin 1 (Ninj 1) [57]. CA attenuated LPS-induced NO production possibly by inhibiting phosphorylation of p38MAPK and JNK1/2, suggesting that CA selectively inhibit different LPS-induced proinflammatory signaling cascades in RAW 264.7 macrophages [58]. Further, CGA showed antiosteoarthritis (anti-OA) properties in IL-1β-stimulated chondrocytes [54]. CGA suppressed the production of NO and PGE2 via downregulating the expression of iNOS and COX-2 which are implicated in the pathogenesis of OA

[59]. In another study, CGA leads to attenuation in TLR4-mediated inflammatory responses such as NO and PGE2 production in LPS-treated RAW 264.7 cells and improves HCl/EtOH-induced acute gastritis symptoms [60].

9. Neuroprotective Activity

Neuroprotection means prevention of nerve cells from dying and usually involves an intervention of drug treatment. It is a mechanism used to protect neuronal injury or degeneration of CNS following acute disorders. The goal of neuroprotection is to limit neuronal dysfunction after injury and attempt to maintain the possible integrity of cellular interactions in the brain resulting in undisturbed neural function. There are wide ranges of natural compounds from plants and in particular PAs have been the focus of research. These compounds may act as free radical scavengers, antiexcitotoxic agents, apoptosis inhibitors, and so forth. Two hydroxycinnamic acids CGA and CA have been shown to be associated with anti-Alzheimer's properties [61]. Mechanistically, these properties could be attributed to inhibition of BChE and AChE activities; thus butyrylcholine breaks down and slows down acetylcholine *in vitro*. Furthermore, CGA and CA decrease the malondialdehyde (MDA) formed due to prooxidants such as FeSO$_4$, sodium nitroprusside, and quinolinic acid. Recent studies demonstrated the novel evidence explaining the neurological effects of CGA. Voltage gated potassium channels (Kv) play crucial role in the electrophysiological processes of sensory neurons and have been identified as potential therapeutic targets for inflammation and neuropathic pain disorders. The effects of CGA on the two main subtypes of Kv in trigeminal ganglion (TG) neurons, namely, the IK,V and IK,A channels, are also highlighted [62]. Upon CGA treatment, activation and inactivation currents of both IK,V and IK,A were significantly shifted toward depolarization, which implies that Kv is triggered at a lower threshold with a prolonged duration thus enhancing Kv activities in both IK,A and IK,V channels. This would gradually decrease the excitability of neurons during trigeminal hyperalgesic conditions in neuropathic and inflammatory pain.

Functional restoration of injured spinal cord by self-assembled nanoparticles composed of FA modified glycol chitosan (FA-GC) has been investigated to a considerable extent [63]. These nanoparticles protected primary neurons from glutamate-induced excitotoxicity *in vitro*. In addition, significant recovery in locomotor function was observed in a spinal cord contusion injury rat model that was intravenously administered FA-GC nanoparticles at 2 h after injury. Further, histological analysis revealed that FA-GC treatment significantly preserved axons and myelin and also reduced cavity volume, inflammatory response, and astrogliosis at the lesion site.

The accumulation of Aβ deposit owing to the metabolic disorders in the brain is key step in the pathogenesis of Alzheimer's disease (AD). Aβ can stimulate chronic neuroinflammation response and worsen the neurological degradation. Two genes, namely, presenilins 1 and 2 (PS1 and PS2) genes, or the amyloid-protein precursor (APP) plays an important role in the processing of Aβ. PCA derived from

Radix Salviae Miltiorrhizae has been found to have a protective effect on improving cognitive deficits in STZ-induced AD rats [64]. The Morris water maze test revealed that PCA (100 mg/kg) significantly prolonged the mean latency time and the path length of AβPP/PS1 mice. PCA reduced the number of Aβ positive expressions in the hippocampus and cerebral cortex of AβPP/PS1 mice by immunocytochemical assay with Congo red staining and decreased remarkably APP expression levels by western blot analysis. In addition, PCA improves the cognitive deficits of AD animal by decreasing the levels of inflammatory cytokines including TNF-α, IL-1β, IL-6, and IL-8.

10. Hepatoprotective Activity

Liver diseases are a major health problem which causes high mortality and morbidity affecting the human of all ages. Liver diseases are classified as autoimmune hepatitis, alcoholic liver disease, and viral hepatitis. Despite advances in modern medicine, still there is lack of effective drug that completely cures liver complications. Therefore, there is urgent need for search of effective drugs to replace current drugs. Natural PAs are undoubtedly valuable as a source of new medicinal agents. Hepatoprotective effect of EA in concanavalin A- (Con A-) induced hepatitis mice model has been evaluated [65]. Pretreatment with EA significantly decreased the expression levels of the toll-like receptor 4 (TLR4) and TLR2 implicated in hepatitis possibly by inflammation. Further, EA decreased the expression of inflammatory cytokines and in turn inhibit the phosphorylation of MAPK and nuclear translocation of NF-κB. This may account for a reduction in TNF-α, IL-6, and IL-1β expression by inhibition of NF-κB-mediated transcriptional activation and IκB-α degradation and prevention of JNK, p38, and ERK MAPK phosphorylation.

Resistin is a hormone implicated in enhanced hepatic steatosis via downregulation of content and activities of mitochondria [38]. EA reduced serum resistin levels and improved hepatic steatosis and serum lipid profile in high-fat fed obese diabetic KK-Ay mice [66]. EA supplementation also improved hepatic steatosis by reducing triglycerides, which play key role in liver steatosis and ameliorated serum HDLC and non-HDLC levels which might be caused by reduced serum resistin levels. Moreover, EA upregulated mRNA levels of PPARa and its target genes including cpt1a suggesting that EA acts as transcriptional activator of PPARa in the liver.

11. Antiaging Activity

Aging is the accumulation of changes over time associated with increasing susceptibility to different diseases and ultimately leading to death. Several hypotheses have been proposed to explain how aging occurs. However, many evidences led to the general acceptance of the oxidative stress theory that the accumulation of molecular damage caused by reactive oxygen species is a major factor in aging. PCA derived from dried fruits of *Alpinia oxyphylla* Miq. showed strong ability to attenuate ageing alterations of antioxidative defense systems in spleen and liver male Sprague-Dawley rats [67]. Intraperitoneal injection of PCA showed

effects on splenic weight, antioxidant enzyme activities, and MDA levels in spleen and liver of rats. PCA isolated from *Veronica peregrine* exhibited significant antiaging effects on *Caenorhabditis elegans* model system [68]. In the presence of PCA, lifespan of the wild-type worms increased in a dose dependent manner. PCA also improved tolerance of worms against heat shock and osmotic and oxidative stress which might result in extension of lifespan. Pharyngeal pumping rate and progeny production are the two factors evidenced for prolonged lifespan and improved longevity. Interestingly, both factors were significantly reduced after PCA exposure. In addition, PCA-treated aged worms showed improved body movement compared to untreated controls suggesting PCA could enhance health span as well as lifespan.

12. Antimicrobial Activity

Illnesses resulting from pathogens and the emergence of resistance to conventional antibiotics are vital concern in public health and demand new antimicrobial compounds [69, 70]. Plants do not possess immune system like animals but instead synthesize phenolic compounds in response to the presence of pathogens, herbivores, and insects [71]. Research on natural products has demonstrated significant progress in the discovery of novel compounds with antimicrobial activity [72–74].

The antibacterial activities of PAs have been demonstrated in various studies on different pathogens. *Veronica montana* L. water extract and its main phenolic constituent, PCA, showed being highly effective against the growth of *Listeria monocytogenes* which causes listeriosis, which occurs mostly in elderly people, immune-compromised patients, and pregnant women [75, 76]. The mechanism of action of PCA towards *L. monocytogenes* appears to be alteration of permeability of bacterial cytoplasmic membrane. Antibacterial activity and mode of action of two phenolic acids have been investigated on *E. coli*, *P. aeruginosa*, *S. aureus*, and *L. monocytogenes*. It was found that FA and GA had antimicrobial activity against the bacteria tested with MIC of 500 mg/mL for *P. aeruginosa*; 1500 mg/mL for *E. coli*; 1750 mg/mL for *S. aureus*; and 2000 mg/mL for *L. monocytogenes* with GA. Similarly, FA showed the antimicrobial activity with MIC of 100 mg/mL for *E. coli* and *P. aeruginosa* and 1100 mg/mL and 1250 mg/mL for *S. aureus* and *L. monocytogenes*, respectively. CGA has been shown to have potent antibacterial and antibiofilm properties against emerging nosocomial pathogen *S. maltophilia*. The minimum inhibitory concentration was shown to be 8 to 16 μg mL^{-1} and dose-dependently reduced the adhesion of *S. maltophilia* to polystyrene plate. Influence of subinhibitory concentrations of CGA on virulence associated factors of enterotoxigenic *S. aureus* has been investigated [77]. At subinhibitory concentrations (1.25 mg/mL), CGA significantly inhibited the hemolysis and coagulase titter. Reduced binding to fibrinogen and decreased production of SEA (an enterotoxin) were observed at concentrations ranging from 1/16MIC to 1/2MIC. Finally, CA markedly inhibited the expression of sea, hla, and agr genes in *S. aureus* [78].

13. Conclusion

The new lifestyles adopted by people have considerably enhanced the risk of acquiring various diseases. Extensive research on natural PAs provides new insight into the comprehension of the cellular and molecular mechanisms responsible for the immense potential therapeutic activity of these compounds against a number of human diseases. However, evidence of such properties has been collected from cellular and animal models, while clinical studies are still lacking. It is worth mentioning that further studies and clinical trials are needed to fully establish the preventive and therapeutic effectiveness of PAs and also to prove their safety for human consumption. Moreover, natural PAs also have the potential to drive the flux of funds to the corporate sector for investment in drug development which eventually may influence the quality of life for many patients. Certainly more intricate molecular mechanisms need to be investigated to further enhance their widespread usage and pharmaceutical potential.

Conflict of Interests

The authors declare that they have no conflict of interests.

Authors' Contribution

Venkata Saibabu and Zeeshan Fatima had equal contribution.

Acknowledgments

Saif Hameed thanks Science and Engineering Research Board (SERB), New Delhi (SR/FT/LS-12/2012), for Young Scientist award. The authors thank Professor Rajendra Prasad, Director of Amity Institute of Biotechnology, for encouragement.

References

[1] T. Odugbemi, "Medicinal plants as antimicrobials," in *Outline and Pictures of Medicinal Plants from Nigeria*, pp. 53–64, University of Lagos Press, 2006.

[2] I. K. Valentine, V. K. Maria, and B. Bruno, "Phenolic cycle in plants and environment," *Journal of Cell & Molecular Biology*, vol. 2, no. 1, pp. 13–18, 2003.

[3] A. A. Elzaawely, T. D. Xuan, and S. Tawata, "Essential oils, kava pyrones and phenolic compounds from leaves and rhizomes of *Alpinia zerumbet* and their antioxidant activity," *Food Chememistry*, vol. 103, no. 2, pp. 486–494, 2007.

[4] A. Piazzon, U. Vrhovsek, D. Masuero, F. Mattivi, F. Mandoj, and M. Nardini, "Antioxidant activity of phenolic acids and their metabolites: synthesis and antioxidant properties of the sulfate derivatives of ferulic and caffeic acids and of the acyl glucuronide of ferulic acid," *Journal of Agricultural and Food Chemistry*, vol. 60, no. 50, pp. 12312–12323, 2012.

[5] A. Cherubini, C. Ruggiero, M. C. Polidori, and P. Mecocci, "Potential markers of oxidative stress in stroke," *Free Radical Biology and Medicine*, vol. 39, no. 7, pp. 841–852, 2005.

[6] S. Roy, S. K. Metya, S. Sannigrahi, N. Rahaman, and F. Ahmed, "Treatment with ferulic acid to rats with streptozotocin-induced diabetes: effects on oxidative stress, pro-inflammatory cytokines, and apoptosis in the pancreatic β cell," *Endocrine*, vol. 44, no. 2, pp. 369–379, 2013.

[7] M. A. Alam, C. Sernia, and L. Brown, "Ferulic acid improves cardiovascular and kidney structure and function in hypertensive rats," *Journal of Cardiovascular Pharmacology*, vol. 61, no. 3, pp. 240–249, 2013.

[8] X. Li, X. Wang, D. Chen, and S. Chen, "Antioxidant activity and mechanism of protocatechuic acid *in vitro*," *Functtional Food in Health and Disease*, vol. 7, pp. 232–244, 2011.

[9] G. Sindhu, E. Nishanthi, and R. Sharmila, "Nephroprotective effect of vanillic acid against cisplatin induced nephrotoxicity in wistar rats: a biochemical and molecular study," *Environmental Toxicology and Pharmacology*, vol. 39, no. 1, pp. 392–404, 2015.

[10] S. M. Nabavi, S. Habtemariam, S. F. Nabavi et al., "Protective effect of gallic acid isolated from *Peltiphyllum peltatum* against sodium fluoride-induced oxidative stress in rat's kidney," *Molecular and Cellular Biochemistry*, vol. 372, no. 1-2, pp. 233–239, 2013.

[11] S. F. Nabavi, S. Habtemariam, A. Sureda, A. Hajizadeh Moghaddam, M. Daglia, and S. M. Nabavi, "In vivo protective effects of gallic acid isolated from peltiphyllum peltatum against sodium fluoride-induced oxidative stress in rat erythrocytes," *Arhives of Industrial Hygiene and Toxicolog*, vol. 64, no. 4, pp. 553–559, 2013.

[12] W. W. Wasserman and W. E. Fahl, "Functional antioxidant responsive elements," *Proceedings of the National Academy of Sciences of the United States of America*, vol. 94, no. 10, pp. 5361–5366, 1997.

[13] R. Vari, M. D'Archivio, C. Filesi et al., "Protocatechuic acid induces antioxidant/detoxifying enzyme expression through JNK-mediated Nrf2 activation in murine macrophages," *Journal of Nutritional Biochemistry*, vol. 22, no. 5, pp. 409–417, 2011.

[14] R. Vari, B. Scazzocchio, C. Santangelo et al., "Protocatechuic acid prevents oxLDL-induced apoptosis by activating JNK/Nrf2 survival signals in macrophages," *Oxidative Medicine and Cellular Longevity*, vol. 2015, Article ID 351827, 11 pages, 2015.

[15] C.-T. Yeh and G.-C. Yen, "Induction of hepatic antioxidant enzymes by phenolic acids in rats is accompanied by increased levels of multidrug resistance-associated protein 3 mRNA expression," *Journal of Nutrition*, vol. 136, no. 1, pp. 11–15, 2006.

[16] A. F. Syam, M. Sadikin, S. I. Wanandi, and A. A. Rani, "Molecular mechanism on healing process of peptic ulcer," *Acta Medica Indonesiana*, vol. 41, no. 2, pp. 95–98, 2009.

[17] K. Asokkumar, S. Sen, M. Umamaheswari, A. T. Sivashanmugam, and V. Subhadradevi, "Synergistic effect of the combination of gallic acid and famotidine in protection of rat gastric mucosa," *Pharmacological Reports*, vol. 66, no. 4, pp. 594–599, 2014.

[18] A. M. S. E. S. Beserra, P. I. Calegari, M. D. C. Souza et al., "Gastroprotective and ulcer-healing mechanisms of ellagic acid in experimental rats," *Journal of Agricultural and Food Chemistry*, vol. 59, no. 13, pp. 6957–6965, 2011.

[19] P. K. Prabhakar and M. Doble, "Synergistic effect of phytochemicals in combination with hypoglycemic drugs on glucose uptake in myotubes," *Phytomedicine*, vol. 16, no. 12, pp. 1119–1126, 2009.

[20] B. Scazzocchio, R. Vari, C. Filesi et al., "Cyanidin-3-O-β-glucoside and protocatechuic acid exert insulin-like effects by upregulating PPARγ activity in human omental adipocytes," *Diabetes*, vol. 60, no. 9, pp. 2234–2244, 2011.

[21] C. N. Vishnu Prasad, T. Anjana, A. Banerji, and A. Gopalakrishnapillai, "Gallic acid induces GLUT4 translocation and glucose

uptake activity in 3T3-L1 cells," *FEBS Letters*, vol. 584, no. 3, pp. 531–536, 2010.

[22] K. W. Ong, A. Hsu, and B. K. H. Tan, "Chlorogenic acid stimulates glucose transport in skeletal muscle via AMPK activation: a contributor to the beneficial effects of coffee on diabetes," *PLoS ONE*, vol. 7, no. 3, Article ID e32718, 2012.

[23] S.-A. Yoon, S.-I. Kang, H.-S. Shin et al., "p-Coumaric acid modulates glucose and lipid metabolism via AMP-activated protein kinase in L6 skeletal muscle cells," *Biochemical and Biophysical Research Communications*, vol. 432, no. 4, pp. 553–557, 2013.

[24] J. W. Baynes, "Role of oxidative stress in development of complications in diabetes," *Diabetes*, vol. 40, no. 4, pp. 405–412, 1991.

[25] N. S. Dhalla, G. N. Pierce, I. R. Innes, and R. E. Beamish, "Pathogenesis of cardiac dysfunction in diabetes mellitus," *Canadian Journal of Cardiology*, vol. 1, no. 4, pp. 263–281, 1985.

[26] K. C. Tomlinson, S. M. Gardiner, R. A. Hebden, and T. Bennett, "Functional consequences of streptozotocin-induced diabetes mellitus, with particular reference to the cardiovascular system," *Pharmacological Reviews*, vol. 44, no. 1, pp. 103–150, 1992.

[27] J. Herlitz, A. Hjalmarson, K. Swedberg, L. Ryden, and F. Waagstein, "Effects on mortality during five years after early intervention with metoprolol in suspected acute myocardial infarction," *Acta Medica Scandinavica*, vol. 223, no. 3, pp. 227–231, 1988.

[28] P.-C. Chao, C.-C. Hsu, and M.-C. Yin, "Anti-inflammatory and anti-coagulatory activities of caffeic acid and ellagic acid in cardiac tissue of diabetic mice," *Nutrition & Metabolism*, vol. 6, article 33, 2009.

[29] G. Davì and C. Patrono, "Platelet activation and atherothrombosis," *The New England Journal of Medicine*, vol. 357, no. 24, pp. 2482–2494, 2007.

[30] P. Aukrust, B. Halvorsen, T. Ueland et al., "Activated platelets and atherosclerosis," *Expert Review of Cardiovascular Therapy*, vol. 8, no. 9, pp. 1297–1307, 2010.

[31] S.-S. Chang, V. S. Y. Lee, Y.-L. Tseng et al., "Gallic acid attenuates platelet activation and platelet-leukocyte aggregation: involving pathways of Akt and GSK3β," *Evidence-Based Complementary and Alternative Medicine*, vol. 2012, Article ID 683872, 8 pages, 2012.

[32] C. Y. Moon, C. R. Ku, Y. H. Cho, and E. J. Lee, "Protocatechuic aldehyde inhibits migration and proliferation of vascular smooth muscle cells and intravascular thrombosis," *Biochemical and Biophysical Research Communications*, vol. 423, no. 1, pp. 116–121, 2012.

[33] L.-Y. Zang, G. Cosma, H. Gardner, X. Shi, V. Castranova, and V. Vallyathan, "Effect of antioxidant protection by p-coumaric acid on low-density lipoprotein cholesterol oxidation," *The American Journal of Physiology—Cell Physiology*, vol. 279, no. 4, pp. C954–C960, 2000.

[34] S.-H. Park, J.-L. Kim, E.-S. Lee et al., "Dietary ellagic acid attenuates oxidized LDL uptake and stimulates cholesterol efflux in murine macrophages," *Journal of Nutrition*, vol. 141, no. 11, pp. 1931–1937, 2011.

[35] P. Yue, Z. Chen, F. Nassir et al., "Enhanced hepatic apoA-I secretion and peripheral efflux of cholesterol and phospholipid in CD36 null mice," *PLoS ONE*, vol. 5, no. 3, Article ID e9906, 2010.

[36] M. Xu, H. Zhou, K. C. B. Tan, R. Guo, S. W. M. Shiu, and Y. Wong, "ABCG1 mediated oxidized LDL-derived oxysterol efflux from macrophages," *Biochemical and Biophysical Research Communications*, vol. 390, no. 4, pp. 1349–1354, 2009.

[37] D. H. Mouhamed, A. Ezzaher, L. Gaha, W. Douki, and M. F. Najjar, "In vitro ffects of salicylic acid on plasma paraoxonase 1 activity," *Journal of Drug Metabolism & Toxicology*, vol. 4, no. 2, article 148, 3 pages, 2013.

[38] L. Zhou, X. Yu, Q. Meng et al., "Resistin reduces mitochondria and induces hepatic steatosis in mice by the protein kinase C/protein kinase G/p65/PPAR gamma coactivator 1 alpha pathway," *Hepatology*, vol. 57, no. 4, pp. 1384–1393, 2013.

[39] S. Kumar, P. Prahalathan, and B. Raja, "Vanillic acid: a potential inhibitor of cardiac and aortic wall remodeling in l-NAME induced hypertension through upregulation of endothelial nitric oxide synthase," *Environmental Toxicology and Pharmacology*, vol. 38, no. 2, pp. 643–652, 2014.

[40] L. H. Opie, P. J. Cammerford, B. J. Gerch, and M. A. Pfeffer, "Controversies in ventricular remodelling," *The Lancet*, vol. 367, no. 9507, pp. 356–367, 2006.

[41] H. C. D. Souza, G. Ballejo, M. C. O. Salgado, V. J. Dias Da Silva, and H. C. Salgado, "Cardiac sympathetic overactivity and decreased baroreflex sensitivity in L-NAME hypertensive rats," *The American Journal of Physiology—Heart and Circulatory Physiology*, vol. 280, no. 2, pp. H844–H850, 2001.

[42] O. Pechánová, I. Bernátová, P. Babál et al., "Red wine polyphenols prevent cardiovascular alterations in L-NAME-induced hypertension," *Journal of Hypertension*, vol. 22, no. 8, pp. 1551–1559, 2004.

[43] S. Mishra and M. Vinayak, "Anti-carcinogenic action of ellagic acid mediated via modulation of oxidative stress regulated genes in Dalton lymphoma bearing mice," *Leukemia & Lymphoma*, vol. 52, no. 11, pp. 2155–2161, 2011.

[44] S. Umesalma and G. Sudhandiran, "Ellagic acid prevents rat colon carcinogenesis induced by 1, 2 dimethyl hydrazine through inhibition of AKT-phosphoinositide-3 kinase pathway," *European Journal of Pharmacology*, vol. 660, no. 2-3, pp. 249–258, 2011.

[45] S. Srigopalram, I. A. Jayraaj, B. Kaleeswaran et al., "Ellagic acid normalizes mitochondrial outer membrane permeabilization and attenuates inflammation-mediated cell proliferation in experimental liver cancer," *Applied Biochemistry and Biotechnology*, vol. 173, no. 8, pp. 2254–2266, 2014.

[46] C.-C. Ho, A.-C. Huang, C.-S. Yu et al., "Ellagic acid induces apoptosis in TSGH8301 human bladder cancer cells through the endoplasmic reticulum stress- and mitochondria-dependent signaling pathways," *Environmental Toxicology*, vol. 29, no. 11, pp. 1262–1274, 2014.

[47] S. Umesalma, P. Nagendraprabhu, and G. Sudhandiran, "Ellagic acid inhibits proliferation and induced apoptosis via the Akt signaling pathway in HCT-15 colon adenocarcinoma cells," *Molecular and Cellular Biochemistry*, vol. 399, no. 1-2, pp. 303–313, 2015.

[48] J. Wu, C. Omene, J. Karkoszka et al., "Caffeic acid phenethyl ester (CAPE), derived from a honeybee product propolis, exhibits a diversity of anti-tumor effects in pre-clinical models of human breast cancer," *Cancer Letters*, vol. 308, no. 1, pp. 43–53, 2011.

[49] C.-S. Kong, C.-H. Jeong, J.-S. Choi, K.-J. Kim, and J.-W. Jeong, "Antiangiogenic effects of *P*-coumaric acid in human endothelial cells," *Phytotherapy Research*, vol. 27, no. 3, pp. 317–323, 2013.

[50] A. Rocha, L. Wang, M. Penichet, and M. Martins-Green, "Pomegranate juice and specific components inhibit cell and molecular processes critical for metastasis of breast cancer," *Breast Cancer Research and Treatment*, vol. 136, no. 3, pp. 647–658, 2012.

[51] L. Wang, W. Li, M. Lin et al., "Luteolin, ellagic acid and punicic acid are natural products that inhibit prostate cancer metastasis," *Carcinogenesis*, vol. 35, no. 10, pp. 2321–2330, 2014.

[52] H.-H. Ho, C.-S. Chang, W.-C. Ho, S.-Y. Liao, C.-H. Wu, and C.-J. Wang, "Anti-metastasis effects of gallic acid on gastric cancer cells involves inhibition of NF-κB activity and downregulation of PI3K/AKT/small GTPase signals," *Food and Chemical Toxicology*, vol. 48, no. 8-9, pp. 2508–2516, 2010.

[53] M.-H. Pan, C.-S. Lai, and C.-T. Ho, "Anti-inflammatory activity of natural dietary flavonoids," *Food and Function*, vol. 1, no. 1, pp. 15–31, 2010.

[54] S. Massberg, C. Schulz, and M. Gawaz, "Role of platelets in the pathophysiology of acute coronary syndrome," *Seminars in Vascular Medicine*, vol. 3, no. 2, pp. 147–161, 2003.

[55] E. Fuentes, J. Caballero, M. Alarcón, A. Rojas, and I. Palomo, "Chlorogenic acid inhibits human platelet activation and thrombus formation," *PLoS ONE*, vol. 9, no. 3, Article ID e90699, 2014.

[56] S. J. Hwang, Y.-W. Kim, Y. Park, H.-J. Lee, and K.-W. Kim, "Anti-inflammatory effects of chlorogenic acid in lipopolysaccharide-stimulated RAW 264.7 cells," *Inflammation Research*, vol. 63, no. 1, pp. 81–90, 2014.

[57] M. C. Búfalo, I. Ferreira, G. Costa et al., "Propolis and its constituent caffeic acid suppress LPS-stimulated pro-inflammatory response by blocking NF-κB and MAPK activation in macrophages," *Journal of Ethnopharmacology*, vol. 149, no. 1, pp. 84–92, 2013.

[58] W.-P. Chen and L.-D. Wu, "Chlorogenic acid suppresses interleukin-1β-induced inflammatory mediators in human chondrocytes," *International Journal of Clinical and Experimental Pathology*, vol. 7, no. 12, pp. 8797–8801, 2014.

[59] R. Studer, D. Jaffurs, M. Stefanovic-Racic, P. D. Robbins, and C. H. Evans, "Nitric oxide in osteoarthritis," *Osteoarthritis and Cartilage*, vol. 7, no. 4, pp. 377–379, 1999.

[60] W. S. Yang, D. Jeong, Y.-S. Yi et al., "IRAK1/4-targeted anti-inflammatory action of caffeic acid," *Mediators of Inflammation*, vol. 2013, Article ID 518183, 12 pages, 2013.

[61] G. Oboh, O. M. Agunloye, A. J. Akinyemi, A. O. Ademiluyi, and S. A. Adefegha, "Comparative study on the inhibitory effect of caffeic and chlorogenic acids on key enzymes linked to Alzheimer's disease and some pro-oxidant induced oxidative stress in rats' brain-in vitro," *Neurochemical Research*, vol. 38, no. 2, pp. 413–419, 2013.

[62] Y. J. Zhang, X. W. Lu, N. Song et al., "Chlorogenic acid alters the voltage-gated potassium channel currents of trigeminal ganglion neurons," *International Journal of Oral Science*, vol. 6, no. 4, pp. 233–240, 2014.

[63] W. Wu, S.-Y. Lee, X. Wu et al., "Neuroprotective ferulic acid (FA)-glycol chitosan (GC) nanoparticles for functional restoration of traumatically injured spinal cord," *Biomaterials*, vol. 35, no. 7, pp. 2355–2364, 2014.

[64] Y. Song, T. Cui, N. Xie, X. Zhang, Z. Qian, and J. Liu, "Protocatechuic acid improves cognitive deficits and attenuates amyloid deposits, inflammatory response in aged AβPP/PS1 double transgenic mice," *International Immunopharmacology*, vol. 20, no. 1, pp. 276–281, 2014.

[65] J. H. Lee, J. H. Won, J. M. Choi et al., "Protective effect of ellagic acid on concanavalin A-induced hepatitis via toll-like receptor and mitogen-activated protein kinase/nuclear factor κB signaling pathways," *Journal of Agricultural and Food Chemistry*, vol. 62, no. 41, pp. 10110–10117, 2014.

[66] Y. Yoshimura, S. Nishii, N. Zaima, T. Moriyama, and Y. Kawamura, "Ellagic acid improves hepatic steatosis and serum lipid composition through reduction of serum resistin levels and transcriptional activation of hepatic *ppara* in obese, diabetic KK-A^y mice," *Biochemical and Biophysical Research Communications*, vol. 434, no. 3, pp. 486–491, 2013.

[67] X. Zhang, G.-F. Shi, X.-Z. Liu, L.-J. An, and S. Guan, "Anti-ageing effects of protocatechuic acid from *Alpinia* on spleen and liver antioxidative system of senescent mice," *Cell Biochemistry and Function*, vol. 29, no. 4, pp. 342–347, 2011.

[68] Y. S. Kim, H. W. Seo, M.-H. Lee, D. K. Kim, H. Jeon, and D. S. Cha, "Protocatechuic acid extends lifespan and increases stress resistance in *Caenorhabditis elegans*," *Archives of Pharmacal Research*, vol. 37, no. 2, pp. 245–252, 2014.

[69] S. Hameed and Z. Fatima, "Novel regulatory mechanisms of pathogenicity and virulence to combat MDR in *Candida albicans*," *International Journal of Microbiology*, vol. 2013, Article ID 240209, 10 pages, 2013.

[70] J. Tanwar, S. Das, Z. Fatima, and S. Hameed, "Multidrug resistance: an emerging crisis," *Interdisciplinary Perspectives on Infectious Diseases*, vol. 2014, Article ID 541340, 7 pages, 2014.

[71] M. M. Cowan, "Plant products as antimicrobial agents," *Clinical Microbiology Reviews*, vol. 12, no. 4, pp. 564–582, 1999.

[72] M. A. Ansari, Z. Fatima, and S. Hameed, "Sesamol: a natural phenolic compound with promising anticandidal potential," *Journal of Pathogens*, vol. 2014, Article ID 895193, 12 pages, 2014.

[73] S. Das, J. Tanwar, S. Hameed, and Z. Fatima, "Antimicrobial potential of epigallocatechin-3-gallate (EGCG): a green tea polyphenol," *Journal of Biochemical and Pharmacological Research*, vol. 2, no. 3, pp. 167–174, 2014.

[74] M. A. Ansari, A. Anurag, Z. Fatima, and S. Hameed, "Natural phenolic compounds: a potential antifungal agent," in *Microbial Pathogens and Strategies for Combating Them: Science, Technology and Education*, vol. 1, pp. 1189–1195, Formatex Research Center, 2013.

[75] D. S. Stojković, J. Živković, M. Soković et al., "Antibacterial activity of *Veronica montana* L. extract and of protocatechuic acid incorporated in a food system," *Food and Chemical Toxicology*, vol. 55, pp. 209–213, 2013.

[76] J. C. Low and W. Donachie, "A review of *Listeria monocytogenes* and listeriosis," *The Veterinary Journal*, vol. 153, no. 1, pp. 9–29, 1997.

[77] A. Karunanidhi, R. Thomas, A. Van Belkum, and V. Neela, "In vitro antibacterial and antibiofilm activities of chlorogenic acid against clinical isolates of *Stenotrophomonas maltophilia* including the trimethoprim/sulfamethoxazole resistant strain," *BioMed Research International*, vol. 2013, Article ID 392058, 7 pages, 2013.

[78] G. Li, M. Qiao, Y. Guo, X. Wang, Y. Xu, and X. Xia, "Effect of subinhibitory concentrations of chlorogenic acid on reducing the virulence factor production by *Staphylococcus aureus*," *Foodborne Pathogens and Disease*, vol. 11, no. 9, pp. 677–683, 2014.

7

BF$_3$·Et$_2$O Catalysed 4-Aryl-3-phenyl-benzopyrones, Pro-SERMs, and Their Characterization

Ambika Srivastava, Pooja Singh, and Rajesh Kumar

Department of Chemistry, Centre of Advanced Study, Faculty of Science, Banaras Hindu University, Varanasi 221005, India

Correspondence should be addressed to Rajesh Kumar; rkr_bhu@yahoo.com

Academic Editor: Todd C. Skaar

We have synthesized the novel 4-(4-hydroxy-benzyl)-3-phenyl-chromen-2-one which is a precursor of SERMs with a smaller number of steps and good yield. Two methodologies for the synthesis have been worked out. Anhydrous BF$_3$·Et$_2$O catalyzed reaction was found to be selective for product formation while anhydrous AlCl$_3$, FeCl$_3$, and SnCl$_4$ catalyzed ones were nonselective.

1. Introduction

Activity of estrogen receptor can be controlled by a class of compounds which is called selective estrogen receptor modulators (SERMs). The modulators have a distinctive feature in different individual tissues by which they can inhibit or stimulate or selectively suppress or excite estrogen-like behavior in different tissues. The structures of few biologically vital SERMs are shown in Figure 1 in which compound A is a polyhydroxy phenyl benzothiophene which has low physiological response when combined with the receptor estrogen in gnawing uterus [1]. Compound A was initially known as Ly156758/keoxifen and its advancement has been stopped for improved action for treatment of breast cancer [2] due to less bioavailability than the required essential dose [3]. But the concept of SERM was shown by compound A due to sustainable property of bone density [4, 5] with restriction in mammary carcinogenesis in rat [6, 7]. Studies on compound A reveal the reduction of risk of osteoporosis [8] and breast cancer in women after menopause [9]. Compound B is a nonhydroxy and typical model compound for SERM which was used clinically for the occupational therapy of breast cancer [10, 11] with the maintained density in bone of women after menopause [12]. The drawback of the treatment by compound B was the increased possibilities of endometrial cancer [13]. Hence, it is clear that there are various factors which are responsible for estrogenic and antiestrogenic properties of

SERM complexes and could be useful in improving targeted therapeutic agents.

Coumarin and its derivatives are important compounds due to their presence in numerous natural products along with their wide ranging applications as drugs, pharmaceuticals, and SERMs. Coumarin based selective estrogen receptor modulators (SERMs) and coumarin-estrogen conjugates have been described as potential anti-breast-cancer agents. Thus, coumarin derivatives acting as SERMs either stimulate or inhibit the estrogen action, thereby generating the possibility of curing estrogen related problems. Coumarins and their derivatives are common in nature [14–18]; among them the 4-substituted coumarins were identified as anticancer and anti-HIV-1 molecules [19, 20].

Among the oxygen heterocycles coumarins are one of them which are present in various naturally [21, 22] occurring motifs. Due to comprehensive and inexhaustible performance of coumarin in biological activities [23–33] such as anti-HIV [34–37], anticoagulation [38], antibiotic [39–42], anticancer [43, 44], anti-inflammatory [45, 46], antioxidant [47–49], antitumor [50–52], antiviral [53], antihypertensive, and antimicrobial activity its chemistry grew up widely. Among the nuclear hormone receptor modulators, *namely*, SERMs, PRMs, and SARMs [54–58], coumarins are also identified with a similar kind of properties. Among the coumarin derivatives more attention is given to 4-substituted coumarins, but there are very few methods known for

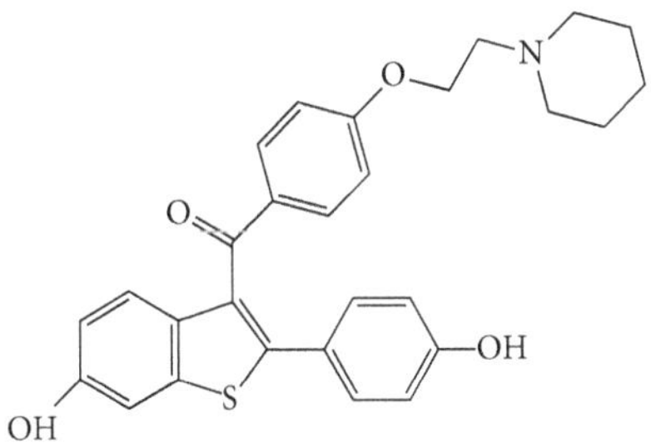

(A) Raloxifene 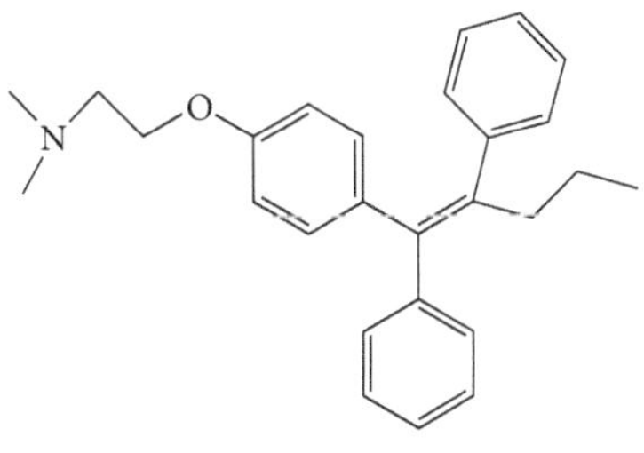   (B) Tamoxifen 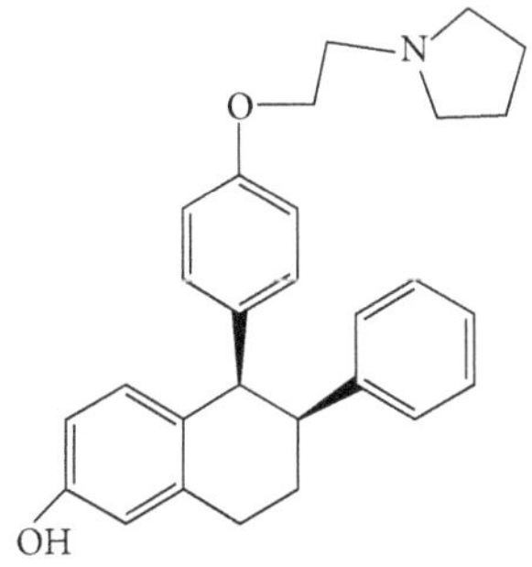   (C) Lasofoxifene

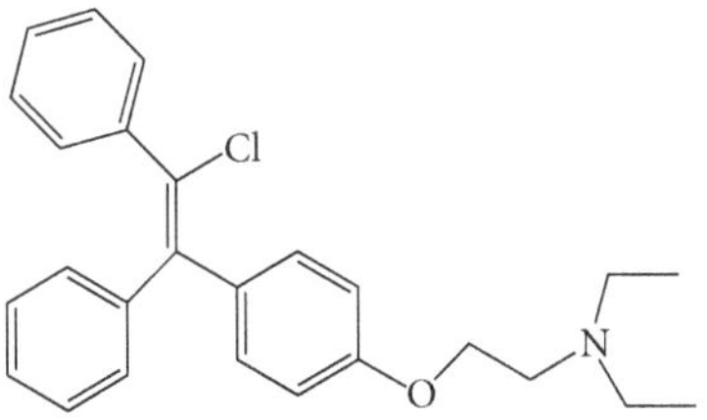

(D) Clomifene 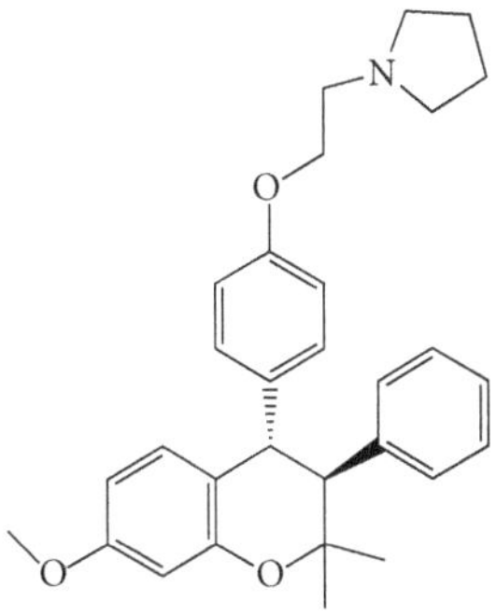   (E) Centchroman

FIGURE 1: Examples of biologically active heterocyclic frameworks.

synthesis. Route 1 (Scheme 1) to coumarins incorporates Pechmann [59, 60], Knoevenagel [61–64], Reformatsky [61–64], Perkin [65], and Wittig [66] condensation reactions. To make these reactions efficacious, several variations in terms of catalyst and reaction conditions have been done. However, the route 1 methodology suffers from laborious multistep procedures, long reaction time, high reaction temperature, nonselectivity, and waste problem. To overcome these, a facile two-step synthesis of 4-aryl-3-phenyl-coumarin-2-one has been reported as shown in Scheme 2, which would be helpful in designing novel SERMs.

2. Results and Discussion

Condensation reactions have been amongst the most useful routes for the synthesis of these compounds, particularly catalyzed by Lewis acids. In Scheme 1, 4-methoxy phenyl acetic acid and phenol were taken as starting material. In the first step, acyl chloride of acid was prepared, where the yield of phenyl acyl chloride obtained was 50%. Further esterification led to some good yield, but the yield was very poorly shed down to 10% with next step reaction, that is, Fries rearrangement. The reaction of ester and AlCl₃ at 145°C led to four products, of which only two (iv-a, iv-b) were important for synthesis purpose. Fries rearrangement with AlCl₃ has no selectivity and gave four products with almost 10% yield, which were separated chromatographically. Then cyclization with phenyl acetyl chloride was carried out with anhydrous K₂CO₃ in dry acetone. There were some shortcomings like low reaction yields and nonselectivity of reaction/more byproduct formation/low atom economic reactions. Hence,

the nonselectivity of reactions (via Scheme 1) and low atom economy demanded the search for a simple, short, and high-yielding alternate process to synthesize substituted coumarin based SERMs precursors.

To decrease the product loss and number of steps, the synthetic strategy was modified and Scheme 2 route was selected in which 4-substituted phenyl acetic acid and substituted phenol were used as starting material and reaction was catalyzed by BF₃·Et₂O which was found to be a very efficient catalyst. In this report, a facile and high-yielding protocol for diverse SERMs precursors through synthesis of functionalized benzylic ketone and further intermolecular cyclization using substituted phenyl acetyl chloride with dry acetone and potassium carbonate under reflux condition has been described. Further, to our ongoing research on novel synthetic methodologies for SERMs precursors synthesis, we commenced our synthetic strategy with environmentally benign phenol, which on coupling with different phenyl acetyl chlorides including p-anisole acetyl chloride, p-phenyl acetyl chloride, and p-hydroxy phenyl acetyl chloride afforded substituted benzylic ketones in good yields. The substituted benzylic ketones (ix (a–i)) on further treatment with substituted phenyl acetyl chloride in the presence of K₂CO₃ and dry acetone led to the formation of various substituted SERMs precursors (4-benzyl-3-phenyl coumarin) (vi (a–i)), in good yields (Scheme 2). Thus, the synthesis of substituted SERMs precursor (4-benzyl-3-phenyl coumarin) was achieved in two steps. Acetylation was regioselective and occurred at ortho position which was the major reaction product. Thus, in just one step, phenol was esterified and the ester readily rearranged to give 4-methoxy phenyl acetyl

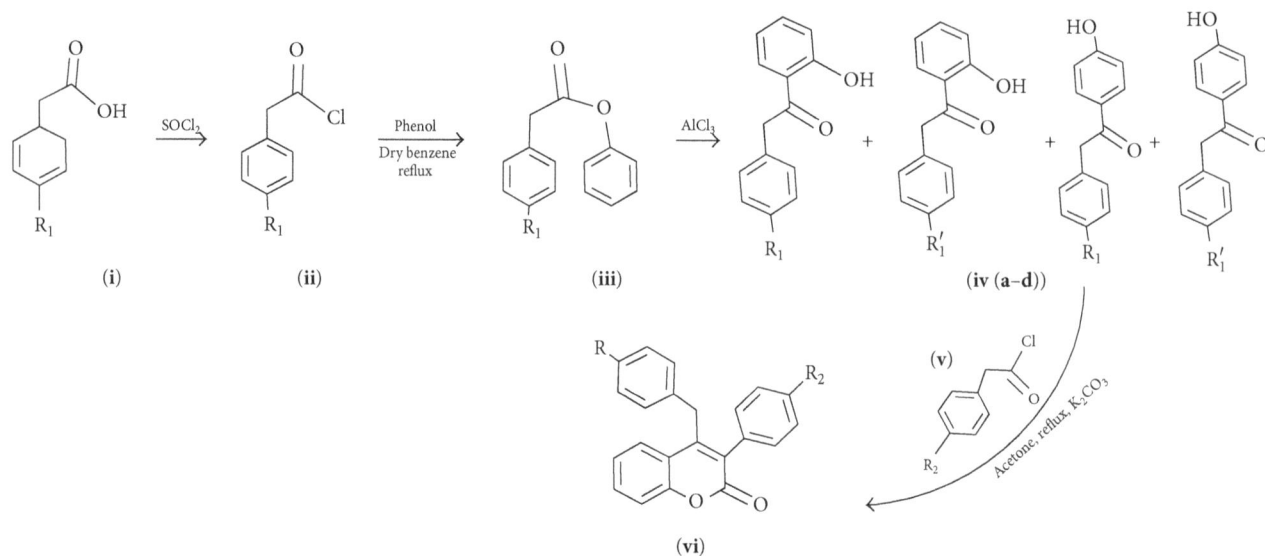

where: R_1 = OCH_3, R_1' = OH, R_2 = H, CH_3, C_2H_5,
OCH_3, R = OCH_3, OH

SCHEME 1: Route 1 for the synthesis of coumarin based SERM's precursors.

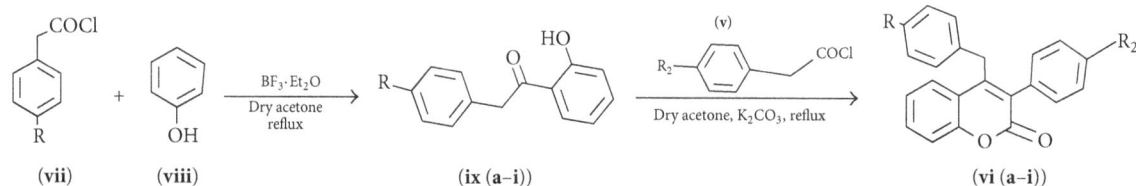

where R = OCH_3, OH, R_2 = H, CH_3, C_2H_5, OCH_3

SCHEME 2: Route 2 for the synthesis of coumarin based SERM's precursors.

group at ortho position of phenol. This stage product was achieved by Scheme 1 after 3 steps with low atom economy and many undesirable products. The intermediate ester (Scheme 2) could not be isolated since $BF_3 \cdot Et_2O$ readily rearranged it to ortho substituted phenol. Thus, the two-step process was reduced to one step, the probable mechanism of which has been given in Figure 2.

In our early attempts, to synthesize the coumarin based SERMs precursors, we were not successful in converting the reactants to products without the catalyst ($BF_3 \cdot Et_2O$). The anhydrous $AlCl_3$, $FeCl_3$, and $SnCl_4$ were not able to give the desired intermediate selectively in quantitative yield. This was possibly due to poor Lewis acid character of $AlCl_3$, $FeCl_3$, and $SnCl_4$ compared to BF_3. The reaction was investigated carefully and it was observed that the intermediate (benzylic ketones (ix (a–i))) formed after the coupling of phenol with substituted phenyl acetyl chloride was sufficiently stable and could be isolated. In the second step intermolecular cyclization was carried out with substituted phenyl acetyl chloride and a base (anhydrous K_2CO_3). The desired product (vi-e) was characterized by ^{1}H NMR (Figure S6(a) in Supplementary Material available online at

http://dx.doi.org/10.1155/2015/527159), which contains additional peaks at δ 6.79 and 6.98 due to benzylic proton and at δ 7.2 and 7.3 due to phenylic protons and one signal at δ 7.15 was due to proton at para position in the phenyl ring. The rest of the protons were the same as in the precursor, that is, ortho substituted phenol (iv-a).

^{13}C NMR (Figure S6(b)) also confirmed the formation of 4-(4-hydroxy-benzyl)-3-phenyl-chromen-2-one; peaks at 119.60, 126.40, 128.38, 129.53, 134.05, and 161.22 show six different types of carbons which are present in 4-aryl-3-phenyl-benzopyrone in addition to the carbons already present in the starting, that is, 2-(4-hydroxy-phenyl)-1-(2-hydroxy phenyl)-ethanone. FTIR spectrum also confirmed the formation of lactone ring; that is, the cyclized product shows carbonyl absorption at a higher wavenumber, that is, at 1707 cm^{-1} (Figure S6(c)), while it was 1633 cm^{-1} in the 2-(4-hydroxy-phenyl)-1-(2-hydroxy-phenyl)-ethanone (Figure S2(a)). Mass spectroscopy shows (m + 1) peak at 343 while the molecular weight of (vi-e) is 342 (Figure S6(d)).

Finally the single crystal diffraction studies showed the space orientation (Figures 3(a) and 3(b)), bond lengths, and bond angles regarding the crystal structure (Table 1). The

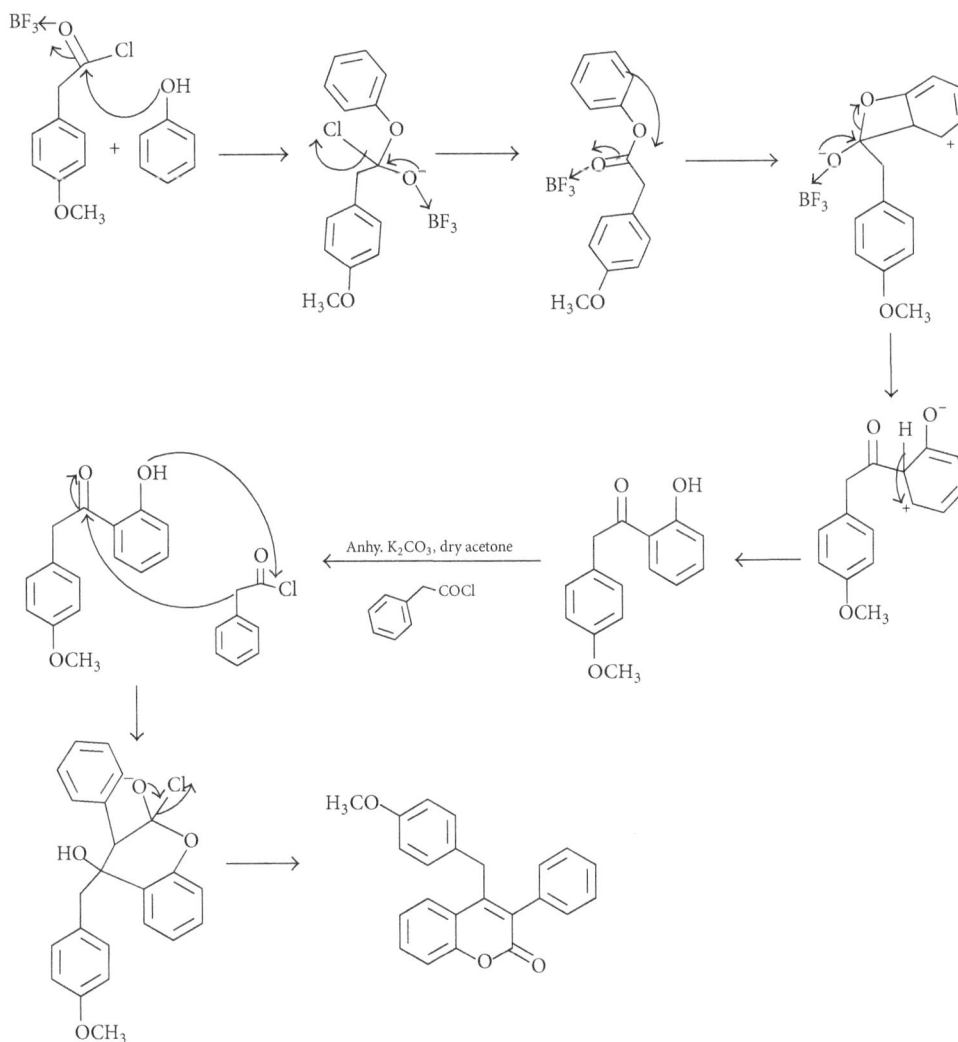

FIGURE 2: Probable mechanism related to Scheme 2.

structure reflects that the coumarin ring is planar, phenyl ring which is attached at position 3 is slightly out of plane, and substituted benzylic group is perpendicular to the ring coumarin (Figure 3(a)). Compound (vi-e) exhibited "Z-" like packing diagram (Figure 3(b)).

This new procedure allows facile introduction of substituents at position 4 of the 4-(4-substituted-benzyl)-3-phenyl-chromen-2-one skeleton and gives the flexibility for the construction of novel precursors.

Various derivatives have been prepared with para substituted benzyl chloride with hydroxyl, methoxy, acetoxy, methyl, and ethyl groups as shown in Table 2. All the derivatives have been prepared smoothly under the same reaction conditions. The reactions are simple, easy to handle, and feasible and have simple workup procedures.

After the establishment of the protocol for the synthesis of substituted SERMs precursors (4-benzyl-3-phenyl coumarins), we shifted our focus towards the role of solvents like CH_2Cl_2, $CHCl_3$, acetone, and toluene upon yield and the reaction time. The results illustrated that the reaction in toluene did not give the desired precursors, whereas the

TABLE 1: Bond lengths and bond angles of (vi-e) have been demonstrated.

S. number	Atoms	Bond lengths	Atoms	Bond angles
1	O3-C20	1.3772(1)	C20-O3-C23	117.76
2	O3-C23	1.3963(1)	C8-O1-C7	121.71
3	O1-C8	1.3848(1)	O3-C20-C21	115.93
4	O1-C7	1.3722(1)	O1-C8-C1	115.40
5	C5-C6	1.3610(1)	O3-C20-C19	124.73
6	C6-C7	1.4647(1)	O1-C7-C6	117.78
7	O2-C7	1.2114(1)	C6-C7-O2	125.71

reaction in $CHCl_3$ was slow and the yield was low. However, for this cyclization, CH_2Cl_2 was found to be good in terms of yield and handling but took a slightly longer time to afford the products. Eventually, acetone appeared as a solvent of choice for intermolecular cyclization in very good yield. Intermolecular cyclization was greatly influenced by the base used; therefore, to find out the appropriate base, we examined K_2CO_3 and triethylamine in the intermolecular cyclization

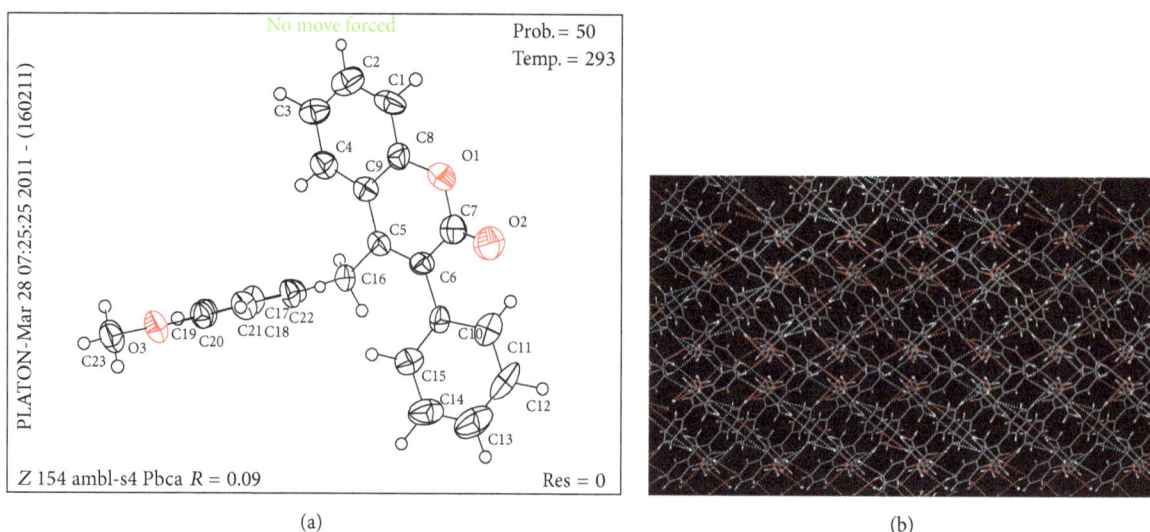

FIGURE 3: (a) ORTEP/PLATON structure of (**vi-e**). (b) Packing structure of (**vi-e**) showing Z-like packing.

TABLE 2: Derivatives of 4-aryl-3-phenyl-coumarin-2-one and their yield (%) for Scheme 2.

S. number	Compound	R	R_2	Time (h)	Yield[a] (%)
1	(**vi-a**)	-OH	H	7	74
2	(**vi-b**)	-OH	-CH$_3$	7	77
3	(**vi-c**)	-OH	-OCH$_3$	6	80
4	(**vi-d**)	-OH	-C$_2$H$_5$	8	70
5	(**vi-e**)	-OCH$_3$	H	7	75
6	(**vi-f**)	-OCH$_3$	-CH$_3$	8	79
7	(**vi-g**)	-OCH$_3$	-OCH$_3$	7	82
8	(**vi-h**)	-OCH$_3$	-C$_2$H$_5$	7	80
9	(**vi-i**)	-OAc	H	6	90

[a]The reaction yield refers to product isolated through column chromatography.

reaction of (**ix-a**) with (**v**) and found that the reaction in the presence of K_2CO_3 afforded the cyclized product (**vi-a**) in 74% yield after 7 h, whereas triethylamine gave this product in 57% yield. We believe that potassium carbonate may be more dissociated in aprotic polar solvents and consequently proved to be more reactive.

3. Conclusion

In conclusion, a simple, efficient, and novel method has been developed for an easy access to synthesis of the 4-(4-hydroxy-benzyl)-3-phenyl-chromen-2-one via Scheme 2 and this has been supported by ^{1}H NMR, FTIR, ^{13}C NMR, mass spectroscopy, and single crystal X-ray data analysis. Synthetic pathway with just 2 steps proved to be the best with less side reactions and greater yield. Thus, the number of steps has been decreased and the yield was increased. Herein we reported some precursors of coumarin based SERMs which could be useful in designing new SERMs. The pure products were obtained by column chromatography.

This methodology presents several advantages including (a) mild reaction conditions, (b) simple workup procedure, (c) moderately high yields of the desired products, (d) the selectivity of the product, and finally (e) economic availability of the reagents making the whole process simple and feasible. Efforts to extend the span of the procedure on SERMs are under progress in our laboratory.

4. Experimental Section

4.1. General Methods. All the required chemicals are purchased since they are commercially available and used as received without further purification. Commercially available acetone and benzene were further purified and dried following the known procedure. Thin-layer chromatography (TLC) was performed using silica gel 60 F254 precoated plates. Column chromatography was carried out on silica gel 60 (100–200 mesh). Infrared (FTIR) spectra were recorded in KBr, and wavelengths (ν) have been reported in cm^{-1}; ^{1}H and ^{13}C NMR spectra were recorded on NMR spectrometers operating at 300 and 75.5 MHz, respectively. Chemical shifts (δ) were given in parts per million (ppm) using the residue solvent peaks as reference relative to TMS. J values have been given in Hz. Mass spectra were recorded using electrospray ionization (ESI) mass spectrometer. The melting points were taken in open capillary and uncorrected.

4.1.1. Procedure for Scheme 1

Compound (ii). To a solution of 4-methoxy phenyl acetic acid (42.5 g, 0.25 mol) in dry benzene (50 mL) was added thionyl chloride (30 mL, 0.25 mol) dropwise with syringe. After the reaction was complete, the reaction mixture was distilled to remove excess thionyl chloride and the solvent benzene. Brown colored liquid was obtained. Yield:- 50%, ^{1}H NMR-(300 MHz, CDCl$_3$): δ 3.77 (s, 3H, -CH$_3$), 4.20 (s, 2H, -CH$_2$), 6.68 (d, J = 7.8 Hz, 2H, Ar-H), 7.10 (d, J = 7.8 Hz, 2H, Ar-H).

Compound (iii). A solution of p-methoxy phenyl acetyl chloride (24 g, 0.13 mol) and phenol (12.2 mL, 0.13 mol) in dry benzene (63 mL) was refluxed for 21 h, till the reaction was complete as monitored by TLC. Then the reaction mixture was washed with 5% aqueous NaOH to remove excess unreacted phenol and then washed with water three times and dried over anhydrous Na_2SO_4 and concentrated over vacuum. Orange colored liquid compound was obtained. Yield:- 70% ^{1}H NMR- (300 MHz, CDCl$_3$): δ 3.54 (s, 2H, -CH$_2$), 3.77 (s, 3H, -CH$_3$), 6.70 (d, J = 7.6 Hz, 2H, -Ar-H), 7.10 (d, J = 7.8 Hz, 2H, -Ar-H), 7.23 (m, 3H, -Ar-H), 7.35 (t, J = 7.9 Hz, 2H, -Ar-H); FTIR (KBr, cm^{-1}): 2937, 2837, 1755, 1600, 1513, 1300, 1248, 1125, 814 (Figure S1(a & b); m/z 242, Elemental Analysis C, 74.36, H, 5.82, O, 19.81.

Compounds (iv (a–d)). A solution of ester (23.6 g, 0.1 mol) and AlCl$_3$ (13.3 g, 0.1 mol) was refluxed at 150°C till completion of reaction (as monitored by TLC). The reaction mixture was cooled, and then 5% cooled aqueous HCl was added till all the excess AlCl$_3$ neutralized. The reaction mixture was extracted with ethyl acetate and the organic layer was collected, dried over Na_2SO_4, and concentrated over vacuum. The residue was chromatographed to obtain the pure compound. Yield:- 12%, (**iv-a**):- ^{1}H NMR- (300 MHz, CDCl$_3$): δ 3.79 (s, 3H, -CH$_3$), 4.24 (s, 2H, -CH$_2$), 6.90 (m, 3H, -Ar-H), 6.99 (s, 1H, -Ar-H), 7.18 (d, J = 8.4 Hz, 2H, -Ar-H), 7.46 (t, J = 7.5 Hz, 1H, -Ar-H), 7.86 (d, J = 6.9 Hz, 1H, -Ar-H); ^{13}C NMR- (75 MHz, CDCl$_3$): δ 44.231, 55.234, 114.219, 118.933, 125.790, 130.390, 136.463, 158.724, 162.870, 204.185; FTIR (KBr, cm^{-1}): 3448, 2914, 2836, 1633, 1504, 1445, 1344, 1248, 844, 791, 751; m/z 242, Elemental Analysis C, 74.36, H, 5.82, O, 19.81 Figure S2(a, b&c); (**iv-b**):- ^{1}H NMR- (300 MHz, CDCl$_3$): 4.23 (s, 2H, -CH$_2$), 6.806 (d, J = 8.4 Hz, 2H, -Ar-H), 6.886 (d, J = 7.5 Hz, 1H, -Ar-H), 6.960 (t, J = 8.4 Hz, 1H, -Ar-H), 7.132 (d, J=8.4 Hz, 2H, -Ar-H), 7.466 (t, J = 7.2 Hz, 1H, -Ar-H), 7.852 (d, J = 7.8 Hz, 1H, Ar-H); FTIR (KBr, cm^{-1}): 3447, 3045, 2909, 1635, 1515, 1483, 1443, 1341, 847, 798, 754 (Figures S3(a) & S3(b)); m/z 328, Elemental Analysis C, 80.47, H, 4.91, O, 14.62.

General Procedure for Compounds (vi (a–h))

Compounds (vi (a–h)). To a solution of ortho substituted phenol (236 mg, 1 mmol) and K$_2$CO$_3$ (690 mg, 5 mmol) in dry acetone (25 mL) was added phenyl acetyl chloride (308 mg, 2 mmol) dropwise. The reaction mixture was refluxed at 100°C for 7 h. After the reaction was completed (as monitored by TLC), the reaction mixture was cooled, filtered, and concentrated. The residue was chromatographed to obtain the pure compound with 20% ethyl acetate-hexane. Yield:- 70%.

4.1.2. Procedure for Scheme 2

Compound (ix-e). To a solution of 4-methoxy phenyl acetic acid (166 mg, 1 mmol) in dry acetone (10 mL) was added BF$_3$·Et$_2$O (0.4 mL, 3 mmol) at 0°C. After 30 minutes, we added phenol (0.1 mL, 1 mmol) and refluxed it till the reaction was completed as monitored by TLC. Then we filtered the reaction mixture and evaporated the solvent in vacuum.

White solid was obtained, recrystallized from ethanol. Yield:- 80%, m.p. 65°C, ^{1}H NMR- (300 MHz, CDCl$_3$): δ 3.79 (s, 3H, -CH$_3$), 4.24 (s, 2H, -CH$_2$), 6.90 (m, 3H, -Ar-H), 6.99 (s, 1H, -Ar-H), 7.18 (d, J = 8.4 Hz, 2H, -Ar-H), 7.46 (t, J = 7.5 Hz, 1H, -Ar-H), 7.86 (d, J = 6.9 Hz, 1H, -Ar-H); FTIR (KBr, cm^{-1}): 3448, 2914, 2836, 1633, 1504, 1445, 1344, 1248, 844, 791, 751. (Figure S2(a, b & c).

Compound (vi-e). Phenyl acetyl chloride (0.13 mL, 1 mmol) was added to a solution of (**ix-e**) (242 mg, 1 mmol) in dry acetone and K$_2$CO$_3$ (552 mg, 4 mmol) and refluxed for 6 h. Then the reaction mixture was filtered and concentrated in vacuum. The obtained crude was recrystallized from ethanol to obtain the pure product. Yield:- 75%.

Procedure for Compound (vi-i). Acetic anhydride (920 mg, 1 mL) was added to a solution of (**vi-a**) (328 mg, 1 mmol) and pyridine (0.25 mL, 9 mmol) and refluxed under nitrogen atmosphere for 6 h at 90°C. After the reaction was completed (as monitored by TLC), solvent was removed under vacuum. The residue was washed with saturated Na$_2$HCO$_3$ until excess pyridine was removed and then it was washed with aqueous HCl and finally with saturated brine solution and dried and chromatographed with 20% ethyl acetate-hexane. Yield: 90%, m.p. 160°C.

Analytical Data for Compounds (vi (a–i))

(**vi-a**). ^{1}H NMR- (300 MHz, CDCl$_3$): δ 4.03 (s, 2H, -CH$_2$), 6.717 (d, J = 8.4 Hz, 2H, Ar-H), 6.932 (d, J = 8.1 Hz, 2H, Ar-H), 7.170 (t, J = 7.5 Hz, 1H, Ar-H), 7.273 (d, J = 8.4 Hz, 2H, Ar-H), 7.384 (d, J = 7.5 Hz, 4H, Ar-H), 7.459 (m, 2H, Ar-H); FTIR (KBr, cm^{-1}): 3484, 3433, 3059, 2931, 1707, 1604, 1564, 1513, 1446, 1267, 1173, 828, 750 Figure S5(a, b & c); m/z 342.13, Elemental Analysis C, 80.68, H, 5.30, O, 14.02; (**vi-b**):- ^{1}H NMR- (300 MHz, CDCl$_3$): δ 3.01 (s, 3H, -CH$_3$), 4.05 (s, 2H, -CH$_2$), 6.722 (d, J = 8.1 Hz, 2H, Ar-H), 6.937 (d, J = 7.2 Hz, 2H, Ar-H), 7.179 (t, J = 7.8 Hz, 1H, Ar-H), 7.266 (d, J = 8.1 Hz, 2H, Ar-H), 7.377 (d, J = 7.8 Hz, 4H, Ar-H), 7.450 (m, 2H, Ar-H); ^{13}C NMR (75 MHz, CDCl$_3$): δ 22.9, 40.2, 115.6, 122.3, 125.2, 126.3, 126.8, 128.0, 129.5, 130.5, 130.9, 132.0, 137.0, 145.1, 150.8, 155.2, 162.1; (**vi-c**):- ^{1}H NMR- (300 MHz, CDCl$_3$): δ 3.75 (s, 3H, -CH$_3$), 4.03 (s, 2H, -CH$_2$), 6.717 (d, J = 8.4 Hz, 2H, Ar-H), 6.932 (d, J = 8.1 Hz, 2H, Ar-H), 7.132 (d, J = 7.5 Hz, 2H, Ar-H), 7.363 (d, J = 7.5 Hz, 2H, Ar-H), 7.459 (m, 4H, Ar-H); ^{13}C NMR (75 MHz, CDCl$_3$): δ 40.1, 56.2, 114.0, 121.3, 122, 125.2, 127.2, 127.8, 128.1, 130.3, 130.6, 144.0, 150.8, 154.3, 161.2, 162.0; (**vi-d**):- ^{1}H NMR- (300 MHz, CDCl$_3$): δ 1.30 (s, 3H, -CH$_3$), 3.51 (s, 2H, -CH$_2$), 4.04 (s, 2H, -CH$_2$), 6.721 (d, J = 8.1 Hz, 2H, Ar-H), 6.938 (d, J = 7.2 Hz, 2H, Ar-H), 7.202 (d, J = 7.5 Hz, 2H, Ar-H), 7.370 (d, J = 7.5 Hz, 2H, Ar-H), 7.459 (m, 4H, Ar-H); ^{13}C NMR (75 MHz, CDCl$_3$): δ 18.1, 28.6, 40.1, 115.6, 121.3, 122, 125.2, 126.4, 126.9, 128.0, 128.4, 130.5, 130.8, 132.3, 139.8, 145.0, 150.9, 155.0, 162.1; (**vi-e**):- ^{1}H NMR- (300 MHz, CDCl$_3$): δ 3.75 (s, 3H, -OCH$_3$), 4.04 (s, 2H, -CH$_2$), 6.79 (d, J = 8.4 Hz, 2H, Ar-H), 6.98 (d, J = 8.4 Hz, 2H, Ar-H), 7.15 (t, J = 7.5 Hz, 1H, Ar-H), 7.30 (s, 2H, -Ar-H), 7.37 (s, 4H, -Ar-H), 7.49 (q, J = 8.1 Hz, 2H, -Ar-H); ^{13}C NMR (75 MHz, CDCl$_3$): δ 34.74, 55.19, 114.19, 116.93, 119.60, 124.22, 126.40, 128.38, 128.47, 128.83, 129.53,

129.79, 131.19, 134.05, 149.06, 153.13, 158.18, 161.22; FTIR (KBr, cm^{-1}): 3075, 2928, 2857, 1707, 1509, 1445, 1384, 1241, 1121, 836, 798; m/z 342.13, Elemental Analysis C, 80.68, H, 5.30, O, 14.02, Figure S6(a, b, c & d); (vi-f):- ^{1}H NMR (300 MHz, CDCl$_3$): δ 2.36 (s, 3H, -CH$_3$), 3.75 (s, 3H, -OCH$_3$), 4.04 (s, 2H, -CH$_2$), 6.79 (d, J = 8.4 Hz, 2H, Ar-H), 6.98 (d, J = 8.4 Hz, 2H, Ar-H), 7.10 (s, 2H, -Ar-H), 7.29 (s, 4H, -Ar-H), 7.49 (q, J = 8.1 Hz, 2H, -Ar-H); ^{13}C NMR (75 MHz, CDCl$_3$): δ 21.0, 40.0, 56.4, 114.1, 121.6, 1222.0, 125.5, 126.1, 126.8, 128.1, 128.4, 129.3, 130.1, 130.6, 132.2, 137.2, 145.1, 150.9, 160.3, 162.0; (vi-g):- ^{1}H NMR (300 MHz, CDCl$_3$): δ 3.75 (s, 3H, -OCH$_3$), 4.04 (s, 2H, -CH$_2$), 6.67 (d, J = 8.4 Hz, 2H, Ar-H), 6.88 (d, J = 8.4 Hz, 2H, Ar-H), 7.15 (s, 2H, -Ar-H), 7.29 (s, 4H, -Ar-H), 7.45 (q, J = 8.1 Hz, 2H, -Ar-H); ^{13}C NMR (75 MHz, CDCl$_3$): δ 40.0, 56.4, 114.0, 115.6, 121.6, 121.8, 125.7, 126.9, 127.6, 127.8, 128.1, 130.0, 130.4, 144.0, 150.9, 156.7, 159.6, 162.1; m/z 358, C, 77.08, H, 5.06, O, 17.86; (vi-h):- ^{1}H NMR (300 MHz, CDCl$_3$): δ 1.30 (s, 3H, -CH$_3$), 3.51 (s, 2H, -CH$_2$), 3.75 (s, 3H, -OCH$_3$), 4.04 (s, 2H, -CH$_2$), 6.67 (d, J = 8.4 Hz, 2H, Ar-H), 6.88 (d, J = 8.4 Hz, 2H, Ar-H), 7.15 (s, 2H, -Ar-H), 7.29 (s, 4H, -Ar-H), 7.45 (q, J = 8.1 Hz, 2H, -Ar-H); ^{13}C NMR (75 MHz, CDCl$_3$): δ 18.1, 29.6, 40.1, 56.0, 114.2, 121.4, 122.3, 125.2, 126.3, 127.8, 128.4, 130.0, 130.2, 132.1, 140.0, 144.0, 151.1, 159.2, 162.0.

(vi-i). ^{1}H NMR- (300 MHz, CDCl$_3$): δ 2.29 (s, 3H, CH$_3$), 4.15 (s, 2H, CH$_2$), 7.01 (d, J = 6.69 Hz, 2H, Ar-H), 7.10 (d, J = 8.64 Hz, 2H, Ar-H), 7.20 (t, J = 1.44 Hz, 1H, Ar-H), 7.30 (m, 2H, Ar-H), 7.43 (m, 4H, Ar-H), 7.53 (m, 2H, Ar-H) (Figure S7); m/z 370.12, Elemental Analysis C, 77.82, H, 4.90, O, 17.28; m/z 370, C, 81.06, H, 5.99, O, 12.96.

Note. Crystallographic information is given in the supporting file with details of refinement and other structural parameters.

Conflict of Interests

The authors declare that there is no conflict of interests regarding the publication of this paper.

Acknowledgments

The authors are thankful to the Department of Chemistry, BHU, for proving NMR, FTIR, and single crystal X-ray data. Financial assistance from CSIR (Grant no. 01(2362)/10/EMR-II), New Delhi, in the form of a project and fellowships to Ambika Srivastava and Pooja Singh and CSIR and UGC, New Delhi, in the form of SRF and UGC Fellowship, respectively, is gratefully acknowledged.

References

[1] L. J. Black, C. D. Jones, and J. F. Falcone, "Antagonism of estrogen action with a new benzothiophene derived antiestrogen," *Life Sciences*, vol. 32, no. 9, pp. 1031–1036, 1983.

[2] A. U. Buzdar, C. Marcus, F. Holmes, V. Hug, and G. Hortobagyi, "Phase II evaluation of LY156758 in metastatic breast cancer," *Oncology*, vol. 45, no. 5, pp. 344–345, 1988.

[3] K. R. Snyder, N. Sparano, and J. M. Malinowski, "Raloxifene hydrochloride," *American Journal of Health-System Pharmacy*, vol. 57, no. 18, pp. 1669–1678, 2000.

[4] V. C. Jordan, E. Phelps, and J. U. Lindgren, "Effects of antiestrogens on bone in castrated and intact female rats," *Breast Cancer Research and Treatment*, vol. 10, no. 1, pp. 31–35, 1987.

[5] L. J. Black, M. Sato, E. R. Rowley et al., "Raloxifene (LY139481 HCI) prevents bone loss and reduces serum cholesterol without causing uterine hypertrophy in ovariectomized rats," *The Journal of Clinical Investigation*, vol. 93, no. 1, pp. 63–69, 1994.

[6] M. M. Gottardis and V. C. Jordan, "Antitumor actions of keoxifene and tamoxifen in the N-nitrosomethylurea-induced rat mammary carcinoma model," *Cancer Research*, vol. 47, no. 15, pp. 4020–4024, 1987.

[7] M. A. Anzano, C. W. Peer, J. M. Smith et al., "Chemoprevention of mammary carcinogenesis in the rat: combined use of raloxifene and 9-cis-retinoic acid," *Journal of the National Cancer Institute*, vol. 88, no. 2, pp. 123–125, 1996.

[8] B. Ettinger, D. M. Black, B. H. Mitlak et al., "Reduction of vertebral fracture risk in postmenopausal women with osteoporosis treated with raloxifene: results from a 3-year randomized clinical trial," *The Journal of the American Medical Association*, vol. 282, no. 7, pp. 637–645, 1999.

[9] S. R. Cummings, S. Eckert, K. A. Krueger et al., "The effect of raloxifene on risk of breast cancer in postmenopausal women: results from the MORE randomized trial," *The Journal of the American Medical Association*, vol. 281, no. 23, pp. 2189–2197, 1999.

[10] M. Clarke, R. Collins, C. Davies, J. Godwin, R. Gray, and R. Peto, "The EBCTCG secretariat, clinical trial service, unit, radcliffe infirmary, Oxford OX2 6HE, UK," *The Lancet*, vol. 351, pp. 1451–1467, 1998.

[11] B. Fisher, J. P. Costantino, D. L. Wickerham et al., "Tamoxifen for prevention of breast cancer: report of the National Surgical Adjuvant Breast and Bowel Project P-1 Study," *Journal of the National Cancer Institute*, vol. 90, no. 18, pp. 1371–1388, 1998.

[12] R. R. Love, R. B. Mazess, H. S. Barden et al., "Effects of tamoxifen on bone mineral density in postmenopausal women with breast cancer," *The New England Journal of Medicine*, vol. 326, no. 13, pp. 852–856, 1992.

[13] V. J. Assikis, P. Neven, V. C. Jordan, and I. Vergote, "A realistic clinical perspective of tamoxifen and endometrial carcinogenesis," *European Journal of Cancer A*, vol. 32, no. 9, pp. 1464–1476, 1996.

[14] E. J. Lederer, "Chemistry and biochemistry of some mammalian secretions and excretions," *Journal of the Chemical Society*, pp. 2115–2125, 1949.

[15] G. G. Freeman, "Isolation of alternariol and alternariol monomethyl ether from *Alternaria dauci* (kühn) groves and skolko," *Phytochemistry*, vol. 5, no. 4, pp. 719–725, 1966.

[16] W. T. L. Sidwell, H. Fritz, and C. Tamm, "Autumnariol und Autumnariniol, zwei neue Dibenzo-α-pyrone aus *Eucomis autumnalis Graeb*. Nachweis einer Fernkopplung über sechs Bindungen in den magnetischen Protonenresonanz—Spektren," *Helvetica Chimica Acta*, vol. 54, no. 1, pp. 207–215, 1971.

[17] L. Farkas, F. Soti, M. Incze, and M. Nogradi, "Synthese natürlicher Dibenzo-α-pyrone, I. Synthese des Autumnariniols und des Autumnariniols," *Chemische Berichte*, vol. 107, no. 12, pp. 3874–3877, 1974.

[18] S. Ghosal, J. P. Reddy, and V. K. Lal, "Shilajit I: chemical constituents," *Journal of Pharmaceutical Sciences*, vol. 65, no. 5, pp. 772–773, 1976.

[19] B. Naser-Hijazi, B. Stolze, and K. S. Zanker, *Second Proceedings of the International Society of the Coumarin Investigators*, Springer, Berlin, Germany, 1994.

[20] R. D. H. Murray, J. Méndez, and S. A. Brown, *The Natural Coumarin: Occurrence, Chemistry and Biochemistry*, John Wiley, Chichester, UK, 1982.

[21] J. D. Hepworth, C. D. Gabbutt, and B. N. Heron, *Comprehensive Heterocyclic Chemistry II*, vol. 5, Pergamon Press, Oxford, UK, 1996.

[22] F. M. Deans, *Naturally Occurring Oxygen Ring Compounds*, Butterworths, London, UK, 1963.

[23] J. A. Joule and K. Mills, Eds., *Heterocyclic Chemistry*, Blackwell Science, Oxford, UK, 4th edition, 2006.

[24] R. D. H. Murray, "Naturally occurring plant coumarins," *Fortschritte der Chemie Organischer Naturstoffe*, vol. 35, pp. 199–249, 1978.

[25] G. R. Geen, J. M. Evans, and A. K. Vong, in *Comprehensive Heterocyclic Chemistry II*, A. R. Katritzky, C. W. Rees, and E. F. V. Scriven, Eds., vol. 5, p. 469, Pergamon Press, Oxford, UK, 1984.

[26] H.-X. Xu and S. F. Lee, "Activity of plant flavonoids against antibiotic-resistant bacteria," *Phytotherapy Research*, vol. 15, no. 1, pp. 39–43, 2001.

[27] J. M. Hamilton-Miller, "Antimicrobial properties of tea (*Camellia sinensis* L.)," *Antimicrobial Agents and Chemotherapy*, vol. 39, no. 11, pp. 2375–2377, 1995.

[28] K. C. Fylaktakidou, D. J. Hadjipavlou-Litina, K. E. Litinas, and D. N. Nicolaides, "Natural and synthetic coumarin derivatives with anti-inflammatory/antioxidant activities," *Current Pharmaceutical Design*, vol. 10, no. 30, pp. 3813–3833, 2004.

[29] J. R. Hwu, R. Singha, S. C. Hong et al., "Synthesis of new benzimidazole-coumarin conjugates as anti-hepatitis C virus agents," *Antiviral Research*, vol. 77, no. 2, pp. 157–162, 2008.

[30] S. Sardari, Y. Mori, K. Horita, R. G. Micetich, S. Nishibe, and M. Daneshtalab, "Synthesis and antifungal activity of coumarins and angular furanocoumarins," *Bioorganic & Medicinal Chemistry*, vol. 7, no. 9, pp. 1933–1940, 1999.

[31] D. Egan, P. James, D. Cooke, and R. O'Kennedy, "Studies on the cytostatic and cytotoxic effects and mode of action of 8-nitro-7-hydroxycoumarin," *Cancer Letters*, vol. 118, no. 2, pp. 201–211, 1997.

[32] P. Valenti, A. Rampa, M. Recanatini et al., "Synthesis, cytotoxicity and SAR of simple geiparvarin analogues," *Anti-Cancer Drug Design*, vol. 12, no. 6, pp. 443–451, 1997.

[33] C. Spino, M. Dodier, and S. Sotheeswaran, "Anti-HIV coumarins from calophyllum seed oil," *Bioorganic and Medicinal Chemistry Letters*, vol. 8, no. 24, pp. 3475–3478, 1998.

[34] L. M. Bedoya, M. Beltran, R. Sancho et al., "4-Phenylcoumarins as HIV transcription inhibitors," *Bioorganic & Medicinal Chemistry Letters*, vol. 15, no. 20, pp. 4447–4450, 2005.

[35] K.-H. Lee, "Current developments in the discovery and design of new drug candidates from plant natural product leads," *Journal of Natural Products*, vol. 67, no. 2, pp. 273–283, 2004.

[36] D. Yu, M. Suzuki, L. Xie, S. L. Morris-Natschke, and K.-H. Lee, "Recent progress in the development of coumarin derivatives as potent anti-HIV agents," *Medicinal Research Reviews*, vol. 23, no. 3, pp. 322–345, 2003.

[37] S. Kirkiacharian, D. T. Thuy, S. Sicsic, R. Bakhchinian, R. Kurkjian, and T. Tonnaire, "Structure–activity relationships of some 3-substituted-4-hydroxycoumarins as HIV-1 protease inhibitors," *Farmaco*, vol. 57, no. 9, pp. 703–708, 2002.

[38] A. G. Kidane, H. Salacinski, A. Tiwari, K. R. Bruckdorfer, and A. M. Seifalian, "Anticoagulant and antiplatelet agents: their clinical and device application(s) together with usages to engineer surfaces," *Biomacromolecules*, vol. 5, no. 3, pp. 798–813, 2004.

[39] K. M. Khan, Z. S. Saify, M. Z. Khan et al., "Synthesis of coumarin derivatives with cytotoxic, antibacterial and antifungal activity," *Journal of Enzyme Inhibition and Medicinal Chemistry*, vol. 19, no. 4, pp. 373–379, 2004.

[40] G. Appendino, E. Mercalli, N. Fuzzati et al., "Antimycobacterial coumarins from the Sardinian giant fennel (*Ferula communis*)," *Journal of Natural Products*, vol. 67, no. 12, pp. 2108–2110, 2004.

[41] N. Hamdi, M. Saoud, and A. Romerosa, "4-Hydroxy coumarine: a versatile reagent for the synthesis of heterocyclic and vanillin ether coumarins with biological activities," in *Bioactive Heterocycles V*, vol. 11 of *Topics in Heterocyclic Chemistry*, pp. 283–301, Springer, Berlin, Germany, 2007.

[42] F. Chimenti, B. Bizzarri, A. Bolasco et al., "Synthesis and in vitro selective anti-Helicobacter pylori activity of N-substituted-2-oxo-2H-1-benzopyran-3-carboxamides," *European Journal of Medicinal Chemistry*, vol. 41, no. 2, pp. 208–212, 2006.

[43] C. Ito, M. Itoigawa, Y. Mishina et al., "Chemical constituents of *Calophyllum brasiliense*. 2. Structure of three new coumarins and cancer chemopreventive activity of 4-substituted coumarins," *Journal of Natural Products*, vol. 66, no. 3, pp. 368–371, 2003.

[44] I. Kostova, "Synthetic and natural coumarins as cytotoxic agents," *Current Medicinal Chemistry—Anti-Cancer Agents*, vol. 5, no. 1, pp. 29–46, 2005.

[45] G. Melagraki, A. Afantitis, O. Igglessi-Markopoulou et al., "Synthesis and evaluation of the antioxidant and anti-inflammatory activity of novel coumarin-3-aminoamides and their alpha-lipoic acid adducts," *European Journal of Medicinal Chemistry*, vol. 44, no. 7, pp. 3020–3026, 2009.

[46] C. A. Kontogiorgis and D. J. Hadjipavlou-Litina, "Synthesis and antiinflammatory activity of coumarin derivatives," *Journal of Medicinal Chemistry*, vol. 48, no. 20, pp. 6400–6408, 2005.

[47] S. Stanchev, V. Hadjimitova, T. Traykov, T. Boyanov, and I. Manolov, "Investigation of the antioxidant properties of some new 4-hydroxycoumarin derivatives," *European Journal of Medicinal Chemistry*, vol. 44, no. 7, pp. 3077–3082, 2009.

[48] C. A. Kontogiorgis and D. J. Hadjipavlou-Litina, "Synthesis and biological evaluation of novel coumarin derivatives with a 7-azomethine linkage," *Bioorganic and Medicinal Chemistry Letters*, vol. 14, no. 3, pp. 611–614, 2004.

[49] C. Xiao, Z.-G. Song, and Z.-Q. Liu, "Synthesis of methyl-substituted xanthotoxol to clarify prooxidant effect of methyl on radical-induced oxidation of DNA," *European Journal of Medicinal Chemistry*, vol. 45, no. 6, pp. 2559–2566, 2010.

[50] O. M. Abdel Hafez, K. M. Amin, N. A. Abdel-Latif, T. K. Mohamed, E. Y. Ahmed, and T. Maher, "Synthesis and antitumor activity of some new xanthotoxin derivatives," *European Journal of Medicinal Chemistry*, vol. 44, no. 7, pp. 2967–2974, 2009.

[51] V. Reutrakul, P. Leewanich, P. Tuchinda et al., "Cytotoxic coumarins from *Mammea harmandii*," *Planta Medica*, vol. 69, no. 11, pp. 1048–1051, 2003.

[52] I. Kempen, D. Papapostolou, N. Thierry et al., "3-Bromophenyl 6-acetoxymethyl-2-oxo-2H-1-benzopyran-3-carboxylate inhibits cancer cell invasion *in vitro* and tumour growth *in vivo*," *British Journal of Cancer*, vol. 88, no. 7, pp. 1111–1118, 2003.

[53] P. O'Kennedy and R. D. Thornes, Eds., *Coumarins: Biology, Applications and Mode of Action*, John Wiley & Sons, Chichester, UK, 1997.

[54] L. Zhi, C. M. Tegley, E. A. Kallel et al., "5-Aryl-1,2-dihydrochromeno[3,4-f]quinolines: a novel class of nonsteroidal human progesterone receptor agonists," *Journal of Medicinal Chemistry*, vol. 41, no. 3, pp. 291–302, 1998.

[55] J. M. Schmidt, G. B. Tremblay, M. Pagé et al., "Synthesis and evaluation of a novel nonsteroidal-specific endothelial cell proliferation inhibitor," *Journal of Medicinal Chemistry*, vol. 46, no. 8, pp. 1289–1292, 2003.

[56] K. Hajela, K. Kapoor, and R. Kapil, "Synthesis and post-coital contraceptive activity of ether and ester analogues of 2,3-diaryl-2H-1-benzopyrans," *Bioorganic & Medicinal Chemistry*, vol. 3, pp. 1417–1420, 1995.

[57] K. Hajela and R. S. Kapil, "Synthesis and post-coital contraceptive activity of a new series of substituted 2,3-diaryl-2H-1-benzopyrans," *European Journal of Medicinal Chemistry*, vol. 32, no. 2, pp. 135–139, 1997.

[58] K. Hajela, J. Pandey, A. Dwivedy et al., "Resolution, molecular structure and biological activities of the D- and L-enantiomers of potent anti-implantation agent, DL-2-[4-(2-piperidinoethoxy)phenyl]-3-phenyl-2H-1-benzopyran," *Bioorganic & Medicinal Chemistry*, vol. 7, no. 9, pp. 2083–2090, 1999.

[59] H. Pechmann and C. Duisberg, "Neue Bildungsweise der Cumarine. Synthese des Daphnetins. I," *Chemische Berichte*, vol. 17, no. 1, pp. 929–936, 1884.

[60] J. Johnson, "The Perkin reaction and related reactions," *Organic Reactions*, vol. 1, pp. 210–265, 1942.

[61] G. Jones, "The Knoevenagel condensation," *Organic Reactions*, vol. 15, pp. 204–599, 1967.

[62] G. Brufola, F. Fringuelli, O. Piermatti, and F. Pizzo, "Simple and efficient one-pot preparation of 3-substituted coumarins in water," *Heterocycles*, vol. 43, no. 6, pp. 1257–1266, 1996.

[63] R. L. Shriner, "The reformatsky reaction," in *Organic Reactions*, vol. 1, pp. 1–58, John Wiley & Sons, 1942.

[64] I. Yavari, R. Hekmat-Shoar, and A. Zonouzi, "A new and efficient route to 4-carboxymethylcoumarins mediated by vinyltriphenylphosphonium salt," *Tetrahedron Letters*, vol. 39, no. 16, pp. 2391–2392, 1998.

[65] J. R. Johnson, "Perkin reaction and related reactions," *Organic Reactions*, vol. 1, p. 210, 1942.

[66] M. H. Elnagdi, S. O. Abdallah, K. M. Ghoneim, E. M. Ebied, and K. N. Kassab, "Synthesis of some Coumarin derivatives as potential LaserDyes," *Journal of Chemical Research, Synopses*, no. 2, pp. 44–45, 1997.

8

Comparative Effect of Lisinopril and Fosinopril in Mitigating Learning and Memory Deficit in Scopolamine-Induced Amnesic Rats

Debasree Deb,[1] **K. L. Bairy,**[2] **Veena Nayak,**[2] **and Mohandas Rao**[3]

[1]*Department of Pharmacology, Melaka Manipal Medical College, Manipal University, Manipal Campus, Manipal 576104, India*
[2]*Department of Pharmacology, Kasturba Medical College, Manipal University, Manipal 576104, India*
[3]*Department of Anatomy, Melaka Manipal Medical College, Manipal University, Manipal Campus, Manipal 576104, India*

Correspondence should be addressed to K. L. Bairy; kl.bairy@manipal.edu

Academic Editor: Masahiro Oike

Lisinopril and fosinopril were compared on scopolamine-induced learning and memory deficits in rats. A total of eighty-four male Wistar rats were divided into seven groups. Group I received 2% gum acacia orally for 4 weeks, group II received normal saline, and group III received scopolamine (2 mg/kg/ip) as single dose. Groups IV and V received lisinopril (0.225 mg/kg and 0.45 mg/kg), while Groups VI and VII received fosinopril (0.90 mg/kg and 1.80 mg/kg), respectively, orally for four weeks, followed by scopolamine (2 mg/kg/ip) given 45 minutes prior to experimental procedure. Evaluation of learning and memory was assessed by using passive avoidance, Morris water maze, and elevated plus maze tests followed by analysis of hippocampal morphology and quantification of the number of surviving neurons. Scopolamine induced marked impairment of memory in behavioral tests which correlated with morphological changes in hippocampus. Pretreatment with fosinopril 1.80 mg/kg was found to significantly ameliorate the memory deficits and hippocampal degeneration induced by scopolamine. Fosinopril exhibits antiamnesic activity, indicating its possible role in preventing memory deficits seen in dementia though the precise mechanism underlying this effect needs to be further evaluated.

1. Introduction

Learning and memory are the most fundamental and closely related processes in the brain. Memory is defined as a change in mental representation caused by an experience, and learning is defined as a process of acquiring memory [1]. During this period of consolidation, memory can be disrupted with a wide variety of amnesia inducing agents. Scopolamine, a muscarinic receptor antagonist, induces memory deficits in rodents and healthy humans, and this effect has been proposed to mimic the cognitive and behavioral deficits seen during aging or in Alzheimer's disease (AD) [2]. Scopolamine produces a reversible impairment in maintaining attention, processing of information, and the acquisition of new knowledge in both rodents [3] and humans [4]. The amnesic action produced by the administration of scopolamine has thus been widely used as an experimental model for the screening and validation of drugs with potential cognitive enhancing ability [5, 6].

Angiotensin converting enzyme inhibitors (ACEIs) are a class of drugs effective in controlling hypertension and treating congestive heart failure, and their use in these patients has been associated with reduced cardiovascular morbidity and mortality [7]. However, in addition to their role in controlling blood pressure, ACE inhibitors have been shown to be effective in preventing cognitive decline and improving cognitive function in patients with hypertension [8, 9]. It has also been suggested that all ACE inhibitors do not prevent dementia in older adults being treated for hypertension but centrally acting ACEIs such as ramipril or perindopril do appear to reduce cognitive decline in older adults [10]. Because all ACEIs share a similar mechanism of action, it can be assumed that all centrally acting ACEIs may possess cognitive enhancing activity like ramipril or perindopril.

The present study was thus undertaken to investigate the effects of two centrally acting ACEIs, namely, lisinopril and fosinopril, for their effect on learning and memory in scopolamine-induced amnesic rats. Further, the effects of scopolamine and test drugs on rat hippocampal morphology were analysed followed by quantification of the number of healthy neurons.

2. Materials and Methods

2.1. Animals. A total of eighty four male Wistar rats weighing 200–250 grams were used in the study. All animals were housed in polypropylene cage with only four animals in each cage to prevent overcrowding. The animals were kept at room temperature ($25 \pm 3°C$) with a 12 h dark/light cycle and were provided with standard laboratory feed (VRK Nutritional Solutions, Pune, India Ltd.) and water *ad libitum*. The experimental protocol was approved by the Institutional Animal Ethical Committee (number IAEC/KMC/36/2011-2012, May 2011) and experiments were conducted in accordance with the CPSCEA guidelines on the use and care of experimental animals.

2.2. Drugs and Doses. Lisinopril and fosinopril powders were obtained as generous gift samples from Torrent Pharmaceuticals Ltd., Ahmedabad, India. Scopolamine hydrobromide was procured from Sigma Aldrich, Mumbai.

Rats equivalent doses in mg/kg body weight of clinical doses were calculated as mg/kg body weight as described by Paget and Barnes [11]. All the drugs except scopolamine were dissolved in 2% gum acacia while scopolamine was dissolved in normal saline.

The experiment was conducted in two stages as follows.

Stage 1. A total of 42 male Wistar rats were randomly divided into seven groups for assessing learning and memory using the elevated plus maze test and passive avoidance test.

Stage 2. A total of 42 male Wistar rats were randomly divided into seven groups for assessing learning and memory using the Morris water maze test.

The seven groups were divided as follows:

Group I: 2 mL/kg of 2% gum acacia (normal control),

Group II: 1 mL/kg of 0.9% normal saline i.p. (saline control),

Group III: 2% gum acacia and scopolamine treatment,

Group IV: lisinopril 0.225 mg/kg and scopolamine treatment,

Group V: lisinopril 0.45 mg/kg and scopolamine treatment,

Group VI: fosinopril 0.90 mg/kg and scopolamine treatment,

Group VII: fosinopril 1.80 mg/kg and scopolamine treatment.

Each of the above groups of animals (except Group II) was treated orally for 4 weeks. Group II received i.p. injection of normal saline 45 minutes before experimental procedures. Scopolamine 2 mg/kg [12, 13] was administered intraperitoneally to the above groups of animals (except Groups I and II) for induction of amnesia, 45 minutes before the behavioural tests.

2.3. Behavioural Tests

2.3.1. Elevated Plus Maze Test. Elevated plus maze serves as the exteroceptive behavioral model to evaluate acquisition and retention of memory in rats. The elevated plus maze for rats consists of two open arms (16 cm × 5 cm) and two covered arms (16 cm × 5 cm × 12 cm) extended from a central platform (5 cm × 5 cm) and is elevated to a height of 25 cm from the floor. Each rat was placed at the end of an open arm, facing away from the central platform. The rats received drug treatment for 4 weeks, followed by administration of scopolamine (2 mg/kg body weight, dissolved in normal saline) for induction of amnesia, 45 minutes before the training trial. Transfer latency (TL) which is the time taken by the rats to move from open arm to closed arm with all four legs in elevated plus maze was noted. The rat was allowed to explore the maze for another 2 min and then allowed to return to its home cage. After 24 hours of acquisition trial, TL was again noted as an index of retrieval [14].

2.3.2. Step-Through Passive Avoidance Test. Passive avoidance test is an exteroceptive behavioural model for testing learning and memory in experimental rodents. The apparatus has a box (27 cm × 27 cm × 27 cm) of three wooden walls and one Plexiglas wall, with a grid floor (made up of 3 mm stainless-steel rods set 8 mm apart) and a platform (10 cm × 7 cm × 1.7 cm) at the centre of the grid floor. The box was kept illuminated with a 15 W bulb during the experiment. Each rat was kept in the larger compartment facing away from the entrance to the dark compartment. Three exploratory trials were given to each rat in which the rat explored the apparatus for 3 minutes. The intertrial interval was 5 minutes. The rat was removed from the cage during the intertrial period. In each trial, the total time taken by the animal to enter the dark compartment was noted using a stopwatch. A decrease in the latency to enter the dark compartment was considered as an index of improved learning. After the third exploratory trial, the rat was kept in the light compartment and when it entered the dark compartment, the sliding door was closed and three foot shocks (50 Hz, 1.5 mA, and 1 s duration) were delivered at 5-second intervals. The retention test was carried out after 24 hours of receiving the aversive stimuli.

Rats received gum acacia or test compounds for 4 weeks; this was followed by scopolamine (2 mg/kg body weight, dissolved in normal saline) for induction of amnesia, 45 minutes before the acquisition trial. After 24 hours of acquisition trials, the rats were again placed in the light compartment. The latency time required for the animal to enter the dark compartment and the total time spent by the animal in the light compartment were recorded. The latency time was recorded as 3 minutes for those animals that did not enter the dark compartment within 3 minutes. Increase in the latency to enter the dark compartment and more time spent in the light compartment indicated positive memory retention [15].

2.3.3. Morris Water Maze Test.

Morris water maze is a behavioural test to evaluate spatial learning and memory in experimental rodents. It is a circular tank (diameter 150 cm and height 45 cm), which was filled with water and maintained at 25°C. The water was made opaque by adding milk. The tank was divided into four equal quadrants (Q1, Q2, Q3, and Q4). A white platform (10 cm^2) centered in one of the four quadrants of the pool was submerged approximately 1 cm below the surface of water. The position of platform and clues were kept consistent throughout the training session. In our study, the target quadrant was considered as Q4. Each animal was subjected to four consecutive acquisition trials on each day with an interval of 5 min, during which rats were allowed to locate the hidden platform and allowed to remain there for 20 sec. If the animal was unable to locate the hidden platform within 60 sec, it was gently guided by hand to the platform and allowed to remain there for 20 sec. During each trial, the latencies of rats to locate the hidden platform were recorded and the latency was considered as an index of acquisition and learning. On the 5th day, the platform was removed and each rat was allowed to explore the pool for 60 s. The latency to enter the target quadrant Q4 and the total time spent in target quadrant Q4 were noted as indices of retrieval. Rats received gum acacia or test compounds for 4 weeks; this was followed by scopolamine (2 mg/kg body weight, dissolved in normal saline) for induction of amnesia. All the animals were tested for spatial memory 45 mins after the scopolamine treatment [16, 17].

2.4. Histological Analysis by Hematoxylin and Eosin (H&E) Staining.

All histological procedures were kept uniform for control and test group animals. At the end of behavioural tests, the rats were sacrificed by cervical dislocation under ether anaesthesia. The animals were perfused with 250 mL 4% paraformaldehyde, followed by 0.01 mol/L phosphate buffered saline (PBS), and the brain was exposed by cutting the skull along the midline. The brain section with hippocampus was carefully dissected out and fixed in 10% buffered formalin (with pH 7.4) for 24 h. The brains were then dehydrated in ascending grades of alcohol: 50% alcohol: 24 hours, 70% alcohol: 24 hours, 90% alcohol: 12 hours, and absolute alcohol: 12 hours. The tissue was cleared in xylene for 1-2 hours, infiltrated with paraffin wax (4 changes of 1 hour each), and embedded in fresh paraffin wax. Five-micron thick paraffin sections were obtained and mounted on clean glass slides, labeled, and stained with hematoxylin and eosin (H&E) according to standard procedure. The hippocampal CA1, CA3, and dentate gyrus regions were studied under a light microscope. To avoid observer's bias, an independent person coded the slides before subjecting them to morphological evaluations.

Quantification of neurons in the subregions of hippocampus (CA1, CA3, and dentate gyrus) was done using the light microscope under 40x (Magnus, Olympus Pvt. Ltd., New Delhi, India). To avoid manual bias slides from different groups were coded while counting. Cell counting was done using an ocular micrometer. The number of surviving or viable neurons (neurons with a distinct nucleus) within a specific measured (using ocular micrometer) area (e.g., 250-micron area) under 40x was counted. Ten sections were counted per rat and the mean was taken. Cells with darkly stained shrunken cell body and cells with fragmented nuclei were excluded from quantification.

2.5. Statistical Analysis.

Data obtained from experiments were expressed as mean ± SE. Statistical differences between the treatment and the control groups were calculated by one-way analysis of variance (ANOVA) followed by Tukey's post hoc test. The data was considered to be statistically significant if the probability had a value of 0.05 or less.

3. Results

3.1. Effects of Lisinopril and Fosinopril on Elevated Plus Maze.

Transfer latency (TL) of control animals decreased on the 2nd day, after 24 hours of training on the elevated plus maze. Administration of scopolamine increased the TL on the 1st and 2nd days, and it was significantly different compared to control ($p < 0.001$). Pretreatment with low and high doses of lisinopril and low dose of fosinopril did not show any significant difference in TL of rats on 1st and 2nd days compared to scopolamine group. Rats which were pretreated with high dose of fosinopril however showed a significant decrease in TL of rats on 1st and 2nd days compared to scopolamine group ($p < 0.001$), as shown in Table 1.

3.2. Effects of Lisinopril and Fosinopril in Passive Avoidance Test.

During the exploratory trials, the latency to enter the dark compartment was decreased in all the groups from first to third trial. The scopolamine treated animals took more time to enter the dark compartment during the three exploration trials (Table 2 and Figure 1). Rats pretreated with lower and higher doses of lisinopril did not show significant difference during the exploration trials compared to scopolamine treated rats. Lower dose of fosinopril also could not significantly ameliorate scopolamine-induced learning impairment as reflected in their latency during the exploratory trials (Table 2 and Figure 1). However, rats pretreated with high dose of fosinopril showed a decreased latency to enter the dark compartment during the exploratory trials and spent more time in the light compartment in each successive trial compared to scopolamine treated rats ($p < 0.05$). This is indicative of positive learning behaviour among fosinopril treated rats.

During the memory retention test, the latency to enter the dark compartment was significantly reduced for scopolamine and lisinopril treated groups compared to normal control rats ($p < 0.001$). Rats which received scopolamine and lisinopril also spent lesser time in the light compartment compared to normal control rats ($p < 0.05$). Pretreatment with higher dose of fosinopril increased the entrance latency time of rats and the difference was statistically significant compared to scopolamine group ($p < 0.001$). Rats pretreated with higher dose of fosinopril also spent more time in the light compartment indicating improved memory retention and

TABLE 1: Effects of lisinopril and fosinopril on the transfer latencies on 1st day and 2nd day in elevated plus maze test.

Treatment	Transfer latency on the 1st day (sec)	Transfer latency on 2nd day after 24 h (sec)
Control	$57.50 \pm 4.32^{**}$	$35.50 \pm 2.15^{**,b}$
Saline control	$61.00 \pm 3.20^{**}$	$37.90 \pm 2.81^{**}$
Scopolamine	92.17 ± 5.57^{b}	94.00 ± 3.55^{b}
Lisinopril (0.225 mg/kg) + scopolamine	83.33 ± 3.81^{b}	75.61 ± 2.75^{b}
Lisinopril (0.45 mg/kg) + scopolamine	$76.16 \pm 5.74^{*,a}$	$55.17 \pm 3.04^{**,a}$
Fosinopril (0.90 mg/kg) + scopolamine	85.33 ± 3.56^{b}	75.67 ± 5.16^{b}
Fosinopril (1.80 mg/kg) + scopolamine	$73.50 \pm 3.34^{**,a}$	$53.00 \pm 3.67^{**}$

Comparisons between control, scopolamine, lisinopril, and fosinopril treated groups in the elevated plus maze test. Values are mean $\pm$ SE, *versus scopolamine ($p < 0.05$), **versus scopolamine ($p < 0.001$), ^{a}versus control ($p < 0.05$), and ^{b}versus control ($p < 0.001$).

TABLE 2: Effects of lisinopril and fosinopril on the exploratory behaviour of scopolamine-induced amnesic rats in passive avoidance test.

Treatment	Exploration trial (day 1)	Exploration trial (day 2)	Exploration trial (day 3)
Control	$19.3 \pm 0.95^{**}$	$17.16 \pm 1.54^{**}$	$12.67 \pm 1.31^{**}$
Saline control	$20.6 \pm 1.28^{**}$	$16.00 \pm 2.71^{**}$	$14.10 \pm 1.92^{**}$
Scopolamine	37.3 ± 2.55^{b}	33.5 ± 1.88^{b}	30.67 ± 1.85^{b}
Lisinopril (0.225 mg/kg) + scopolamine	39.5 ± 2.91^{b}	38.22 ± 1.03^{b}	27.50 ± 2.46^{b}
Lisinopril (0.45 mg/kg) + scopolamine	34.75 ± 1.88^{b}	31.00 ± 2.71^{b}	$25.21 \pm 1.18^{b,*}$
Fosinopril (0.90 mg/kg) + scopolamine	35.75 ± 2.78^{b}	36.0 ± 2.92^{b}	$25.50 \pm 1.08^{b,*}$
Fosinopril (1.80 mg/kg) + scopolamine	34.00 ± 3.02^{b}	$28.75 \pm 2.45^{a,*}$	$19.75 \pm 1.26^{a,*}$

Comparison between control, scopolamine, lisinopril, and fosinopril during the exploration trials in passive avoidance test. Values are mean $\pm$ SE, *versus scopolamine ($p < 0.05$), **versus scopolamine ($p < 0.001$), ^{a}versus control ($p < 0.05$), and ^{b}versus control ($p < 0.001$).

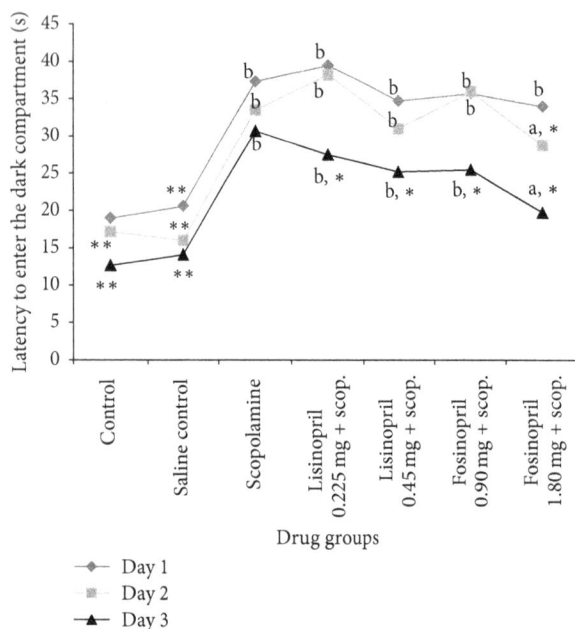

FIGURE 1: Effect of lisinopril and fosinopril in scopolamine-induced amnesic rats during the exploration trials in passive avoidance test. Comparison between control, scopolamine, lisinopril, and fosinopril during the exploration trials in passive avoidance test. Values are mean $\pm$ SE, *versus scopolamine ($p < 0.05$), **versus scopolamine ($p < 0.001$), ^{a}versus control ($p < 0.05$), and ^{b}versus control ($p < 0.001$).

the difference was significant compared to rats that received only scopolamine ($p < 0.001$), as shown in Table 3.

3.3. Effects of Lisinopril and Fosinopril during Morris Water Maze Test.

Control rats which received gum acacia and saline rapidly learned the location of the hidden platform as reflected by a decrease in their latencies from day 1 to day 4, indicating normal acquisition behaviour (Table 4 and Figure 2). Rats which received scopolamine showed an increased latency to locate the hidden platform during the acquisition trials, the difference being statistically significant compared to control rats ($p < 0.001$). This indicates impairment of acquisition in the scopolamine treated rats. Further, scopolamine treated rats showed a significant increase in the latency to locate the target quadrant (Q4) compared to control rats ($p < 0.001$), which indicates impaired memory (Table 4 and Figure 2).

Rats treated with lisinopril (0.225 mg/kg and 0.45 mg/kg) and low dose fosinopril (0.90 mg/kg) could not ameliorate the scopolamine-induced impairment in both the learning and memory retention parameters of water maze tests (Tables 4 and 5). This was evident by increased latency to locate the hidden platform during the acquisition trials and greater time spent to locate the target quadrant (Q4) during the memory retention trial. Higher dose of fosinopril (1.80 mg/kg) showed a decrease in the latencies from day 1 to day 4 during the acquisition trials. Pretreatment with fosinopril in higher dose demonstrated a reversal of amnesia, as indicated by decreased

TABLE 3: Effects of lisinopril and fosinopril on memory retention behaviour of scopolamine-induced amnesic rats in passive avoidance test.

Treatment	Latency to enter the dark compartment (sec) 24 h after receiving foot shock	Total time spent in light compartment (sec) 24 h after receiving foot shock
Control	$51.83 \pm 2.71^{**}$	$114.50 \pm 3.87^{**}$
Saline control	$49.29 \pm 2.21^{**}$	$109.78 \pm 2.55^{**}$
Scopolamine	14.83 ± 1.05^b	57.33 ± 4.23^b
Lisinopril (0.225 mg/kg) + scopolamine	25.68 ± 2.34^b	63.00 ± 5.45^b
Lisinopril (0.45 mg/kg) + scopolamine	27.81 ± 4.78^b	73.67 ± 2.24^a
Fosinopril (0.90 mg/kg) + scopolamine	$29.83 \pm 4.09^{*,b}$	88.66 ± 8.59^b
Fosinopril (1.80 mg/kg) + scopolamine	$36.33 \pm 2.89^{**,a}$	$98.17 \pm 3.54^{**}$

Comparisons between control, scopolamine, lisinopril, and fosinopril during the retention trial in passive avoidance test. Values are mean ± SE, [*]versus scopolamine ($p < 0.05$), [**]versus scopolamine ($p < 0.001$), [a]versus control ($p < 0.05$), and [b]versus control ($p < 0.001$).

TABLE 4: Effects of lisinopril and fosinopril during acquisition trials in Morris water maze test.

Treatment	Latency (sec) to locate the hidden platform on day 1	Latency (sec) to locate the hidden platform on day 4	Mean swim speed (seconds)
Control	$44.89 \pm 1.42^{**}$	$17.24 \pm 0.88^{**}$	$0.166 \pm 0.12^{**}$
Saline control	$41.20 \pm 1.88^{**}$	$16.18 \pm 1.71^{**}$	$0.172 \pm 0.22^{**}$
Scopolamine	53.08 ± 1.56^b	38.42 ± 2.59^b	0.387 ± 0.18^b
Lisinopril (0.225 mg/kg) + scopolamine	50.47 ± 1.45^b	33.64 ± 1.90^b	0.307 ± 0.07^b
Lisinopril (0.45 mg/kg) + scopolamine	46.53 ± 2.08^a	35.93 ± 1.43^b	0.268 ± 0.20^b
Fosinopril (0.90 mg/kg) + scopolamine	47.08 ± 2.58^a	37.42 ± 1.23^b	0.294 ± 0.17^b
Fosinopril (1.80 mg/kg) + scopolamine	49.87 ± 0.89^a	$33.10 \pm 1.45^{*,a}$	$0.198 \pm 0.18^{a,*}$

Comparisons between control, scopolamine, lisinopril, and fosinopril treated groups during acquisition trials on day 1 and day 4, and on the mean swim speed during the Morris water maze test. Values are mean ± SE, [*]versus scopolamine ($p < 0.05$), [**]versus scopolamine ($p < 0.001$), [a]versus control ($p < 0.05$), and [b]versus control ($p < 0.001$).

TABLE 5: Effects of lisinopril and fosinopril in the probe trial on day 5 of Morris water maze test.

Treatment	Latency to enter the target quadrant (sec)	Total time spent in target quadrant (sec)
Control	$14.59 \pm 1.54^{**}$	$26.11 \pm 0.54^{**}$
Saline control	$17.11 \pm 1.62^{**}$	$29.20 \pm 1.66^{**}$
Scopolamine	27.48 ± 2.00^b	12.58 ± 0.42^b
Lisinopril (0.225 mg/kg) + scopolamine	23.90 ± 1.37^b	12.28 ± 0.37^b
Lisinopril (0.45 mg/kg) + scopolamine	22.83 ± 1.96^b	14.75 ± 0.96^b
Fosinopril (0.90 mg/kg) + scopolamine	22.29 ± 1.91^b	14.37 ± 0.91^b
Fosinopril (1.80 mg/kg) + scopolamine	$20.18 \pm 0.85^{*,a}$	$19.25 \pm 1.85^{*,a}$

Comparison between control, scopolamine, lisinopril, and fosinopril treated groups in the probe trial of Morris water maze test in which no platform was present. Values are mean ± SE, [*]versus scopolamine ($p < 0.05$), [**]versus scopolamine ($p < 0.001$), [a]versus control ($p < 0.05$), and [b]versus control ($p < 0.001$).

latency to reach the target quadrant and increased time spent in target quadrant, the difference being significant compared to scopolamine ($p < 0.05$).

3.4. Effects of Lisinopril and Fosinopril on Hippocampal Morphology and Degree of Neuronal Survival.

In hematoxylin and eosin stained sections of hippocampal CA3 (Figure 3), CA1 (Figure 4), and dentate gyrus regions (Figure 5), cells with lightly stained nucleus, healthy cell membrane, and clear cytoplasm were considered as normal neurons while flame-shaped cells with pyknotic cell bodies, homogenous cytoplasm, and intense basophilic appearance were considered as damaged cells. Control rats and rats treated with higher dose of fosinopril demonstrated healthy neurons in all the three regions of the hippocampus compared to scopolamine treated rats which showed damaged neuronal cells. However, treatment with lower and higher doses of lisinopril could not markedly reverse the scopolamine-induced morphological changes produced in the hippocampus as demonstrated in Figures 3, 4, and 5.

Quantification of healthy neurons in the CA3, CA1, and dentate gyrus (DG) regions revealed a significant decrease in the mean number of neurons in the scopolamine group compared to control rats (Figure 6). The mean number of healthy surviving neurons in the CA3, CA1, and DG of control group was found to be 35.00 ± 1.29, 29.50 ± 1.55, and 35.75 ± 1.10, respectively. This was reduced to 13.30 ± 1.37, 11.0 ± 1.68, and 17.5 ± 3.12 for CA3, CA1, and DG regions, respectively. ANOVA test revealed a significant difference in the mean values of control group compared to scopolamine group ($^{**}p < 0.001$) as shown in Figure 6. In rats pretreated

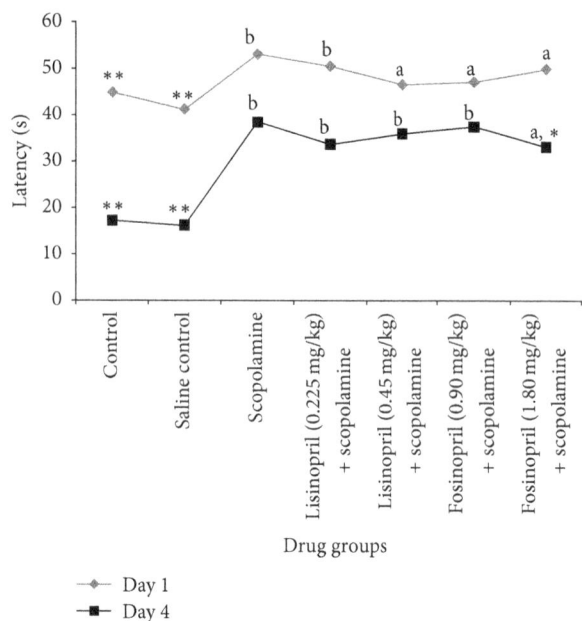

FIGURE 2: Effect of lisinopril and fosinopril in scopolamine-induced amnesic rats during the acquisition trials in Morris water maze test. Comparison between control, scopolamine, lisinopril, and fosinopril treated groups during the acquisition trials on day 1 and day 4 of Morris water maze test. Values are mean ± SE, *versus scopolamine ($p < 0.05$), **versus scopolamine ($p < 0.001$), [a]versus control ($p < 0.05$), and [b]versus control ($p < 0.001$).

with higher dose of lisinopril (0.45 mg/kg), the mean number of surviving neurons was 25.75 ± 1.79, 22.78 ± 1.69, and 27.75 ± 0.85 in the CA3, CA1, and DG regions, respectively, while for rats that received higher dose of fosinopril (1.80 mg/kg), the mean number of surviving neurons was 28.0 ± 1.49, 23.76 ± 1.68, and 30.15 ± 1.04 in CA3, CA1, and DG regions, respectively. Higher dose of lisinopril and fosinopril showed a significantly increased number of healthy neurons compared to scopolamine group but the numbers were not significantly increased compared to control rats ([b]$p < 0.001$ and [a]$p < 0.05$ for lisinopril and fosinopril, resp.) as shown in Figure 6.

4. Discussion

The present study was carried out using rats for investigation of learning and memory tasks. Passive avoidance is a fear-aggravated task used to assess memory or retention in animal models of CNS disorders, particularly dementia. Rats, as a part of their normal behaviour, generally avoid bright illumination and prefer dim illumination. When placed in a brightly illuminated compartment connected with a dark enclosure, they rapidly enter the dark compartment and remain there [15]. Once they receive an aversive consequence (foot shock) in the dark compartment, the animals modify their behaviour to avoid a noxious event by suppressing the learned habits of staying in the dark compartment and remain in the bright compartment. Since there is punishment to the natural exploratory drive of a rodent with a pulsating electric foot shock, this is clearly an aversive task. In our present study,

administration of scopolamine clearly produced memory deficits (amnesia) in rat performance in passive avoidance test as indicated by their shorter latency to enter into the dark compartment in the memory retention test compared to the control group. The mean latency of rats treated with high dose of fosinopril (1.80 mg/kg) was significantly higher compared to scopolamine group, indicating reversal of amnesia. This showed that scopolamine treated rats after being exposed to aversive stimulation in the passive avoidance task failed to remember the task on the following day, but this effect could be attenuated following treatment with fosinopril at a dose of 1.80 mg/kg, indicating that fosinopril has a positive effect on memory retention.

The Morris water maze (MWM) test is a well-established model for evaluating hippocampal dependent memory deficits in experimental animals and has been used for the evaluation of drugs with neurocognitive enhancing ability [18]. In the MWM task, the animal learns to swim in a water tank, guided by external cues, and climbs up to a submerged platform [16]. Based upon spatial information, this animal learns how to escape to a platform. Rats and mice are natural swimmers, but in this task they just want to get out of the water and escape into the platform. In our study, administration of scopolamine produced severe deficits in both the acquisition and the memory retention trials as indicated by their longer latencies to escape into the submerged platform. Scopolamine treated animals also spent lesser time in the target quadrant during the retention trial compared to control rats. Treatment with fosinopril 1.80 mg/kg could attenuate the scopolamine-induced memory deficits in the water maze test, demonstrated by their shorter latencies to locate the hidden platform during the acquisition and longer time spent in the target quadrant during the retention, thus indicating its potential memory enhancing effects.

The elevated plus maze test has been considered as an indicator of short-term memory [14]. In this test, scopolamine treated rats showed a significant decrease in transfer latencies on 1st day and 2nd day which could be markedly attenuated by pretreatment with fosinopril 1.80 mg/kg.

Data generated from the present study demonstrated that administration of scopolamine induces profound memory deficits in rat performance in all the three paradigms of learning and memory tasks. This change in behaviour was found to be associated with signs of neurodegeneration in the hippocampus as evident by the deeply stained and shrunken neuronal cells in CA3, CA1, and dentate gyrus regions of the hippocampus. Administration of 1.80 mg/kg fosinopril was found to arrest the scopolamine-induced degenerative changes in the hippocampus, as reflected by the decreased number of damaged neuronal cells in all the three regions of the hippocampus. Although the degeneration of cells in the hippocampus induced by scopolamine was decreased in all the groups, marked differences were noted only in rats that were treated with higher dose (1.80 mg/kg) of fosinopril.

Our study is the first of its kind that has investigated the effect of fosinopril on behavioural paradigms of memory retention. The beneficial effect of fosinopril on memory retention could be partly attributed to its ability to suppress angiotensin-II (Ang-II) mediated inhibition of acetylcholine

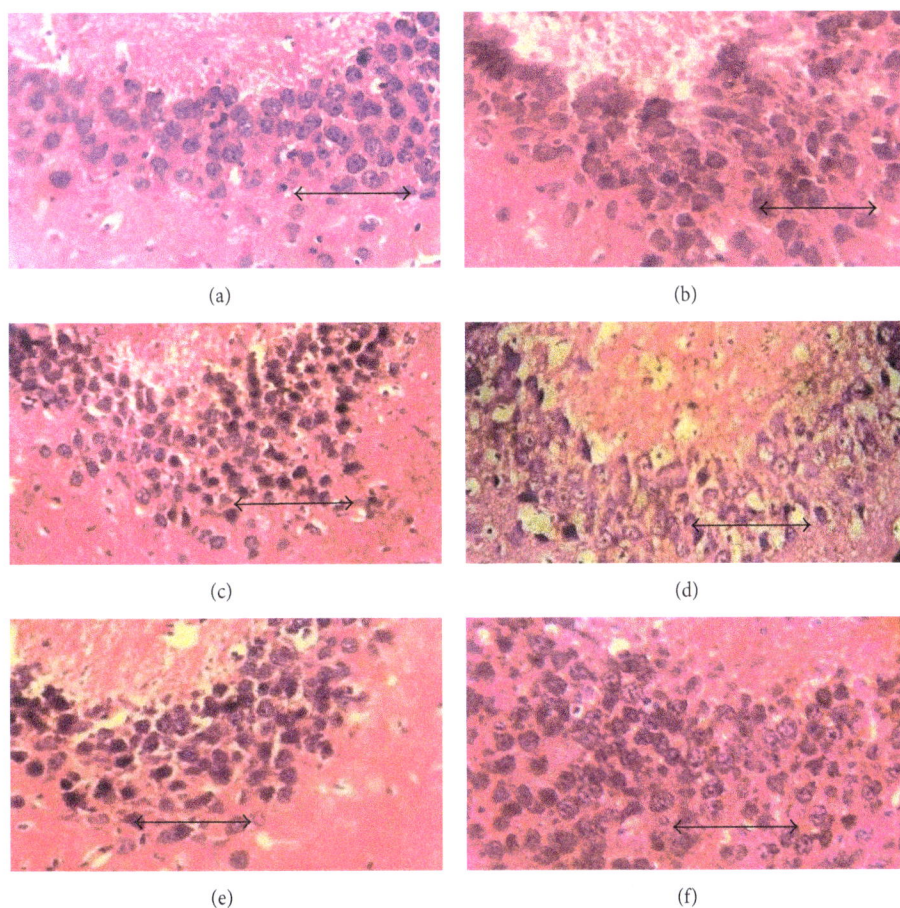

FIGURE 3: Effect of lisinopril and fosinopril on the morphology of CA3 region of hippocampus in scopolamine-induced amnesic rats. Light photomicrographs of CA3 layer of hippocampus in (a) control rats, (b) scopolamine, (c) lisinopril (0.225 mg/kg) + scop., (d) lisinopril (0.45 mg/kg) + scop., (e) fosinopril (0.90 mg/kg) + scop., and (f) fosinopril (1.80 mg/kg) + scop. Scale bar represents $1\,\mu$.

(ACh) release in the brain [19]. The brain is known to possess an intrinsic renin angiotensin system (RAS) that is involved in memory and cognition [20] and the brain Ang-II is involved in inhibiting release of ACh. ACh is the primary neurotransmitter involved in learning and memory [19] and reductions in brain ACh level have been found to strongly correlate with the degree of cognitive impairment in patients with AD [21]. The integrity of cholinergic system is essential to learning and memory, and scopolamine, a muscarinic receptor antagonist, can produce learning and memory defects by disrupting the functional integrity of the cholinergic system through competitive receptor blockade [2]. Thus, a drug such as fosinopril that can reverse scopolamine-induced behavioural deficits by enhancing cholinergic transmission is likely to offer beneficial effects which may improve debilitated patient's condition in AD.

The memory deficits produced by scopolamine in the behavioral tasks could also be due to the altered functioning of neurons in both the hippocampal and the amygdala. It is well-established that structural abnormalities of hippocampus, cortex, and medial temporal lobe structures along with a decrease in hippocampal volume are associated with the severity of deficits in learning and memory [22, 23].

In our study, the hematoxylin and eosin staining of the hippocampal region in scopolamine group clearly showed damaged neuronal cells indicating the degenerative changes in these areas. Further, scopolamine treated rats showed lesser number of healthy neurons compared to control and drug treated groups, indicating loss of neuronal function. The exact mechanism responsible for this degeneration is not clear but it could be due to the generation of reactive oxygen species. In previous reports, scopolamine has been shown to trigger the induction of ROS and cause free radical injuries associated with reduced activity of antioxidant enzymes like superoxide dismutase glutathione peroxidase in the brain [24]. In the current study, fosinopril was able to attenuate the hippocampal damage caused by scopolamine as reflected by an increase in the number of healthy neurons and decrease in the number of damaged neuronal cells in the CA3 and dentate gyrus regions. Although the precise mechanism by which fosinopril has produced these beneficial effects is not known, it could be attributed to its effect on ACh release or to its antioxidant property. A study by Hayek et al. [25] reported that ACEIs exhibit antioxidant properties and block LDL oxidation, lipid peroxidation, and the generation of MDA and 4-HNE. Furthermore, ACE inhibitors such as captopril and

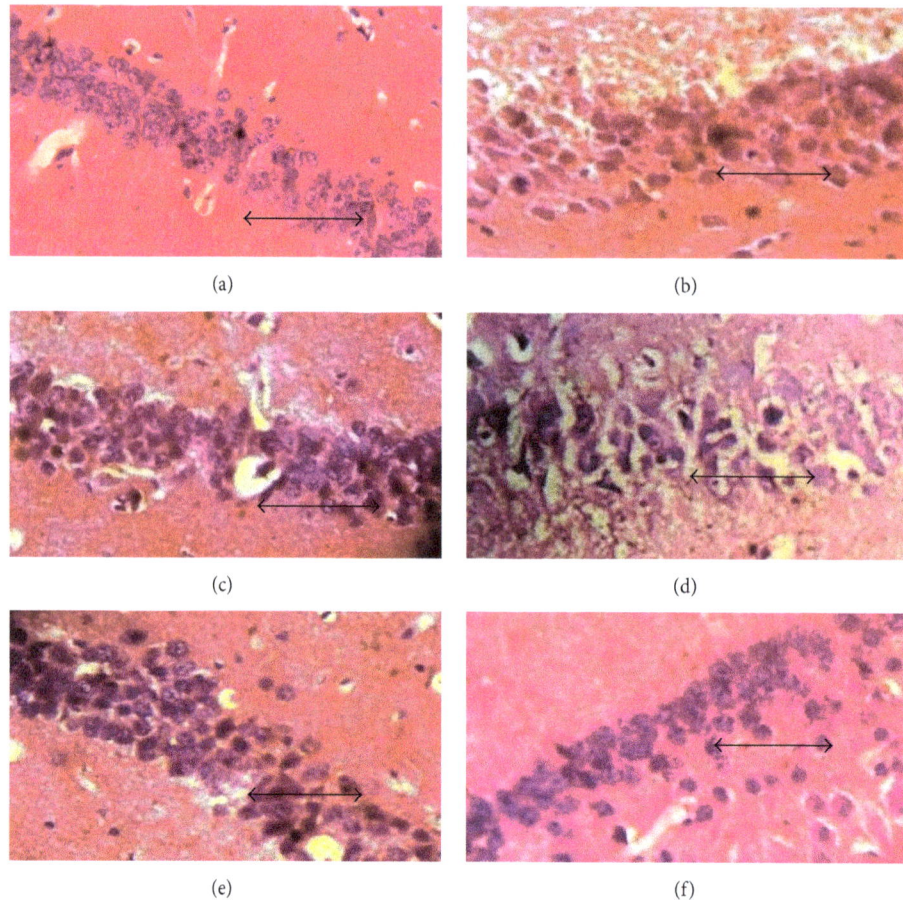

FIGURE 4: Effect of lisinopril and fosinopril on the morphology of CA1 region of hippocampus in scopolamine-induced amnesic rats. Light photomicrographs of CA1 layer of hippocampus in (a) control rats, (b) scopolamine, (c) lisinopril (0.225 mg/kg) + scop., (d) lisinopril (0.45 mg/kg) + scop., (e) fosinopril (0.90 mg/kg) + scop., and (f) fosinopril (1.80 mg/kg) + scop. Scale bar represents $1\,\mu$.

fosinopril have been found to exhibit a potent antiatherogenic effect in apoE−/− mice due to their protective effect against LDL oxidation [25, 26]. An improvement in cerebral blood flow could also be a factor involved in mediating the memory enhancing effects by fosinopril though other putative mechanisms cannot be ruled out.

The present study thus showed that, among the two centrally acting ACEIs, fosinopril but not lisinopril exhibits antiamnesic activity. Lack of significant antiamnesic activity with lisinopril could be due to its poor lipophilicity, resulting in their lesser concentration in the brain [27]. Both fosinopril and lisinopril are centrally acting ACEIs with an ability to cross the blood brain barrier [28, 29]. However, differences in lipophilicity between lisinopril and fosinopril could be responsible for the differences in their degree of penetration into the brain. Lipophilicity is an important physicochemical property that governs the passage of drugs across cells and tissues. Higher the lipophilicity of the drug, better the tissue and cell penetration. Differences in lipophilicity between lisinopril and fosinopril could be attributed to their heterogeneous chemical structure [30]. Lisinopril, like enalapril, contains pyrrolidone ring of proline, whereas fosinopril contains a bicyclic ring that accounts for

its higher lipophilicity. Fosinopril which is more lipophilic exhibits a plasma protein binding of more than 90% whereas lisinopril which is least lipophilic exhibits minimal protein binding. The more lipophilic compound exhibits a greater degree of plasma protein binding, which in turn increases its ACE inhibitory activity in various tissues [30]. Thus, better efficacy seen with fosinopril could be due to its ability to penetrate the brain to a greater degree than lisinopril though other factors need to be evaluated. Differences in pharmacological and physicochemical properties such as lipophilicity, tissue penetration, absolute bioavailability, and plasma half-life extend to differences in the efficacy among various ACEIs [31]. Thus, members of a drug class although having a common mechanism of action, they may not be identical in their pharmacodynamic efficacies due to marked differences in their chemical structure and pharmacokinetic features.

In a previous study, lisinopril has been shown to reverse the memory deficits in streptozotocin-induced experimental dementia [32]. In contrast, *in vitro* findings from an earlier report suggested that the ACEI lisinopril could interfere with the ability of ACE to inhibit the aggregation of Aβ and reduce Aβ mediated toxic effects in rat cells, further worsening

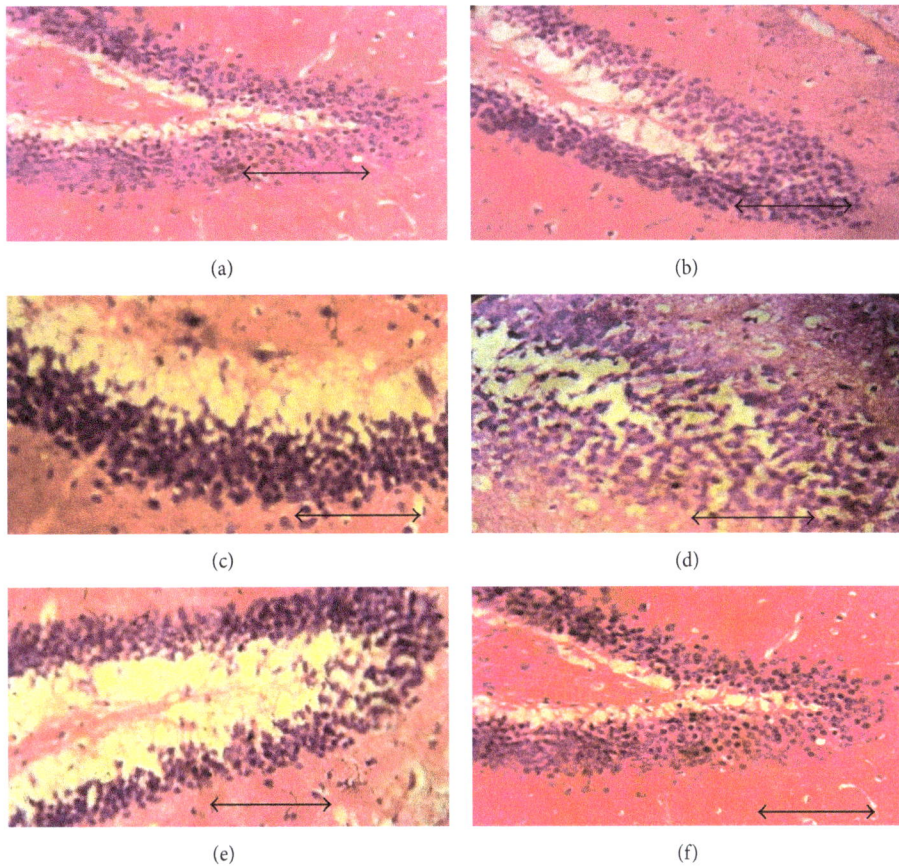

FIGURE 5: Effect of lisinopril and fosinopril on the morphology of dentate gyrus region of hippocampus in scopolamine-induced amnesic rats. Light photomicrographs of dentate gyrus layer of hippocampus in (a) control rats, (b) scopolamine, (c) lisinopril (0.225 mg/kg) + scop., (d) lisinopril (0.45 mg/kg) + scop., (e) fosinopril (0.90 mg/kg) + scop., and (f) fosinopril (1.80 mg/kg) + scop. Scale bar represents $1\,\mu$.

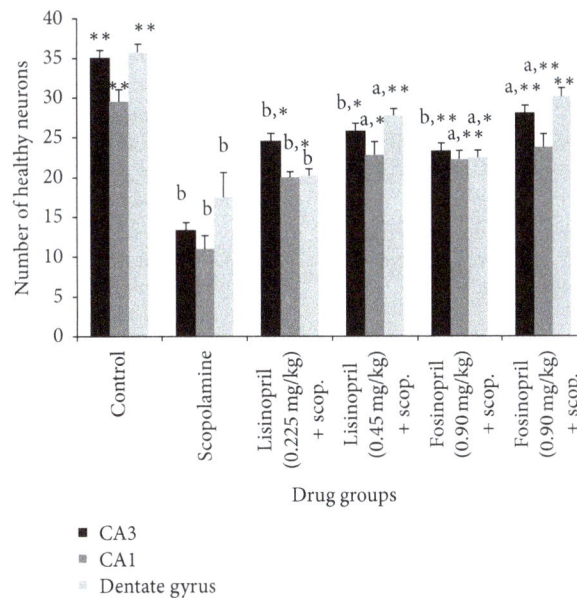

FIGURE 6: Number of healthy neurons at CA3, CA1, and dentate gyrus regions of the hippocampus of scopolamine treated amnesic rats following treatment with lisinopril and fosinopril. Comparison between control, scopolamine, lisinopril, and fosinopril treated groups in the probe trial of Morris water maze test in which no platform was present. Values are mean ± SE, *versus scopolamine ($p < 0.05$), **versus scopolamine ($p < 0.001$), [a]versus control ($p < 0.05$), and [b]versus control ($p < 0.001$).

the memory deficits in rats [33]. The differences in responses remain unexplained, but it could be due to differences in experimental designs between the studies such as the age of the animal and the period for which the treatment was received or due to differences in the species involved.

In conclusion, our study demonstrated that centrally acting ACEI such as fosinopril has potent memory, enhancing effects against scopolamine-induced amnesic mice. Since ACEIs are one of the commonly used drugs for hypertension, treatment with fosinopril may be particularly beneficial in preventing the memory deficits in elderly patients with both hypertension and dementia. However, further studies will be required to investigate the other putative mechanisms by which fosinopril may exert its beneficial effect on cognition.

Conflict of Interests

The authors report no conflict of interests. The authors alone are responsible for the content and writing of this paper.

Acknowledgment

This work was supported by a grant (BMS-58/34/2011) from the Indian Council of Medical Research, Government of India, New Delhi, India.

References

[1] H. Okano, T. Hirano, and E. Balaban, "Learning and memory," *Proceedings of the National Academy of Sciences of the United States of America*, vol. 97, no. 23, pp. 12403–12404, 2000.

[2] D. A. Drachman and J. Leavitt, "Human memory and the cholinergic system: a relationship to aging?" *Archives of Neurology*, vol. 30, no. 2, pp. 113–121, 1974.

[3] C. Bejar, R.-H. Wang, and M. Weinstock, "Effect of rivastigmine on scopolamine-induced memory impairment in rats," *European Journal of Pharmacology*, vol. 383, no. 3, pp. 231–240, 1999.

[4] R. W. Jones, K. A. Wesnes, and J. Kirby, "Effects of NMDA modulation in scopolamine dementia," *Annals of the New York Academy of Sciences*, vol. 640, pp. 241–244, 1991.

[5] U. Ebert and W. Kirch, "Scopolamine model of dementia: electroencephalogram findings and cognitive performance," *European Journal of Clinical Investigation*, vol. 28, no. 11, pp. 944–949, 1998.

[6] W. W. Beatty, N. Butters, and D. S. Janowsky, "Patterns of memory failure after scopolamine treatment: implications for cholinergic hypotheses of dementia," *Behavioral and Neural Biology*, vol. 45, no. 2, pp. 196–211, 1986.

[7] N. J. Brown and D. E. Vaughan, "Angiotensin-converting enzyme inhibitors," *Circulation*, vol. 97, no. 14, pp. 1411–1420, 1998.

[8] T. Ohrui, N. Tomita, T. Sato-Nakagawa et al., "Effects of brain-penetrating ACE inhibitors on Alzheimer disease progression," *Neurology*, vol. 63, no. 7, pp. 1324–1325, 2004.

[9] L. Rozzini, B. V. Chilovi, E. Bertoletti et al., "Angiotensin converting enzyme (ACE) inhibitors modulate the rate of progression of amnestic mild cognitive impairment," *International Journal of Geriatric Psychiatry*, vol. 21, no. 6, pp. 550–555, 2006.

[10] G. Yang, O. C. Ronan, H. Liam et al., "Effects of centrally acting ACE inhibitors on the rate of cognitive decline in dementia," *BMJ Open*, vol. 3, no. 7, Article ID e002881, 2013.

[11] G. E. Paget and J. M. Barnes, "Evaluation of drug activities," in *Pharmacometrics*, D. R. Lawrence and A. L. Bacharcach, Eds., vol. 1, p. 161, Academic Press, New York, NY, USA, 1964.

[12] A. Zanotti, L. Valzelli, and G. Toffano, "Reversal of scopolamine-induced amnesia by phosphatidylserine in rats," *Psychopharmacology*, vol. 90, no. 2, pp. 274–275, 1986.

[13] J. Wang, X. Wang, B. Lv et al., "Effects of fructus akebiae on learning and memory impairment in a scopolamine-induced animal model of dementia," *Experimental and Therapeutic Medicine*, vol. 8, no. 2, pp. 671–675, 2014.

[14] A. C. Sharma and S. K. Kulkarni, "Evaluation of learning and memory mechanisms employing elevated plus-maze in rats and mice," *Progress in Neuropsychopharmacology and Biological Psychiatry*, vol. 16, no. 1, pp. 117–125, 1992.

[15] J. Bures, O. Buresova, and J. P. Huston, *Techniques and Basic Experiments for the Study of Brain and Behavior*, Elsevier Science, New York, NY, USA, 2nd edition, 1983.

[16] R. Morris, "Developments of a water-maze procedure for studying spatial learning in the rat," *Journal of Neuroscience Methods*, vol. 11, no. 1, pp. 47–60, 1984.

[17] A. V. Dhwaj and R. Singh, "Reversal effect of *Asparagus racemosus* wild (Liliaceae) root extract on memory deficits of mice," *International Journal of Drug Development and Research*, vol. 3, no. 2, pp. 314–323, 2011.

[18] R. D'Hooge and P. P. De Deyn, "Applications of the Morris water maze in the study of learning and memory," *Brain Research Reviews*, vol. 36, no. 1, pp. 60–90, 2001.

[19] E. Savaskan, "The role of the brain renin-angiotensin system in neurodegenerative disorders," *Current Alzheimer Research*, vol. 2, no. 1, pp. 29–35, 2005.

[20] H. K. Hamdi and R. Castellon, "A genetic variant of ACE increases cell survival: a new paradigm for biology and disease," *Biochemical and Biophysical Research Communications*, vol. 318, no. 1, pp. 187–191, 2004.

[21] N. R. Sims, D. M. Bowen, S. J. Allen et al., "Presynaptic cholinergic dysfunction in patients with dementia," *Journal of Neurochemistry*, vol. 40, no. 2, pp. 503–509, 1983.

[22] G. B. Frisoni, N. C. Fox, C. R. Jack Jr., P. Scheltens, and P. M. Thompson, "The clinical use of structural MRI in Alzheimer disease," *Nature Reviews Neurology*, vol. 6, no. 2, pp. 67–77, 2010.

[23] E. Moria, Y. Yoneda, H. Yamashitaa, N. Hironoa, M. Ikedaa, and A. Yamadoric, "Medial temporal structures relate to memory impairment in Alzheimer's disease: an MRI volumetric study," *Journal of Neurology, Neurosurgery & Psychiatry*, vol. 63, pp. 214–221, 1997.

[24] Y. Fan, J. Hu, J. Li et al., "Effect of acidic oligosaccharide sugar chain on scopolamine-induced memory impairment in rats and its related mechanisms," *Neuroscience Letters*, vol. 374, no. 3, pp. 222–226, 2005.

[25] T. Hayek, J. Attias, R. Coleman et al., "The angiotensin-converting enzyme inhibitor, fosinopril, and the angiotensin II receptor antagonist, losartan, inhibit LDL oxidation and attenuate atherosclerosis independent of lowering blood pressure in apolipoprotein E deficient mice," *Cardiovascular Research*, vol. 44, no. 3, pp. 579–587, 1999.

[26] T. Hayek, J. Attias, J. Smith, J. L. Breslow, and S. Keidar, "Antiatherosclerotic and antioxidative effects of captopril in apolipoprotein E-deficient mice," *Journal of Cardiovascular Pharmacology*, vol. 31, no. 4, pp. 540–544, 1998.

[27] K. M. Raizada, I. M. Phillips, and C. Sumners, "Tissue renin angiotensin systems," in *Cellular and Molecular Biology of the Renin—Angiotensin System*, I. M. Phillips, E. Speakman, and B. Kimura, Eds., chapter 4, p. 97, CRC Press, New York, NY, USA, 1993.

[28] D. W. Cushman, F. L. Wang, W. C. Fung, C. M. Harvey, and J. M. DeForrest, "Differentiation of angiotensin-converting enzyme (ACE) inhibitors by their selective inhibition of ACE in physiologically important target organs," *American Journal of Hypertension*, vol. 2, no. 4, pp. 294–306, 1989.

[29] K. M. Sink, X. Leng, J. Williamson et al., "Angiotensin-converting enzyme inhibitors and cognitive decline in older adults with hypertension: results from the cardiovascular health study," *Archives of Internal Medicine*, vol. 169, no. 13, pp. 1195–1202, 2009.

[30] C. M. White, "Pharmacologic, pharmacokinetic, and therapeutic differences among ACE inhibitors," *Pharmacotherapy*, vol. 18, no. 3, pp. 588–599, 1998.

[31] B. Singh, B. Sharma, A. S. Jaggi, and N. Singh, "Attenuating effect of lisinopril and telmisartan in intracerebroventricular streptozotocin induced experimental dementia of Alzheimer's disease type: possible involvement of PPAR-γ agonistic property," *Journal of the Renin-Angiotensin-Aldosterone System*, vol. 14, no. 2, pp. 124–136, 2013.

[32] K. Zou, H. Yamaguchi, H. Akatsu et al., "Angiotensin-converting enzyme converts amyloid β-protein 1–42 (Aβ_{1-42}) to Aβ_{1-40}, and its inhibition enhances brain Aβ deposition," *Journal of Neuroscience*, vol. 27, no. 32, pp. 8628–8635, 2007.

[33] J. M. Barnes, N. M. Barnes, B. Costall et al., "Angiotensin-converting enzyme inhibition, angiotensin, and cognition," *Journal of Cardiovascular Pharmacology*, vol. 19, no. 6, pp. S63–S71, 1992.

9

Methanolic Extract of Ceplukan Leaf (*Physalis minima* L.) Attenuates Ventricular Fibrosis through Inhibition of TNF-α in Ovariectomized Rats

Bayu Lestari,[1,2] **Nur Permatasari,**[2] **and Mohammad Saifur Rohman**[3]

[1]*Biomedical Sciences, Medical Faculty, Brawijaya University, Malang 65145, Indonesia*
[2]*Department of Pharmacology, Medical Faculty, Brawijaya University, Malang 65145, Indonesia*
[3]*Department of Cardiology and Vascular Medicine, Medical Faculty, Brawijaya University, Saiful Anwar General Hospital, Malang 65145, Indonesia*

Correspondence should be addressed to Nur Permatasari; nungky.permatasari@gmail.com

Academic Editor: Masahiro Oike

The increase of heart failure prevalence on menopausal women was correlated with the decrease of estrogen level. The aim of this study is to investigate the effects of ceplukan leaf (*Physalis minima* L.), which contains phytoestrogen physalin and withanolides, on ventricular TNF-α level and fibrosis in ovariectomized rats. Wistar rats were divided into six groups (control (—); OVX 5: 5-week ovariectomy (OVX); OVX 9: 9-week ovariectomy; treatments I, II, and III: 9-weeks OVX + 4-week ceplukan leaf's methanolic extract doses 500, 1500, and 2500 mg/kgBW, resp.). TNF-α levels were measured with ELISA. Fibrosis was counted as blue colored tissues percentage using Masson's Trichrome staining. This study showed that prolonged hypoestrogen increases ventricular fibrosis ($p < 0.05$). Ceplukan leaf treatment also resulted in a decrease of ventricular fibrosis and TNF-α level in dose dependent manner compared to without treatment group ($p < 0.05$). Furthermore, the TNF-α level was normalized in 2500 mg/kgBW *Physalis minima* L. ($p < 0.05$) treatment. The reduction of fibrosis positively correlated with TNF-α level ($p < 0.05$, $r = 0.873$). Methanolic extract of ceplukan leaf decreases ventricular fibrosis through the inhibition of ventricular TNF-α level in ovariectomized rats.

1. Introduction

Incidences of heart failure increase on postmenopausal women related to hypoestrogen condition [1, 2]. Previous study also showed an increase in inflammatory response and myocardial fibrosis in an animal model of menopause, at least in part, via TNF-α pathway [2–4]. Estrogen possessed anti-inflammatory properties through transcription rate inhibition of several proinflammatory cytokines and cardioprotective effects [4].

Phytoestrogen is a group of substances originated from plants which have similar structure and functionality with estrogen [5]. The aim of this study is to investigate the effect of ceplukan leaf's methanolic extract (*Physalis minima* L.), which contains phytoestrogen physalin and withanolides [6–8], on ventricular TNF-α level and fibrosis in ovariectomized Wistar rats.

2. Materials and Methods

2.1. Animals. Three-month female Wistar rats (*Rattus norvegicus*) were kept in cages made of a plastic with a lid made of woven wire cage, with a cycle of 12 hours light/dark, fed, and watered by ad libitum. After 7 days of acclimatization, Wistar rats were divided into six groups (K1: normal; K2: 5-week ovariectomy (OVX); K3: 9-week ovariectomy (OVX), K4, K5, and K6: 9-week OVX + 4-week ceplukan leaf's methanolic extract doses 500, 1500, and 2500 mg/kgBW, resp.). The dosage of methanolic extract of ceplukan leaf was determined based on preliminary study (unpublished data). All procedures were approved by Health Research Ethics Committee of Brawijaya University.

2.2. Sample Preparation. Ceplukan leaves were obtained from *Balai Tanaman Obat Materia Medica*, Batu, Indonesia.

TABLE 1: Measurements of heart morphometric.

Parameters	Control (−)	OVX 5	OVX 9	Treatment I	Treatment II	Treatment III	ANOVA
BW (gram)	236.5 ± 14.2	280.8 ± 33.4	264.3 ± 20.0	237.0 ± 19.9	250.8 ± 16.5	252.5 ± 34.6	0.124^{*}
LVW (mg)	501 ± 16.2	$578.8 \pm 54.6^{\#}$	547 ± 41.6	502.6 ± 25.1	519.2 ± 40.3	514.5 ± 30.8	0.026^{**}
RVW (mg)	127 ± 15.6	136.6 ± 22.0	119.7 ± 16.9	125.4 ± 24.9	121.8 ± 16.9	119.3 ± 8.3	0.706
AW (mg)	82.9 ± 3.4	88.9 ± 10.0	81.5 ± 5.05	88.8 ± 2.9	84.4 ± 5.5	80.3 ± 1.7	0.174
LVW/HW ratio	0.705	0.720	0.731	0.704	0.716	0.720	0.298
HW/BW ratio	3.01×10^{-3}	2.87×10^{-3}	2.85×10^{-3}	3.03×10^{-3}	2.90×10^{-3}	2.85×10^{-3}	0.757

*Statistical analysis for body weight using Kruskal-Wallis test as post hoc test. **$p < 0.05$ using one-way ANOVA analysis. #$p < 0.05$ compared with control (−) using Tukey's test as post hoc test.
BW: body weight; LVW: left ventricular weight; RVW: right ventricular weight; AW: atrial weight; OVX 5: 5-week ovariectomy; OVX 9: 9-week ovariectomy; Treatments I, II, and III: 9-week ovariectomy with 500, 1500, and 2500 mg/kgBW ceplukan leaf's methanolic extract, respectively.

Ceplukan leaves (dry powder) were weighed and wrapped in filter paper, inserted in funnel extraction, and then soaked with methanol to obtain the compounds. The solution from immersion process was then collected and precipitated. The solution was separated and collected from the precipitated product and then dried in rotator evaporator at 70–80°C to obtain the thick extract. The product was then heated in oven at 70°C to remove the remaining methanol.

2.3. Ovariectomy Procedure.
Ovariectomy procedure was performed as previously described [9]. The rats were anaesthetized by intraperitoneal (IP) injection of ketamine (40 mg/kg). Ventral hair was shaved approximately 1 cm above the imaginary line ovaries. The site was then cleaned with povidone-iodine and alcohol 70%. The paralumbar lateral incision was made using a sharp knife and the ovaries were removed. The wound was sutured using catgut and covered by sterile gauze. Each rat was injected with gentamicin (60–80 mg/kg, IM) and cleaned with povidone iodine for 3 days after surgery to prevent postoperative infection.

2.4. Heart Morphometric Measurements.
The separated heart organ from the pulmonary artery, pulmonary vein, aorta, and vena cava was cleaned from blood using saline solution. Heart organ was continuously cleaned optimally from vein and artery. An atrial part was separated from the whole heart organ carefully. Mitral and tricuspid valve was left for ventricular weight measurements. Right ventricle was separated carefully from the left ventricle. Septum interventricular was left for left ventricular measurements. Atrial weight, right ventricular weight, and left ventricular weight were measured using the digital analytic weighing machine at Pharmacology Laboratory, Faculty of Medicine, Brawijaya University.

2.5. TNF-α Level Measurements.
TNF-α level was measured as previously described [10]. Briefly, heart ventricle was taken off approximately 100 mg and washed with distilled water and 1 mL PBS. The tissue protein was extracted by homogenizing the tissue in lysis buffer PMSF (containing Tris base, 0.1211 g; EDTA, 0.0074 g; NaCl, 0.8775 g; PMSF, 0.009 g; NP 40, 0.125 mL; deionized water, 100 mL; protease inhibitor cocktail, 50 μL) for about 2 minutes. The mixture was then incubated for 30 minutes at 4°C and cold centrifuged at 6000 rpm for 10 minutes. The supernatant was taken to measure TNF-α levels using Quantikine Rat TNF-α kit (R&D Systems, USA, and Canada) according to the manufacturer instructions.

2.6. Ventricular Fibrosis Measurements.
Ventricular fibrosis was measured as previously described [11]. Briefly, left ventricle that had been separated from the whole heart organ and analyzed for morphometric measurements was fixed in formalin 10% solution. After the fixation process for at least 1 day, ventricular tissue was blocked in paraffin and then sliced for histologic preparation using microtome. Histologic preparations of left ventricular tissue were stained with Masson's Trichrome. Ventricular fibrosis percentage was measured by counting the percentage of blue colored cells using software ImageJ. Fibrosis percentage was measured in 3 fields of view (40x ocular magnification) randomly at the midmyocardium area. This method was done to avoid both large artery and vein at epicardium area and artifact caused by compression/slicing process. Histologic preparation had been conducted at Pathologic Anatomy Laboratory, Faculty of Medicine, Brawijaya University.

2.7. Statistical Analysis.
The results were expressed as means ± SD. Multiple comparisons were analyzed by one-way analysis of variance (ANOVA) followed by Tukey as post hoc test. The relationship between the two variables was examined using Pearson's correlation method. The level of significance was $p < 0.05$. All statistical tests were performed by SPSS 17.00.

3. Results

3.1. Heart Morphometric.
Heart weight, right and left ventricular weight, and atrial weight had been measured as shown in Table 1. There were no significant differences among six groups based on heart weight, right ventricular weight, and atrial weight. Interestingly, this study showed significant differences of left ventricular weight between groups (ANOVA, $p = 0.026$). Furthermore, post hoc test revealed a significant increase of left ventricular weight (LVW) in 5-week ovariectomized rats (OVX 5) treatment placebo as compared to rats without treatment (negative control), suggesting that, after 5 weeks, ovariectomy procedure successfully induced hypertrophy in left ventricular. However,

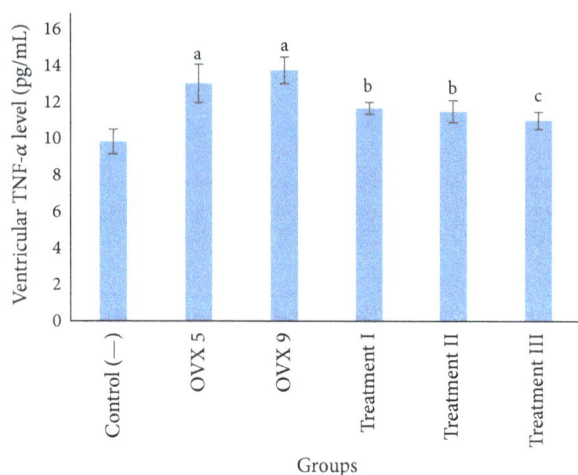

FIGURE 1: Mean of ventricular TNF-α level in each group (pg/mL).
[a]$p < 0.05$ compared to control (−) group and treatment groups;
[b]$p < 0.05$ compared to control (−) and OVX groups; [c]$p < 0.05$ compared to OVX groups. OVX 5: 5-week ovariectomy; OVX 9: 9-week ovariectomy. Treatments I, II, and III reflected 9-week ovariectomy treated with 500, 1500, and 2500 mg/kgBW ceplukan leaf's methanolic extract, respectively.

left ventricular hypertrophy in 9-week ovariectomized rats did not show any statistical differences compared to negative control or 5-week ovariectomized rats treatment. Treatment with 500 mg/kg body weight of ceplukan leaf' methanolic extract (treatment I) significantly decreased LVW similar to control (−). However, there was also no significant decrease of LVW in 1500 and 2500 mg/kgBW treated rats (treatment II and treatment III) compared to ovariectomized rats.

3.2. Ventricular TNF-α Level. Ventricular TNF-α level of each group had been measured as shown in Figure 1. Ovariectomy procedure of both 5 weeks (OVX 5) and 9 weeks (OVX 9) significantly increased ventricular TNF-α level compared to negative control. However, there were no significant differences of ventricular TNF-α level between 5-week and 9-week ovariectomized rats. Treatment with either 500 or 1500 mg/kgBW (treatment I and treatment II) methanolic extract of ceplukan leaves successfully decreased ventricular TNF-α level compared to placebo treated ovariectomized rats. Interestingly, ventricular TNF-α level was normalized in 2500 mg/kgBW ceplukan leaf's methanolic extract treated rats. Pearson correlation test showed a strong negative correlation between the dose of ceplukan leaf's methanolic extract and ventricular TNF-α level ($p = 0.000, r = -0.888$).

3.3. Ventricular Fibrosis. Ventricular fibrosis presented in blue colored tissues using Masson's Trichrome staining shown in Figure 2. Semiquantitative measurements of ventricular fibrosis using ImageJ were done as shown in Figure 3. Ovariectomy procedure of both 5 weeks (OVX 5) and 9 weeks (OVX 9) significantly increases ventricular fibrosis, suggesting that hypoestrogenic condition induces fibrosis formation of ventricular tissue. Furthermore, 9-week ovariectomy procedure significantly increases ventricular fibrosis compared

to 5-week ovariectomy procedure. All variant dose resulted in a significant decrease of ventricular fibrosis compared to 9-week ovariectomized rats. However, ventricular fibrosis was not normalized even with the highest dose of 2500 mg/kgBW ceplukan leaf's methanolic extract. Pearson correlation test showed a strong negative correlation between the dose of ceplukan leaf's methanolic extract and ventricular fibrosis percentage ($p = 0.000, r = -0.860$).

3.4. Correlation of Ventricular TNF-α Level and Fibrosis. Pearson's correlation test showed a strong positive correlation between ventricular TNF-α level and fibrosis ($p = 0.000, r = 0.873$). This result suggested that there was a causative correlation between inflammation (particularly TNF-α level) and fibrosis formation in ventricular tissue.

4. Discussion

4.1. Ovariectomy and Left Ventricular Hypertrophy, TNF-α Level, and Fibrosis. This study showed that left ventricular weight was elevated in 5-week ovariectomized rats compared to negative control. Ovariectomy-induced hypoestrogenic state also resulted in the elevation of TNF-α in 5-week and 9-week ovariectomized rats. The results in accordance with the previous study reported about the correlation of depleted estrogen (caused by either ovariectomy or knockout of ERβ) and cardiac hypertrophy [12–14]. Hypertrophied myocardium is usually accompanied with interstitial fibrosis which is characterized by the increase of collagen genes expression [15] which could affect coordinated excitation-contraction coupling of cardiomyocytes and induce diastolic stiffness and impairing cardiac output [16, 17].

Moreover, ovariectomized rats model also showed an elevated secretion of various proinflammatory cytokines such as TNF-α in hypoestrogenic state and animal model of menopause [2, 18, 19]. As previously studied, there was a correlation between estrogen depletion and inflammation marked by elevated TNF-α level [20, 21].

There was also elevated ventricular fibrosis in 5-week and 9-week ovariectomized rats compared to negative control group. Moreover, in 9-week ovariectomized rats treatment, there was a significant elevated fibrosis compared to 5-week ovariectomized rats. Interestingly, further increase of fibrosis in 9-week ovariectomized rats was not in line with further increase of TNF-α. These results indicate that inflammation alone did not cause ventricular fibrosis. Previous study showed that ovariectomy without estrogen replacement was associated with elevated expression of proapoptotic, proinflammatory, and profibrotic genes [22].

Cardiac fibrosis formation in ovariectomized rats could be triggered by myocardial cell apoptosis (both intrinsic and extrinsic) [4] and angiotensin II-induced fibrosis [23]. Extrinsic apoptosis pathway was induced by TNF-α as a ligand which in turn leads to heart remodeling marked by fibrosis [24, 25]. Otherwise, angiotensin II could increase TNF expression regulation through NF-κB (nuclear factor kappa B) dependent pathway [24–26]. ER-β knockout on mice showed an elevated transcription of cardiac proapoptotic genes [13]. In hypertensive ovariectomized rat model,

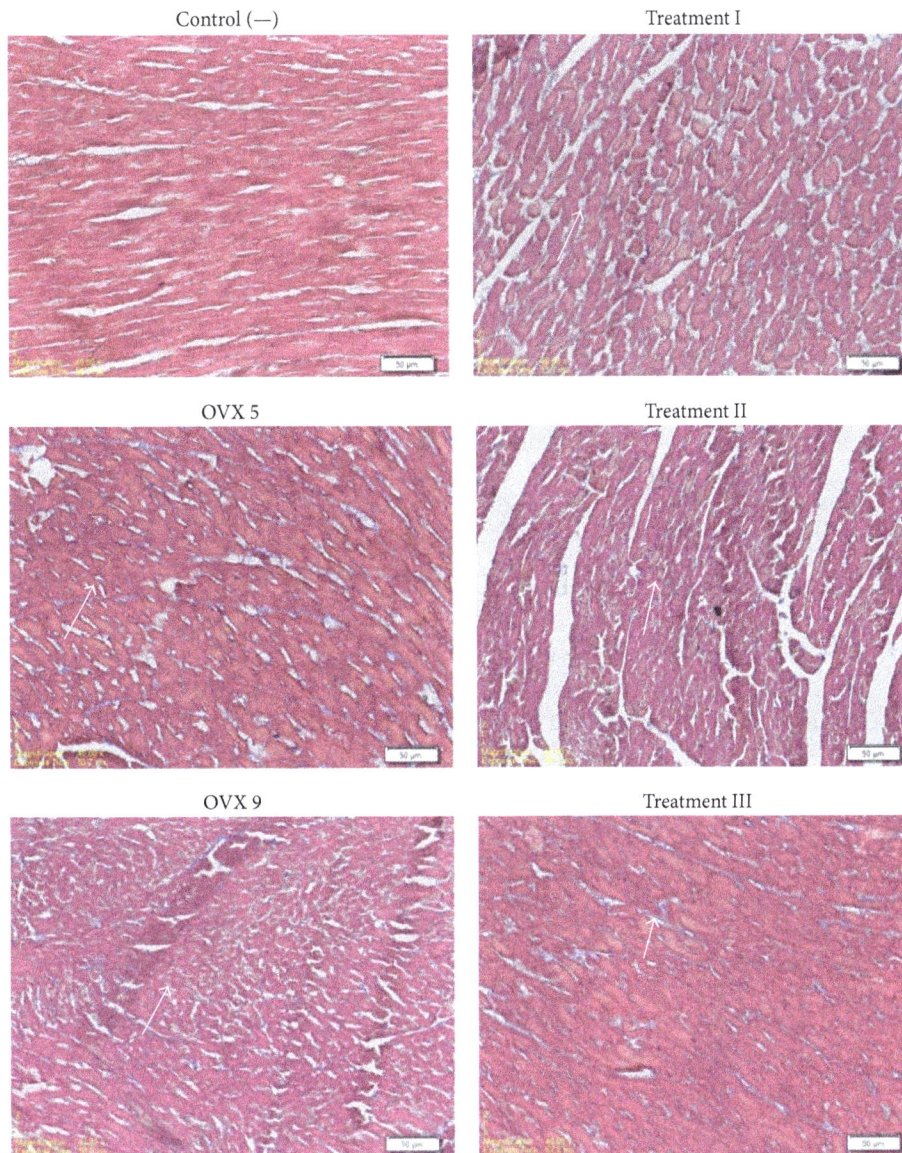

FIGURE 2: Masson's Trichrome staining of ventricular histologic preparation (ocular magnification 4x). Blue color indicates ventricular fibrosis (marked with white arrows).

hypoestrogenic condition is able to augment cardiac inflammation and oxidative stress and it thus aggravates myocardial fibrosis and diastolic dysfunction [27].

In accordance with the previous study, the results showed that TNF-α strongly correlated with fibrosis, suggesting that inflammation process triggered fibrosis formation and is macroscopically represented by left ventricular hypertrophy. However, this study needs further investigation on the impact of hypoestrogenic duration on ventricular inflammation, apoptosis, RAAS, fibrosis, and also left ventricular functionality.

4.2. Ceplukan Leaf's Methanolic Extract Treatment and Left Ventricular Hypertrophy, TNF-α Level, and Fibrosis. Gilles and colleagues [28] reported that ceplukan leaf contains 13,14-seco-16,24-cyclosteroid called physalin. Physalin consists of several compounds such as physalin A, physalin C, physalin D, 5β-6β epoxyphysalin, dihydroxyphysalin B, whitaphysalin A, whitaphysalin B, and whitaphysalin C [5]. Besides physalin, *Physalis minima* L. also contains withanolides, molecule that also possessed estrogenic activity and had been studied for its antifibrotic activities [7, 8].

Treatment with 500 mg/kgBW of ceplukan leaf's methanolic extract significantly decreases left ventricular hypertrophy compared to 5-week ovariectomized rats. The effect of estrogen and phytoestrogen on heart morphometric revealed controversy results. Previous study demonstrated that estradiol administration did not significantly affect heart morphometric compared with 3.5-week ovariectomized rats [19]. Conversely, Tang and colleagues reported that estradiol

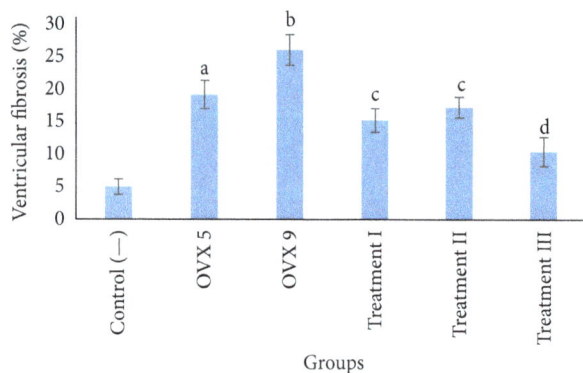

FIGURE 3: Mean of ventricular fibrosis in each group (%). $^a p < 0.05$ compared to control (—), OVX 9, treatment III groups; $^b p < 0.05$ compared to all other groups; $^c p < 0.05$ compared to control (—) and OVX 9; $^d p < 0.05$ compared to OVX and control (—). OVX 5: 5-week ovariectomy; OVX 9: 9-week ovariectomy. Treatments I, II, and III reflected 9-week ovariectomy treated with 500, 1500, and 2500 mg/kgBW ceplukan leaf's methanolic extract, respectively.

administration significantly decreases heart weight and heart weight/body weight ratio compared to ovariectomized rats, but phytoestrogen genistein did not show similar results [29]. In chronic volume overload model, either estradiol or phytoestrogen administration decreased ventricular remodeling [30, 31].

Estrogen via ER-β has been found to attenuate cardiac hypertrophy [32]. Several mechanisms have been proposed to explain the effect of estrogen administration on cardiac hypertrophy such as the mitigation of Ang-II signaling [33] and increased degradation of calcineurin as hypertrophic factor [34].

Treatment with ceplukan leaf's methanolic extract also significantly decreases TNF-α level and was normalized in the highest dose treatment (2500 mg/kgBW). Furthermore, the decreased ventricular TNF-α level evidently inhibits ventricular fibrosis in ceplukan leaf's methanolic extract treated rats. Interestingly, normalized TNF-α level in 2500 mg/kgBW ceplukan leaf's methanolic extract was not followed by normalized fibrosis, suggesting that fibrosis signaling was not independently caused by TNF-α.

Estrogen possessed anti-inflammation properties through the downregulation of several proinflammatory cytokines such as TNF-α [20, 35, 36] and cardioprotective effects through the upregulation of eNOS (endothelium-derived nitric oxide) [37] and cardiac biopterins [38]. Previous study also reported that estradiol binds to ER-β which inhibits TNF-α expression in rat's aortic smooth muscle cell culture via dependent pathway [39] and heart fibrosis pathway through the inhibition of downstream activity caused by Angiotensin II-induced TGF-β (Transforming Growth Factor-β) [40]. Angiotensin II is an important molecule in neonatal cardiac fibroblast proliferation [40, 41] and collagen deposition [41] and this process could be inhibited by estradiol administration [40–42].

The effect of phytoestrogen administration on ventricular inflammation and fibrosis had been previously studied using genistein. Genistein administration in human umbilical vascular endothelial cells (HUVECs) culture decreased monocyte adhesion induced by TNF-α [43]. Another study reported that the combination of herbs which contains withanolides showed antiapoptotic and cardioprotective effects in acute myocardial infarct model [8].

Our study showed a positive correlation between cardiac inflammation and fibrosis, and we hypothesized that methanolic extract of *Physalis minima* which contains phytoestrogen could inhibit cardiac inflammation, thereby inhibiting cardiac fibrosis. This finding was in accordance with the previous study which reported that proinflammatory cytokines are critically involved in modulating the initial myocardial remodeling suggesting that a reduction or prevention of an inflammatory response by phytoestrogenic compounds attenuates the development of adverse ventricular dilatation [44].

However, this study did not investigate the effects of ceplukan leaf's methanolic extract on myocardial apoptosis. This pathway should be confirmed with more advanced research. Furthermore, fibrosis pathway is not only triggered by TNF-α, but also triggered by several pathways such as TGF-β signaling that in turn induced various intracellular protein kinase signaling for fibrosis formation. To investigate this pathway, further studies are needed.

5. Conclusion

We concluded that ceplukan leaf's methanolic extract could decrease the ventricular fibrosis through the inhibition of TNF-α in ovariectomized rats. The duration of hypoestrogen increases ventricular fibrosis but not TNF-α level.

Conflict of Interests

The authors declare that there is no conflict of interests regarding the publication of this paper.

Acknowledgment

This work was supported by Grants from BOPTN, The Operational Funding Assistance for State Universities, University of Brawijaya, Indonesia (DIPA-023.04.2414 989/2013).

References

[1] I. Dumitru, "Heart Failure," July 2014, http://www.emedicine.com.

[2] P. Bhupathy, C. D. Haines, and L. A. Leinwand, "Influence of sex hormones and phytoestrogens on heart disease in men and women," *Women's Health*, vol. 6, no. 1, pp. 77–95, 2010.

[3] R. S. Vasan, L. M. Sullivan, R. Roubenoff et al., "Inflammatory markers and risk of heart failure in elderly subjects without prior myocardial infarction: the Framingham Heart Study," *Circulation*, vol. 107, no. 11, pp. 1486–1491, 2003.

[4] S.-D. Lee, W.-W. Kuo, Y.-J. Ho et al., "Cardiac Fas-dependent and mitochondria-dependent apoptosis in ovariectomized rats," *Maturitas*, vol. 61, no. 3, pp. 268–277, 2008.

[5] L. Pilsková, I. Riecanský, and F. Jagla, "The physiological actions of isoflavone phytoestrogens," *Physiological Research*, vol. 59, no. 5, pp. 651–664, 2010.

[6] D. L. Chothani and H. U. Vaghasiya, "A phyto-pharmacological overview on *physalis minima linn*," *Indian Journal of Natural Products and Resources*, vol. 3, no. 4, pp. 477–482, 2012.

[7] N. Permatasari, Nurdiana, and S. Karyono, "Efek non genomik dan genomik ekstrak daun ceplukan (*Physalis minima* L) pada kultur sel endotel manusia (HUVECs)," *Jurnal Ilmu-Ilmu Hayati*, vol. 22, pp. 14–19, 2010.

[8] R. P. Machin, A. S. Veleiro, V. E. Nicotra, J. C. Oberti, and J. M. Padrón, "Antiproliferative activity of withanolides against human breast cancer cell lines," *Journal of Natural Products*, vol. 73, no. 5, pp. 966–968, 2010.

[9] A. Lasota and D. Danowska-Klonowska, "Experimental osteoporosis—different methods of ovariectomy in female white rats," *Roczniki Akademii Medycznej w Białymstoku*, vol. 49, pp. 129–131, 2004.

[10] G. Torre-Amione, S. Kapadia, J. Lee et al., "Tumor necrosis factor-α and tumor necrosis factor receptors in the failing human heart," *Circulation*, vol. 93, no. 4, pp. 704–711, 1996.

[11] S.-H. Cherng, C.-Y. Huang, W.-W. Kuo et al., "GABA tea prevents cardiac fibrosis by attenuating TNF-α and Fas/FasL-mediated apoptosis in streptozotocin-induced diabetic rats," *Food and Chemical Toxicology*, vol. 65, pp. 90–96, 2014.

[12] M. van Eickels, C. Grohé, J. P. M. Cleutjens, B. J. Janssen, H. J. J. Wellens, and P. A. Doevendans, "17β-Estradiol attenuates the development of pressure-overload hypertrophy," *Circulation*, vol. 104, no. 12, pp. 1419–1423, 2001.

[13] D. Fliegner, C. Schubert, A. Penkalla et al., "Female sex and estrogen receptor-β attenuate cardiac remodeling and apoptosis in pressure overload," *American Journal of Physiology—Regulatory Integrative and Comparative Physiology*, vol. 298, no. 6, pp. R1597–R1606, 2010.

[14] F. A. Babiker, D. Lips, R. Meyer et al., "Estrogen receptor β protects the murine heart against left ventricular hypertrophy," *Arteriosclerosis, Thrombosis, and Vascular Biology*, vol. 26, no. 7, pp. 1524–1530, 2006.

[15] I. Manabe, T. Shindo, and R. Nagai, "Gene expression in fibroblasts and fibrosis: involvement in cardiac hypertrophy," *Circulation Research*, vol. 91, no. 12, pp. 1103–1113, 2002.

[16] B. C. Berk, K. Fujiwara, and S. Lehoux, "ECM remodeling in hypertensive heart disease," *Journal of Clinical Investigation*, vol. 117, no. 3, pp. 568–575, 2007.

[17] D. L. Mann, "Pathophysiology of heart failure," in *Braunwald's Heart Disease*, pp. 541–560, Saunders, 8th edition, 2008.

[18] I. Mercier, M. Pham-Dang, R. Clement et al., "Elevated mean arterial pressure in the ovariectomized rat was normalized by ET$_A$ receptor antagonist therapy: absence of cardiac hypertrophy and fibrosis," *British Journal of Pharmacology*, vol. 136, no. 5, pp. 685–692, 2002.

[19] M. Jankowski, G. Rachelska, W. Donghao, S. M. McCann, and J. Gutkowska, "Estrogen receptors activate atrial natriuretic peptide in the rat heart," *Proceedings of the National Academy of Sciences of the United States of America*, vol. 98, no. 20, pp. 11765–11770, 2001.

[20] A. S. Pechenino, L. Lin, F. N. Mbai et al., "Impact of aging vs. estrogen loss on cardiac gene expression: estrogen replacement and inflammation," *Physiological Genomics*, vol. 43, no. 18, pp. 1065–1073, 2011.

[21] K. L. Hamilton, L. Lin, Y. Wang, and A. A. Knowlton, "Effect of ovariectomy on cardiac gene expression: inflammation and changes in SOCS gene expression," *Physiological Genomics*, vol. 32, no. 2, pp. 254–263, 2008.

[22] M. W. Carr, S. J. Roth, E. Luther, S. S. Rose, and T. A. Springer, "Monocyte chemoattractant protein 1 acts as a T-lymphocyte chemoattractant," *Proceedings of the National Academy of Sciences of the United States of America*, vol. 91, no. 9, pp. 3652–3656, 1994.

[23] A. Patel, E. E. Spangenburg, and S. Witkowski, "Ovariectomy induces early changes in cardiac fibrosis and angiotensin II gene expression," Paper 124, UMass Center for Clinical and Translational Science Research Retreat, 2014, http://escholarship.umassmed.edu/.

[24] D. L. Mann, "Inflammatory mediators and the failing heart: past, present, and the foreseeable future," *Circulation Research*, vol. 91, no. 11, pp. 988–998, 2002.

[25] S. B. Haudek, G. E. Taffet, M. D. Schneider, and D. L. Mann, "TNF provokes cardiomyocyte apoptosis and cardiac remodeling through activation of multiple cell death pathways," *Journal of Clinical Investigation*, vol. 117, no. 9, pp. 2692–2701, 2007.

[26] A. Deswal, N. J. Petersen, A. M. Feldman, J. B. Young, B. G. White, and D. L. Mann, "Cytokines and cytokine receptors in advanced heart failure: an analysis of the cytokine database from the Vesnarinone trial (VEST)," *Circulation*, vol. 103, no. 16, pp. 2055–2059, 2001.

[27] T. Mori, H. Kai, H. Kajimoto et al., "Enhanced cardiac inflammation and fibrosis in ovariectomized hypertensive rats: a possible mechanism of diastolic dysfunction in postmenopausal women," *Hypertension Research*, vol. 34, no. 4, pp. 496–502, 2011.

[28] P. Gilles, M. Phillipe, and D. Louis, "Plant Extracts and Methods of Treating Skin Therewith," 2003, http://www.freepatentsonline.com/y2003/0175366.html.

[29] Y. B. Tang, Q. L. Wang, B. Y. Zhu, H. L. Huang, and D. F. Liao, "Phytoestrogen genistein increases eNOS and decrease caveolin-1 expression in ovariectomized rat hearts," *Acta Physiologica Sinica*, vol. 57, no. 3, pp. 373–378, 2005.

[30] J. D. Gardner, G. L. Brewer, and J. S. Janicki, "Effects of dietary phytoestrogens on cardiac remodeling secondary to chronic volume overload in female rats," *Journal of Applied Physiology*, vol. 99, no. 4, pp. 1378–1383, 2005.

[31] J. D. Gardner, G. L. Brower, and J. S. Janicki, "Gender differences in cardiac remodeling secondary to chronic volume overload," *Journal of Cardiac Failure*, vol. 8, no. 2, pp. 101–107, 2002.

[32] A. A. Knowlton and A. R. Lee, "Estrogen and the cardiovascular system," *Pharmacology and Therapeutics*, vol. 135, no. 1, pp. 54–70, 2012.

[33] A. Pedram, M. Razandi, D. Lubahn, J. Liu, M. Vannan, and E. R. Levin, "Estrogen inhibits cardiac hypertrophy: role of estrogen receptor-β to inhibit calcineurin," *Endocrinology*, vol. 149, no. 7, pp. 3361–3369, 2008.

[34] C. Donaldson, S. Eder, C. Baker et al., "Estrogen attenuates left ventricular and cardiomyocyte hypertrophy by an estrogen receptor-dependent pathway that increases calcineurin degradation," *Circulation Research*, vol. 104, no. 2, pp. 265–275, 2009.

[35] R. Pacifici, L. Rifas, R. McCracken et al., "Ovarian steroid treatment blocks a postmenopausal increase in blood monocyte interleukin 1 release," *Proceedings of the National Academy of Sciences of the United States of America*, vol. 86, no. 7, pp. 2398–2402, 1989.

[36] J. Pfeilschifter, R. Köditz, M. Pfohl, and H. Schatz, "Changes in proinflammatory cytokine activity after menopause," *Endocrine Reviews*, vol. 23, no. 1, pp. 90–119, 2002.

[37] A. Pósa, R. Szabó, A. Csonka et al., "Endogenous estrogen-mediated heme oxygenase regulation in experimental menopause," *Oxidative Medicine and Cellular Longevity*, vol. 2015, Article ID 429713, 7 pages, 2015.

[38] J. A. Jessup, H. Wang, L. M. Macnamara et al., "Estrogen therapy, independent of timing, improves cardiac structure and function in oophorectomized mRen2.Lewis rats," *Menopause*, vol. 20, no. 8, pp. 860–868, 2013.

[39] D. Xing, W. Feng, A. P. Miller et al., "Estrogen modulates TNF-α-induced inflammatory responses in rat aortic smooth muscle cells through estrogen receptor-β activation," *American Journal of Physiology—Heart and Circulatory Physiology*, vol. 292, no. 6, pp. H2607–H2612, 2007.

[40] A. Pedram, M. Razandi, F. O'Mahony, D. Lubahn, and E. R. Levin, "Estrogen receptor-β prevents cardiac fibrosis," *Molecular Endocrinology*, vol. 24, no. 11, pp. 2152–2165, 2010.

[41] L. Zhou, Y. Shao, Y. Huang, T. Yao, and L.-M. Lu, "17β-Estradiol inhibits angiotensin II-induced collagen synthesis of cultured rat cardiac fibroblasts via modulating angiotensin II receptors," *European Journal of Pharmacology*, vol. 567, no. 3, pp. 186–192, 2007.

[42] A. K. Natoli, T. L. Medley, A. A. Ahimastos et al., "Sex steroids modulate human aortic smooth muscle cell matrix protein deposition and matrix metalloproteinase expression," *Hypertension*, vol. 46, no. 5, pp. 1129–1134, 2005.

[43] Z. Jia, P. V. A. Babu, H. Si et al., "Genistein inhibits TNF-α-induced endothelial inflammation through the protein kinase pathway A and improves vascular inflammation in C57BL/6 mice," *International Journal of Cardiology*, vol. 168, no. 3, pp. 2637–2645, 2013.

[44] G. Baumgarten, P. Knuefermann, D. Kalra et al., "Load-dependent and -independent regulation of proinflammatory cytokine and cytokine receptor gene expression in the adult mammalian heart," *Circulation*, vol. 105, no. 18, pp. 2192–2197, 2002.

10

Antileishmanial Effect of 5,3′-Hydroxy-7,4′-dimethoxyflavanone of *Picramnia gracilis* Tul. (Picramniaceae) Fruit: *In Vitro* and *In Vivo* Studies

Sara M. Robledo,[1] **Wilson Cardona,**[2] **Karen Ligardo,**[1] **Jéssica Henao,**[1] **Natalia Arbeláez,**[1] **Andrés Montoya,**[1] **Fernando Alzate,**[3] **Juan M. Pérez,**[2] **Victor Arango,**[4] **Iván D. Vélez,**[1] **and Jairo Sáez**[2]

[1]*PECET, Medical Research Institute, School of Medicine, University of Antioquia (UdeA), Calle 70, No. 52-21, A.A. 1226, Medellín, Colombia*

[2]*Chemistry of Colombian Plants, Institute of Chemistry, Exact and Natural Sciences School, University of Antioquia (UdeA), Calle 70, No. 52-21, A.A. 1226, Medellín, Colombia*

[3]*Botanical Studies, Institute of Biology, Exact and Natural Sciences School, University of Antioquia (UdeA), Calle 70, No. 52-21, A.A. 1226, Medellín, Colombia*

[4]*Pharmacy School, University of Antioquia (UdeA), Calle 70, No. 52-21, A.A. 1226, Medellín, Colombia*

Correspondence should be addressed to Sara M. Robledo; sara.robledo@udea.edu.co

Academic Editor: Eduardo Munoz

Species of *Picramnia* genus are used in folk medicine to treat or prevent skin disorders, but only few species have been studied for biological activity and chemical composition. *P. gracilis* Tul. is a native species from Central and South America and although its fruits are edible, phytochemical analysis or medicinal uses of this species are not known. In the search of candidates to antileishmanial drugs, this work aimed to evaluate the antileishmanial activity of *P. gracilis* Tul. in *in vitro* and *in vivo* studies. Only ethanolic extract of fruits showed leishmanicidal activity. The majoritarian metabolite was *5,3′-hydroxy-7,4′-dimethoxyflavanone* ether that exhibited high activity against *L. (V.) panamensis* (EC$_{50}$ 17.0 + 2.8 mg/mL, 53.7 μM) and low toxicity on mammalian U-937 cells, with an index of selectivity >11.8. *In vivo* studies showed that the flavanone administered in solution (2 mg/kg/day) or cream (2%) induces clinical improvement and no toxicity in hamsters with CL. In conclusion, this is the first report about isolation of *5,3′-hydroxy-7,4′-dimethoxyflavanone* of *P. gracilis* Tul. The leishmanicidal activity attributed to this flavanone is also reported for the first time. Finally, the *in vitro* and *in vivo* leishmanicidal activity reported here for *5,3′-hydroxy-7,4′-dimethoxyflavanone* offers a greater prospect towards antileishmanial drug discovery and development.

1. Introduction

Leishmaniasis is a tropical disease caused by *Leishmania* parasites that affects about 12 million people in 99 countries. Approximately, 350 million people are at risk of infection and two million new cases occur yearly [1]. Despite high morbidity, therapeutic alternatives are very few and have serious drawbacks associated mainly with use of high doses and prolonged administration resulting in moderate to severe toxicity [2]. The presence of severe toxic reactions to conventional medication indicates the need for new therapies that cure leishmaniasis. Natural products of plant origin are potential tools for these discoveries and have been used for centuries to treat empirically parasitic diseases for people around the world, stimulating clinical and laboratory research [3].

Picramnia species (Picramniaceae, previously Simaroubaceae) are commonly used in folk medicine to treat or prevent dermatosis, external ulcers (sores), and skin irritations [4]. Phytochemical investigation in some of these *Picramnia*

species resulted in isolation of several metabolites [5, 6], mainly triterpenes [7–9], anthrones and anthraquinone glycosides [10–14], and oxanthrones [10–12, 15] with cytotoxic, antimicrobial, antifungal, or antiparasitic activities [16–18]. *Picramnia gracilis* Tul. is a native species of the Andean region in South and Central America [19]. Although fruits of *P. gracilis* Tul. are edible [20], reports about phytochemical analysis or medicinal uses of this species are not known. Moreover, there are no reports about antileishmanial activity of any of *Picramnia* species.

Motivated by the presence of metabolites with antiparasitic activity previously demonstrated in several *Picramnia* species and their traditional use in skin problems, this study aimed to discover antileishmanial activity and cytotoxicity in extracts and metabolites of leaves and fruits of *P. gracilis* Tul. Here, the presence of *5,3′-hydroxy-7,4′-dimethoxyflavanone* in *P. gracilis* Tul. fruits and its antileishmanial activity *in vitro* and *in vivo* are reported for the first time.

2. Materials and Methods

2.1. General Experimental Procedures. ^{1}HNMR and ^{13}C NMR spectra (all in $CDCl_3$) were recorded on Bruker AMX 300 NMR spectrometers, using TMS as internal standard. Silica gel 60 (Merck, 0.063–0.200 mesh) was used for column chromatography, and precoated silica gel plates (Merck, 60 F_{254}, 0.2 mm) were used for TLC.

2.2. Plant Material. Plant material was collected in the village of Santa Elena, "Sector Silletero," municipality of Medellin, department of Antioquia (Colombia), in January 2011 at 2540 m.o.s.l. A voucher specimen was deposited in the Herbarium of the University of Antioquia (number 4588, F. Alzate).

2.3. Preparation of Extracts and Partial Purification. Material was dried in an oven at 35°C for 48 hours. Powdered leaves (86 g) of *P. gracilis* Tul. were extracted successively with hexane, then dichloromethane and ethyl acetate, and finally ethanol in a percolator at room temperature and concentrated in vacuum to give the corresponding extract (2.35 (2.7%), 5.63 g (6.5%), 4.59 g (5.3%), and 9.59 g (5.3%), resp.). On the other hand, 37.34 g of dried fruits was extracted with ethanol only and after concentration a dark brown paste was obtained, 7.88 g (21%). Presence of major compound was observed by TLC (mobile phase, dichloromethane). Then, extract was subjected to silica gel column chromatography eluting with a step gradient of *n*-hexane-ethylacetate (100 : 0, 90 : 10, 80 : 20, 70 : 30, 60 : 40, 50 : 50, 40 : 60, 30 : 70, 20 : 80, 10 : 90, and 0 : 100, each 200 mL) to obtain 20 fractions (F1–F20) collected on the basis of their TLC profiles. Fractions F4–F10 were recognized as the most interesting ones, due to the appearance of red spots after spraying with anisaldehyde reagent. Flavanone (350 mg, 4.4%) was isolated from this fraction by preparative TLC using *n*-hexane-ethyl acetate (4 : 1) mixture.

5,3′-Hydroxy-7,4′-dimethoxyflavanone. ^{1}HNMR (CDCl₃, 300 MHz): δ 2.83 (H-3β, dd, *J* = 3.1, 17.2 Hz), 3.12 (H-3α, dd, *J* = 12.9, 17.2 Hz), 3.85 (s, OCH₃), 3.96 (s, OCH₃), 5.37 (H-2, dd, *J* = 3.1, 12.9 Hz), 5.78 (OH), 6.09 (H-8, d, *J* = 2.3 Hz), 6.12 (H-6, d, *J* = 2.3 Hz), 6.92 (H-5′, d, *J* = 8.3 Hz), 6.98 (H-6′, dd, *J* = 1.9, 8.3 Hz), 7.09 (H-2′, d, *J* = 1.9 Hz); 12.07 (OH). ^{13}C NMR (CDCl₃, 75 MHz): δ 43.21 (C-3), 55.71 (OCH₃), 56.07 (OCH₃), 78.94 (C-2), 94.27 (C-8), 95.13 (C-6), 103.17 (C-10), 110.69 (C-5′), 112.70 (C-2′), 118.18 (C-6′), 131.56 (C-1′), 145.96 (C-3′), 147.03 (C-4′), 162.87 (C-9), 164.14 (C-5), 168.00 (C-7), 196.02 (C=O) (see Supplementary Data of the Supplementary Material available online at http://dx.doi.org/10.1155/2015/978379).

2.4. Studies In Vitro of Cytotoxicity. Cytotoxic activity of all extracts and pure compound was evaluated in the human U937 cell line by MTT method, as described previously [21, 22]. In brief, cells were cultured in RPMI 1640 medium supplemented with 10% fetal bovine serum (FBS), and 1% of antibiotics (penicillin-streptomycin (10.000 U/mL) at 100.000 cells/mL and six concentrations of each product (200, 100, 50, 25, 12.5, and 6.25 µg/mL). Cells cultured in medium alone were used as negative control (no toxicity) while cells exposed to amphotericin B (AmB) were positive control (toxicity). Cells were incubated at 37°C, 5% CO_2 for 72 hours; then, the effect of each product on the viability of cells was determined incubating exposed and unexposed cells for 3 hours with 10 µL of *3-(4,5-dimethylthiazol-2-yl)-2,5-diphenyltetrazolium bromide*. The MTT was reduced by succinate mitochondrial dehydrogenase to purple formazan that was then solubilized with 100 µL/well isopropanol 50% and SDS 10% and its concentration was determined by optical density at 570 nm in a spectrometer (Benchmark BioRad). Each concentration of the product and unexposed cells was tested in triplicate in at least two different experiments.

The *in vitro* cytotoxicity was determined as the percentage of viability and growth inhibition obtained from the optical densities (O.D.) for each experimental condition using the formula: viability (%) = (O.D. treated cells/O.D. untreated cells) × 100, where O.D. of untreated cells correspond to 100% viability. In turn, growth inhibition (%) is calculated as 100 − % viability. Growth inhibition (%) data obtained for each experimental condition was used to calculate the lethal concentration 50 (LC_{50}) by Probit analysis [23]. Compounds were classified using an arbitrary scale as follows: potentially toxic: LC_{50} < 100 µg/mL; moderately toxic: LC_{50} > 100 and < 200 µg/mL; and potentially nontoxic: LC_{50} > 200 µg/mL.

2.5. Studies In Vitro of Antileishmanial Activity. The activity of each extract or metabolite obtained from *P. gracilis* Tul. was determined on Phorbol 12-myristate 13-acetate-differentiated U-937 cells infected with intracellular amastigotes of *L. (V.) panamensis* expressing the green fluorescent protein gene (MHOM/CO/87/UA140pIR-GFP) [24, 25]. One mL of cells was dispensed into each well of 24-well plate (300.000 cell/mL RPMI 1640 medium and 100 ng/mL). Plates were incubated at 37°C, 5% CO_2 during 72 hours and then washed twice with phosphate buffer saline (PBS). U-937 cells were then infected with stationary phase promastigotes of *L. (V.) panamensis* in a proportion of 35 : 1 (parasites : cell). Plates were incubated for 3 hours at 34°C, 5% CO_2 and after incubation cells were washed twice with PBS and incubated again for 24 hours at 37°C, 5% CO_2. Infected cells were exposed to four serial concentration dilutions of each product (100, 25, 6.25, and 1.56 μg/mL RPMI 1640 medium). In parallel, cells incubated in medium alone were used as control of infection (negative control) and cells exposed to AmB were used as control of leishmanicidal activity (positive control). After 72 hours of incubation at 37°C, 5% CO_2 cells were removed using trypsin/EDTA solution and washed twice with PBS by centrifuging 10 min at 1100 rpm, 4°C. Then, cells were analyzed in an Argon laser flow cytometer (Cytomics FC 500MPL) by reading at 488 nm excitation and 525 nm emission. Ten thousand events were counted from each well. The percentage of infected cells was determined by dot plot analysis while the parasitic load was calculated by the mean fluorescence intensity using histogram analysis. Each concentration was assessed in triplicate in at least two independent experiments.

In vitro antileishmanial activity was determined as percentage of infection (viable parasites inside infected cells) according to the MFI units from flow cytometry analysis for each experimental condition using the formula: % infection = (FMI treated infected cells/FMI untreated infected cells) × 100, where FMI of untreated infected cells corresponds to 100% viable parasites. Then, % of reduction of infection was calculated using the formula: % inhibition = 100 − % infection. The % inhibition obtained for each experimental condition was used to calculate the effective concentration 50 (EC_{50}) by Probit analysis [23]. Compounds were classified according to their antileishmanial activity using an arbitrary scale as follows: active: $EC_{50} < 20$ μg/mL; moderately active: $EC_{50} > 20$ and <50 μg/mL; or potentially nonactive: $EC_{50} > 50$ μg/mL. The index of selectivity (IS) was calculated by correlating cytotoxicity with antileishmanial activity using the formula: $IS = LC_{50}/EC_{50}$.

2.6. Evaluation of Therapeutic Response and Toxicity of 5,3'-Hydroxy-7,4'-dimethoxyflavanone In Vivo. The therapeutic response of flavanone was tested in the hamster (*Mesocricetus auratus*) model for CL [26]. Briefly, previously anesthetized (ketamine 40 mg/kg and xylazine 5 mg/kg) hamsters were inoculated in the dorsal skin with promastigotes of *L. (V.) braziliensis* (MHOM/CO/88/UA301-EpiR-GFP) (5×10^8 parasites/100 μL PBS). Three experimental groups ($n = 8$ each), consisting of four males and four females, were coded accordingly: A: flavanone pure, B: 2% flavanone cream, and C: MA (positive control). Treatment with flavanone pure (40 μL per dose), flavanone cream (40 mg per dose), or MA (200 μg per dose) was initiated immediately after development of a typical ulcer (4–6 weeks after infection). Flavanone (groups A and B) was applied topically daily for 28 days. In turn, MA (20 μL, 10 mg/mL) was applied intralesionally, also every day for 28 days. Animal welfare was supervised daily during the study. Both areas of the ulcer and body weight were measured every two weeks from the beginning of the treatments to the end of the study (three months after completion of treatment). The overall time points of evaluation were pretreatment day (TD0), end

of treatment (PTD0), and posttreatment days 30, 60, and 90 (PTD30, PTD60, and PTD90, resp.). At the end of the study, hamsters were humanely sacrificed and, after necropsy, liver and kidney biopsies were taken for histopathological studies. A skin biopsy (from the site where the injury occurred) was also taken to determine parasite load by qPCR.

The effectiveness of each treatment was assessed comparing the lesion sizes prior to and after treatments. Treatment outcome at the end of study was recorded as *cure* (healing of 100% of the area and complete disappearance of the lesion); *clinical improvement* (reducing the size of the lesion in >30% of the area); *failure* (increasing the size of the lesion); or *relapse* (reactivation of lesion after initial cure). To compare the effectiveness among groups of treatments an arbitrary score was assigned to each treatment: 3 = cure, 2 = clinical improvement, 1 = relapse, and 0 = failure.

The toxicity of flavanone pure, flavanone cream, or MA was evaluated according to hepatic and renal functions of hamsters in treated and untreated animals as described previously [26]. At day TD0 and day 8 of treatment (TD8), blood was drawn from the heart and serum was separated by centrifugation at 5000 ×g for 2-3 min. The serum was stored at −80°C until use. Hepatic and renal functions were assessed by measuring the levels of alanine amino transferase (ALT), blood urea nitrogen (BUN), and creatinine using commercially available kits (Biosystems, Spain). The hepatic and renal functions were also evaluated in healthy (uninfected and untreated) hamsters. Toxicity of treatments was determined by comparing serum levels of ALT, BUN, and creatinine and postmortem histological changes in liver and kidney. Severity of histological changes was also graded as severe, moderate, or mild.

2.7. Quantification of Parasite Load. Quantification of parasites present in the lesions was based on amplification of a single copy gene of *Leishmania* DNA polymerase (housekeeping gene) using quantitative real time PCR (qPCR) and a standard curve as described elsewhere [27]. Initially, a 600 bp fragment of DNA of *L. (V.) panamensis* was amplified by conventional PCR (T1000 thermocycler, BioRad) and purified using QIAquick Gel Extraction Kit according to the manufacturer's instructions and product was ligated to InsTAclone pTZ57R/T vector. Then, DH5 alpha cells (Invitrogen, USA) were transformed with the construct. The construct was purified and, then, qRT-PCR was set to amplify a 120 bp fragment within the 600 bp sequence initially cloned. The number of copies per plasmid was determined based on the size of the cloned fragment and the size of the insert. A standard curve ranging from 1 to 1 million parasites in log increases from 10 was established. The QuantiFast SYBR Green qRT-PCR kit (Qiagen Inc., USA) was used for qPCR. The PCR amplifications were performed in a SmartCycler II (Cepheid, Sunnyvale, CA, USA) using a final volume of 25 μL containing 100 ng of DNA, 12.5 μL of the reaction mix, 100 nmol/L of each primer, and nuclease-free water. The amplification efficiency of each was measured using the PCR program LinReg. Tissue samples were weighted and lysed with 500 mL of lysis buffer (100 mM

Table 1: *In vitro* cytotoxicity and antileishmanial activity of *Picramnia gracilis* Tul.

Product	Biological activity (μg/mL)		IS
	LC$_{50}$	EC$_{50}$	
E-EtOH-le	>200.0	>100.0	>2
E-He-le	22.4 ± 5.4	>22.4	<1
E-DiCl-Me-le	29.1 ± 9.0	>29.1	<1
E-EtAc-le	>200.0	>100.0	>2
E-EtOH-fr	>200.0	35.7 ± 1.3	>2
5,3′-Hydroxy-7,4′-dimethoxyflavanone	>200.0	17.0 ± 2.8 (53.7 μM)	>11.8
Amphotericin B	37.5 ± 7.6	0.06 ± 0.004	625.0
Meglumine antimoniate	>1000.0	6.8 + 0.5	>147.1

Data represent the mean value ± SD of cytotoxicity in terms of 50% lethal concentration (LC$_{50}$) and leishmanicidal activity in terms of 50% effective concentration (EC$_{50}$). E-EtOH-fr: ethanolic extract from fruit; E-EtOH-le: ethanolic extract from leaves; E-DiClMe-le: dichloromethane extract from leaves; E-He-le: hexane extract from leaves; and E-EtAc-le: ethyl acetate extract from leaves. IS (index of selectivity) = LC$_{50}$/EC$_{50}$.

NaCl, 10 mM Tris-HCl, 25 mM EDTA, and 0.5% SDS, pH 8.0) and 0.1 mg/mL proteinase K by incubation in a water-bath for 4 hours at 56°C. Then, DNA was extracted with one mL of phenol : chloroform : isoamylic alcohol (25 : 24 : 1). After centrifugation for 10 min at 1700 rpm, the aqueous layer was carefully removed, washed with 90% ethanol, centrifuged 2 min at 500 ×g, and dried at room temperature. The pellet was resuspended in 300 μL of autoclaved nuclease-free water. DNA was quantified using NanoDrop 1000 (Thermo Scientific, NH, USA) at 260 nm of absorbance and stored at −20°C until further use.

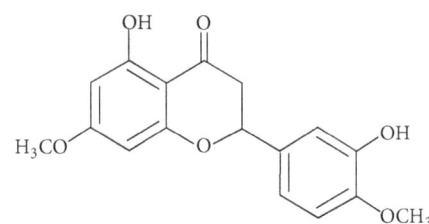

Figure 1: Chemical structure of *5,3′-hydroxy-7,4′-dimethoxyflavanone* isolated from fruits of *Picramnia gracilis* Tul.

2.8. Data Analysis. For each parameter, average values with standard deviations (mean ± SD) were calculated. Data were analyzed by a two-way ANOVA. Differences were considered significant if $P < 0.05$. Statistical analysis was performed with Prism 6.0 (Graphpad Prism, San Diego, CA, USA).

3. Results

A majoritarian compound (4.4% yield) was identified as *5,3′-hydroxy-7,4′-dimethoxyflavanone*, after NMR analysis and high resolution mass (Figure 1).

Ethanolic and ethyl acetate extracts from leaves (E-EtOH-1 and E-EtAc-le) and ethanol extract from fruit (E-EtOH-fr) were potentially nontoxic for U-937 cells (LC$_{50}$ > 200 μg/mL) (Table 1) while hexane and dichloromethane extracts from leaves (E-He-le and E-DiClMe-le, resp.) were highly cytotoxic (LC$_{50}$ 22.4 and 29.1 μg/mL, resp., as shown in Table 1). AmB, which is a highly cytotoxic drug, showed a LC$_{50}$ of 37.5 μg/mL, while MA was nontoxic on U-937 (LC$_{50}$ > 1000.0 μg/mL). The *5,3′-hydroxy-7,4′-dimethoxyflavanone* did not exhibit cytotoxicity on human macrophages (LC$_{50}$ > 200 μg/mL).

Data represent the mean value ± SD of cytotoxicity in terms of 50% lethal concentration (LC$_{50}$) and leishmanicidal activity in terms of 50% effective concentration (EC$_{50}$): E-EtOH-fr: ethanolic extract from fruit; E-EtOH-le: ethanolic extract from leaves; E-DiClMe-le: dichloromethane extract from leaves; E-He-le: hexane extract from leaves; E-EtAc-le:

ethyl acetate extract from leaves; IS (index of selectivity) = LC$_{50}$/EC$_{50}$.

The E-EtOH-fr showed moderate leishmanicidal activity on intracellular amastigotes of *L. (V.) panamensis* (EC$_{50}$ 35.7 μg/mL) (Table 1), while E-EtOH-le and E-EtAc-le were nonactive against intracellular amastigotes of *L. (V.) panamensis* (EC$_{50}$ > 100 μg/mL). Unfortunately, E-He-le and E-DiClMe-le (EC$_{50}$ > 22.4 and > 29.1 μg/mL, resp.) had leishmanicidal activity at concentrations that are toxic to cells that are the host cells for *Leishmania* parasites. As expected, AmB and MA were highly active against intracellular amastigotes of *L. (V.) panamensis* (EC$_{50}$ 0.06 and 6.8 μg/mL, resp.). The *5,3′-hydroxy-7,4′-dimethoxyflavanone* showed high antileishmanial activity (EC$_{50}$ 17.0 μg/mL, 53.7 μM). This biological activity of *5,3′-hydroxy-7,4′-dimethoxyflavanone* was highly selective with an IS > 11.8 while in extracts from fruit and leaves the IS was <2.0 (Table 1). AmB and MA had an IS of 625.0 and >147.1, respectively.

Treatment of *L. (V.) braziliensis* 40 μL/2 mg/kg body weight/day/for 28 days with flavanone (group A) resulted in clinical improvement in 4/6 hamsters with 40 to 80% of reduction in their lesion sizes, failure in 1/6 hamsters, and relapse in 1/6 hamsters. Parasite load in this group of animals was 392.3 + 192.7 parasites/mg of tissue. On the other hand, treatment with 40 mg/2% flavanone cream/day/for 28 days (group B) produced cure in 2/6 hamsters (with 100% reduction of lesion size); clinical improvement (>80% of reduction in their lesion size) was observed in 2/6 hamsters

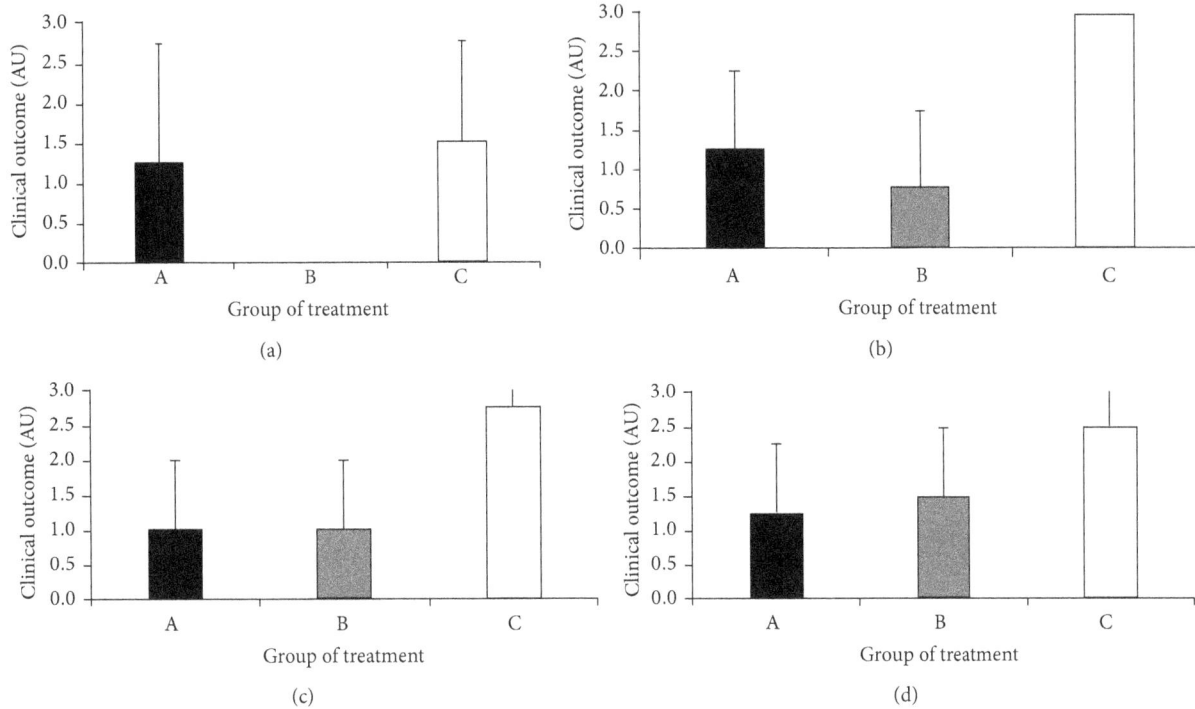

FIGURE 2: Clinical outcome after treatment with topical *5,3'-hydroxy-7,4'-dimethoxyflavanone* isolated from *P. gracilis* Tul. fruit. Bars represent the mean value ± SD of clinical outcome in arbitrary units scored at the end of the treatment (a), PTD30 (b), PTD60 (c), and PTD90 (d). Axis *x*: group treated with flavanone solution (group A); group treated with 2% flavanone cream (group B); and group treated with trademark meglumine antimoniate (group C). Axis *y*: score of 0 = failure; 1 = relapse; 2 = clinical improvement; and 3 = cure.

and relapse was in 2/8 hamsters (reactivation of ulcer after initial cure at PTD45 or PTD75). In this group parasite load was 2405.0 ± 4312.6 parasites/mg of tissue. Finally, treatment with intralesion injection of MA 200 μg/day/twice a week/28 days (group C) cured 5/6 hamsters and 1/6 hamster experienced relapse, 15 days after treatment. The amount of parasites in hamsters cured was 218.5 ± 393.7 parasites per mg of tissue. The parasite load in hamsters treated with flavanone solution (group A) was similar to that detected in hamsters treated with MA (group C), while it was different from that detected in hamsters treated with flavanone cream ($P < 0.005$).

Differences in treatment effectiveness were based on results obtained in each of the different stages of evaluation: end of treatment (PTD0) and PTD30, PTD60, and PTD90, using the arbitrary scale as described in the Materials and Methods. The mean value of treatment outcomes obtained at each time point for each treatment group is summarized in Figure 2. Effectiveness of topical treatment with topical flavanone pure (group A) was similar to that observed with intralesion injection of MA (group C) at any time point during follow-up except at PTD90 where response was higher in group C. Differences were not statistically significant ($P > 0.05$). On the other hand, the effectiveness of topical flavanone cream (group B) was higher than flavanone pure at PTD90. These differences were not statistically significant ($P > 0.05$).

Some animals in each treatment group experienced weight loss < 10%. Thus, loss weight was not associated with toxic effects of treatment with *5,3'-hydroxy-7,4'-dimethoxy-flavanone*. Levels of serum ALT for liver dysfunction and BUN and creatinine for renal dysfunction, measured 8 days upon treatment with this flavanone, as well as uninfected and untreated hamsters demonstrated increased levels of the serum of ALT and BUN after treatment with flavanone formulation, while creatinine levels were mildly increased after treatment with MA. However these levels were similar to those observed in hamsters infected but untreated (Table 2). Differences were not statistically significant ($P > 0.05$).

On the other hand, no histological alterations attributable to treatment were observed in animals treated with *5,3'-hy-droxy-7,4'-dimethoxyflavanone*. In contrast, hamsters treated with MA induced the following changes, which were observed in the liver: cloudiness, vacuolar and fat degeneration, karyomegaly, binucleation, and pigmentation. These occurred in moderate to severe degree. MA treatment also induced changes in kidney, including vacuolar and fat degeneration and binucleation in mild to moderate degree.

4. Discussion

Cutaneous leishmaniasis is an infectious disease that can cause serious psychologic and social stigma, especially when face and other visible areas of the body are compromised.

TABLE 2: Blood levels of ALT, BUN, and creatinine in hamsters treated with *5,3'-hydroxy-7,4'-dimethoxyflavanone*.

Group	ALT (U/L)	BUN (mg/dL)	Creatinine (mg/dL)
(A) TD0			
Healthy ($n = 5$)	64.4 ± 5.6	15.9 ± 2.6	0.4 ± 0.1
Infected/untreated ($n = 3$)	73.9 ± 2.8	18.2 ± 1.9	0.4 ± 0.14
Flavanone solution ($n = 6$)	67.8 ± 3.2	18.0 ± 4.9	0.5 ± 0.1
Flavanone cream ($n = 6$)	65.8 ± 17.6	17.4 ± 1.3	0.3 ± 0.02
MA (i.l) ($n = 6$)	57.0 ± 6.1	20.9 ± 6.9	0.4 ± 0.1
(B) TD8			
Flavanone solution ($n = 6$)	76.8 ± 3.7	20.0 ± 2.2	0.4 ± 0.03
Flavanone cream ($n = 6$)	77.1 ± 7.6	22.9 ± 6.4	0.3 ± 0.1
MA (i.l) ($n = 6$)	62.0 ± 8.5	23.8 ± 2.2	0.8 ± 0.1

Data represent the mean values ± SD of n animals per group of treatment.

Hereby, in the search of new or better drugs to treat CL, antileishmanial activity and cytotoxicity products derived from leaves and fruit of *P. gracilis* Tul. were tested *in vitro*. Only ethanolic extract of fruit had moderate leishmanicidal activity on intracellular amastigotes of *L. (V.) panamensis* and no cytotoxicity on macrophages and the antileishmanial activity and toxicity of the majoritarian compound of this extract was validated *in vivo*.

The majoritarian compound was identified as follows. This same flavanone was previously isolated from *Chromolaena odorata* (L.) (Asteraceae) [28], *Artemisia campestris* subsp. *maritima* (Asteraceae) [29], and *Heliotropium glutinosum* Phil. (Heliotropiceae) [30] and named *eriodictyol-7,4'-dimethyl ether*. However, the presence of *5,3'-hydroxy-7,4'-dimethoxyflavanone* as a majoritarian compound in one species of the Picramniaceae family is reported for the first time. Additionally, activity of *5,3'-hydroxy-7,4'-dimethoxyflavanone* against *L. (V.) panamensis* and *L. (V.) braziliensis* is reported also for the first time. Other flavanones have been reported having activities against *Leishmania* species and *T. cruzi*; thus, for example, *5,6,7-trihydroxy-4-methoxyflavanone* isolated from methanol extract of *Baccharis retusa* (Asteraceae) showed activity against promastigotes of *L. (V.) braziliensis*, *L. (L.) amazonensis*, and *L. (L.) chagasi* (IC_{50} 49.0, 53.0, and 57.0 µg/mL, resp.) and intracellular amastigotes of *L. (L.) chagasi* (IC_{50} 45.0 µg/mL). This *5,6,7-trihydroxy-4-methoxyflavanone* was also active on trypomastigotes of *T. cruzi* (IC_{50} 20.4 µg/mL) without cytotoxicity to mouse peritoneal macrophages but with considerable toxicity to rhesus monkey kidney cells (LLC-MK2) and tumoral monocyte THP-1 cells (LC_{50} 31.0 and 49.0 µg/mL, resp.) [31, 32]. Similarly, *5,4'-dihydroxy-7-methoxyflavanone* (sakuranetin-2) isolated also from *B. retusa* was active against promastigotes of *L. (L.) amazonensis*, *L. (V.) braziliensis*, *L. (L.) major*, and *L. (L.) chagasi* (IC_{50} 51.9, 45.1, 52.6, and 38.4 µg/mL, resp.). This flavanone was also active against intracellular amastigotes of *L. (L.) chagasi* with an IC_{50} value of 43.7 µg/mL. No toxicity to Balb/c mice peritoneal macrophages was observed. However, this compound showed considerable toxicity to kidney cells LLC-MK2 and human monocytes THP-1 cells (IC_{50} 25.9 and 39.5 µg/mL,

resp.). This flavanone also was active on *T. cruzi* trypomastigotes (IC_{50} 20.2 µg/mL) [33].

In addition, *5,3'-hydroxy-7,4'-dimethoxyflavanone* reported here was active on intracellular amastigotes but inactive on axenic amastigotes of *L. (V.) panamensis* (data not shown). This result suggests that the flavanone may require metabolization after internalization by the host cell to produce the metabolite responsible for the leishmanicidal activity, as is seen with pentavalent antimony [33]. Although the possibility of metabolization by the host cell remains to be determined, antileishmanial activity of *5,3'-hydroxy-7,4'-dimethoxyflavanone* on intracellular parasite may be related to its ability to chelate iron (Fe), depriving this essential nutrient from the intracellular forms [34].

The *5,3'-hydroxy-7,4'-dimethoxyflavanone* administered at 2 mg/kg body weight/day (solution) or 2% (cream) during 28 days was able to induce cure or clinical improvement of CL in hamsters experimentally infected with *L. (V.) braziliensis*. Although effectiveness of flavanone was lower than MA in terms of treatment outcome at the end of the study, parasite load was similar in both groups of treatments. These results confirm that *5,3'-hydroxy-7,4'-dimethoxyflavanone* is able to kill intracellular amastigotes of *L. (V.) braziliensis* present in the ulcer, but the efficiency is affected not only by dose but also by pharmaceutical formulation. None of the treatments produced detrimental effect on the body weight, histological morphology, or blood levels of ALT, BUN, and creatinine attributed to toxic effects of flavanone. Because the levels observed after treatment were similar to those in infected/untreated hamsters, variations are probably associated with *Leishmania* infection process. Moreover, nitrogen compounds may be increased due to the high degradation of amino acids or high-protein diets and are not always associated with an alteration in the kidney [35].

5. Conclusion

Hereby, the *5,3'-hydroxy-7,4'-dimethoxyflavanone* is reported for the first time in one species of the Picramniaceae family. The activity against *L. (V.) panamensis* and *L. (V.) braziliensis* is also reported for the first time. Overall, bioassay testing results observed in this investigation indicate that *5,3'-hydroxy-7,4'-dimethoxyflavanone* isolated from *P. gracilis* Tul. represents promising antiprotozoal leads for further development of drugs to treat CL. Therapeutic response of this flavanone would be improved by increasing the amount of the active ingredient in the formulation, increasing the frequency of administration or extending the days of treatment. Finally, this work contributes with new knowledge chemical composition and novel biological activity of *P. gracilis* Tul., a native species from Central and South America.

Abbreviations

CL: Cutaneous leishmaniasis
LC_{50}:   Lethal concentration 50
EC_{50}:   Effective concentration 50
IS: Index of selectivity.

Ethical Approval

The Institutional Ethical Committee for Animal Experimentation endorsed all procedures (Act no. 77-2012).

Conflict of Interests

The authors declare no conflict of interests.

Acknowledgments

Authors thank CV Mesa, for her help in biological assays. To Colciencias (CT-357-2011) and University of Antioquia (Cidepro and Estrategia de Sostenibilidad 2013-2014). They also thank Ms. A. Alvarez for language review.

References

[1] J. Alvar, I. D. Vélez, C. Bern et al., "Leishmaniasis worldwide and global estimates of its incidence," *PLoS ONE*, vol. 7, no. 5, Article ID e35671, 2012.

[2] World Health Organisation, "Control of the leishmaniases," WHO Technical Report Series: Report of a Meeting of the WHO Expert Committee on the Control of Leishmaniases 949, World Health Organisation, Geneva, Switzerland, 2010, http://whqlibdoc.who.int/trs/WHO_TRS_949_eng.pdf.

[3] D. J. Newman and G. M. Cragg, "Natural products as sources of new drugs over the 30 years from 1981 to 2010," *Journal of Natural Products*, vol. 75, no. 3, pp. 311–335, 2012.

[4] E. S. Fernando and C. J. Quinn, "Picramniaceae, a new family, and a recircumscription of *Simaroubaceae*," *Taxon*, vol. 44, no. 2, pp. 177–181, 1995.

[5] A. Cortadi, L. Andriolo, M. N. Campagna et al., "Morphoanatomy of leaves barks and wood of Argentinean Simaroubaceae *sensu latu*. Part I: *Alvaradoa subovata* Cronquist, *Picramnia parvifolia* Engl., Picramnia sellowii Planch. and *Castela coccinea* Griseb," *Boletin Latinoamericano y del Caribe de Plantas Medicinales y Aromaticas*, vol. 9, no. 1, pp. 38–55, 2010.

[6] H. Jacobs, "Comparative phytochemistry of *Picramnia* and *Alvaradoa*, genera of the newly established family Picramniaceae," *Biochemical Systematics and Ecology*, vol. 31, no. 7, pp. 773–783, 2003.

[7] L. Balderrama, A. Braca, E. Garcia, M. Melgarejo, C. Pizza, and N. De Tommasi, "Triterpenes and anthraquinones from *Picramnia sellowii* Planchon in Hook (Simaroubaceae)," *Biochemical Systematics and Ecology*, vol. 29, no. 3, pp. 331–333, 2001.

[8] W. Herz, P. S. Santhanam, and I. Wahlberg, "3-epi-betulinic acid, a new triterpenoid from *Picramnia pentandra*," *Phytochemistry*, vol. 11, no. 10, pp. 3061–3063, 1972.

[9] T. Rodríguez-Gamboa, J. B. Fernandes, E. Rodrigues Filho et al., "Triterpene benzoates from the bark of *Picramnia teapensis* (Simaroubaceae)," *Journal of the Brazilian Chemical Society*, vol. 12, no. 3, pp. 386–390, 2001.

[10] T. Rodríguez-Gamboa, S. R. Victor, J. B. Fernandes et al., "Anthrone and oxanthrone C,O-diglycosides from *Picramnia teapensis*," *Phytochemistry*, vol. 55, no. 7, pp. 837–841, 2000.

[11] F. Diaz, H.-B. Chai, Q. Mi et al., "Anthrone and oxanthrone c-glycosides from *Picramnia latifolia* collected in Peru," *Journal of Natural Products*, vol. 67, no. 3, pp. 352–356, 2004.

[12] T. Rodríguez-Gamboa, J. B. Fernandes, E. R. Fo, M. F. Das G. F. Da Silva, P. C. Vieira, and C. O. Castro, "Two anthrones and one oxanthrone from *Picramnia teapensis*," *Phytochemistry*, vol. 51, no. 4, pp. 583–586, 1999.

[13] P. N. Solis, A. G. Ravelo, A. G. Gonzalez, M. P. Gupta, and J. D. Phillipson, "Bioactive anthraquinone glycosides from *Picramnia antidesma* ssp. fessonia," *Phytochemistry*, vol. 38, no. 2, pp. 477–480, 1995.

[14] M. D. R. Hernández-Medel and R. Pereda-Miranda, "Cytotoxic anthraquinone derivatives from *Picramnia antidesma*," *Planta Medica*, vol. 68, no. 6, pp. 556–558, 2002.

[15] M. D. R. Hernandez-Medel, O. Lopez-Marquez, R. Santillan, and A. Trigos, "Mayoside, an oxanthrone from *Picramnia hirsuta*," *Phytochemistry*, vol. 43, no. 1, pp. 279–281, 1996.

[16] M. D. R. Camacho, J. D. Phillipson, S. L. Croft, P. N. Solis, S. J. Marshall, and S. A. Ghazanfar, "Screening of plant extracts for antiprotozoal and cytotoxic activities," *Journal of Ethnopharmacology*, vol. 89, no. 2-3, pp. 185–191, 2003.

[17] S. L. de Castro, M. C. Pinto, and A. V. Pinto, "Screening of natural and synthetic drugs against *Trypanosoma cruzi*. 1. Establishing a structure/activity relationship," *Microbios*, vol. 78, no. 315, pp. 83–90, 1994.

[18] M. L. Martínez, M. L. Travaini, M. V. Rodriguez et al., "Tripanocide and antibacterial activity of *Alvaradoa subovata* Cronquist extracts," *Boletin Latinoamericano y del Caribe de Plantas Medicinales y Aromaticas*, vol. 12, no. 3, pp. 302–312, 2013.

[19] 2015, http://www.tropicos.org.

[20] F. J. Morton, *Atlas of Medicinal Plants of Middle America—Bahamas to Yucatan*, Charles Thomas Publisher, Springfield, Ill, USA, 1981.

[21] S. Robledo, E. Osorio, D. Muñoz et al., "In vitro and in vivo cytotoxicities and antileishmanial activities of thymol and hemisynthetic derivatives," *Antimicrobial Agents and Chemotherapy*, vol. 49, no. 4, pp. 1652–1655, 2005.

[22] B. Insuasty, J. Ramírez, D. Becerra et al., "An efficient synthesis of new caffeine-based chalcones, pyrazolines and pyrazolo[3,4-b][1,4]diazepines as potential antimalarial, antitrypanosomal and antileishmanial agents," *European Journal of Medicinal Chemistry*, vol. 93, no. C, pp. 401–413, 2015.

[23] J. D. Finney, *Statistical Method in Biological Assay*, Griffin, London, UK, 1978.

[24] S. A. Pulido, D. L. Muñoz, A. M. Restrepo et al., "Improvement of the green fluorescent protein reporter system in *Leishmania* spp. for the *in vitro* and *in vivo* screening of antileishmanial drugs," *Acta Tropica*, vol. 122, no. 1, pp. 36–45, 2012.

[25] M. R. E. Varela, D. L. Muñoz, S. M. Robledo et al., "*Leishmania (Viannia) panamensis*: an *in vitro* assay using the expression of GFP for screening of anti-leishmanial drug," *Experimental Parasitology*, vol. 122, no. 2, pp. 134–139, 2009.

[26] S. M. Robledo, L. M. Carrillo, A. Daza et al., "Cutaneous leishmaniasis in the dorsal skin of hamsters: a useful model for the screening of antileishmanial drugs," *Journal of Visualized Experiments*, no. 62, p. 3533, 2012.

[27] L. M. Carrillo-Bonilla, A. Montoya, N. Arbeláez, H. Cadena, J. Ramírez, and S. M. Robledo, "Migration of *Leishmania (Viannia) panamensis* and its persistence in healthy skin of hamster," *Revista U.D.C.A Atualidade y Divulgação Científica*, vol. 17, no. 4, pp. 341–350, 2014.

[28] S. K. Ling, M. M. Pisar, and S. Man, "Platelet-activating factor (PAF) receptor binding antagonist activity of the methanol extracts and isolated flavonoids from *Chromolaena odorata* (L.) King and Robinson," *Biological and Pharmaceutical Bulletin*, vol. 30, no. 6, pp. 1150–1152, 2007.

[29] J. M. J. Vasconcelos, A. M. S. Silva, and J. A. S. Cavaleiro, "Chromones and flavanones from *Artemisia campestris* subsp. Maritima," *Phytochemistry*, vol. 49, no. 5, pp. 1421–1424, 1998.

[30] B. Modak, M. Rojas, R. Torres, J. Rodilla, and F. Luebert, "Antioxidant activity of a new aromatic geranyl derivative of the resinous exudates from *Heliotropium glutinosum* Phil.," *Molecules*, vol. 12, no. 5, pp. 1057–1063, 2007.

[31] S. S. Grecco, J. Q. Reimão, A. G. Tempone et al., "Isolation of an antileishmanial and antitrypanosomal flavanone from the leaves of *Baccharis retusa* DC. (Asteraceae)," *Parasitology Research*, vol. 106, no. 5, pp. 1245–1248, 2010.

[32] S. D. S. Grecco, J. Q. Reimão, A. G. Tempone et al., "In vitro antileishmanial and antitrypanosomal activities of flavanones from *Baccharis retusa* DC. (Asteraceae)," *Experimental Parasitology*, vol. 130, no. 2, pp. 141–145, 2012.

[33] P. Shaked-Mishant, N. Ulrich, M. Ephros, and D. Zilberstein, "Novel intracellular Sb-V reducing activity correlates with antimony susceptibility in *Leishmania donovani*," *The Journal of Biological Chemistry*, vol. 276, no. 6, pp. 3971–3976, 2001.

[34] G. Sen, S. Mukhopadhyay, M. Ray, and T. Biswas, "Quercetin interferes with iron metabolism in *Leishmania donovani* and targets ribonucleotide reductase to exert leishmanicidal activity," *Journal of Antimicrobial Chemotherapy*, vol. 61, no. 5, pp. 1066–1075, 2008.

[35] D. E. García, L. J. Cova, S. Briceño et al., "Metabolitos nitrogenados en el hámster dorado alimentado a base de harina de lombriz (*Eisenia* spp.)," *Archivos de Zootecnia*, vol. 61, no. 234, pp. 163–174, 2012.

11

Antihyperglycemic Activity of *Eucalyptus tereticornis* in Insulin-Resistant Cells and a Nutritional Model of Diabetic Mice

Alis Guillén,[1] **Sergio Granados,**[2] **Kevin Eduardo Rivas,**[1] **Omar Estrada,**[3]
Luis Fernando Echeverri,[4] **and Norman Balcázar**[1,2]

[1]*Molecular Genetics Group, University of Antioquia, Calle 70, No. 52-21, A.A. 1226, Medellín, Colombia*
[2]*Department of Physiology and Biochemistry, School of Medicine, University of Antioquia, Calle 70, No. 52-21, A.A. 1226, Medellín, Colombia*
[3]*Laboratory of Cellular Physiology, Center of Biophysic and Biochemistry, IVIC, Carretera Panamericana km 11, Altos de Pipe, Caracas, Venezuela*
[4]*Group of Organic Natural Product Chemistry, Faculty of Natural and Exact Sciences, University of Antioquia, Calle 70, No. 52-21, A.A. 1226, Medellín, Colombia*

Correspondence should be addressed to Norman Balcázar; norman.balcazar@udea.edu.co

Academic Editor: Masahiro Oike

Eucalyptus tereticornis is a plant used in traditional medicine to control diabetes, but this effect has not been proved scientifically. Here, we demonstrated through *in vitro* assays that E. tereticornis extracts increase glucose uptake and inhibit their production in insulin-resistant C2C12 and HepG2 cells, respectively. Furthermore, in a nutritional model using diabetic mice, the administration of ethyl acetate extract of E. tereticornis reduced fasting glycaemia, improved tolerance to glucose, and reduced resistance to insulin. Likewise, this extract had anti-inflammatory effects in adipose tissue when compared to control diabetic mice. Via bioguided assays and sequential purification of the crude extract, a triterpenoid-rich fraction from ethyl acetate extracts was shown to be responsible for the biological activity. Similarly, we identified the main compound responsible for the antihyperglycemic activity in this extract. This study shows that triterpenes found in E. tereticornis extracts act as hypoglycemic/antidiabetic compounds and contribute to the understanding of their use in traditional medicine.

1. Introduction

Type 2 diabetes mellitus (T2DM) is characterized because pancreatic β cells cannot synthesize adequate amounts of insulin to satisfy the metabolic demand of peripheral tissues such as skeletal muscle, adipose tissue, and liver [1, 2]. There is a strong association between T2DM and obesity; for instance, increase in body mass index (BMI), especially in the abdominal region, is related to increase in insulin resistance and in the risk of developing T2DM [3, 4]. Consequently, obesity is found in 90% of T2DM patients. In obesity, as calorie intake increases, adipocyte hypertrophy increases because of an increase in stored triacylglycerol (TAG) [5]. When the hypertrophy reaches a threshold and remains over time, the endocrine function of adipocytes is altered and a special microenvironment is established. This induces oxidative stress, inflammation, and the release of nonesterified free fatty acids (FFAs), which are phenomena involved in generating insulin resistance (IR), both in adipose tissue and in peripheral organs. It is also the greatest risk factor in developing T2DM.

Currently, there are a variety of T2DM treatments, but the presence of side effects, limited therapeutic effects, and intravenous administration has led to a worldwide search for new and better therapeutic agents [6]. Regarding this issue, traditional medicine is particularly valuable for the development of new treatments with the advantage that information exists about its safe therapeutic effect *in vivo* [7]. Colombia has notable biodiversity and a great cultural tradition in the therapeutic use of plants. Nevertheless, the scientific analysis of these medicinal plants remains unexplored.

Previous studies identified *Eucalyptus globulus* compounds that reduce oxidative stress in diabetic rats [8], and ursolic acid isolated from *E. tereticornis* avoids the accumulation of lipids in hepatic rat cells [9]. In Swiss Webster mice, raw extracts from *E. tereticornis* presented antihyperglycemic activity evaluated through an oral glucose tolerance test (OGTT) [10]. The experimental models developed in the studies previously mentioned simulate more type 1 diabetes mellitus than type 2. The latter is more prevalent and accounts for about 90% to 95% of all diagnosed cases of diabetes.

On the other hand, it is relevant to use animal models derived from genetic and environmental factors [11, 12] that simulate type 2 diabetic patients, to study their pathophysiological events and to evaluate the actions or the mechanisms of the new therapeutic agents.

In this study, we investigated the effect of *E. tereticornis* on insulin sensitivity in mice and in HepG2 and C2C12 insulin-resistant cell lines. Streptozotocin (STZ) treated and high-fat diet-fed C57BL/6J mice were selected as diabetic animal models because of their close similarities to type 2 diabetic patients. Effectively, extracts and a pure compound from *E. tereticornis* displayed an antihyperglycemic effect in both *in vitro* and *in vivo* assays.

2. Materials and Methods

2.1. Chemical and Reagents.
All solvents used for extraction and fractionations, methanol, ethanol, ethyl acetate, *n*-hexane, and dichloromethane, were previously distilled from commercial sources. Thin layer chromatography (TLC) was run in aluminum-backed F_{254} silica gel chromatoplates (Merck, Darmstadt, Germany). Column chromatography was performed with Sephadex LH-20 (Sigma, St. Louis, MO, USA) and glass columns (60 × 7 cm) filled with silica gel 60H (Merck) as well as with glass columns (40 × 3 cm). ^{1}H and ^{13}C-NMR and two-dimensional spectra were obtained in an AMX 300 spectrometer (Bruker BioSpin GmbH, Rheinstetten, Germany) operating at 300 MHz for ^{1}H and 75.0 for ^{13}C using CDCl$_3$ or DMSO d$_6$. Shifts are reported in δ units (ppm) and coupling constants (J) in Hz.

PBS 1x (Gibco, Carlsbad, CA, USA), low glucose Dulbecco's Modified Eagle Medium (DMEM), fetal bovine serum (FBS), penicillin-streptomycin (P/S) 10,000 U/mL, glutamine, bovine serum albumin (BSA), sodium lactate, sodium pyruvate, sodium bicarbonate, sodium palmitate and streptozotocin (STZ, Sigma, St. Louis, MO, USA), and 100 IU/mL insulin were used.

Plasma glucose level was measured using a commercial glucose oxidase-peroxidase kit (BioSystems, Bogotá DC, Colombia); plasma insulin level was measured using an enzyme-linked immunosorbent assay (ELISA) kit (Mercodia AB, Uppsala, Sweden); viability of the cells was measured by methyl thiazole tetrazolium (MTT, Amresco, Solon, OH, USA) assay. All measurements were performed using a Varioskan Flash spectrophotometer (Thermo, Waltham, MA, USA) at 500 or 570 nm. Glycaemia in mice was measured with the GlucoQuick Glucometer (Procaps, Barranquilla, Colombia).

2.2. Preparation of the Extract and Chromatographic Fractionation.
E. tereticornis leaves were collected in Valledupar (Colombia) in 2011. A specimen was deposited in the Herbarium of the University of Antioquia with # 178511. The dried leaves (2 kg) were extracted with 2 L 96% methanol at room temperature for 24 h and then filtered and concentrated to dryness at 38°C under reduced pressure to yield 120 g of crude methanol extract (crude extract). This extract was dissolved in 250 mL of a water-methanol mixture (1:1, v/v) and then partitioned with 400 mL (4 × 100 mL) petroleum ether and subsequently with 400 mL (4×100 mL) ethyl acetate, to afford to produce extracts F1 (48.0 g) and F2 (17.0 g), respectively.

Subsequently, 4.0 g ethyl acetate extract (from now on, designated F2) was fractionated on a Sephadex LH-20 column using hexane-dichloromethane-methanol 2:1:1 (v/v) as eluent and monitoring by silica gel TLC in hexane-ethyl acetate 1:1 (v/v); eight fractions were collected (F2-1 to F2-8), which were analyzed for the *in vitro* glucose uptake. Fractions F2-3 and F2-4 showed similar compositions, but the latter fraction (300 mg) contained several triterpenes, as revealed by TLC, and provoked high hypoglycemia activity.

The compounds contained in the active fraction F2-4 (300 mg) were separated on a silica gel column, eluted with a hexane-ethyl acetate 9:1 (v/v) mixture, which increased in polarity to finish with pure ethyl acetate; a total of 26 fractions were collected. From this new column, the *in vitro* active fractions 21 and 26 (F2-21 and F2-26) showed the presence of three compounds by TLC in hexane-ethyl acetate (1:1, v/v) that were separated by preparative chromatography in the same system (three runs). In this way, 20 mg of the active compound **1** with hypoglycemic activity was obtained. The other two substances could not be identified due to low yield and complexity of the NMR spectra.

2.3. Cell Cultures.
The C2C12 (ATCCCRL-1772) mouse muscle cells and HepG2 (ATCC HB-8065) human liver carcinoma cells were purchased from ATCC (Manassas, VA, USA). The cells were cultured and maintained at 37°C and 5% CO$_2$ in DMEM culture medium with 10% fetal bovine serum (FBS), 2 mM glutamine, penicillin, and 1% streptomycin (Sigma-Aldrich, St. Louis, MO, USA). When the C2C12 cells reached 80 to 90% confluence, they were differentiated into myotubes, using low glucose DMEM (5.5 mM) supplemented with 5% horse serum (HS) [13].

2.4. Insulin-Resistant Cell Model.
To develop a model of insulin-resistant cells, 4-day differentiated myotubes and HepG2 cells were preincubated for 2 h in DMEM with 5.5 mM glucose without FBS and supplemented with 1% BSA and then incubated for 18 h in DMEM with 5.5 mM glucose without FBS, 1% BSA, 0.75 mM palmitate, and 200 mM insulin [13, 14].

C2C12 myotubes were incubated for 4 h in 500 μL DMEM, 5.5 mM glucose, and various chromatographic fractions or extracts. After 4 h of incubation, 500 μL of supernatant was collected, and glucose concentration was measured using the glucose oxidase/peroxidase technique with a commercial kit. To calculate glucose utilization, the remaining glucose in the culture medium after incubation with controls and extracts or fractions was subtracted from the initial amount of glucose (5.5 mM).

HepG2 cells were washed three times with PBS to remove glucose, incubated for 4 h in 1 mL glucose production medium (glucose and phenol red-free DMEM supplemented with 20 mM sodium lactate and 2 mM sodium pyruvate) and in the presence of 1 nM insulin during the last 3 h. Medium (300 μL) was sampled to measure glucose concentration using the Amplex Red Glucose/Glucose Oxidase Assay Kit (Invitrogen, MA, USA). Commercial metformin (100 mg; Laboratorio Memphis, Bogotá DC, Colombia) was pulverized, dissolved in cultured media, and used as positive control in both cell lines.

2.5. Glucose and Insulin Tolerance Test in the Mouse Model of T2DM. C57BL/6J male mice (Charles Rivers Laboratories, Wilmington, MA, USA) over 4 weeks old were used in this study. The mice were housed at 22 $\pm$ 2°C with a 12 : 12 h light dark cycle with free access to food and water for 8 weeks. They were then randomly divided into three groups. A control group (n = 10) was fed a normal diet (ND, 14% fat/54% carbohydrates/32% protein). A high-fat diet (HFD) + STZ group (n = 10) and an HFD + STZ + F2 group (n = 10) were fed a high-fat diet (HFD, 42% fat, 42% carbohydrates, and 15% proteins) and received 3 doses of STZ at a low concentration (25 mg/kg) at the same time every day, after 4-hour fasting. The HFD + STZ + F2 group received 10 intraperitoneal doses, one dose every two days of F2 300 mg/kg. All animal studies were approved by the Institutional Animal Care and Use Committee of the University of Antioquia (Protocol number 65). Before and after treatment with F2, an intraperitoneal glucose tolerance test (IPGTT) was performed on the mice by administering a glucose load of 2.0 g/kg body weights. An insulin tolerance test (ITT) was performed after overnight fast. Initial blood glucose levels were determined, followed by injection (IP) of human insulin 0.75 U/kg. Blood glucose levels were measured via tail vein blood at 0, 30, 60, and 120 min after the injection using a GlucoQuick Glucometer (Procaps, Barranquilla, Colombia). Zero time was measured just before glucose injection. After glucose metabolism studies, mice were sacrificed and blood, liver, and adipose tissue were collected for further analyses.

2.6. RNA Extraction and Real-Time PCR. Total RNA was extracted from liver and visceral white adipose tissue with the RNeasy kit (QIAGEN, Valencia, CA), and the reverse transcription reaction was performed with 500 ng total RNA, 50 ng/μL random hexamers, 10 mM dNTP Mix, 20 mM Tris-HCl pH 8.4, 50 nM KCl, 2.5 mM MgCl$_2$, 40 U/μL RNaseOut, and 200 U/μL SuperScript III RT (Invitrogen, MA, USA) according to the manufacturers' instructions.

Real-time quantitative PCR (qPCR) analyses were performed with 50 ng cDNA and 100 nM sense and anti-sense primers (Integrated DNA Technologies, Coralville, IA, USA) in a final reaction volume of 25 μL using the Maxima SYBR Green/ROX qPCR Master Mix (Thermo Scientific, Waltham, MA, USA) and the CFX96 real-time PCR detection system (Bio-Rad, Hercules, CA, USA). Specific primer sequences are provided in supporting

information Table 1 (see Supplementary Material available online at http://dx.doi.org/10.1155/2015/418673). Relative quantification of each gene was calculated after normalization to GAPDH RNA by using the comparative CT method. The program for thermal cycling was 10 min at 95°C, followed by 40 cycles of 15 s at 95°C, 30 s at 60°C, and 30 s at 72°C.

2.7. Statistical Analysis. The results are expressed as means $\pm$ SEM. Student t-tests were used to compute individual pairwise comparisons of least square means. The trapezoidal rule was used to determine the area under the curve (AUC). Differences were considered to be significant at $p < 0.05$. All analyses were performed with the Prism 4 (GraphPad software Inc., La Jolla, CA, USA) statistical software.

3. Results

3.1. Hypoglycemic Effect of F2 on C2C12 and HepG2 Insulin-Resistant Cells. Figure 1 shows the effect of crude methanol extract and different extracts, F1, F2, and F3, on glucose uptake and production in cells previously exposed to palmitate. Figure 1(a) demonstrates that the glucose concentration in response to insulin in cells pretreated with palmitate was reduced by 14.8% compared with its control (Control R). Comparatively, when cells had not been treated previously with palmitate and were exposed to insulin (Ins 100 nM), the reduction of glucose concentration in the supernatant compared to its control (Control) was 23%. This means that palmitate induced a 35.7% reduction of the effect of insulin showing that C2C12 cells were insulin resistant. Likewise, under conditions of insulin resistance, the effect of crude extract (100 μg/mL) and its different extracts (gray bars in Figure 1(a)) on glucose uptake was determined. After testing various crude extract concentrations (data not shown), it was determined that there was a greater increase of glucose uptake at 100 μg/mL and that it was 17.1% in comparison with its control (Control R). Nevertheless, this response was lower than the one obtained with a positive control (Metf 1 mM). Regarding the fraction involved in response to the extract, F2 treatment showed a similar glucose uptake compared to the extract. No significant difference was found between this condition and the control (Control R).

On the other hand, the inhibition of glucose production in response to insulin was measured in control conditions using HepG2 cells pretreated with palmitate. Figure 1(b) shows a 36% inhibition of glucose production when insulin is present (Ins 100 nM) in comparison with control cells. Nevertheless, when the cells were pretreated with palmitate and stimulated with insulin (Ins R), this inhibition was reduced to 7% when compared with its control (Control R) indicating a state of resistance to the hormone. The effect of crude extract with its respective solvent extracts F1, F2, and F3 (gray bars in Figure 1(b)) was evaluated for 4 h in insulin-resistant cells. Crude extract at 150 μg/mL inhibited 82% of the glucose production in comparison with its control (Control R, Figure 1(b)). This value was greater than the percentage of inhibition obtained with the positive control (Metf 1 mM). It is also shown that the fraction involved in the

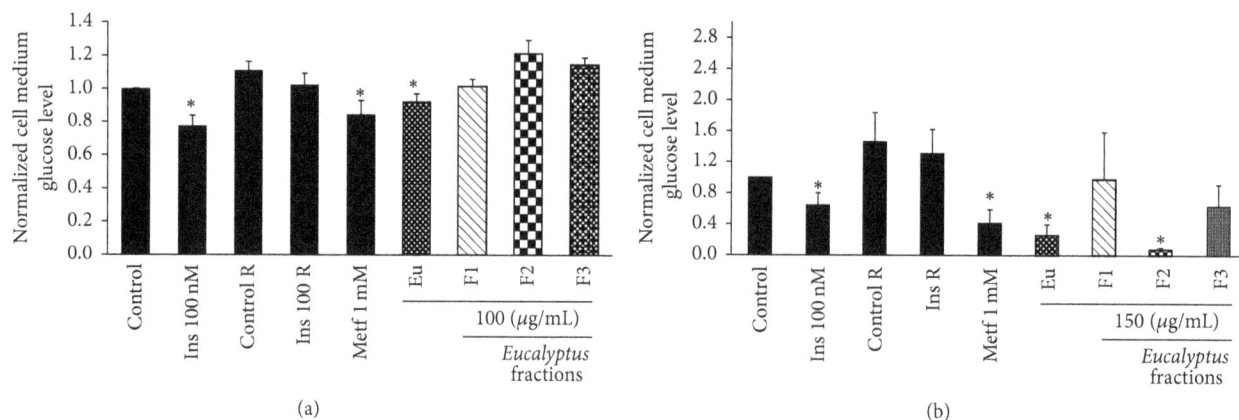

FIGURE 1: Effect of raw extract and fractions from *E. tereticornis* on insulin-resistant C2C12 and HepG2 cells. Glucose uptake in insulin-resistant C2C12 cells (a) and glucose production in insulin-resistant HepG2 cells (b). Cells were treated with different concentrations of the fractions or raw extract and glucose was measured in cultured supernatant after 4 h of treatment by the glucose oxidase technique. Eu, crude methanol extract; Ins (100 nM insulin); Control R, insulin-resistant C2C12 myotubes as controls; Ins 100 R, insulin-resistant C2C12 myotubes treated with 100 nM insulin; Metf, metformin 1 mM positive control. Bar values correspond to the arithmetic mean of glucose concentration for each treatment/control glucose concentration, $n = 6$ (C2C12) and $n = 3$ (HepG2). *Ins 100 nM versus control. *Treatment versus control R. $p < 0.05$, Student t-test. Error bars represent SEM.

response obtained with the extract is F2 with a 95% inhibition in comparison with its control (Control R).

3.2. F2 Improved Carbohydrate Metabolism in the Type 2 Diabetes Mouse Model.

To determine glucose tolerance and insulin resistance of diabetic mice and diabetic mice treated with F2, IPGTT and ITT were conducted. The results were analyzed as the total area under the curve (AUC) between 0 and 120 min or 0 and 90 min in Figures 2(a) and 2(c), respectively. The results obtained in the IPGTT (Figures 2(a) and 2(b)) show a decrease in glucose tolerance in diabetic mice (HFD + STZ) in comparison with the controls (normal diet). Treatment with F2 (HFD + STZ + F2) significantly increased glucose tolerance (Figures 2(a) and 2(b)). The ITT showed that treatment with HFD + STZ caused insulin resistance and that it is reverted when mice were treated with F2 (Figures 2(c) and 2(d)).

The fasting glucose concentration in the three animal groups of the study is presented in Figure 2(e). Diabetic mice (HFD + STZ) have glycaemia almost twice as high as the controls (normal diet). F2 treatment reverted fasting hyperglycemia. Figure 2(f) shows plasma insulin concentration; insulin level decreases in the diabetic group in comparison with the control, just as expected. Nevertheless, this value did not increase in the group treated with F2 (Figure 2(e)).

3.3. F2 Reduced Proinflammatory Cytokine mRNA Expression in Adipose Tissue from Diabetic Mice.

To determine if F2 improved the inflammation process caused by the HFD diet, we evaluated the mRNA expression of four proinflammatory cytokines, MCP-1, TNF-α, IL-1, and IL-6, in adipose tissue of diabetic mice (HFD + STZ) and diabetic mice treated with F2 (HFD + STZ + F2) including their respective controls. In Figure 3, we observe a significant increase, from 3 to 8 times,

of the expression of the four cytokines in diabetic mice in comparison with their respective controls. This alteration was reverted in mice that received 10 doses of F2.

3.4. F2 Reduced Glucose-6-Phosphatase (G6Pase) mRNA Expression in Liver from Diabetic Mice.

To evaluate the influence of F2 on gluconeogenesis, we evaluated the expression of the G6Pase gene in the liver of mice of the three study groups. In Figure 4, a rising trend ($p = 0.06$) of G6Pase expression in diabetic mice is visible in comparison with mice fed a normal diet; nevertheless, this increase was significantly reduced to 37.7% in diabetic mice treated with F2.

3.5. Structure of Compound 1 with Hypoglycemic Effects.

The ^{1}H NMR spectra (300 MHz, CDCl$_3$) showed signs of methyl groups at δ 0.83 (s), 0.95 (d, $J = 6.0$), 1.03 (s), 1.05 (d, $J = 6.0$), 1.10 (s, 3H), 1.20 (s), and 1.29 (s) and a dd in 3.25 (1H), a triplet in 4.26 (1H, disappeared adding D$_2$O), a dd (1H, $J = 3.0$ y 10.0) in 5.75, and doublet (1H, $J = 10.0$).

^{13}C RMN (DEPT 135, 75.0 MHz, and CDCl$_3$) spectrum showed the following signals, δ 14.95 (q), 16.13 (q), 17.70 (t), 17.85 (q), 17.93 (q), 18.91 (q), 19.19 (q), 22.82 (t), 25.55 (t), 27.02 (t), and 27.79 (q), and the following doublets, 30.83, 31.23, 31.33, 38.14, 38.30, 40.27, 53.04, 54.76, 60.58, 78.85, 128.82, and 133.50. Moreover, there were signals of quaternary carbons (singlets) at δ 36.37, 38.02, 38.80, 38.94, 40.02, 41.70, 41.95, 89.75, and 180.00.

Through experiments, COSY ^{1}H-^{1}H, HMQC, and HMBC, the complete structure of bioactive compound 1 was assigned as shown in Figure 5(c) and corresponds to 3β-hydroxy-urs-11-en-28,13β-olide. This compound was previously described from this plant [15].

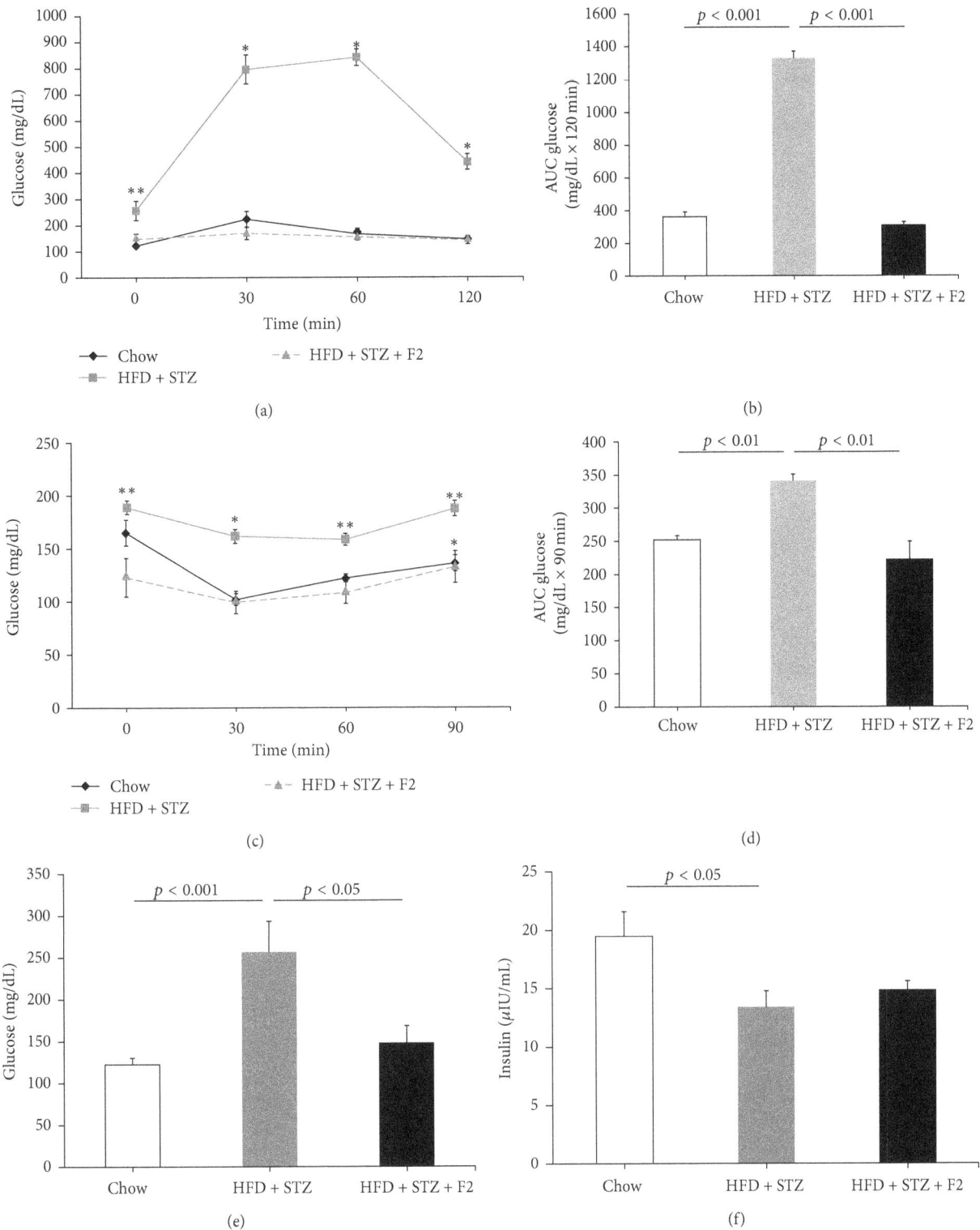

FIGURE 2: Glucose tolerance test (IPGTT) (a), insulin tolerance test (ITT) (c), fasting blood glucose levels (e), and fasting blood insulin levels (f) in F2 treated diabetic mice. All assays were performed after 10 IP treatment doses. ((b) and (d)) Area under the curve (AUC) values, calculated using data obtained in (a) and (c). HFD + STZ: diabetic control group and HFD + STZ + F2: diabetic group given 10 IP doses of ethyl acetate fraction (F2). ($n = 6$.) $^*p < 0.05$ and $^{**}p < 0.001$, Student t-test. Values are expressed as mean ± SEM.

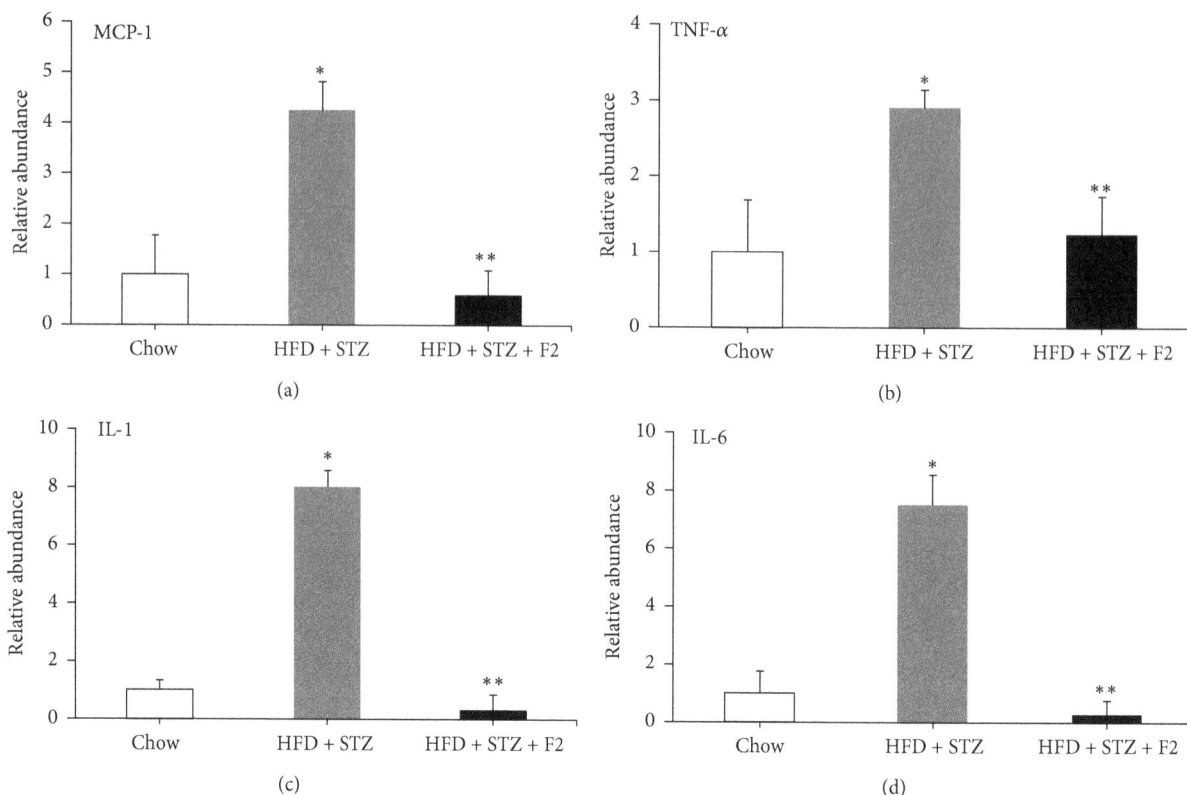

FIGURE 3: Effect of F2 on adipose expression of proinflammatory cytokine genes. mRNA expression levels by qRT-PCR of MCP-1 (a), TNF-α (b), IL-1β (c), and IL-6 (d) in adipose tissues of F2 treated diabetic mice. HFD + STZ: diabetic control group and HFD + STZ + F2: diabetic group given 10 IP doses of ethyl acetate fraction (F2). ($n = 6$.) $^*p < 0.05$ versus control and $^{**}p < 0.05$ versus HFD + STZ group. Values are expressed as mean ± SEM.

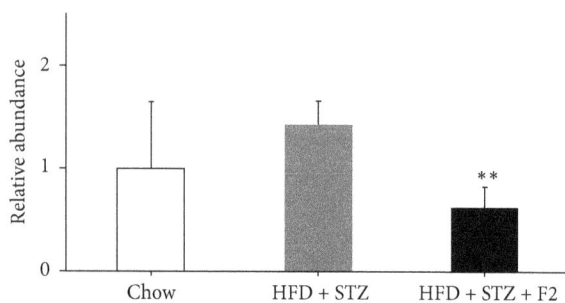

FIGURE 4: Effect of F2 on hepatic gluconeogenic gene. mRNA expression levels by qRT-PCR of glucose-6-phosphatase (G6P) in hepatic tissue of ethyl acetate fraction (F2) treated diabetic mice. HFD + STZ: diabetic control group and HFD + STZ + F2: diabetic group given 10 IP doses of F2. ($n = 6$.) $^{**}p < 0.05$ versus HFD + STZ group. Values are expressed as mean ± SEM.

4. Discussion

In this study, we evaluated the effect of the methanolic extract from *E. tereticornis* leaves and ethyl acetate extract (F2) in two *in vitro* models (C2C12 and HepG2 insulin-resistant cell lines) and an *in vivo* model (C57BL/6J diabetic mice). Our findings can be summarized as follows. (1) Crude extract increased glucose uptake in C2C12 cells and inhibited

glucose production in HepG2 cells, both insulin-resistant cells. (2) F2 improved glucose and insulin tolerance in a type 2 diabetes mouse model. (3) F2 had anti-inflammatory activity when evaluated on the adipose tissue of obese mice. (4) Identification of an F2 molecule could be responsible for the activity in this extract in C2C12 cells.

In mammals, skeletal muscle represents approximately 70% of their body mass, and it is the main tissue implicated in insulin-stimulated glucose uptake. It has been well established that muscle glucose uptake is reduced in T2DM [16]. Here we used a C2C12 mouse cell line that produces myotubes that have been used as a skeletal muscle glucose uptake model [17, 18].

One of the relevant aspects of this study is the establishment of models of insulin-resistant myotubes and hepatic cells. This implies a decrease in muscle glucose uptake and a decrease in hepatic gluconeogenesis inhibition. Moreover, in T2DM, low glycogen synthesis and high gluconeogenesis and glycogenolysis are important mechanisms responsible for fasting hyperglycemia [19].

Crude extract increased glucose uptake by 17% in comparison with an insulin-resistant control (Figure 1(a)). However, the uptake percentage was lower than the one obtained from normal cells (23% versus 17%, see supplementary Figure S1), showing that the signaling pathways involved in glucose uptake have been impaired by the chronic action of palmitate.

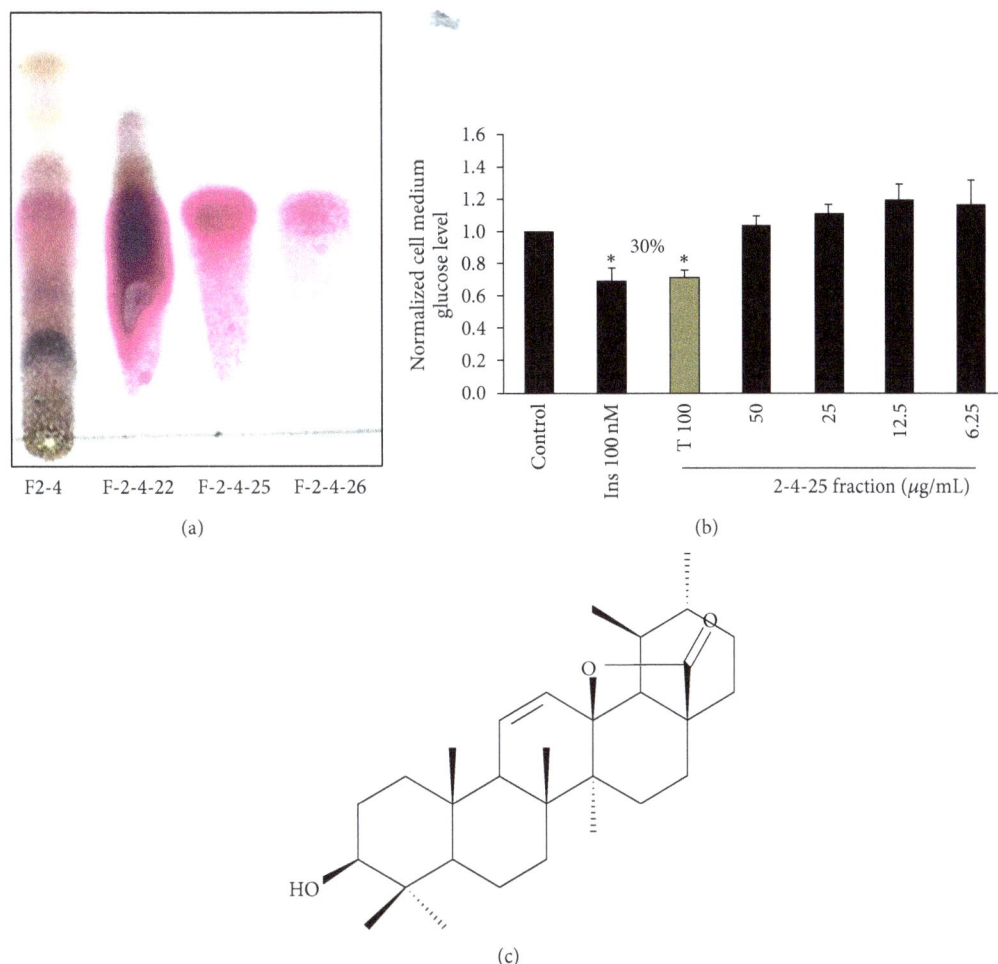

FIGURE 5: Effect of the fraction 2-4-25 enriched in compound **1** on glucose uptake in C2C12 cells. (a) Thin-layer chromatography. Fraction F2-4 was separated again on a silica gel column. Subfraction 22 shows a large amount of triterpenes; pure compound **1** obtained from subfractions 25 and 26 after TLC. (b) 2-4-25 fraction rich in compound **1** increases glucose uptake. $n = 3$. $^{*}p < 0.05$ versus control, Student t-test. (c) Structure of compound **1**: 3β-hydroxy-urs-11-en-28,13β-olide.

On the other hand, glucose production was evaluated in the HepG2 cell line. Insulin inhibited gluconeogenesis in comparison with controls and the addition of palmitate impaired this response (36% control versus 7% resistance), showing that the cells were insulin resistant (Figure 1(b)).

Crude extract reverted the effect of insulin resistance induced by palmitate by 82% in comparison with resistance control. As for the different solvent extracts, F2 was the fraction involved in such response, obtaining even a greater percentage of inhibition (95%) than the one obtained with pure extract. This demonstrated that the molecule or molecules involved in inhibition of glucose production in the *in vitro* system were mostly located in the F2. In order to validate the results obtained *in vitro*, we decided to evaluate the effect of F2, in a T2DM murine model.

Here, we used a T2DM nutritional model developed on C57BL/6J mice. Taking into account the etiology of the disease caused by a combination of multiple factors, we integrated an environmental component (mice fed with a high-fat diet) with the impairment of a mice's capability to

secrete insulin by pancreatic β cells using multiple doses at a low STZ concentration, which produces DNA alkylation and increases ROS (reactive oxygen species) production. The latter could facilitate an increase of the glucolipotoxicity in the pancreatic cells of mice fed a HFD. Furthermore, it has been reported that low doses of STZ induce low percentages of β cell destruction as observed in T2DM [20, 21]. This is a great difference when comparing this model to others used in which a sole dose is given at a high STZ concentration (100–200 mg/kg) or alloxan (65–150 mg/kg) producing the total destruction of β cells, which is characteristic of type 1 diabetes [21, 22].

As expected, this diabetic mice model showed an increase in fasting glucose in comparison to control mice (Figure 2(e)). After administering 10 IP doses of F2, a clear decrease in fasting glucose levels (Figure 2(e)) and an increase in glucose tolerance (Figures 2(a) and 2(b)) were observed. In other words, mechanisms related to the maintenance of glucose homeostasis are most effective because there is greater glucose uptake by peripheral tissues or a lower glucose hepatic production. In mice treated with F2, we also observed a reversion of insulin resistance (Figure 2(d)). Likewise, the molecules present in F2 could be acting in the liver activating routes that favor the inhibition of glucose production, as an insulin pathway, or activating proteins such as AMPK ($5'$ adenosine monophosphate-activated protein kinase) that inhibit the expression of key genes of gluconeogenesis as in the case of G6Pase. We confirmed that F2 treatment leads to a significant decrease in the expression of the G6Pase gene in liver (Figure 4). Jung et al. (2012) [23] observed a similar mechanism in a study where diabetic mice fed with a diet supplemented with persimmon (Diospyros spp.) extract showed lower glycaemia, lipaemia, and less fat accumulation related to a decrease in G6Pase activity.

On the other hand, it is important to highlight the fact that there was a significant decrease in the insulin level in fasting diabetic mice in comparison with controls (Figure 2(f)), indicating pancreatic β cell damage of this group. Since the group treated with 10 IP doses of F2 did not increase plasma insulin levels, it is possible that the compounds of F2 did not act in the pancreas or that treatment was insufficient to observe an improvement or an increase of β cells that could reflect an increase in insulin levels. These results agree with the ones obtained in vitro, where there was no evidence of insulin secretion stimulated by glucose, in MIN6 cells (mouse insulinoma cell line) treated with an F2 (data not shown).

In T2DM, an increase in the expression of proinflammatory cytokines such as TNF-α (tumor necrosis factor), IL-6 (interleukin-6), IL-1 (interleukin-1), and MCP-1 chemokine (monocyte chemotactic protein 1) has been demonstrated [24]. MCP-1 is secreted by preadipocytes and adipocytes and participates in recruiting monocytes and macrophages implicated in a chronic low inflammation condition observed in obesity. Once the macrophages have been infiltrated in adipose tissue, they can secrete cytokines that favor the development and/or the deterioration of insulin resistance. The TNF-α gene is expressed constitutively in adipose tissue where its expression increases principally due to the infiltration of macrophages. mRNA expression in adipose tissue of the TNF-α of obese subjects is 2.5 times greater than in subjects with normal weight, and this high expression level is greatly correlated with hyperinsulinemia. It is an important event in the physiopathology of insulin resistance and T2DM [24, 25].

We evaluated the expression of 4 proinflammatory cytokines in the adipose tissue of the three groups used in the murine model. In Figure 3, an increase in MCP-1, TNF-α, IL-1, and IL-6 expression of diabetic mice (fed simultaneously with HFD + STZ) is visible in comparison with controls (normal diet); we clearly noticed that treatment with F2 (HFD + STZ + F2) reduced mRNA levels of all the cytokines. This suggests that F2 compounds reduce the proinflammatory condition of adipose tissue in diabetic mice.

According to the NMR spectra, the ethyl acetate extract (F2) is rich in triterpenes. These molecules are secondary metabolites found in plants distributed around the world. Phytochemical researches have implicated triterpenes as one of the most important chemical groups in which biological

activity lies [26]. In vitro and in vivo studies have demonstrated the potential use of these types of molecules (e.g., lupeol, betulinic, ursolic, and oleanolic acids) to prevent and treat a wide spectrum of diseases including cancer, infectious diseases, diabetes, and cardiovascular and rheumatic diseases [27, 28]. Interestingly, the triterpenes studied so far have demonstrated an immunomodulatory activity, which turns them into very promising molecules for treatment of type 2 diabetes [28].

Lupeol is found in various edible vegetable and fruit species as olives, mango, pear, ginseng oil, red fruits, carrots, peppers, tomatoes, guavas, and tea among others. It has been reported that, among all the properties related to these types of molecules, lupeol modulates the expression of various proinflammatory molecules including TNF-α, IL-1β, prostaglandin E2 (PGE2), IL-2, IL-4, IL-6, and myeloperoxidase [29]. Oleanolic acid (OA) is a pentacyclic triterpene found in a large variety of plants that has a very wide range of pharmacological and biochemical properties including anti-inflammatory, antioxidant, antihyperlipidemic, and hypoglycemic effects [30, 31]. OA reduces insulin resistance related to obesity and hyperlipidemia and protects against endothelial dysfunction [32, 33]. Studies by de Melo et al. (2010) [34] reported that administering 50 mg/dL OA daily to animals fed a high-fat diet significantly reduces abdominal fat making it a candidate to evaluate its anti-inflammatory and antioxidant properties in adipose tissue of obese animals.

Due to the fact that the ethyl acetate extract F2 showed high in vitro and in vivo activity, it was further fractionated by Sephadex LH-20 column chromatography using a mixture of three eluents to yield eight fractions (F2-1 to F2-8). These fractions were then tested in C2C12 cells using the same methodology as the previous glucose uptake assays. Fraction F2-4 was further fractionated by silica gel column. Preliminary results with fraction F2-4-25 (Figure 5(a)), rich in compound 1 in glucose uptake in C2C12 cells, suggest that this molecule is involved in E. tereticornis hypoglycemia effects (Figure 5(b)). The structure shown in Figure 5(c) corresponds to 3β-hydroxy-urs-11-en-28,13β-olide, a molecule previously described in E. tereticornis with antimicrobial activity [15] and in E. camaldulensis, showing an antiproliferative effect on ovarian cancer lines [35]. Despite the large number of pharmacological actions that are attributed to Eucalyptus spp., among them antidiabetic, this is the first time we determine one of the potential compounds responsible for such activity.

On the other hand, this molecule is related structurally to other triterpene glycosides isolated from Boussingaultia baselloides (syn. Anredera baselloides) [36] that have intense hypoglycemic activity and, as such, are used in traditional medicine. Likewise, the treatment with extracts of a plant of the same genus, Boussingaultia gracilis Miers var. pseudobaselloides, can regulate the expression of genes involved in lipogenesis and lipolysis [37].

Finally, in this study, we demonstrate that F2 reduces the expression levels of proinflammatory cytokines in adipose tissue. This allows us to suggest that the systemic effects of this fraction on the metabolism of carbohydrates could be due to its action in an inflammation established in adipose tissue of mice with obesity-related T2DM. Now we aim to identify the action mechanisms of plant extracts and their active molecules to be able to contribute to the development of new therapeutic strategies that cut the connection between inflammation and oxidative stress and the development of important pathologies in public health such as T2DM. In addition, the next step is to clarify the action mechanisms of compound 1 in the liver, muscles, and adipose tissue and to determine effects of triterpene mixtures as well as possible synergism among them.

5. Conclusions

E. tereticornis has potential as hypoglycemic when it is used in insulin-resistant cell models. Furthermore, F2 reduces the expression of proinflammatory cytokines in a T2DM mouse model, which could contribute to improving the cell-signaling pathways in target organs such as muscles and the liver. It results in an increase in glucose tolerance and an improvement of insulin resistance. 3β-Hydroxy-urs-11-en-28,13β-olide is one of the main molecules of the bioactive F2 extract and is responsible for the antihyperglycemic effects.

Conflict of Interests

The authors declare no conflict of interests.

Authors' Contribution

Alis Guillén, Sergio Granados, and Kevin Eduardo Rivas helped with bioassay, separation process, and data collection; Omar Estrada contributed to some separation process; Norman Balcázar and Luis Fernando Echeverri were responsible for study conception and design, data analysis, and writing of the paper.

Acknowledgment

The authors thank COLCIENCIAS (Colombia) for funding the Project no. 111551929137 and an M.S. scholarship for Alis Guillén.

References

[1] M. Stumvoll, B. J. Goldstein, and T. W. van Haeften, "Type 2 diabetes: principles of pathogenesis and therapy," *The Lancet*, vol. 365, no. 9467, pp. 1333–1346, 2005.

[2] S. E. Kahn, R. L. Hull, and K. M. Utzschneider, "Mechanisms linking obesity to insulin resistance and type 2 diabetes," *Nature*, vol. 444, no. 7121, pp. 840–846, 2006.

[3] S. Colagiuri, "Diabesity: therapeutic options," *Diabetes, Obesity and Metabolism*, vol. 12, no. 6, pp. 463–473, 2010.

[4] Á. J. Ruiz, P. J. Aschner, M. F. Puerta, and R. Alfonso-Cristancho, "IDEA study (international day for the evaluation of abdominal obesity): primary care study of the prevalence of abdominal obesity and associated risk factors in Colombia," *Biomedica*, vol. 32, no. 4, pp. 610–616, 2012.

[5] K. J. Strissel, Z. Stancheva, H. Miyoshi et al., "Adipocyte death, adipose tissue remodeling, and obesity complications," *Diabetes*, vol. 56, no. 12, pp. 2910–2918, 2007.

[6] P. J. Phillips and S. M. Twigg, "Oral hypoglycaemics: a review of the evidence," *Australian Family Physician*, vol. 39, no. 9, pp. 651–653, 2010.

[7] S. Granados, N. Balcázar, A. Guillén, and F. Echeverri, "Evaluation of the hypoglycemic effects of flavonoids and extracts from *Jatropha gossypifolia* L.," *Molecules*, vol. 20, no. 4, pp. 6181–6193, 2015.

[8] A. Nakhaee, M. Bokaeian, M. Saravani, A. Farhangi, and A. Akbarzadeh, "Attenuation of oxidative stress in streptozotocin-induced diabetic rats by *Eucalyptus globulus*," *Indian Journal of Clinical Biochemistry*, vol. 24, no. 4, pp. 419–425, 2009.

[9] B. Saraswat, P. K. S. Visen, and D. P. Agarwal, "Ursolic acid isolated from *Eucalyptus tereticornis* protects against ethanol toxicity in isolated rat hepatocytes," *Phytotherapy Research*, vol. 14, no. 3, pp. 163–166, 2000.

[10] I. M. Villaseñor and M. R. A. Lamadrid, "Comparative antihyperglycemic potentials of medicinal plants," *Journal of Ethnopharmacology*, vol. 104, no. 1-2, pp. 129–131, 2006.

[11] M. J. Reed, K. Meszaros, L. J. Entes et al., "A new rat model of type 2 diabetes: the fat-fed, streptozotocin-treated rat," *Metabolism: Clinical and Experimental*, vol. 49, no. 11, pp. 1390–1394, 2000.

[12] D. Chen and M.-W. Wang, "Development and application of rodent models for type 2 diabetes," *Diabetes, Obesity and Metabolism*, vol. 7, no. 4, pp. 307–317, 2005.

[13] C. Schmitz-Peiffer, D. L. Craig, and T. J. Biden, "Ceramide generation is sufficient to account for the inhibition of the insulin-stimulated PKB pathway in C2C12 skeletal muscle cells pretreated with palmitate," *The Journal of Biological Chemistry*, vol. 274, no. 34, pp. 24202–24210, 1999.

[14] J.-Y. Lee, H.-K. Cho, and Y. H. Kwon, "Palmitate induces insulin resistance without significant intracellular triglyceride accumulation in HepG2 cells," *Metabolism: Clinical and Experimental*, vol. 59, no. 7, pp. 927–934, 2010.

[15] W. Hongcheng and Y. Fujimotot, "Triterpene esters from *Eucalyptus tereticornis*," *Phytochemistry*, vol. 33, no. 1, pp. 151–153, 1993.

[16] M. A. Abdul-Ghani and R. A. DeFronzo, "Pathogenesis of insulin resistance in skeletal muscle," *Journal of Biomedicine and Biotechnology*, vol. 2010, Article ID 476279, 19 pages, 2010.

[17] Y.-T. Deng, T.-W. Chang, M.-S. Lee, and J.-K. Lin, "Suppression of free fatty acid-induced insulin resistance by phytopolyphenols in C_2C_{12} mouse skeletal muscle cells," *The Journal of Agricultural and Food Chemistry*, vol. 60, no. 4, pp. 1059–1066, 2012.

[18] M. van Huyssteen, P. J. Milne, E. E. Campbell, and M. van de Venter, "Antidiabetic and cytotoxicity screening of five medicinal plants used by traditional african health practitioners in the nelson mandela metropole, South Africa," *African Journal of Traditional, Complementary and Alternative Medicines*, vol. 8, no. 2, pp. 150–158, 2011.

[19] J. L. Treadway, P. Mendys, and D. J. Hoover, "Glycogen phosphorylase inhibitors for treatment of type 2 diabetes mellitus," *Expert Opinion on Investigational Drugs*, vol. 10, no. 3, pp. 439–454, 2001.

[20] E. R. Gilbert, Z. Fu, and D. Liu, "Development of a non-genetic mouse model of type 2 diabetes," *Experimental Diabetes Research*, vol. 2011, Article ID 416254, 12 pages, 2011.

[21] M. Zhang, X.-Y. Lv, J. Li, Z.-G. Xu, and L. Chen, "The characterization of high-fat diet and multiple low-dose streptozotocin induced type 2 diabetes rat model," *Experimental Diabetes Research*, vol. 2008, Article ID 704045, 2008.

[22] T. Szkudelski, "The mechanism of alloxan and streptozotocin action in B cells of the rat pancreas," *Physiological Research*, vol. 50, no. 6, pp. 537–546, 2001.

[23] U. J. Jung, Y. B. Park, S. R. Kim, and M.-S. Choi, "Supplementation of persimmon leaf ameliorates hyperglycemia, dyslipidemia and hepatic fat accumulation in type 2 diabetic mice," *PLoS ONE*, vol. 7, no. 11, Article ID e49030, 2012.

[24] N. Ouchi, J. L. Parker, J. J. Lugus, and K. Walsh, "Adipokines in inflammation and metabolic disease," *Nature Reviews Immunology*, vol. 11, no. 2, pp. 85–97, 2011.

[25] K. Sun, C. M. Kusminski, and P. E. Scherer, "Adipose tissue remodeling and obesity," *The Journal of Clinical Investigation*, vol. 121, no. 6, pp. 2094–2101, 2011.

[26] M. Saleem, "Lupeol, a novel anti-inflammatory and anti-cancer dietary triterpene," *Cancer Letters*, vol. 285, no. 2, pp. 109–115, 2009.

[27] H. R. Siddique and M. Saleem, "Beneficial health effects of lupeol triterpene: a review of preclinical studies," *Life Sciences*, vol. 88, no. 7-8, pp. 285–293, 2011.

[28] H. Sheng and H. Sun, "Synthesis, biology and clinical significance of pentacyclic triterpenes: a multi-target approach to prevention and treatment of metabolic and vascular diseases," *Natural Product Reports*, vol. 28, no. 3, pp. 543–593, 2011.

[29] E. L. Nguemfo, T. Dimo, A. B. Dongmo et al., "Anti-oxidative and anti-inflammatory activities of some isolated constituents from the stem bark of *Allanblackia monticola* Staner L.C (Guttiferae)," *Inflammopharmacology*, vol. 17, no. 1, pp. 37–41, 2009.

[30] S. Jäger, H. Trojan, T. Kopp, M. N. Laszczyk, and A. Scheffler, "Pentacyclic triterpene distribution in various plants—rich sources for a new group of multi-potent plant extracts," *Molecules*, vol. 14, no. 6, pp. 2016–2031, 2009.

[31] D. Gao, Q. Li, Y. Li et al., "Antidiabetic and antioxidant effects of oleanolic acid from *Ligustrum lucidum* Ait in alloxan-induced diabetic rats," *Phytotherapy Research*, vol. 23, no. 9, pp. 1257–1262, 2009.

[32] K. Yunoki, G. Sasaki, Y. Tokuji et al., "Effect of dietary wine pomace extract and oleanolic acid on plasma lipids in rats fed high-fat diet and its DNA microarray analysis," *Journal of Agricultural and Food Chemistry*, vol. 56, no. 24, pp. 12052–12058, 2008.

[33] R. Rodriguez-Rodriguez, M. D. Herrera, M. A. de Sotomayor, and V. Ruiz-Gutierrez, "Effects of pomace olive oil-enriched diets on endothelial function of small mesenteric arteries from spontaneously hypertensive rats," *British Journal of Nutrition*, vol. 102, no. 10, pp. 1435–1444, 2009.

[34] C. L. de Melo, M. G. R. Queiroz, S. G. C. Fonseca et al., "Oleanolic acid, a natural triterpenoid improves blood glucose tolerance in normal mice and ameliorates visceral obesity in mice fed a high-fat diet," *Chemico-Biological Interactions*, vol. 185, no. 1, pp. 59–65, 2010.

[35] G. Topu, G. Yapar, Z. Türkmen et al., "Ovarian antiproliferative activity directed isolation of triterpenoids from fruits of *Eucalyptus camaldulensis* Dehnh," *Phytochemistry Letters*, vol. 4, no. 4, pp. 421–425, 2011.

[36] A. Espada and R. Riguera, "Boussingoside E, a new triterpenoid saponin from the tubers of *Boussingaultia baselloides*," *Journal of Natural Products*, vol. 60, no. 1, pp. 17–19, 1997.

[37] D. K. Burdi, S. Qureshi, and A. B. Ghanghro, "An overview of available hypoglycemic triterpenoids and saponins to cure diabetes mellitus," *Advanced Life Sciences*, vol. 1, no. 3, pp. 119–128, 2014.

12

Involvement of Inflammatory Cytokines in Antiarrhythmic Effects of Clofibrate in Ouabain-Induced Arrhythmia in Isolated Rat Atria

Somayeh Moradi,[1] Vahid Nikoui,[2,3] Muhammad Imran Khan,[4] Shayan Amiri,[1,5] Farahnaz Jazaeri,[1] and Azam Bakhtiarian[1,5]

[1]Department of Pharmacology, School of Medicine, Tehran University of Medical Sciences, Tehran, Iran
[2]Razi Institute for Drug Research, Iran University of Medical Sciences, Tehran, Iran
[3]Department of Pharmacology, Faculty of Medicine, Iran University of Medical Sciences, Tehran, Iran
[4]Department of Pharmacology, School of Medicine, International Campus, Tehran University of Medical Sciences, Tehran, Iran
[5]Experimental Medicine Research Center, Tehran University of Medical Sciences, Tehran, Iran

Correspondence should be addressed to Azam Bakhtiarian; bakhtiar@tums.ac.ir

Academic Editor: Masahiro Oike

Considering the cardioprotective and anti-inflammatory properties of clofibrate, the aim of the present experiment was to investigate the involvement of local and systemic inflammatory cytokines in possible antiarrhythmic effects of clofibrate in ouabain-induced arrhythmia in rats. Rats were orally treated with clofibrate (300 mg/kg), and ouabain (0.56 mg/kg) was administered to animals intraperitoneally. After induction of anesthesia, the atria were isolated and the onset of arrhythmia and asystole was recorded. The levels of inflammatory cytokines in atria were also measured. Clofibrate significantly postponed the onset of arrhythmia and asystole when compared to control group ($P \leq 0.05$ and $P \leq 0.01$, resp.). While ouabain significantly increased the atrial beating rate in control group ($P \leq 0.05$), same treatment did not show similar effect in clofibrate-treated group ($P > 0.05$). Injection of ouabain significantly increased the atrial and systemic levels of all studied inflammatory cytokines ($P \leq 0.05$). Pretreatment with clofibrate could attenuate the ouabain-induced elevation of IL-6 and TNF-α in atria ($P \leq 0.01$ and $P \leq 0.05$, resp.), as well as ouabain-induced increase in IL-6 in plasma ($P \leq 0.05$). Based on our findings, clofibrate may possess antiarrhythmic properties through mitigating the local and systemic inflammatory factors including IL-6 and TNF-α.

1. Background

The fibrate class of hypolipidemic drugs is used extensively in treatment of metabolic syndrome in which hyperlipidemia and hypertension are most prominent manifestations of this disorder. Fibrates are ligands of the peroxisome proliferator-activated receptors (PPARs) [1, 2]. These receptors are ligand-dependent transcription factors and belong to the nuclear steroid/thyroid/retinoic acid receptor superfamily [3, 4]. PPARs consisted of three isotypes including α, β, and γ. PPAR-α possesses an important role in lipid metabolism [5]. PPAR-α is predominantly expressed in tissues with high fatty acid oxidation rate including heart, liver, and kidney [6]. It has been shown that fibrates protect heart against experimental ischemia/reperfusion injury in animals through PPARs [7, 8]. Interestingly, previous studies have shown that cardioprotective effects of fibrates are not observed in PPAR-α knockout mice, indicating that PPAR-α plays a critical role in cardioprotective effects of fibrates [7, 8]. Since majority of hyperlipidemic patients are suffering from comorbid cardiovascular diseases, it is clear that many of the cardiovascular patients use clofibrate. It has been demonstrated that PPAR-α agonists have anti-inflammatory properties [9–12], and inflammatory cytokines have been reported to be involved in atrial and ventricular arrhythmias [13–15]. Therefore, the aim of present study was to investigate

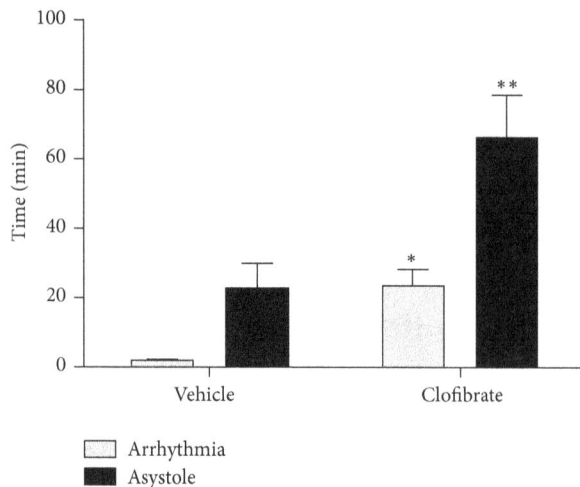

FIGURE 1: Time of onset of arrhythmia and asystole after ouabain incubation in vehicle- and clofibrate-treated groups. Data are shown as mean ± SEM. Six rats were used in each group. $^*P \leq 0.05$ compared to arrhythmia of vehicle group; $^{**}P \leq 0.05$ compared to asystole of vehicle group.

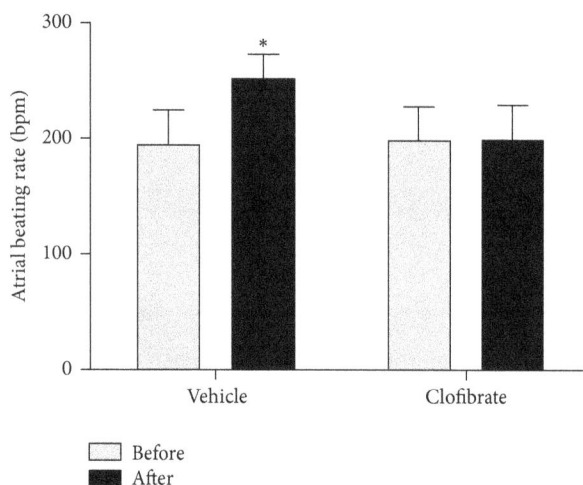

FIGURE 2: Atrial beating rates before and after incubation of ouabain in vehicle- and clofibrate-treated groups. Data are shown as mean ± SEM. Six rats were used in each group. $^*P \leq 0.05$ compared to before time of vehicle group.

the effects of clofibrate on ouabain-induced arrhythmia in isolated rat atria and involvement of local and systemic inflammatory cytokines.

2. Material and Methods

2.1. Animals. Male Wistar albino rats (body weight 250–280 g) were obtained from the Department of Pharmacology and Comparative Biology Unit (Tehran University of Medical Sciences). Animals were housed under the standard laboratory conditions, temperature 22 ± 2°C, humidity 70%–80%, and 12 h light-dark cycle, and have *ad libitum* access to food and water. All experiments were conducted in

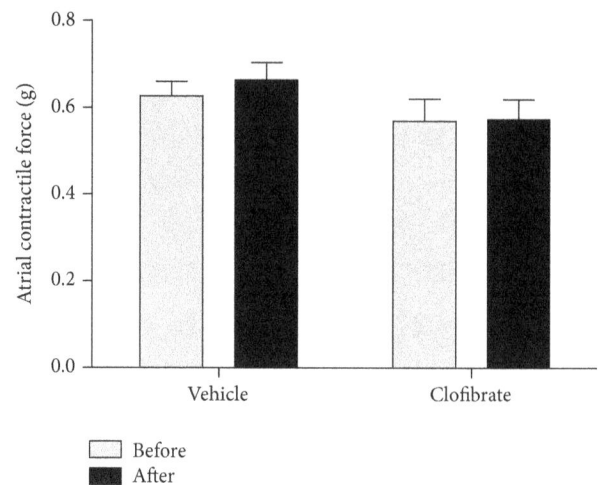

FIGURE 3: Contractile force before and after incubation of ouabain in vehicle- and clofibrate-treated groups. Data are shown as mean ± SEM. Six rats were used in each group.

Tehran University of Medical Sciences in accordance with the recommendations of the ethics committee on animal experimentation of the medical school.

2.2. Chemicals. All materials were purchased from Merck (Germany), unless noted otherwise. Clofibrate was a gift from Zahravi Pharmaceutical Company, Iran. Ouabain and enzyme-linked immunosorbent assay (ELISA) kit for measurement of IL-6 and TNF-α were provided from Sigma-Aldrich (St. Louis, MO, USA). ELISA kit for measurement of IL-1β was purchased from Abcam, UK.

2.3. Experimental Plan. In order to study the isolated atria, 12 rats were randomly divided into 2 equal groups. First group (treatment) received clofibrate (300 mg/kg dissolved in olive oil 1 mL/kg, orally) once daily for 14 days, while the second group (control) received only olive oil (1 mL/kg, orally) once daily for 14 days. For measuring the inflammatory cytokines, 12 rats were divided into three equal groups. First 2 groups received only olive oil (1 mL/kg, orally) once daily for 14 days, while third group was given clofibrate (300 mg/kg, dissolved in olive oil 1 mL/kg, orally) once daily for 14 days. From the days 12th to 14th, first group received normal saline, 1 mL/kg, intraperitoneally (i.p.) once daily, whereas the second and third groups were injected by ouabain dissolved in normal saline at the dose of 0.56 mg/kg [16] once daily (i.p.) for three consecutive days.

2.4. Preparation of Isolated Atria. After induction of anesthesia with ketamine (80 mg/kg, Alfasan, Netherlands) and diazepam (2 mg/kg, Caspian Tamin, Iran) (i.p.), heart was rapidly removed and atria were carefully dissected from the ventricles, attached to a tissue holder, and then were immersed in a tissue bath containing 25 mL of carbogenated (95% O_2 and 5% CO_2) modified Krebs solution at 37°C and pH 7.4. The composition of the solution was as follows (mM): NaCl 118.0, KCl 4.7, $CaCl_2$ 2.6, $MgCl_2$ 1.2, NaH_2PO_4 1.0,

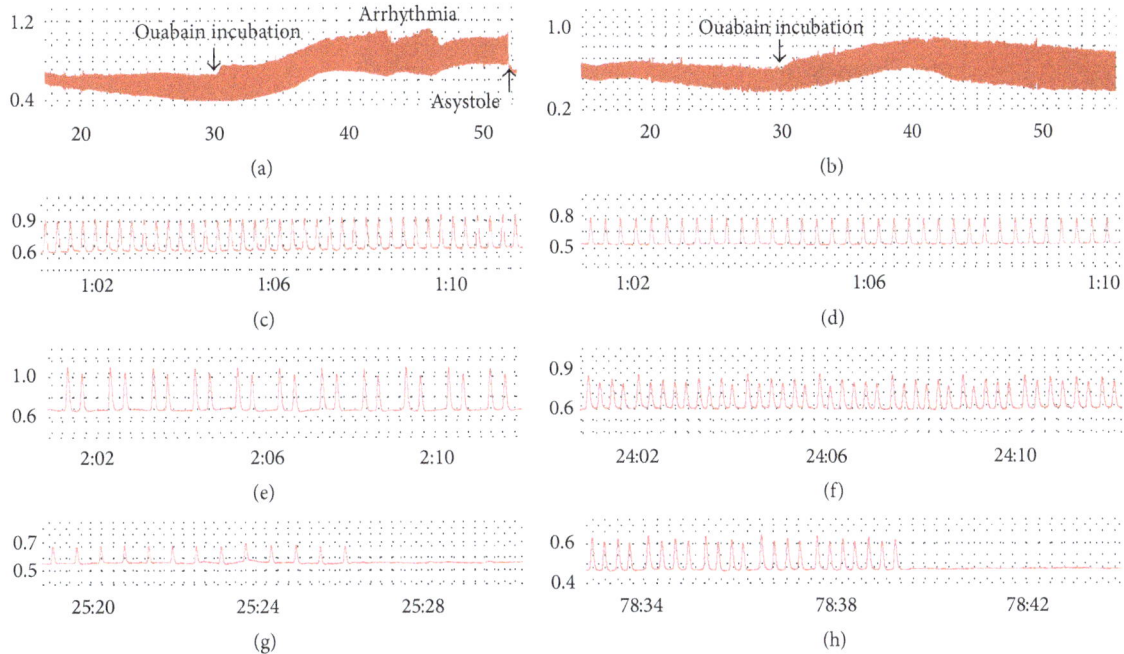

FIGURE 4: A general comparison in chronotropic and inotropic features between vehicle- and clofibrate-treated groups. Complete records of isolated atrial beats of vehicle-treated (a) and clofibrate-treated (b) groups. In vehicle-treated group (a), ouabain-induced arrhythmia is obvious and asystole happens after arrhythmia. The severity of arrhythmia in clofibrate-treated group is lesser and, in some samples (b), no asystole was seen until several hours. Atrial beatings before incubation of ouabain in vehicle-treated (c) and clofibrate-treated (d) groups. As shown, atrial beatings and contractile force are similar in both groups. Ouabain-induced arrhythmia in vehicle-treated (e) and clofibrate-treated (f) groups. The shape of arrhythmia in vehicle-treated group is bigeminy (twin spikes with strong force), which is the typical manifestation of ouabain-induced arrhythmia (a). In clofibrate-treated group (b), spikes of arrhythmia are weak and irregular, and it happens much later than vehicle-treated group. Ouabain-induced asystole in vehicle-treated (g) and clofibrate-treated (h) groups. Time of onset of asystole in clofibrate-treated group (h) is later than vehicle-treated group.

$NaHCO_3$ 25.0, glucose 11.1, EDTA 0.004, and ascorbic acid 0.11. A preload tension of 1000 mg was applied to the atria and tissues were allowed to equilibrate for 30 min [17]. The rate and force of spontaneous contractions were recorded by the isometric force transducer of PowerLab system (ADInstrument, Australia). Atrial beats and contractile forces were calculated using the LabChart software.

2.5. Measurement of IL-1β, IL-6, and TNF-α in Atria and Plasma. The levels of inflammatory cytokines in atria and plasma were measured by specific ELISA kits. Briefly, each atrium was homogenized in 1 mL of phosphate buffered saline (PBS, pH 7.4) and then centrifuged at 10000 g for 15 min at 4°C. For measurement of plasma levels of cytokines, blood samples were taken and centrifuged at 4000 g for 15 min at 4°C. IL-1β, IL-6, and TNF-α levels were measured by adding the sample supernatant and kit reagents to plate wells. Absorbance was read at 450 nm using a plate reader (Synergy HT, Biotek, USA), and the contents of IL-1β, IL-6, and TNF-α in atria and plasma were calculated and reported as ng/mL.

2.6. Statistical Analysis. Statistical analyses were carried out using GraphPad Prism 5 software (San Diego, CA, USA). The results are presented as mean ± SEM. Unpaired Student's *t*-test was carried out to compare the time of onset of arrhythmia or asystole as well as atrial beating rate and contractile force between treatment and control groups. Paired Student's *t*-test was used to detect the effects of ouabain on atrial beating rate and contractile force within groups. Comparison of inflammatory cytokines between three groups was done by one-way analysis of variance (ANOVA) followed by Tukey's *post hoc* test. P values less than 0.05 were considered statistically significant.

3. Results

3.1. Study of Isolated Atria. Clofibrate significantly postponed time of onset of arrhythmia (23.57 ± 4.69 min) rather than control group (2.04 ± 0.27 min, $P \leq 0.05$). Also, we detected a significant increase in the onset time of asystole in the treatment group (66.19 ± 12.33 min), while this time for control group was 22.77 ± 7.17 min ($P \leq 0.01$, Figure 1).

Treating with ouabain significantly increased the atrial beating rate in the control group (194 before and 251 beats per min after ouabain incubation, $P \leq 0.05$), while such effect was not observed in treatment group (198 before and 199 beats per min after ouabain incubation, $P > 0.05$, Figure 2).

Treatment with ouabain had no effect on contractile force in both groups (0.627 g before and 0.663 g after ouabain incubation for the control group, $P > 0.05$, and 0.569 g before and 0.573 g after ouabain incubation for the treatment group, $P > 0.05$, Figure 3). There was also no significant

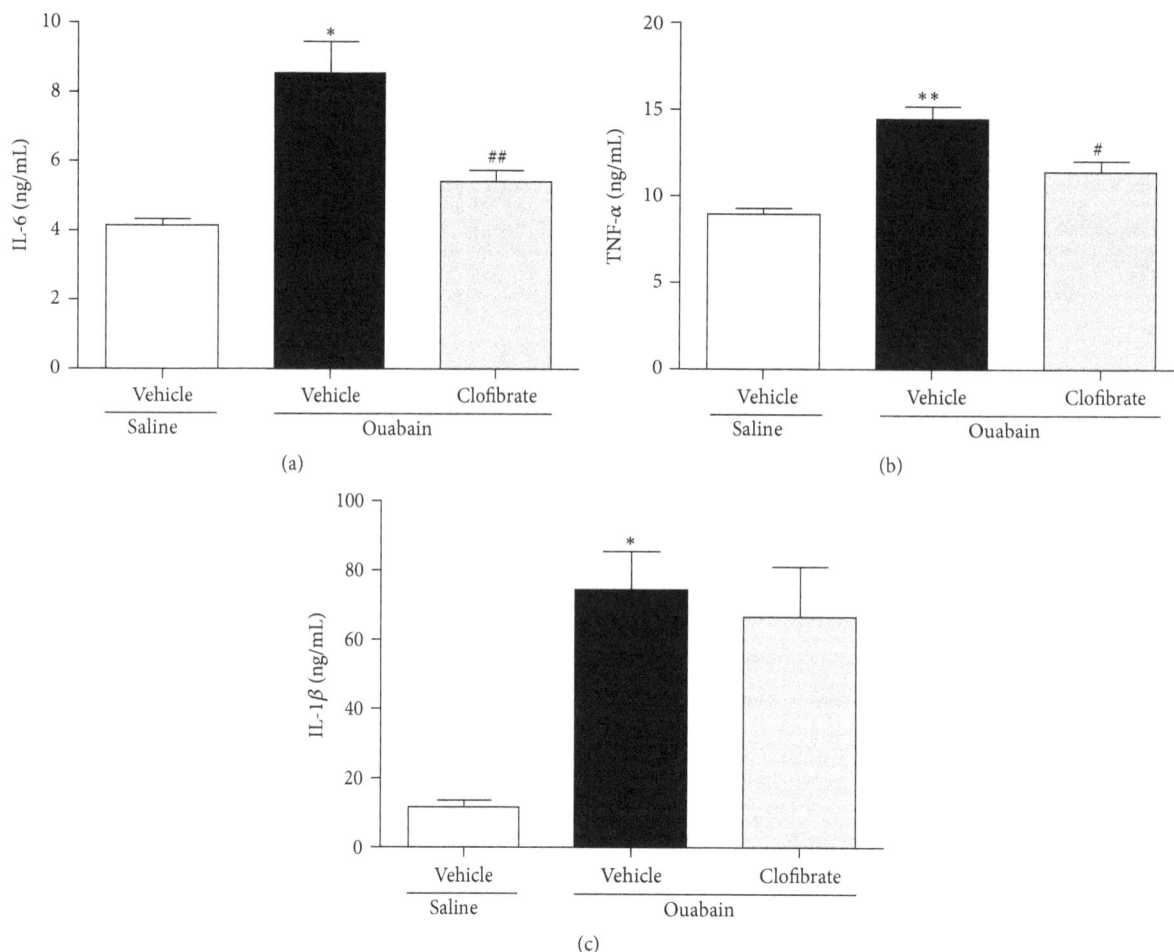

FIGURE 5: Atrial levels of IL-6 (a), TNF-α (b), and IL-1β (c) in saline- and ouabain-injected vehicle- and clofibrate-treated groups. Data are shown as mean $\pm$ SEM. Four rats were used in each group. $^*P \leq 0.01$ and $^{**}P \leq 0.001$ compared to saline-injected vehicle-treated group; $^\#P \leq 0.05$ and $^{\#\#}P \leq 0.01$ compared to ouabain-injected vehicle-treated group.

difference in atrial beating rate and contractile force between the two groups before incubation with ouabain ($P > 0.05$ for atrial beating rate, Figure 2, and $P > 0.05$ for contractile force, Figure 3). Figure 4 represents a general comparison in chronotropic and inotropic features between both groups, but the intensity of arrhythmia in the control group (a) was greater than the treatment group (b). Time of onset of asystole was also observed earlier in control group (a). The shapes of the spikes were normal in both groups before incubation of ouabain (c, d). Figure 4(e) obviously shows the ouabain-induced arrhythmia in control group, while the severity of this arrhythmia is smaller in treatment group (f).

3.2. Levels of IL-1β, IL-6, and TNF-α in Atria and Plasma. As shown in Figure 5, injection of ouabain significantly increased the atrial levels of all studied inflammatory cytokines ($P \leq 0.01$ for IL-1β and IL-6 and $P \leq 0.001$ for TNF-α). Pretreatment with clofibrate attenuated the ouabain-induced elevation of IL-6 and TNF-α in atria ($P \leq 0.01$ and $P \leq 0.05$, resp., Figures 5(a) and 5(b)), while it failed to decrease the ouabain-induced elevation in IL-1β ($P > 0.05$, Figure 5(c)).

Similarly, ouabain boosted the plasma levels of all inflammatory cytokines significantly ($P \leq 0.001$, $P \leq 0.05$, and $P \leq 0.01$ for IL-1β, IL-6, and TNF-α, resp., Figure 6). Nevertheless, pretreatment with clofibrate could only reverse the ouabain-induced elevation of IL-6 in plasma ($P \leq 0.05$, Figure 6(a)), whereas it did not reduce the ouabain-induced increase in TNF-α and IL-1β levels in plasma ($P > 0.05$, Figures 6(b) and 6(c)).

4. Discussion

Cardiac arrhythmias are life-threatening medical conditions. As most antiarrhythmic drugs have serious adverse effects, finding safer antiarrhythmic agents with less side effects has been suggested in the literature. In the present study, we investigated the effects of clofibrate on ouabain-induced arrhythmia in isolated rat atria. For this purpose, induction of arrhythmia and measurement of inflammatory cytokines were performed in rats given ouabain or vehicle. Our results showed that clofibrate, as a PPAR-α agonist, succeeded to induce antiarrhythmic effects by delaying the onset and reducing the intensity of ouabain-induced arrhythmias and

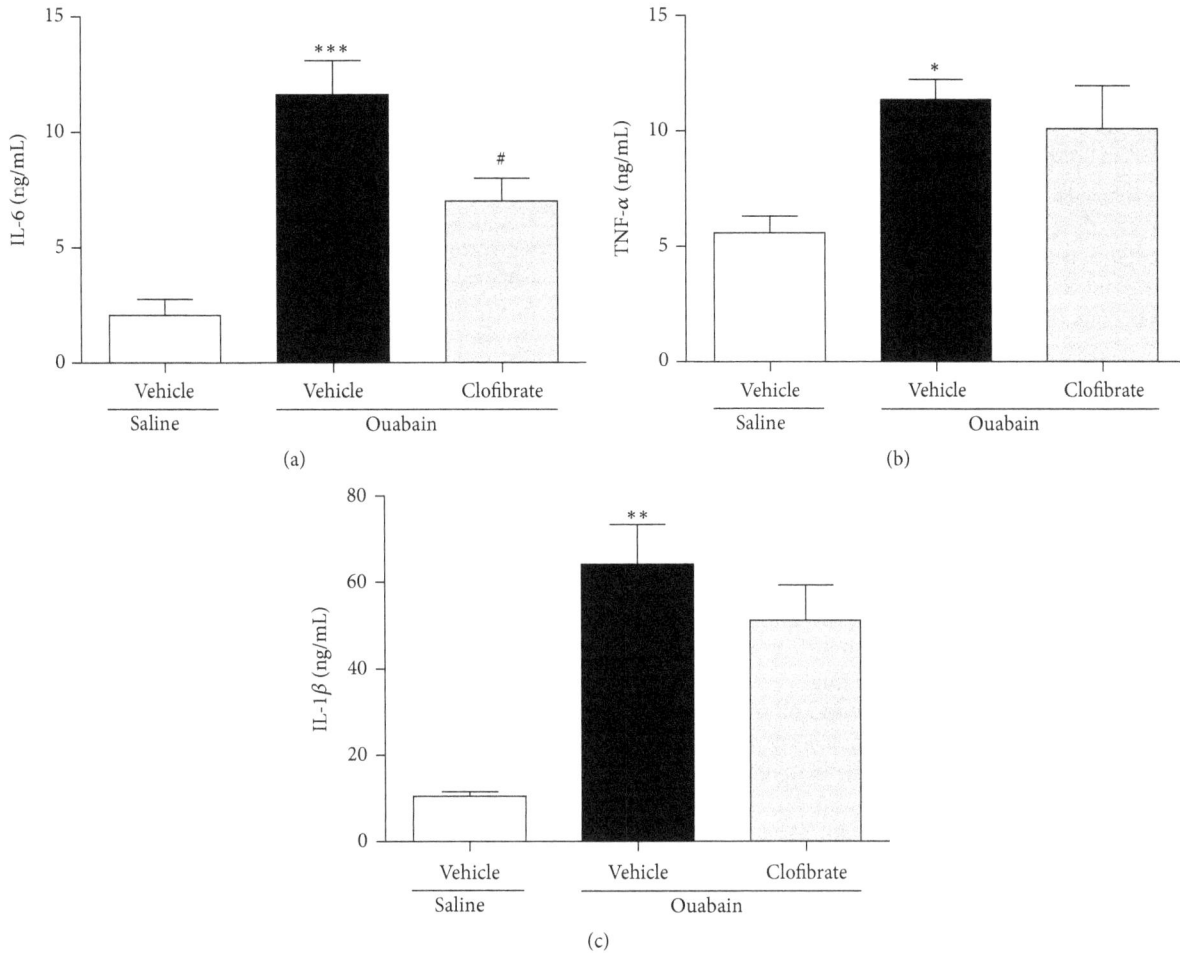

FIGURE 6: Plasma levels of IL-6 (a), TNF-α (b), and IL-1β (c) in saline- and ouabain-injected vehicle- and clofibrate-treated groups. Data are shown as mean ± SEM. Four rats were used in each group. $^*P \leq 0.05$, $^{**}P \leq 0.01$, and $^{***}P \leq 0.001$ compared to saline-injected vehicle-treated group; $^#P \leq 0.05$ compared to ouabain-injected vehicle-treated group.

reduction of ouabain-induced elevation of inflammatory cytokines especially IL-6 in isolated rat atria. In addition, clofibrate alleviated the positive chronotropic effect of ouabain.

It has been reported that ouabain induces the production of proinflammatory cytokines. For example, Matsumori et al. showed that incubation of ouabain increased the levels of IL-1α, IL-1β, and IL-6 in cultured human peripheral blood mononuclear cells [18]. They also reported that ouabain is able to increase the production of TNF-α [19]. In line with previous studies, we showed that ouabain increased proinflammatory cytokines (IL-1β, IL-6, and TNF-α in both of atria and plasma, Figures 5 and 6), in the atria of treated rats. Furthermore, we demonstrated that clofibrate decreased the inflammatory cytokines in atria (IL-6 and TNF-α, Figures 5(a) and 5(b)) and plasma (IL-6, Figure 6(a)). In this regard, Jiang et al. reported that PPAR-γ agonists could suppress phorbol ester-induced elevation of IL-1β, IL-6, and TNF-α [20]. Additionally, it has been shown that PPAR-γ agonists improve insulin resistance through inhibiting the effect of TNF-α in adipocytes [21]. Although these reports mentioned

the protective effects of PPAR-γ receptor agonists against inflammatory cytokines, we found such effects in case of PPAR-α receptor agonist.

Inflammatory cytokines play a key role in mediating the inflammatory responses under pathologic conditions. TNF-α and IL-1 stimulate the release of other inflammatory cytokines such as IL-6 [22]. Evidence indicates that atrial fibrillation after coronary artery bypass grafting is associated with increase in IL-6 in patients [23, 24]. Similar studies have reported that atrial fibrillation results in sequestration of inflammatory cytokines in the heart [13, 14]. With IL-6, there are numerous published studies that suggest that TNF-α (and to some extent IL-1β) possess arrhythmogenic properties. In this context, TNF-α and IL-1β have been reported to boost susceptibility to arrhythmia in rat ventricular myocytes through increase of calcium leakage from the sarcoplasmic reticulum [15]. Moreover, it is frequently reported that overexpression of TNF-α in transgenic animals causes various atrial and ventricular arrhythmias [25–28]. Recent evidence suggests that inflammatory factors, mainly TNF-α, contribute to pathophysiology of ventricular arrhythmias [29]. These findings justify the results of the present study and strengthened our hypothesis that local and systemic inhibition of inflammatory cytokines modulate antiarrhythmic properties of PPAR-α agonist, clofibrate. It seems that the role of IL-6 in mediating the antiarrhythmic properties of clofibrate is more prominent than TNF-α, because clofibrate reduced IL-6, locally and systemically, while it only decreased the local elevation of TNF-α. On the other hand, the local antiarrhythmic effects of clofibrate appear superior to systemic antiarrhythmic properties.

Several lines of research have indicated that there is a high rate of atrial fibrillation and other kinds of cardiac arrhythmias in metabolic syndrome and lipid metabolism disorders [30, 31]. Evidence shows that pretreatment with PPAR-α agonist, clofibrate, can reduce the experimental myocardial infarct size up to 43% in rats [32], and it is well established that cardiac infarction and ischemia can cause the most types of arrhythmias. Tabernero et al. and Yue et al. have also reported that PPAR-α agonists protect the heart against the ischemia-reperfusion injury [7, 8]. Since clofibrate modulates lipid metabolism, this effect might also partly explain its antiarrhythmic properties, which could be investigated in future studies. Although we did not use ischemia-reperfusion model for induction of arrhythmia in the present study, clofibrate could significantly postpone the time of onset of arrhythmia and asystole in ouabain-induced arrhythmias.

5. Conclusions

It is concluded that clofibrate might possess antiarrhythmic properties in reducing the cardiac arrhythmias. It seems that clofibrate shows this beneficial effect through the modulation of some local and systemic inflammatory cytokines including IL-6 and TNF-α.

Conflict of Interests

None of the authors of this paper has a financial or personal relationship with other people or organizations that could inappropriately influence or bias the content of the paper.

Authors' Contribution

Somayeh Moradi and Vahid Nikoui contributed equally to this work.

Acknowledgment

This research has been supported by Tehran University of Medical Sciences (TUMS) Grant no. 90-03-30-15062.

References

[1] B. M. Forman, J. Chen, and R. M. Evans, "Hypolipidemic drugs, polyunsaturated fatty acids, and eicosanoids are ligands for peroxisome proliferator-activated receptors alpha and delta," *Proceedings of the National Academy of Sciences of the United States of America*, vol. 94, no. 9, pp. 4312–4317, 1997.

[2] T. M. Willson and W. Wahli, "Peroxisome proliferator-activated receptor agonists," *Current Opinion in Chemical Biology*, vol. 1, no. 2, pp. 235–241, 1997.

[3] R. M. Evans, "The steroid and thyroid hormone receptor superfamily," *Science*, vol. 240, no. 4854, pp. 889–895, 1988.

[4] N. J. McKenna, R. B. Lanz, and B. W. O'Malley, "Nuclear receptor coregulators: cellular and molecular biology," *Endocrine Reviews*, vol. 20, no. 3, pp. 321–344, 1999.

[5] A. Chawta, J. J. Repa, R. M. Evans, and D. J. Mangelsdorf, "Nuclear receptors and lipid physiology: opening the x-files," *Science*, vol. 294, no. 5548, pp. 1866–1870, 2001.

[6] O. Braissant, F. Foufelle, C. Scotto, M. Dauça, and W. Wahli, "Differential expression of peroxisome proliferator-activated receptors (PPARs): tissue distribution of PPAR-α, -β, and -γ in the adult rat," *Endocrinology*, vol. 137, no. 1, pp. 354–366, 1996.

[7] A. Tabernero, K. Schoonjans, L. Jesel, I. Carpusca, J. Auwerx, and R. Andriantsitohaina, "Activation of the peroxisome proliferator-activated receptor α protects against myocardial ischaemic injury and improves endothelial vasodilatation," *BMC Pharmacology*, vol. 2, article 10, 2002.

[8] T.-L. Yue, W. Bao, B. M. Jucker et al., "Activation of peroxisome proliferator-activated receptor-α protects the heart from ischemia/reperfusion injury," *Circulation*, vol. 108, no. 19, pp. 2393–2399, 2003.

[9] D. S. Straus and C. K. Glass, "Anti-inflammatory actions of PPAR ligands: new insights on cellular and molecular mechanisms," *Trends in Immunology*, vol. 28, no. 12, pp. 551–558, 2007.

[10] X. R. Chen, V. C. Besson, B. Palmier, Y. Garcia, M. Plotkine, and C. Marchand-Leroux, "Neurological recovery-promoting, anti-inflammatory, and anti-oxidative effects afforded by fenofibrate, a PPAR alpha agonist, in traumatic brain injury," *Journal of Neurotrauma*, vol. 24, no. 7, pp. 1119–1131, 2007.

[11] I. P. Torra, P. Gervois, and B. Staels, "Peroxisome proliferator-activated receptor alpha in metabolic disease, inflammation, atherosclerosis and aging," *Current Opinion in Lipidology*, vol. 10, no. 2, pp. 151–160, 1999.

[12] P. Gelosa, C. Banfi, A. Gianella et al., "Peroxisome proliferator-activated receptor α agonism prevents renal damage and the oxidative stress and inflammatory processes affecting the brains of stroke-prone rats," *Journal of Pharmacology and Experimental Therapeutics*, vol. 335, no. 2, pp. 324–331, 2010.

[13] G. M. Marcus, L. M. Smith, K. Ordovas et al., "Intracardiac and extracardiac markers of inflammation during atrial fibrillation," *Heart Rhythm*, vol. 7, no. 2, pp. 149–154, 2010.

[14] M. D. M. Engelmann and J. H. Svendsen, "Inflammation in the genesis and perpetuation of atrial fibrillation," *European Heart Journal*, vol. 26, no. 20, pp. 2083–2092, 2005.

[15] D. J. Duncan, Z. Yang, P. M. Hopkins, D. S. Steele, and S. M. Harrison, "TNF-α and IL-1β increase Ca^{2+} leak from the sarcoplasmic reticulum and susceptibility to arrhythmia in rat ventricular myocytes," *Cell Calcium*, vol. 47, no. 4, pp. 378–386, 2010.

[16] S. Rodrigues-Mascarenhas, N. F. D. Santos, and V. M. Rumjanek, "Synergistic effect between ouabain and glucocorticoids for the induction of thymic atrophy," *Bioscience Reports*, vol. 26, no. 2, pp. 159–169, 2006.

[17] V. Nikoui, S. Ejtemaei Mehr, F. Jazaeri et al., "Prostaglandin $F_{2\alpha}$ modulates atrial chronotropic hyporesponsiveness to cholinergic stimulation in endotoxemic rats," *European Journal of Pharmacology*, vol. 748, pp. 149–156, 2015.

[18] A. Matsumori, K. Ono, R. Nishio, Y. Nose, and S. Sasayama, "Amlodipine inhibits the production of cytokines induced by ouabain," *Cytokine*, vol. 12, no. 3, pp. 294–297, 2000.

[19] A. Matsumori, K. Ono, R. Nishio et al., "Modulation of cytokine production and protection against lethal endotoxemia by the cardiac glycoside ouabain," *Circulation*, vol. 96, no. 5, pp. 1501–1506, 1997.

[20] C. Jiang, A. T. Ting, and B. Seed, "PPAR-γ agonists inhibit production of monocyte inflammatory cytokines," *Nature*, vol. 391, no. 6662, pp. 82–86, 1998.

[21] M. Shibasaki, K. Takahashi, T. Itou, H. Bujo, and Y. Saito, "A PPAR agonist improves TNF-α-induced insulin resistance of adipose tissue in mice," *Biochemical and Biophysical Research Communications*, vol. 309, no. 2, pp. 419–424, 2003.

[22] S. Wan and A. P. C. Yim, "Cytokines in myocardial injury: impact on cardiac surgical approach," *European Journal of Cardiothoracic Surgery*, vol. 16, supplement 1, pp. S107–S111, 1999.

[23] K. Ishida, "Relation of inflammatory cytokines to atrial fibrillation after off-pump coronary artery bypass grafting," *European Journal of Cardio-Thoracic Surgery*, vol. 29, no. 4, pp. 501–505, 2006.

[24] S. N. Psychari, T. S. Apostolou, L. Sinos, E. Hamodraka, G. Liakos, and D. T. Kremastinos, "Relation of elevated C-reactive protein and interleukin-6 levels to left atrial size and duration of episodes in patients with atrial fibrillation," *The American Journal of Cardiology*, vol. 95, no. 6, pp. 764–767, 2005.

[25] B. London, L. C. Baker, J. S. Lee et al., "Calcium-dependent arrhythmias in transgenic mice with heart failure," *The American Journal of Physiology—Heart and Circulatory Physiology*, vol. 284, no. 2, pp. H431–H441, 2003.

[26] S. E. Sawaya, Y. S. Rajawat, T. G. Rami et al., "Downregulation of connexin40 and increased prevalence of atrial arrhythmias in transgenic mice with cardiac-restricted overexpression of tumor necrosis factor," *American Journal of Physiology—Heart and Circulatory Physiology*, vol. 292, no. 3, pp. H1561–H1567, 2007.

[27] H. Xiao, Z. Chen, Y. Liao et al., "Positive correlation of tumor necrosis factor-α early expression in myocardium and ventricular arrhythmias in rats with acute myocardial infarction," *Archives of Medical Research*, vol. 39, no. 3, pp. 285–291, 2008.

[28] P. S. Petkova-Kirova, B. London, G. Salama, R. L. Rasmusson, and V. E. Bondarenko, "Mathematical modeling mechanisms of arrhythmias in transgenic mouse heart overexpressing TNF-α," *The American Journal of Physiology—Heart and Circulatory Physiology*, vol. 302, no. 4, pp. H934–H952, 2012.

[29] M. Kowalewski, M. Urban, B. Mroczko, and M. Szmitkowski, "Proinflammatory cytokines (IL-6, TNF-alpha) and cardiac troponin I (cTnI) in serum of young people with ventricular arrhythmias," *Polskie Archiwum Medycyny Wewnętrznej*, vol. 108, no. 1, pp. 647–651, 2002.

[30] E. L. Onuchina, O. V. Solov'ev, O. V. Mochalova, S. K. Kononov, and S. G. Onuchin, "Metabolic syndrome and chronic persistent atrial fibrillation," *Klinicheskaia Meditsina*, vol. 89, no. 1, pp. 26–31, 2011.

[31] A. O. Badheka, A. Rathod, M. A. Kizilbash et al., "Impact of lipid-lowering therapy on outcomes in atrial fibrillation," *The American Journal of Cardiology*, vol. 105, no. 12, pp. 1768–1772, 2010.

[32] N. S. Wayman, B. L. Ellis, and C. Thiemermann, "Ligands of the peroxisome proliferator-activated receptor-PPAR-α reduce myocardial infarct size," *Medical Science Monitor*, vol. 8, no. 7, pp. BR243–BR247, 2002.

13

Drug Efflux Transporters Are Overexpressed in Short-Term Tamoxifen-Induced MCF7 Breast Cancer Cells

Desak Gede Budi Krisnamurti,[1] **Melva Louisa,**[2] **Erlia Anggraeni,**[3] **and Septelia Inawati Wanandi**[4]

[1]*Department of Medical Pharmacy, Faculty of Medicine, University of Indonesia, Jakarta 10430, Indonesia*
[2]*Department of Pharmacology and Therapeutics, Faculty of Medicine, University of Indonesia, Jakarta 10430, Indonesia*
[3]*Master Program in Biomedicine, Faculty of Medicine, University of Indonesia, Jakarta 10430, Indonesia*
[4]*Department of Biochemistry and Molecular Biology, Faculty of Medicine, University of Indonesia, Jakarta 10430, Indonesia*

Correspondence should be addressed to Desak Gede Budi Krisnamurti; gek_noy@yahoo.com

Academic Editor: Carlos Tirapelli

Tamoxifen is the first line drug used in the treatment of estrogen receptor-positive (ER+) breast cancer. The development of multidrug resistance (MDR) to tamoxifen remains a major challenge in the treatment of cancer. One of the mechanisms related to MDR is decrease of drug influx via overexpression of drug efflux transporters such as P-glycoprotein (P-gp/MDR1), multidrug resistance associated protein (MRP), or BCRP (breast cancer resistance protein). We aimed to investigate whether the sensitivity of tamoxifen to the cells is maintained through the short period and whether the expressions of several drug efflux transporters have been upregulated. We exposed MCF7 breast cancer cells with tamoxifen $1\,\mu M$ for 10 passages (MCF7 (T)). The result showed that MCF7 began to lose their sensitivity to tamoxifen from the second passage. MCF7 (T) also showed a significant increase in all transporters examined compared with MCF7 parent cells. The result also showed a significant increase of CC50 in MCF7 (T) compared to that in MCF7 ($97.54\,\mu M$ and $3.04\,\mu M$, resp.). In conclusion, we suggest that the expression of several drug efflux transporters such as P-glycoprotein, MRP2, and BCRP might be used and further studied as a marker in the development of tamoxifen resistance.

1. Introduction

Tamoxifen has been used as first line treatment for estrogen receptor alpha- (ERα-) positive breast tumors in women for many years [1–3]. However, resistance to tamoxifen occurs in many patients, although ERα expression is maintained in most tumors that acquire resistance [4].

Many factors contribute to tamoxifen-acquired resistance, involving a number of profound changes in the expression of genes, including multidrug resistance (MDR) phenomenon [5–7]. Several mechanisms have been proposed to explain MDR, one of which is decreased intracellular drug accumulation which resulted from a decrease of drug influx via overexpression of drug efflux transporters such as P-glycoprotein (P-gp/MDR1), multidrug resistance associated protein (MRP), or BCRP (breast cancer resistance protein)

[8, 9]. Studies have shown that the overexpression of multidrug resistance (MDR) played an important role in the development of cancer resistance to tamoxifen [8, 10, 11].

Tamoxifen-acquired resistance cell lines have been obtained by researchers by adding tamoxifen to cell lines for months and years [10–12]. Although these cell-based studies of MDR have been an important source of understanding about the mechanism of resistance, no data showed whether overexpression of drug efflux transporters, which leads to resistance to tamoxifen, occurs in a much shorter regimen. In this study, we used a short-term tamoxifen treatment to MCF7 cells and determined whether the sensitivity of drugs to the cells is maintained through the short period and whether the expression of several drug efflux transporters has been upregulated.

2. Materials and Methods

2.1. Materials. MCF7 cell line for breast cancer was a kind gift from the Laboratory of the Agency for the Assessment and Application Technology (BPPT), Serpong, Indonesia. Tamoxifen and DMSO were purchased from Sigma-Aldrich (Singapore). Dulbecco Minimal Essential Medium (DMEM), Fetal Bovine Serum (FBS), Penicillin/Streptomycin, Gentamicin, Fungizone, Dulbecco Phosphate Buffer Solution (D-PBS), and Triple Express were obtained from Gibco, Ltd. (Singapore). Tripure Isolation Reagents were from Roche Diagnostics (Singapore), primers were from 1st BASE Ltd., Singapore, and qRT-PCR kit used was KAPA SYBR FAST One-Step qRT-PCR Kit Universal from KAPA Biosystem, USA. MTS assay kit was obtained from Promega, USA.

2.2. Cell Culture. MCF7 cells were cultured in DMEM supplemented with 10% heat-inactivated fetal bovine serum, 2 mM L-glutamine, 100 IU/mL penicillin, 100 μg/mL streptomycin, and 1% Fungizone. Medium was routinely changed every day. The cells were subcultured when reaching 80–90% confluence.

2.3. Tamoxifen-Induced MCF7 Cells. MCF7 cells were grown in a medium containing tamoxifen 1 μM, continuously up to 10 passages (44 days). When reaching confluence, cells were subcultured and counted using trypan blue exclusion method. For the purpose of cell viability counting, we normalized the data to DMSO, as control, and show the data as % viability over control. Cells from passage 1 (day 5) and passage 10 (day 44) were subjected to RNA isolation and qRT-PCR for drug efflux transporters (P-glycoprotein, MRP2, and BCRP).

2.4. Cell Morphology. MCF7 and MCF7 (T) cells morphology were photographed under confocal microscope (Olympus Fluoview FV1200 Confocal Laser Scanning Microscope, Olympus, Japan). Photo observation is done using gray scale, Pseudo 3D DIC by Transmitted Nomarski System.

2.5. RNA Isolation. Total RNA was isolated using Tripure Isolation Reagents (Roche) according to the manufacturer's protocol. Quantity and purity of RNA were determined by measuring 260/280 absorbance using NanoDrop spectrophotometer. RNA obtained then was subjected to quantitative real-time reverse transcription polymerase chain reactions (qRT-PCR).

2.6. qRT-PCR. mRNA expressions of the following drug transporter were quantified: P-glycoprotein, MRP2 (multidrug resistance protein-2), and BCRP (breast cancer resistance protein). Quantitative real-time reverse transcription polymerase chain reaction (qRT-PCR) was performed using KAPA SYBR FAST One-Step qRT-PCR Kit on Universal Biorad Chromo 4 Real-Time PCR Detection System. β2-microglobulin was used as reference gene. The sequences of the primers were β2mg F: CCAGCAGAGAATGGAAAG-TC; β2mg R: CATGTCTCGATCCCACTTAAC. Primers used for the determination of drug efflux transporters were described previously [13]: P-glycoprotein, P-gp F: CCC-ATCATTGCAATAGCAGG; P-gp R: TGTTCAAACTTC-TGCTCCTGA; MRP2, MRP2 F: ACAGAGGCTGGTGGC-AACC; MRP2 R: ACCATTACCTTGTCACTGTCCATGA; BCRP, BCRP F: AGATGGGTTTCCAAGCGTTCAT; BCRP R: CCAGTCCCAGTACGACTGTGACA. Primers used to determine the mRNA expressions of Caspase-3 and Caspase-9 were described previously by Iwao et al. [14] with sequence as follows: Cas-3 F: TTCAGAGGGGATCGTTGTAGA-AGTC; Cas-3 R: CAAGCTTGTCGGCATACTGTTTCAG; Cas-9 F: ATGGACGAAGCGGATCGGCGGCTCC; Cas-9 R: GCACCACTGGGGGGTAAGGTTTTCTAG. Primers used to determine the mRNA expression of progesterone receptor were used previously by Shanker et al. [15]: PR F: GGCGGATCCGTCAAGTGGTCTAAATCATTG; PR R: GGCGAATTCCTGGGTTTGACTTCGTAGCCC. Relative changes in mRNA transporter expression levels were calculated using Livak method [16].

2.7. MTS Assay (Cell Proliferation Assay). Cytotoxicity concentration of tamoxifen to MCF7 cells before and after 44-day treatment of tamoxifen was determined using MTS assay (Promega). Cells were plated at a density of 2000 cells per well in 96-well plates. At 70–80% confluence, cells were incubated with tamoxifen for 24 h at 37°C. After 24 h drug treatment, 20 μL of MTS solution was then added into each well and incubated for 2 h before reading at a wavelength of 490 nm. CC50 values were calculated from linear regression equation of dose-response curves.

2.8. Statistical Analysis. Data were presented in the form of means ± standard deviation (SD). Graphs were created using GraphPad Prism software 6 (GraphPad, USA). Statistical significance was calculated using t-test or ANOVA One-Way followed by post hoc test, with $p < 0.05$ considered as significant.

3. Results

Cell morphology of MCF7 cells treated with tamoxifen continuously is shown on Figure 1.

Our result showed that cancer cells maintained their sensitivity towards tamoxifen only in the first passage. Cells began to lose their sensitivity to drug from the second passage (or about 9 days of tamoxifen treatment). Afterwards, MCF7 treated with tamoxifen had stable overgrowth compared with MCF7 cells treated with DMSO only (Figure 2).

After 10 passages (44 days) of treatment, we checked the cytotoxicity concentrations of tamoxifen in MCF7 and MCF7 (T). We found a significant increase of CC50 in MCF7 (T) compared to that in MCF7 (97.54 μM and 3.04 μM, resp.) (Figure 3).

In order to show whether the apoptosis process is still active in MCF7 cells treated continuously with tamoxifen, we measured Caspase-3 and Caspase-9 mRNA expressions at passage 4 after drug treatment (Figure 4). We found that Caspase-3 and Caspase-9 expressions were significantly

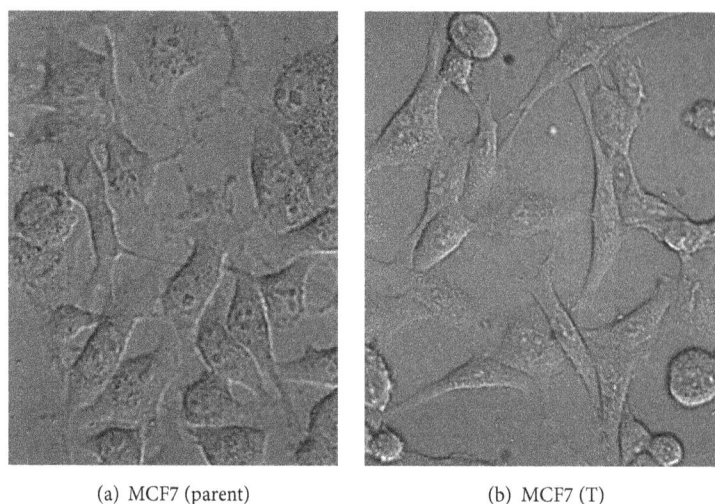

(a) MCF7 (parent)

(b) MCF7 (T)

FIGURE 1: (a) Cell morphology of MCF7 cells (parent). (b) MCF7 (T) cells treated with tamoxifen 1 μM for 10 passages (44 days). Photographed under confocal microscope.

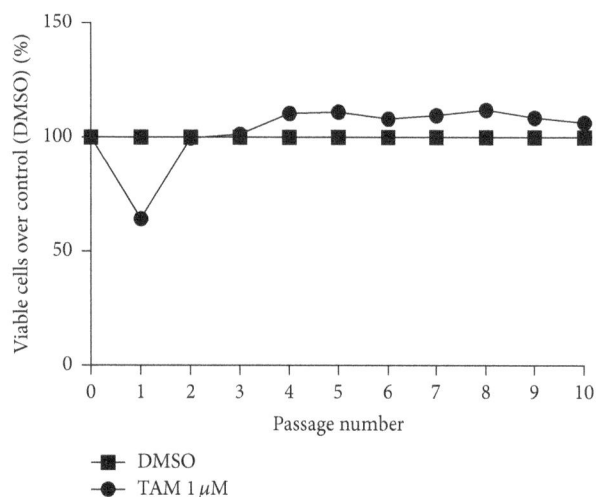

FIGURE 2: Percentage of viable cells over control (DMSO) after treatment with tamoxifen 1 μM or DMSO.

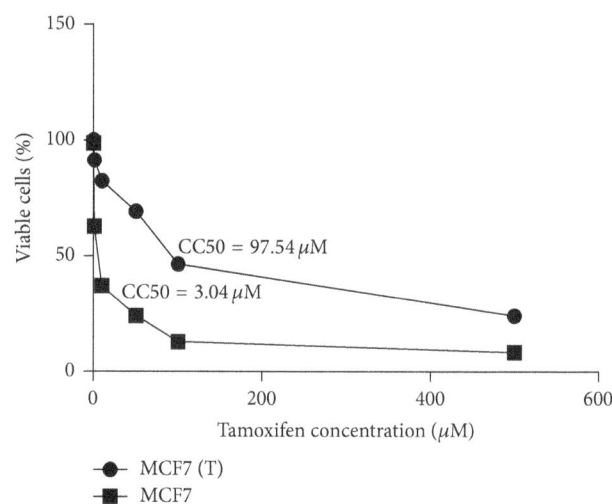

FIGURE 3: Cytotoxicity concentrations 50 (CC50) of tamoxifen in MCF7 or MCF7 (T) cells.

increased compared with parent cells, which proved that apoptosis process, which were still in place.

We found that PR receptor expression was significantly downregulated in MCF7 (T) compared to MCF7 parent cells as shown in Figure 5.

We measure the expressions of P-gp, MRP2, and BCRP in MCF7 parent cells, MCF7-P1 (MCF1 passage 1), and MCF7 (T). The result showed that the expressions of P-gp, MRP2, and BCRP had been elevated from the first passage. MCF7 (T) showed a significant increase in all transporters examined compared with MCF7 parent cells (Figure 6).

4. Discussion

Tamoxifen currently is still the mainstay of endocrine therapies for ERα-positive breast tumors [1]. Unfortunately, majority of patients treated with tamoxifen eventually develop resistance, leading to disease progression and death [5]. Tamoxifen-resistant breast cancer cells often overexpress drug efflux transporter, which lower the effective drug concentration in a cell by pumping out tamoxifen out of the cells [6].

Acquired resistance to anticancer mostly occurred after long-term exposure to drugs [17]. To our knowledge, this is the first to describe the expressions of several drug transporters after short period of tamoxifen treatment. Previous studies had described the development of resistance of breast cancer cells to tamoxifen by exposing the drug for years [8, 11, 18, 19]. In this study, we use 1 μM tamoxifen as a treatment in breast cancer cells, as also used by Motahari and Lykkesfeldt [12, 19]. Fewer studies had used lower dose of tamoxifen compared to this study [20]. Our own preliminary result (data not shown) using tamoxifen 0.1 μM and 0.25 μM had resulted in about 90% viability over control during the first passage.

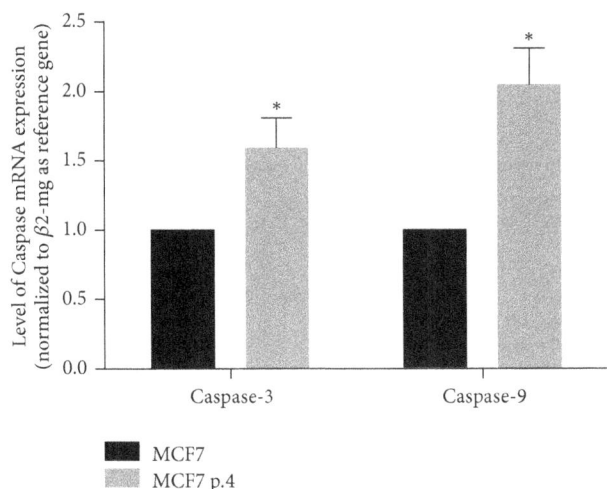

FIGURE 4: Level of Caspase-3 and Caspase-9 mRNA expressions after treatment with tamoxifen $1\,\mu$M at passage 4. Results were shown as mean $\pm$ SD (N = 4). ($*$) Significant difference versus MCF7 parent cells at $p < 0.05$.

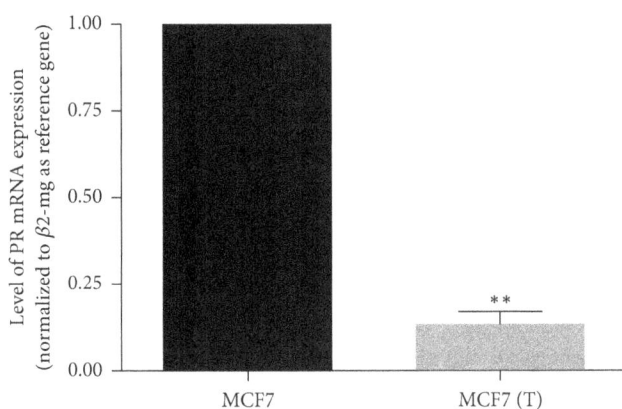

FIGURE 5: Level of progesterone receptor expressions after 44 days of treatment with tamoxifen $1\,\mu$M MCF7 (T). Results were shown as mean $\pm$ SD (N = 4). ($**$) Significant difference versus MCF7 parent cells at $p < 0.001$.

Therefore, we thought tamoxifen in lower dosages had little effect on cell viability and thus would result differently in selection of cells to induce resistance.

After 10 passages of tamoxifen treatment, photographs using confocal microscope indicate that there might be slight changes in cell morphology. We found more mesenchymal-like cells in MCF7 (T) compared to MCF7 parents cells which showed more cobblestone-like cells. Other studies had shown that epithelial-mesenchymal transition process played significant roles in the development of tamoxifen resistance [21–23]. In this study, we did not confirm the markers of EMT, as we mainly aimed to determine drug efflux expressions in tamoxifen-resistant cells.

Our result showed that downstream regulation of ER had occurred, as confirmed with downregulation of progesterone receptor. This is in accordance with previous results that tamoxifen resistance is accompanied with the reduced

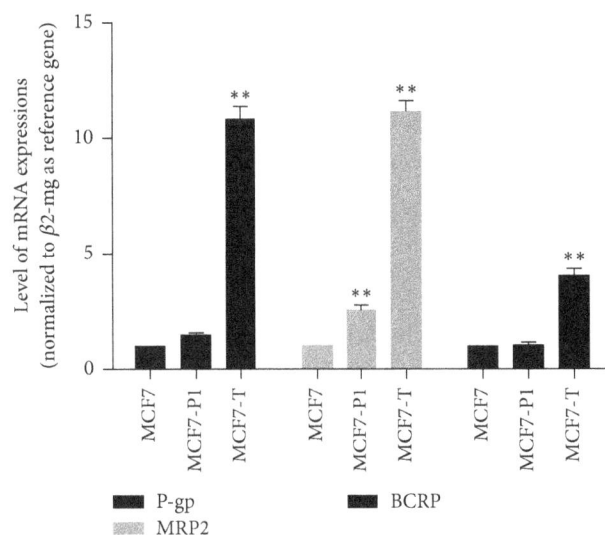

FIGURE 6: Level of mRNA expressions of P-glycoprotein, MRP2, and BCRP after 5 days of treatment (MCF7-P1) or 44 days of treatment (MCF7-T) with tamoxifen $1\,\mu$M. Results were shown as mean $\pm$ SD (N = 4); ($**$) Significant difference versus MCF7 parent cells at $p < 0.001$.

expressions of both ER and PR. In his study, Johnston et al. had also used ER/PR ratio as prognostic markers to tamoxifen resistance [24].

In this study, we showed that reduced sensitivity of cancer cells to tamoxifen developed very early, followed by stable growth up to 10 passages. Tamoxifen had failed to suppress cancer cell growth as early as second passage. We found that apoptosis process was still ongoing in passage 4 as shown by increased expressions of Caspase-3 and Caspase-9. Previous studies using MCF7 and MDA-MB-231 had also shown that tamoxifen, apart from its actions on ER, is able to induce apoptosis process trough cleavage of retinoblastoma (Rb) protein and activation of Caspase-3 [25].

We evaluate the role of drug efflux transporter inhibitors in the parent cells, in first passage (which still showed anticancer activity), and at MCF7 (T). Our result suggests that tamoxifen dramatically increased mRNA expressions of P-glycoprotein, MRP2, and BCRP. The expressions of the three drug transporters mRNA had even began to increase from first passage. Mechanism of modulation of P-glycoprotein and BCRP expressions is reported by Chen and Nie, which suggests that upregulation of mRNA P-glycoprotein and BCRP by tamoxifen occurs through the activation of pregnane X receptor, master regulator of MDR in cancers [26]. Another study by Nagaoka reported that tamoxifen activates CYP3A4 and MDR1/P-glycoprotein genes through steroid and xenobiotic receptor (SXR), a member of nuclear hormone receptors, which may affect tamoxifen metabolism and transport in breast cancer cells [27].

Tamoxifen strongly affects MRP2 expressions in MCF7 cells. Our result is in accordance with Choi et al. who found that tamoxifen-resistant MCF7 cells expressed a very higher level of MRP2 than control MCF7 cells [10]. Choi also found that pregnane X receptor (PXR) was persistently activated in tamoxifen-resistant MCF7 cells [10]. As PXR activates both P-glycoprotein and MRP2, presumably PXR have significant contribution to the development of tamoxifen-resistant breast cancer cells [28].

After 10 passages of treatment with tamoxifen, we found there is 32-fold increase in CC50 of MCF7 (T) compared with that in parent cells. This is a very large magnitude of increase considering a short period of tamoxifen treatment.

Our result suggests that resistance of breast cancer cells to tamoxifen might develop very early, only after a short period of treatment. We suggest that the expression of several drug efflux transporters such as P-glycoprotein, MRP2, and BCRP might be used and further studied as a marker in the development of tamoxifen resistance.

Conflict of Interests

The authors declare that there is no conflict of interests regarding the publication of this paper.

Acknowledgments

This study was supported by the Directorate of Research and Public Service, University of Indonesia, under the grant of Hibah Riset Madya 2012. Confocal microscope was performed at UI-Olympus Bioimaging Center (UOBC), an open user microscopy facility for bioimaging purpose located at Integrated Laboratory and Research Center (ILRC) of Universitas Indonesia.

References

[1] S. P. Gampenrieder, G. Rinnerthaler, and R. Greil, "Neoadjuvant chemotherapy and targeted therapy in breast cancer: past, present, and future," *Journal of Oncology*, vol. 2013, Article ID 732047, 12 pages, 2013.

[2] S. Germano and L. O'Driscoll, "Breast cancer: understanding sensitivity and resistance to chemotherapy and targeted therapies to aid in personalised medicine," *Current Cancer Drug Targets*, vol. 9, no. 3, pp. 398–418, 2009.

[3] V. C. Jordan and B. W. O'Malley, "Selective estrogen-receptor modulators and antihormonal resistance in breast cancer," *Journal of Clinical Oncology*, vol. 25, no. 36, pp. 5815–5824, 2007.

[4] S. Ali and R. C. Coombes, "Endocrine-responsive breast cancer and strategies for combating resistance," *Nature Reviews Cancer*, vol. 2, no. 2, pp. 101–112, 2002.

[5] M. Droog, K. Beelen, S. Linn, and W. Zwart, "Tamoxifen resistance: from bench to bedside," *European Journal of Pharmacology*, vol. 717, no. 1–3, pp. 47–57, 2013.

[6] M. J. Higgins and V. Stearns, "Understanding resistance to tamoxifen in hormone receptor-positive breast cancer," *Clinical Chemistry*, vol. 55, no. 8, pp. 1453–1455, 2009.

[7] R. B. Riggins, R. S. Schrecengost, M. S. Guerrero, and A. H. Bouton, "Pathways to tamoxifen resistance," *Cancer Letters*, vol. 256, no. 1, pp. 1–24, 2007.

[8] C.-H. Choi, "ABC transporters as multidrug resistance mechanisms and the development of chemosensitizers for their reversal," *Cancer Cell International*, vol. 5, article 30, 2005.

[9] E. K. Hoffmann and I. H. Lambert, "Ion channels and transporters in the development of drug resistance in cancer cells,"

Philosophical Transactions of the Royal Society of London Series B: Biological Sciences, vol. 369, no. 1638, Article ID 20130109, 2014.

[10] H. K. Choi, J. W. Yang, S. H. Roh, C. Y. Han, and K. W. Kang, "Induction of multidrug resistance associated protein 2 in tamoxifen-resistant breast cancer cells," *Endocrine-Related Cancer*, vol. 14, no. 2, pp. 293–303, 2007.

[11] F. Farabegoli, C. Barbi, E. Lambertini, and R. Piva, "(-)-epigallocatechin-3-gallate downregulates estrogen receptor alpha function in MCF-7 breast carcinoma cells," *Cancer Detection and Prevention*, vol. 31, no. 6, pp. 499–504, 2007.

[12] Z. Motahari, M. Etebary, and E. Azizi, "Studying the role of P-glycoprotein in resistance to Tamoxifen in humen breast cancer T47D cells by immunocytochemistry," *International Journal of Pharmacology*, vol. 1, no. 2, pp. 112–117, 2005.

[13] N. Albermann, F. H. Schmitz-Winnenthal, K. Z'graggen et al., "Expression of the drug transporters MDR1/ABCB1, MRP1/ABCC1, MRP2/ABCC2, BCRP/ABCG2, and PXR in peripheral blood mononuclear cells and their relationship with the expression in intestine and liver," *Biochemical Pharmacology*, vol. 70, no. 6, pp. 949–958, 2005.

[14] K. Iwao, Y. Miyoshi, C. Egawa, N. Ikeda, and S. Noguchi, "Quantitative analysis of estrogen receptor-β mRNA and its variants in human breast cancers," *International Journal of Cancer*, vol. 88, no. 5, pp. 733–736, 2000.

[15] Y. G. Shanker, S. C. Sharma, and A. J. Rao, "Expression of progesterone receptor mRNA in the first trimester human placenta," *Biochemistry and Molecular Biology International*, vol. 42, no. 6, pp. 1235–1240, 1997.

[16] K. J. Livak and T. D. Schmittgen, "Analysis of relative gene expression data using real-time quantitative PCR and the $2^{-\Delta\Delta C_T}$ method," *Methods*, vol. 25, no. 4, pp. 402–408, 2001.

[17] C. Wong and S. Chen, "The development, application and limitations of breast cancer cell lines to study tamoxifen and aromatase inhibitor resistance," *Journal of Steroid Biochemistry and Molecular Biology*, vol. 131, no. 3–5, pp. 83–92, 2012.

[18] F. Farabegoli, A. Papi, G. Bartolini, R. Ostan, and M. Orlandi, "(-)-epigallocatechin-3-gallate downregulates Pg-P and BCRP in a tamoxifen resistant MCF-7 cell line," *Phytomedicine*, vol. 17, no. 5, pp. 356–362, 2010.

[19] A. E. Lykkesfeldt, M. W. Madsen, and P. Briand, "Altered expression of estrogen-regulated genes in a tamoxifen-resistant and ICI 164,384 and ICI 182,780 sensitive human breast cancer cell line, MCF-7/TAMR-1," *Cancer Research*, vol. 54, no. 6, pp. 1587–1595, 1994.

[20] F. Karami-Tehrani and S. Salami, "Cell kinetic study of tamoxifen treated MCF-7 and MDA-MB 468 breast cancer cell lines," *Iranian Biomedical Journal*, vol. 7, no. 2, pp. 51–56, 2003.

[21] S. Hiscox, W. G. Jiang, K. Obermeier et al., "Tamoxifen resistance in MCF7 cells promotes EMT-like behaviour and involves modulation of β-catenin phosphorylation," *International Journal of Cancer*, vol. 118, no. 2, pp. 290–301, 2006.

[22] X.-P. Shi, S. Miao, Y. Wu et al., "Resveratrol sensitizes tamoxifen in antiestrogen-resistant breast cancer cells with epithelial-mesenchymal transition features," *International Journal of Molecular Sciences*, vol. 14, no. 8, pp. 15655–15668, 2013.

[23] M. Faronato, Y. Lombardo, and R. C. Coombes, "Endocrine therapy resistance and epithelial to mesenchymal transition are driven by Nicastrin and Notch4 cooperation in MCF7 breast cancer cells," *Cancer Cell & Microenvironment*, vol. 1, no. 3, article e356, 2014.

[24] S. R. D. Johnston, G. Saccani-Jotti, I. E. Smith et al., "Changes in estrogen receptor, progesterone receptor, and pS2 expression in tamoxifen-resistant human breast cancer," *Cancer Research*, vol. 55, no. 15, pp. 3331–3338, 1995.

[25] C. L. Fattman, B. An, L. Sussman, and Q. P. Dou, "p53-independent dephosphorylation and cleavage of retinoblastoma protein during tamoxifen-induced apoptosis in human breast carcinoma cells," *Cancer Letters*, vol. 130, no. 1-2, pp. 103–113, 1998.

[26] Y. Chen and D. Nie, "Pregnane X receptor and its potential role in drug resistance in cancer treatment," *Recent Patents on Anti-Cancer Drug Discovery*, vol. 4, no. 1, pp. 19–27, 2009.

[27] R. Nagaoka, T. Iwasaki, N. Rokutanda et al., "Tamoxifen activates CYP3A4 and MDR1 genes through steroid and xenobiotic receptor in breast cancer cells," *Endocrine*, vol. 30, no. 3, pp. 261–268, 2006.

[28] E. Qiao, M. Ji, J. Wu et al., "Expression of the PXR gene in various types of cancer and drug resistance," *Oncology Letters*, vol. 5, no. 4, pp. 1093–1100, 2013.

14

Effects of Curcumin on Parameters of Myocardial Oxidative Stress and of Mitochondrial Glutathione Turnover in Reoxygenation after 60 Minutes of Hypoxia in Isolated Perfused Working Guinea Pig Hearts

Ermita I. Ibrahim Ilyas,[1] Busjra M. Nur,[1] Sonny P. Laksono,[1] Anton Bahtiar,[1] Ari Estuningtyas,[2] Caecilia Vitasyana,[2] Dede Kusmana,[3] Frans D. Suyatna,[2] Muhammad Kamil Tadjudin,[4] and Hans-Joachim Freisleben[5]

[1]Department of Physiology, Faculty of Medicine, University of Indonesia, Jakarta 10430, Indonesia
[2]Department of Pharmacology and Therapeutics, Faculty of Medicine, University of Indonesia, Jakarta 10430, Indonesia
[3]National Cardiovascular Center, Harapan Kita Hospital and Department of Cardiology and Vascular Medicine, University of Indonesia, Jakarta 10430, Indonesia
[4]Department of Medical Biology, Faculty of Medicine, University of Indonesia, Jakarta 10430, Indonesia
[5]Medical Research Unit, Faculty of Medicine, University of Indonesia, Jakarta 10430, Indonesia

Correspondence should be addressed to Ermita I. Ibrahim Ilyas; ermitailyas@yahoo.com and Hans-Joachim Freisleben; hj.freisleben@t-online.de

Academic Editor: Thérèse Di Paolo-Chênevert

In cardiovascular surgery ischemia-reperfusion injury is a challenging problem, which needs medical intervention. We investigated the effects of curcumin on cardiac, myocardial, and mitochondrial parameters in perfused isolated working Guinea pig hearts. After preliminary experiments to establish the model, normoxia was set at 30 minutes, hypoxia was set at 60, and subsequent reoxygenation was set at 30 minutes. Curcumin was applied in the perfusion buffer at 0.25 and $0.5\,\mu M$ concentrations. Cardiac parameters measured were afterload, coronary and aortic flows, and systolic and diastolic pressure. In the myocardium histopathology and AST in the perfusate indicated cell damage after hypoxia and malondialdehyde (MDA) levels increased to 232.5% of controls during reoxygenation. Curcumin protected partially against reoxygenation injury without statistically significant differences between the two dosages. Mitochondrial MDA was also increased in reoxygenation (165% of controls), whereas glutathione was diminished (35.2%) as well as glutathione reductase (29.3%), which was significantly increased again to 62.0% by $0.05\,\mu M$ curcumin. Glutathione peroxidase (GPx) was strongly increased in hypoxia and even more in reoxygenation (255% of controls). Curcumin partly counteracted this increase and attenuated GPx activity independently in hypoxia and in reoxygenation, $0.25\,\mu M$ concentration to 150% and $0.5\,\mu M$ concentration to 200% of normoxic activity.

In memoriam Professor Dr. Guido Zimmer (1932–2014), formerly Johann-Wolfgang-Goethe University Frankfurt am Main, Germany

1. Introduction

Ischemia-reperfusion injury causes challenging problems in cardiovascular surgery [1–3]. Hypoxia and reoxygenation as a model for ischemia and reperfusion [4] have mainly been studied in isolated perfused rat hearts. Neely et al. [5] modified the original Langendorff preparation [6] into the working rat heart model, which we used to investigate the phenomenon of ischemia-reperfusion injury [7]. Now, we changed the rat heart model into isolated perfused working Guinea pig hearts.

Many chemicals used for cardio protection exert severe unwanted side effects. For this reason, natural and more moderate compounds are screened for their protective efficacy against ischemia-reperfusion injury [8]. Curcumin may be a suitable candidate [9] because it has a wide range of clinical activities [10] and structural similarities to antioxidants, for example, tocopherols and cardio protective compounds like flavonoids.

We present a first set of data about cardio protective effects of curcumin using the perfused isolated working Guinea pig heart model. The aims of this study were to find the appropriate experimental conditions for our model and to investigate effects of curcumin under these experimental conditions. In the future, we intend to use this model for the screening of extracts from Indonesian medicinal plants and to study their effects on hypoxia/ischemia-reoxygenation/reperfusion injury.

2. Materials and Methods

The complete isolated working heart perfusion device was established and all experiments were conducted at the Department of Physiology, Faculty of Medicine, Universitas Indonesia. Young adult Guinea pigs, aged one year and weighing 300–400 g, were obtained from the Animal Breeding Department of the Agricultural University of Bogor, Indonesia. All substances used (if not indicated differently) were purchased from Merck, Darmstadt, Germany, via their Indonesian subsidiary in Jakarta or from Sigma-Aldrich at highest purity available.

2.1. The Model. The arrangement of the perfusion apparatus had been described and schematically depicted by Deisinger and Freisleben [11]. Each Guinea pig was neck-fractured by rapid cervical dislocation, the heart was excised, and the aorta immediately connected to the aortic cannula of the apparatus and was perfused retrogradely as known from the Langendorff preparation. Subsequently, the perfusion cannula was connected anterogradely to the left atrium for normoxic perfusion with Krebs-Henseleit buffer [12] gassed with carbogen (O_2 95%/CO_2 5%). During hypoxia, hearts were perfused with the same buffer gassed with N_2 95%/CO_2 5%. In reoxygenation, conditions were readjusted to "normoxia," that is, anterograde perfusion with carbogen-gassed buffer [7]. Normoxia and reoxygenation lasted 30 min, each, whereas hypoxic perfusion varied from 15 to 60 min.

For perfusion of the myocardium, it is important that the cannulation of the aorta does not disturb the access to the coronary arteries. The perfusate flows back to the right atrium mainly via the *sinus coronarius* and drops from the heart via the open pulmonary artery and *venae cavae* into a glass vessel, from where it flows back into the buffer circulation. Coronary flow was measured by the volume of perfusate that dropped per minute from the heart into a graduated glass vessel.

Afterload was measured as the height (cm) of the buffer column, which could be maintained by the aortic pressure.

Aortic flow was determined as the volume (mL) per minute at a fixed afterload of 75 cm buffer column (Figure 1).

To measure systolic and diastolic pressure and heart rate a Nikon Kohden Polygraph was connected. This device also recorded the electrocardiogram, that is, initial arrhythmias; however, further electrocardiographic records were not in an interpretable quality (not shown). Hence, cardiograms were only used to decide about inclusion-exclusion criteria.

2.2. Experimental Procedures: Preliminary Experiments. We conducted preliminary experiments in order to

(i) set up the model and the sequential course of normoxia, hypoxia, and reoxygenation with 15 or 30 min of normoxic perfusion, 15, 30, or 60 min of hypoxia, and subsequent reoxygenation up to 30 min. In these experiments the excised hearts were examined for suitability, that is, stability over the time course in this model,

(ii) determine inclusion-exclusion criteria and find out sensitive parameters for measurements in this model. Afterload was first determined in preliminary experiments and then adjusted to 75 cm water column in the main experiments (Figure 1),

(iii) find appropriate concentrations of curcumin in this model. We applied 0.25, 0.5, and 1 μM concentrations, given into the perfusate at 15 min of normoxia. After a first set of experiments, application of 1 μM concentration was discontinued because we did not see dose-dependent effects and lower concentrations (0.25 and 0.5 μM) were even more effective in our model (not shown).

In our preliminary experiments hematoxylin-eosin staining and histopathological examination were conducted using Olympus light microscope at 1000x magnification and compared to aspartate aminotransferase (AST) measurements. For the latter Merck kit (Cat. number 14829) with solution A containing Tris HCl pH 7.8, L-aspartate, malate dehydrogenase, and lactate dehydrogenase and solution B containing 2-oxoglutarate and NADH was used according to the manufacturer's manual with slight modification. One mL of solution A was mixed with 0.25 mL of solution B and incubated for 30 min. To 1 mL of this mixture 0.2 mL of perfusate was added and the absorption measured at 340 nm in Shimadzu spectrophotometer at 1, 2, and 3 min. In our preliminary experiments, we had tested the volumes needed for measurement of the low AST concentrations in the perfusate. The units per liter perfusate were then correlated to the weight of heart tissue and expressed as $U \times L^{-1} \times g^{-1}$ heart tissue.

In the main experiments, histopathological examination was not continued, because histopathology correlated well with AST measurements and myocardial tissue was rather needed for the isolation of mitochondria and all other experimental procedures.

For statistical evaluation one-way ANOVA was used (normal parametric distribution); for nonparametric evaluation *post hoc* Tukey and Wilcoxon-Mann-Whitney U tests were

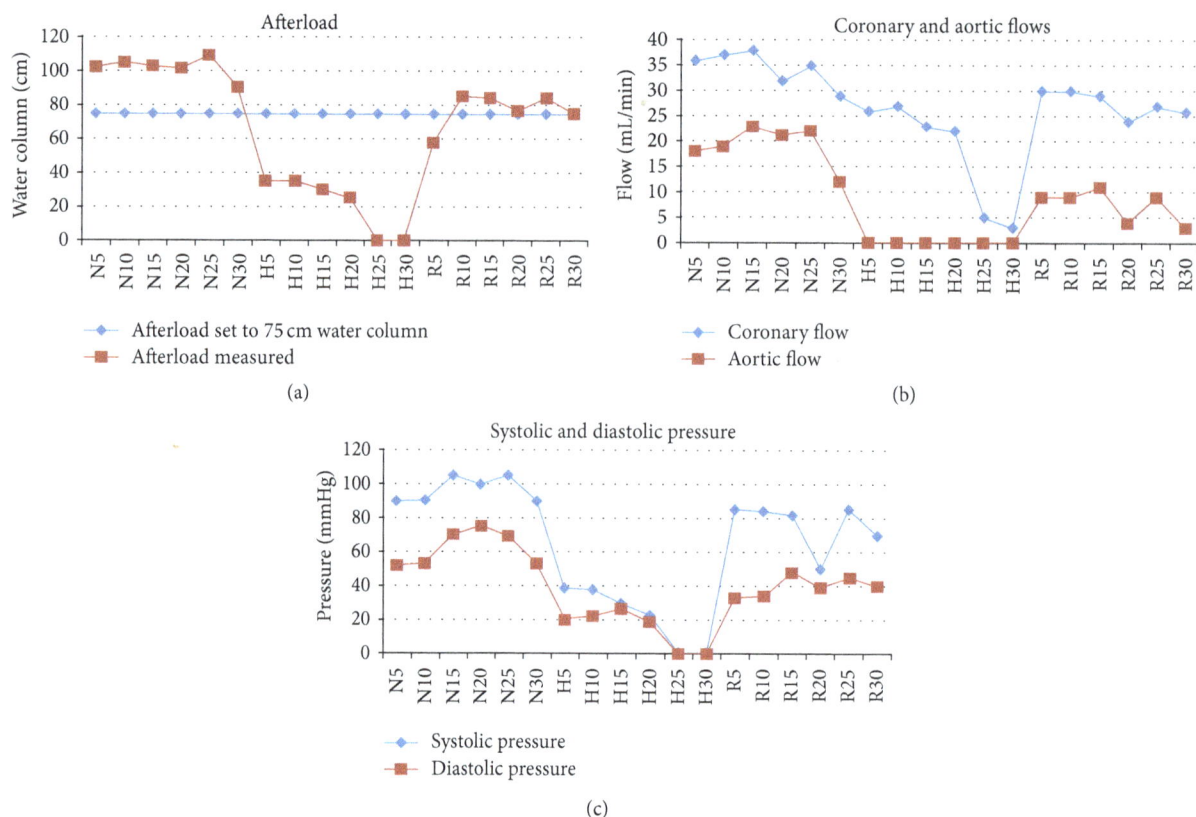

FIGURE 1: Parameters measured in preliminary experiments: (a) Afterload measured (red squares) during the course of 30 min of normoxia (about 100 cm water column) immediately dropped within 5 min of hypoxia to about 35 cm water column and then slowly decreased to zero between 10 and 25 min of hypoxia. In reoxygenation, afterload immediately improved again to 60 cm water column within 5 min and recovered to around 80 cm water column between 10 and 30 min of reoxygenation (red squares). To set up the "working" heart model, afterload was constantly set to 75 cm water column (blue diamond line). In subsequent experiments, the heart muscle had to pump against this pressure in its cardiac output (systolic phase). (b) Due to our model, aortic flow (red squares) was zero during hypoxia; it was around 20 mL/min in normoxia and recovered to about 10 mL/min (about 50% of normoxia) during the first 15 min of reoxygenation and then started to fluctuate and slowly decreased to almost zero by the end of experimental reoxygenation (R30). Coronary flow (blue diamonds) slowly decreased during normoxia and hypoxia from 35–40 mL/min to 3–5 mL/min by the end of hypoxia and then recovered rapidly to 30 mL/min in the beginning of reoxygenation and subsequently decreased slightly to 25 mL/min within 30 min of reoxygenation. (c) Systolic pressure (blue diamonds) was 90–100 mmHg in normoxia, dropped to 40 mmHg within 5 min of hypoxia, and further decreased to zero in 25 min of hypoxia. Within 5 min of reoxygenation, systolic pressure immediately recovered to 80–85 mmHg for 15 min and then started to fluctuate between 50 and 85 mmHg until the end of the experimental reoxygenation (R30). Diastolic pressure (red squares) showed similar course at a lower level with normoxic pressure of 55–75 mmHg, decreased to 20–25 mmHg in hypoxia, and dropped to zero after 20–25 min of hypoxia. Recovery during reoxygenation was stable between 35 and 45 mmHg until the end of experimental reoxygenation. These data in preliminary experiments served as the basis of setting up our model in subsequent main experiments with 60 min of hypoxia.

applied. Results are presented as mean values ± standard deviation (SD); statistical significance is set to $p < 0.05$. Furthermore, the means of all normoxic values are set to 100% and the results of hypoxia, reoxygenation, curcumin 0.25 μM, and curcumin 0.5 μM concentrations expressed as percentage.

2.3. Inclusion-Exclusion Criteria. Our animal housing and experimental procedures strictly followed the Helsinki and Tokyo regulations on animal studies in their actual versions. Guinea pigs were kept in small groups of 3–5 animals with *ad libitum* access to food and water, in an acclimatized room with a window and thus natural day-and-night light fluctuations. Inclusion criteria for the main experiments were young adult

Guinea pigs, aged one year; body weight 300–400 g; heart rate of the isolated perfused heart between 150 and 250 beats per minute; and coronary flow of the isolated perfused heart during normoxia between 20 and 50 mL.

Exclusion criteria for the main experiments were time between excision of the heart and retrograde perfusion more than 3 min; initial arrhythmias after cannulation longer than 3 min; and afterload = aortic pressure performance: less than 75 cm water column in normoxia.

2.4. Main Experiments. Conditions in the main experiments are indicated where necessary. Protein was measured according to Lowry et al. [13]; thiobarbituric acid-reactive substances (TBARS) were determined according to Chirico

[14] using Waters HPLC device with a Spherisorb 5ODS2-C18 column. TBARS are expressed as malondialdehyde (MDA) throughout the text. Glutathione (GSH) was determined with the method of Ellman [15].

Mitochondria were prepared as described by Mela and Seitz [16] omitting nagarse. Relative specific activity of succinate dehydrogenase (SDH) was measured for control: $40 \mu L$ of the sample was added into a cuvette containing a mixture of $120 \mu L$ NaP$_i$ 800 mM, pH 7.6; $120 \mu L$ KCN 10 mM; $240 \mu L$ sodium succinate 100 mM; $48 \mu L$ 2,6-dichlorophenolindophenol 1 mM; and 632 μL distilled water. The absorption at $\lambda = 600$ nm was followed for 5 min at 37°C in a Shimadzu spectrophotometer equipped with a thermostat cuvette holder. We measured relative specific SDH activities between 7.89 and 12.72 to characterize our mitochondrial preparations [17].

Enzyme activity of glutathione peroxidase (GPx) and glutathione reductase (GR) were measured as described by Flohé and Günzler [18] with slight modifications: our reaction mixture contained $200 \mu L$ GSH 20 mM; $200 \mu L$ sodium azide 20 mM; $200 \mu L$ EDTA 20 mM; $200 \mu L$ NADPH 1 mM; and $100 \mu L$ NaP$_i$ 0.1 M, pH 7.0. For measurement of GPx activity, $20 \mu L$ glutathione reductase 1 U was added and incubated with $60 \mu L$ isolation buffer at 37°C for 10 min. Subsequently, $20 \mu L$ of mitochondrial preparation was added and absorption followed for 5 min at $\lambda = 340$ nm. For measurement of glutathione reductase, instead of $20 \mu L$ glutathione reductase 1 U, glutathione peroxidase was added, accordingly. All photometric measurements were accomplished in a Shimadzu spectrophotometer equipped with a thermostat cuvette holder.

3. Results

3.1. Preliminary Experiments. The time course of our model with normoxia, hypoxia, and reoxygenation, 30 min each, is depicted in Figure 1. In our preliminary experiments, hypoxia varied, 15, 30, or 60 min; throughout the main experiments hypoxia was set to 60 min.

Heart rate was between 173 and 217 beats per minute and turned out to be a stable parameter in our experimental setting: it recovered after 15 and 30 min of hypoxia in reoxygenation to 100.5% and 98.9%, respectively, without curcumin, and to 97.1% and 101.7%, respectively, with 0.25 and 0.5 μM curcumin. Differences between all these values were statistically not significant indicating that the hearts were stable over the experimental course of our model.

For measurement of systolic pressure a water column in our device [7, 11] with normoxic values up to 100 cm was used corresponding to and exceeding the constant afterload water column of 75 cm, against which the isolated heart had to perform its work. In addition, systolic and diastolic pressure were measured using a mercury manometer (Figure 1(c)).

3.1.1. Histopathology and Aspartate Aminotransferase (AST). Histopathological changes depended on the duration of hypoxia: in hypoxia up to 15 min we did not observe changes in tissue ultrastructure; however, changes became visible at 30 min and, particularly after 60 min, destruction of the myocardium was obvious (not shown). This result mirrored the measurement of AST activity in the perfusate: with only after 60 min of hypoxia, AST activity increased significantly during reoxygenation indicating tissue damage and release of AST from cardiomyocytes into the perfusate.

3.2. Main Experiments. For the main experiments, the following experimental settings were chosen: normoxia 30 min, hypoxia 60 min, and subsequent reoxygenation 30 min. Curcumin was injected into the perfusion buffer at 0.25 μM or 0.5 μM concentrations after 15 min of normoxic perfusion.

3.2.1. Cardiac Parameters. Cardiac parameters measured were systolic pressure, aortic flow, and coronary flow (Table 1).

3.2.2. Myocardial Tissue. Myocardial tissue parameters measured are shown in Table 2.

(1) Aspartate Aminotransferase (AST). After 60 min of hypoxia, AST activity increased significantly during reoxygenation indicating tissue damage and release of AST from cardiomyocytes into the perfusate (Table 2). Curcumin, at 0.25 μM concentration, protected the myocardium from AST release significantly from 139.9% in reoxygenation to normoxic values. This protective effect was significant with 0.25 μM ($p < 0.05$) but not with 0.5 μM concentration (Table 2).

(2) Thiobarbituric Acid-Reactive Substances (TBARS)/Malondialdehyde (MDA). Lipid peroxidation (LPO) is considered a major reason of membrane destruction; LPO is often determined via thiobarbiturate reaction and expressed through its byproduct malondialdehyde (MDA). As can be seen in Table 2, MDA increased to 232.5% of normoxia (8.33 $\pm$ 5.30 nmol $\times$ g^{-1} tissue, 100%) during reoxygenation (19.37 $\pm$ 8.31 nmol $\times$ g^{-1} tissue) after 60 min of hypoxia. Although during hypoxia 0.5 μM concentration of curcumin had a stronger effect than 0.25 μM, both concentrations equally reduced MDA levels to 150% in reoxygenation.

3.2.3. Mitochondrial Parameters. The mitochondrial parameters measured are presented in Table 3.

(1) Thiobarbituric Acid-Reactive Substances (TBARS). Mitochondrial TBARS levels are expressed as nmol MDA per g mitochondrial protein ($n = 6$). We found higher levels in normoxic mitochondria than in myocardial tissue if correlated to mitochondrial protein, 17.85 $\pm$ 2.79 (100%). During hypoxia the increase to 119% was only moderate but significant in reoxygenation, 165.4% ($p < 0.05$ versus N). Curcumin diminished mitochondrial MDA levels to normoxia at 0.25 μM concentration (R versus R$_{0.25}$; $p < 0.05$), whereas 0.5 μM concentration of curcumin was less effective (Table 3).

(2) Reduced Glutathione (GSH). Mitochondrial GSH decreased from 40.6 $\pm$ 10.9 nmol $\times$ mg^{-1} protein in normoxia (100%) to 56.4% in hypoxia ($p = 0.011$ versus N) and 35.2% in reoxygenation ($p < 0.001$ versus N). During hypoxia,

TABLE 1: Cardiac parameters.

	Normoxia	Hypoxia 60 min	Reoxygenation
	Systolic pressure: cm H_2O ($n = 9$; mean $\pm$ SD)		
	94.61 ± 9.38	0	52.31 ± 6.12 (55.3%) $p < 0.05$
Curc. 0.25 μM	92.73 ± 10.06	0	83.37 ± 7.96 (89.9%)
Curc. 0.5 μM	95.12 ± 11.0	0	77.78 ± 10.24 (83.2%)
Normoxia (mean = 94.15 = 100%)			73.2%
Curc. 0.25 μM			85.6%
Curc. 0.5 μM			88.1%
	Aortic flow: mL $\times$ min^{-1} ($n = 9$; mean $\pm$ SD)		
	14.13 ± 4.70	0	4.37 ± 3.85 (30.9%) $p = 0.05$
Curc. 0.25 μM	12.20 ± 3.75	0	6.10 ± 3.34 (50.0%)
Curc. 0.5 μM	14.27 ± 4.73	0	6.73 ± 4.33 (47.2%)
Normoxia (mean = 13.5 = 100%)			32.4%
Curc. 0.25 μM			45.2%
Curc. 0.5 μM			49.9%
	Coronary flow: mL $\times$ min^{-1} ($n = 9$; mean $\pm$ SD)		
	9.53 ± 3.04	0	15.97 ± 7.39 (167.6%)
Curc. 0.25 μM	10.53 ± 2.5	0	13.6 ± 3.56 (129.2%)
Curc. 0.5 μM	8.9 ± 6.48	0	13.27 ± 7.19 (149.1%)
Normoxia (mean = 9.65 = 100%)			165.5%
Curc. 0.25 μM			140.9%
Curc. 0.5 μM			137.5%

TABLE 2: Myocardial tissue parameters.

	Normoxia	Hypoxia	Reoxygenation
	Aspartate aminotransferase (AST)		
	AST: U $\times$ L^{-1} $\times$ g^{-1} heart tissue ($n = 5$; mean $\pm$ SD)		
	2.934 ± 1.451 (100%)	3.249 ± 1.119 (110.7%)	4.105 ± 1.917 (139.9%) N versus R $p = 0.05$
Curc. 0.25 μM		3.382 ± 2.149 (115.3%)	2.397 ± 0.901 (81.7%) R versus R$_{0.25}$ $p < 0.05$
Curc. 0.5 μM		3.671 ± 1.446 (125.1%)	3.192 ± 1.516 (108.8%)
	TBARS, expressed as malondialdehyde (MDA)		
	MDA: nmol $\times$ g^{-1} heart tissue ($n = 6$; mean $\pm$ SD; N versus R and H versus H$_{0.5}$ $p < 0.05$)		
	8.33 ± 5.30 (100%)	9.36 ± 6.24 (112.4%)	19.37 ± 8.31 (232.5%; N versus R $p < 0.05$)
Curc. 0.25 μM		8.86 ± 0.48 (106.4%)	12.46 ± 10.30 (149.6%)
Curc. 0.5 μM		5.88 ± 5.85 (70.6%) H versus H$_{0.5}$ ($p < 0.05$)	12.52 ± 6.85 (150.3%)

The activity of AST was measured in the perfusate as U $\times$ L^{-1} and then correlated to the weight of the heart (= g heart tissue). TBARS, thiobarbituric acid reactive substances; N, normoxia; H, hypoxia; R, reoxygenation; R$_{0.25}$, reoxygenation with curcumin (curc.) 0.25 μM; H$_{0.5}$, hypoxia with 0.5 μM curc.

curcumin did not have much effect, but in reoxygenation it significantly increased GSH at both concentrations (Table 3).

(3) Glutathione Peroxidase (GPx). Glutathione peroxidase activity was 324.1 ± 115.0 nmol $\times$ min^{-1} $\times$ mg^{-1} protein in normoxia (100%). During hypoxia GPx activity increased slightly to 121.1% and in reoxygenation significantly to 255.2%. Curcumin, at 0.25 μM concentration, attenuated GPx activity to about 150% and at 0.5 μM concentration to about 200%, both during hypoxia and reoxygenation (Table 3).

(4) Glutathione Reductase (GR). Glutathione reductase activity was 77.2 ± 15.7 nmol $\times$ min^{-1} $\times$ mg^{-1} protein in normoxia (100%). During hypoxia GR activity decreased moderately to 58.8% and in reoxygenation significantly to 29.3% ($p < 0.05$). During hypoxia, curcumin did not have a significant effect on GR activity, but, in reoxygenation, 0.25 μM concentration increased GR activity to 46.8% and 0.5 μM concentration significantly increased GR activity to 62.0% (R versus R$_{0.5}$ $p = 0.006$). Interestingly, values with curcumin were almost the same during hypoxia and reoxygenation,

TABLE 3: Mitochondrial parameters.

	Normoxia	Hypoxia	Reoxygenation
MDA: nmol $\times$ mg^{-1} mitochondrial protein ($n = 6$; mean $\pm$ SD; N versus R and R versus R$_{0.25}$ $p < 0.05$)			
	17.85 ± 2.79 (100%)	21.24 ± 3.53 (119.0%)	29.52 ± 9.47 (165.4%; N versus R; $p < 0.05$)
Curc. 0.25 μM		17.68 ± 4.40 (99.1%)	16.47 ± 1.99 (92.3%; R versus R$_{0.25}$; $p < 0.05$)
Curc. 0.5 μM		19.93 ± 3.62 (111.7%)	24.45 ± 3.24 (137.0%)
GSH: nmol $\times$ mg^{-1} protein ($n = 6$ in each group; mean $\pm$ SD)			
	40.6 ± 10.9 (100%)	22.9 ± 10.7 (56.4%) N versus H ($p = 0.011$)	14.3 ± 4.3 (35.2%) N versus R ($p < 0.001$)
Curc. 0.25 μM		19.5 ± 7.1 (48.0%)	27.0 ± 11.2 (66.5%) R versus R$_{0.25}$ ($p < 0.05$)
Curc. 0.5 μM		23.2 ± 7.0 (57.1%)	28.3 ± 8.0 (69.7%) R versus R$_{0.5}$ ($p < 0.05$)
GPx: nmol $\times$ min^{-1} $\times$ mg^{-1} protein ($n = 6$ in each group; mean $\pm$ SD)			
	324.1 ± 115.0 (100%)	392.2 ± 150.1 (121.1%) H versus R ($p < 0.05$)	826.1 ± 268.0 (255.2%) N versus R ($p < 0.05$)
Curc. 0.25 μM		513.3 ± 59.4 (158.6%)	498.6 ± 44.5 (153.8%) R versus R$_{0.25}$ ($p < 0.05$)
Curc. 0.5 μM		664.4 ± 206.3 (205.3%)	665.0 ± 219.1 (205.7%)
GR: nmol $\times$ min^{-1} $\times$ mg^{-1} protein ($n = 6$ in each group; mean $\pm$ SD)			
	77.2 ± 15.7 (100%)	45.3 ± 17.1 (58.8%)	22.2 ± 9.6 (29.3%; N versus R $p < 0.05$)
Curc. 0.25 μM		36.9 ± 16.9 (48.8%)	35.4 ± 16.0 (46.8%)
Curc. 0.5 μM		47.3 ± 18.6 (62.5%)	46.9 ± 18.5 (62.0%; R versus R$_{0.5}$ $p = 0.006$)

MDA, malondialdehyde; GSH, reduced glutathione; GPx, glutathione peroxidase; GR, glutathione reductase; N, normoxia; H, hypoxia; R, reoxygenation; R$_{0.25}$, reoxygenation with 0.25 μM curcumin (curc.); R$_{0.5}$, reoxygenation with 0.5 μM curc.

48.8% and 46.8% at 0.25 μM concentration, 62.5% and 62.0% at 0.5 μM concentration (Table 3).

4. Discussion

In our experiments Guinea pig hearts were more stable than rat hearts over the experimental time course of one hour and thus more suitable to our experimental conditions in Jakarta. The discussion about the stability of the performance of isolated perfused hearts goes back almost four decades; isolated perfused Guinea pig hearts had been considered more stable than rat hearts by some working groups, whereas others could not confirm any differences, which may strongly depend on the experimental conditions [19–26]. We do not want to go into the discussion about differences in metabolic pathways (e.g., endogenous synthesis of ascorbic acid) and whether environmental (e.g., tropical) conditions may play a role. However, we state from our own experience that the slightly bigger Guinea pig hearts make it easier to fix them to the cannulas of the apparatus and thus reduce initial complications such as arrhythmias.

4.1. Main Experiments: Cardiac Parameters. In the main experiments hypoxia was set to 60 min and systolic pressure, aortic flow, and coronary flow were measured as cardiac parameters. Two concentrations of curcumin in the reoxygenation buffer were applied, 0.25 μM and 0.5 μM, but, generally, 0.5 μM curcumin did not exert higher effects than 0.25 μM concentration (after we had already ruled out 1 mM concentration of curcumin in our preliminary experiments).

Systolic pressure recovered during reoxygenation by 55-56%, under 0.25 μM curcumin between 85% and 90% and under 0.5 μM curcumin between 83% and 88%. Aortic flow recovered to 31-32% during reoxygenation, under 0.25 μM curcumin between 45% and 50% and under 0.5 μM curcumin between 47% and 50%.

Coronary flow exerted an overshooting reaction of almost 170% during reoxygenation. This overshoot might depend on the experimental setting of the isolated heart. Coronary flow was measured as the amount of buffer dropping down from the heart's perfused coronary arteries and *sinus coronarius*. Hence, the "coronary flow" especially during reoxygenation might be a mixture of coronary perfusion and leakiness of coronary vessels. The increase of about 70% over the normoxic value was certainly due to the leakiness of the coronary blood vessels after 60 minutes of hypoxia.

Leakiness of blood vessels is a well-known and dreadful reoxygenation/reperfusion phenomenon often causing considerable edema in tissues as part of ischemia-reperfusion injury [1–3]. Hence, the influence of curcumin in lowering this overshoot can be considered a positive therapeutic effect. Curcumin, at 0.25 μM concentration, reduced the overshoot to roughly 140% and at 0.5 μM concentration to about 138%. Thus, coronary flow under the aspect of ischemia-reperfusion injury did not improve much better with 0.5 μM than with 0.25 μM concentration of curcumin.

4.2. Myocardial Tissue. After 60 min of hypoxia lipid per-oxidation destroyed cell membranes and cardiomyocytes became leaky and released AST into the perfusate, where its enzymatic activity increased during reoxygenation; in parallel, also MDA increased to about 233%. During reoxy-genation curcumin reduced AST activity significantly at 0.25 μM ($p < 0.05$), but not at 0.5 μM concentration ($p > 0.05$). Curcumin reduced MDA significantly during hypoxia only at 0.5 μM, but not at 0.25 μM concentration, whereas both concentrations reduced equally MDA tissue levels from 233% in reoxygenation to about 150%.

Thiobarbiturate is the mostly used reagent to measure lipid peroxidation (LPO) and the result is expressed as TBARS (thiobarbituric acid-reactive substances) or as one of the major byproducts of LPO, MDA. These parameters are widely used as markers of oxidative stress and tissue damage. Recently, discussions have been extended about the concept of oxidative damage and the value of LPO and MDA as generalized markers of oxidative stress in cells, tissues, and body fluids. We do not go into this discussion here; however, one point of criticism often raised is that the markers are not determined at the place of origin. Hence, we tried to overcome this point by differentiating MDA as a parameter of tissue damage, measured from myocardium, and MDA measured from mitochondria as a parameter of LPO in mitochondrial membranes.

In general, 0.5 μM curcumin did not exert higher effects on myocardial tissue parameters (AST, MDA) than 0.25 μM concentration.

4.3. Mitochondrial Parameters. Mitochondrial MDA level was only decreased significantly during reoxygenation by 0.25 μM curcumin, but not by 0.5 μM concentration. At both concentrations, curcumin increased significantly mitochon-drial GSH content during reoxygenation, whereas, during hypoxia, no significant effects on MDA and glutathione were observed. We were interested in the activities of glutathione reductase and glutathione peroxidase under the same con-ditions: The activity of glutathione reductase mirrored well the content of reduced glutathione. During reoxygenation curcumin exerted a significantly stimulating effect on GR at 0.5 μM, but not at 0.25 μM concentration. At either concen-tration, GR activity was almost the same during hypoxia and reoxygenation.

Glutathione peroxidase was slightly increased in hypoxia, but during reoxygenation its activity was tremendously high, 255% of normoxic control values. Curcumin, at 0.25 μM concentration, attenuated GPx to about 154% ($p < 0.05$) and at 0.5 μM to 206% ($p > 0.05$). Interestingly, at both concentrations, GPx had the same activity in hypoxia and reoxygenation of about 150% (0.25 μM curcumin) and 200% (0.5 μM curcumin) of normoxic values. Hence, curcumin,

in two concentrations used in our experiments, appeared to be an independent attenuator of both GR and GPx during hypoxia and reoxygenation. Interestingly, on GR 0.5 μM curcumin had a stronger effect than 0.25 μM concentration, whereas the overshoot of GPx activity in reoxygenation was downregulated more strongly by 0.25 than by 0.5 μM of curcumin.

Protective effects through enhanced GPx during hypoxia and reoxygenation in other organs have been reported [27–29]; in human plasma GPx-3 isoenzyme was threefold increased over normal expression during hypoxia [30]. On the contrary, Manikandan et al. [31] reported decreased GPx activity during isoprenaline induced myocardial ischemia in rats. Curcumin at 15 mg × kg^{-1} body weight (pre- and postischemic application) managed to normalize GPx activ-ity, whereas curcumin administered either pre- or postis-chemically had much lower effects.

Animal and organ distribution of cGPx was reported to be low in Guinea pig hearts [32] and less than one-third of the activity found in isolated mouse heart atria was detected in Guinea pigs [33]. On the other hand, overex-pression of PHGPx protected a guinea pig cell line from LPO-mediated injury [34]. In mitochondria, two isoforms out of various GPx isoenzymes [35, 36] appear to exist, for example, cGPx (GPx-1) and PHGPx (GPx-4) [37, 38], and GPx-1 was reported to protect mouse heart mitochon-dria against hypoxia/reoxygenation injury [28]. Transgenic mice overexpressing cGPx were protected against cerebral ischemia/reperfusion injury and apoptosis induced by it, whereas cGPx-mutant mice and nontransgenic control ani-mals were more susceptible [39]. In this context, selenium dependence of GPx isoenzymes should be considered, which differs "hierarchically" between isoforms [32] and we suggest that it should be the scope of future studies with our isolated perfused working guinea pig heart model [40].

During reoxygenation GPx was considerably increased to 255% of control values. Increased GPx activity consumes more GSH and produces GSSG; GR activity is needed to replenish reduced GSH, but diminished GR activity will lead to GSH depletion in hypoxia and reoxygenation. Attenuation of GPx activity by curcumin and concomitant slight stimula-tion of GR activity, as observed in our model, would help to prevent rapid GSH depletion.

At higher concentration up to 2.5 μM curcumin was reported to protect rat liver mitochondria against *tert*-butyl-hydroxyperoxide- (*t*-BHP-) induced mitochondrial dysfunc-tion, such as breakdown of transmembrane potential and swelling [17, 41]. On the other hand, at these concentrations curcumin was suspected to consume reduced glutathione [41]. It was assumed that curcumin participates in phenoxyl-radical recycling mechanisms as demonstrated for tocopherol and other phenolic compounds [42–44]. Such reductive "recycling" mechanisms involve reduced GSH [43, 44] and may consume glutathione at higher concentrations of cur-cumin (and other phenolic antioxidants) and thus contribute to GSH depletion during oxidative stress [17, 45]. Although these mechanisms still need further clarification, they may be the reason for prooxidant effects at higher concentrations; we had to rule out 1 μM curcumin in our preliminary experimentation and did not see a clear advantage of 0.5 μM over 0.25 μM concentration in some results of our main experiments.

In literature, curcumin concentrations differ considerably between experimental settings. Hence, it is difficult to compare results, especially since pharmacokinetic data are often missing. Pan et al. [46] investigated pharmacokinetic parameters of curcumin in mice: one mg $\times$ kg^{-1} body weight peaked in 0.5 μM plasma concentration, 50% of which was metabolized within 8 h. The concentrations in our perfusion buffer correlated to these data. In a Langendorff rat heart model [8] GPx was not much influenced by curcumin, whereas GR was stimulated. The differences with our results on GPx activity may be due to different animals and the experimental model. In the Langedorff preparation the isolated heart is perfused retrogradely, whereas in our model the isolated working heart is perfused anterogradely and its mechanical work is closer to physiological conditions. Their study, which only presented one value for ischemia-reperfusion (I/R) observed a decrease in GR activity during I/R to almost 47% [8]. Their value is very close to the average (about 44%) of our values in hypoxia (58.8%) and reoxygenation (29.3%). This decrease of GR during I/R can only be considered as an enzymatic or metabolic dysregulation, because the low GR activity cannot replenish higher GSH consumption by the oxidative stress during hypoxia/ischemia-reoxygenation/reperfusion, including the overshoot of GPx. Metabolic dysregulations (e.g., calcium paradox) have been observed in the scenario of ischemia-reperfusion injury [1–3].

Curcumin appeared to be an independent regulator of GR and GPx activities under our experimental conditions. In hypoxia and in reoxygenation, 0.25 μM concentration of curcumin attenuated GPx activity to 150% and 0.5 μM concentration of curcumin attenuated GPx to 200% of normoxic activity and, thus, moderately reduced the overshoot of GPx activity during reoxygenation. Concomitantly, curcumin attenuated GR during reoxygenation through moderate upregulation with 0.25 μM curcumin and significant upregulation with 0.5 μM concentration; in other words, towards GR 0.5 μM curcumin was more effective than the lower concentration. This attenuating effect on GR activity by curcumin was also observed in the Langendorff preparation by the before-mentioned study [8].

These considerations demonstrate that the concentration of curcumin is crucial to its metabolic effects; that is, the dosage of curcumin determines whether it exerts therapeutic activity. Moreover, the therapeutic efficacy of curcumin appears to go beyond its antioxidant effects [47, 48]: curcumin exerts regulatory effects on expression and activity of the enzymes involved in mitochondrial glutathione turnover.

5. Conclusion

In our experimental setting of the isolated perfused working Guinea pig heart curcumin exerts protection against hypoxia-reoxygenation injury at 0.25 μM and 0.5 μM concentrations on cardiac parameters and myocardial tissue damage and on mitochondrial GSH turnover. The higher concentration did not exert advantages over the lower one on cardiac parameters and myocardial tissue. On parameters of mitochondrial GSH turnover measured in our study, 0.5 μM concentration was only advantageous towards GR. In clinical cardio protective dose determination it should be considered that curcumin appears to have an upper dose limitation towards cardiac ischemia-reperfusion injury.

Conflict of Interests

The authors declare that there is no conflict of interests regarding the publication of this paper.

Acknowledgments

The authors are especially thankful to Professor Zimmer, posthumously, who had donated the entire perfusion device to the Medical Faculty at Universitas Indonesia. His Guest Professorship in Jakarta, in 1998, was supported by the German Academic Exchange Service (DAAD). Financial support to this research project by the URGE Program of the Indonesian Government and assistance by the Deutsch-Indonesische Gesellschaft für Medizin (DIGM e.V.) as well as the Indonesian Society For Free Radical Research (INA-SFRR) are also gratefully acknowledged. Furthermore, the authors want to express their gratitude to Dr. Gordon McDonald for proofreading the paper.

References

[1] H.-J. Freisieben, "Lipoate ameliorates ischemia-reperfusion in animal models," *Clinical Hemorheology and Microcirculation*, vol. 23, no. 2–4, pp. 219–224, 2000.

[2] A. Hanselmann, F. Beyersdorf, G. Matheis et al., "Verminderung des Postischämie-Syndroms nach akutem peripherem Gefäßverschluß durch Modifikation der initialen Reperfusion unter Berücksichtigung des Kalziumgehaltes des Reperfusates," *Zeitschrift für Herz-, Thorax- und Gefäßchirurgie*, vol. 4, pp. 13–20, 1990 (German).

[3] Z. Mitrev, F. Beyersdorf, R. Hallmann et al., "Reperfusion in skeletal muscle: controlled limb reperfusion reduces local and systemic complications after prolonged ischemia," *Cardiovascular Surgery*, vol. 2, no. 6, pp. 737–748, 1994.

[4] K. Ytrehus, "The ischemic heart—experimental models," *Pharmacological Research*, vol. 42, no. 3, pp. 193–203, 2000.

[5] J. R. Neely, H. Liebermeister, E. J. Battersby, and H. E. Morgan, "Effect of pressure development on oxygen consumption by isolated rat heart," *American Journal of Physiology*, vol. 212, no. 4, pp. 804–814, 1967.

[6] O. Langendorff, "Untersuchungen am überlebenden Säugetierherzen," *Pflüger, Archiv für die Gesammte Physiologie des Menschen und der Thiere*, vol. 61, no. 6, pp. 291–332, 1895.

[7] H.-J. Freisleben, H. Kriege, C. Clarke, F. Beyersdorf, and G. Zimmer, "Hemodynamic and mitochondrial parameters during hypoxia and reoxygenation in working rat hearts," *Arzneimittel-Forschung/Drug Research*, vol. 41, no. 1, pp. 81–88, 1991.

[8] A. González-Salazar, E. Molina-Jijón, F. Correa et al., "Curcumin protects from cardiac reperfusion damage by attenuation of oxidant stress and mitochondrial dysfunction," *Cardiovascular Toxicology*, vol. 11, no. 4, pp. 357–364, 2011.

[9] W. Wongcharoen and A. Phrommintikul, "The protective role of curcumin in cardiovascular diseases," *International Journal of Cardiology*, vol. 133, no. 2, pp. 145–151, 2009.

[10] A. Goel, A. B. Kunnumakkara, and B. B. Aggarwal, "Curcumin as 'Curecumin': from kitchen to clinic," *Biochemical Pharmacology*, vol. 75, no. 4, pp. 787–809, 2008.

[11] B. Deisinger and H.-J. Freisleben, "Animal models in hypoxia/reoxygenation and ischemia/reperfusion: II. Perfusion procedures," *The Indonesian Journal of Vascular Surgery*, vol. 2, no. 1, pp. 1–12, 1998.

[12] H. A. Krebs and K. Henseleit, "Untersuchungen über die Harnstoffbildung im Tierkörper," *Biological Chemistry Hoppe-Seyler*, vol. 210, pp. 33–66, 1932 (German).

[13] O. H. Lowry, N. J. Rosenbrough, A. L. Farr, and R. J. Randall, "Protein measurement with the Folin phenol reagent," *The Journal of Biological Chemistry*, vol. 193, no. 1, pp. 265–275, 1951.

[14] S. Chirico, "High-performance liquid chromatography-based thiobarbituric acid tests," *Methods in Enzymology*, vol. 234, pp. 314–318, 1994.

[15] G. L. Ellman, "Tissue sulfhydryl groups," *Archives of Biochemistry and Biophysics*, vol. 82, no. 1, pp. 70–77, 1959.

[16] L. Mela and S. Seitz, "Isolation of mitochondria with emphasis on heart mitochondria from small amount of tissue," *Methods in Enzymology*, vol. 55, pp. 39–46, 1979.

[17] S. Susilowati, F. D. Suyatna, and A. Setiawati, "The prevention of curcumin against rat liver mitochondrial swelling induced by tert-butylhydroperoxide," *Medical Journal of Indonesia*, vol. 15, no. 3, pp. 131–136, 2006.

[18] L. Flohé and W. A. Günzler, "Assays of glutathione peroxidase," *Methods in Enzymology*, vol. 105, pp. 114–121, 1984.

[19] R. Bünger, F. J. Haddy, A. Querengässer, and E. Gerlach, "An isolated guinea pig heart preparation with in vivo like features," *Pflügers Archiv—European Journal of Physiology*, vol. 353, no. 4, pp. 317–326, 1975.

[20] R. Bünger, O. Sommer, G. Walter, H. Stiegler, and E. Gerlach, "Functional and metabolic features of an isolated perfused guinea pig heart performing pressure-volume work," *Pflügers Archiv*, vol. 380, no. 3, pp. 259–266, 1979.

[21] R. Bünger, B. Swindall, D. Brodie, D. Zdunek, H. Stiegler, and G. Walter, "Pyruvate attenuation of hypoxia damage in isolated working guinea-pig heart," *Journal of Molecular and Cellular Cardiology*, vol. 18, no. 4, pp. 423–438, 1986.

[22] S. B. Flynn, R. W. Gristwood, and D. A. A. Owen, "Characterization of an isolated, working guinea-pig heart including effects of histamine and noradrenaline," *Journal of Pharmacological Methods*, vol. 1, no. 3, pp. 183–195, 1978.

[23] B. Gessner, E. R. Müller-Ruchholtz, and H. Reinauer, "Regulation der pyruvatdehydrogenaseaktivität und dynamik des isoliert perfundierten meerschweinchenherzens im thiaminmangel," *Pflügers Archiv*, vol. 334, no. 4, pp. 327–344, 1972.

[24] H. L. Maddock, K. J. Broadley, A. Bril, and N. Khandoudi, "Effects of adenosine receptor agonists on guinea-pig isolated working hearts and the role of endothelium and NO," *Journal of Pharmacy and Pharmacology*, vol. 54, no. 6, pp. 859–867, 2002.

[25] S. Soboll, R. Buenger, M. Müller, and O. Sommer, "Compartmentation of adenine nucleotides in the isolated working guinea pig heart stimulated by noradrenaline," *Biological Chemistry Hoppe-Seyler*, vol. 362, no. 2, pp. 125–132, 1981.

[26] R. R. Suwito, *Die langzeitstabilität isolierter, unterschiedlich belasteter, arbeitender rattenherzen bei zusatz von pyruvat zum perfusionsmedium [Dissertation]*, Freie Universität Berlin, Berlin, Germany, 1983 (German).

[27] D. A. Lepore, T. A. Shinkel, N. Fisicaro et al., "Enhanced expression of glutathione peroxidase protects islet β cells from hypoxia-reoxygenation," *Xenotransplantation*, vol. 11, no. 1, pp. 53–59, 2004.

[28] V. T. Thu, H. K. Kim, S. H. Ha et al., "Glutathione peroxidase 1 protects mitochondria against hypoxia/reoxygenation damage in mouse hearts," *Pflügers Archiv*, vol. 460, no. 1, pp. 55–68, 2010.

[29] C. W. White, J. H. Jackson, I. F. McMurtry, and J. E. Repine, "Hypoxia increases glutathione redox cycle and protects rat lungs against oxidants," *Journal of Applied Physiology*, vol. 65, no. 6, pp. 2607–2616, 1988.

[30] C. Bierl, B. Voetsch, R. C. Jin, D. E. Handy, and J. Loscalzo, "Determinants of human plasma glutathione peroxidase (GPx-3) expression," *The Journal of Biological Chemistry*, vol. 279, no. 26, pp. 26839–26845, 2004.

[31] P. Manikandan, M. Sumitra, S. Aishwarya, B. M. Manohar, B. Lokanadam, and R. Puvanakrishnan, "Curcumin modulates free radical quenching in myocardial ischaemia in rats," *The International Journal of Biochemistry & Cell Biology*, vol. 36, no. 10, pp. 1967–1980, 2004.

[32] R. Brigelius-Flohé, "Tissue-specific functions of individual glutathione peroxidases," *Free Radical Biology and Medicine*, vol. 27, no. 9-10, pp. 951–965, 1999.

[33] M. Floreani, E. Napoli, and P. Palatini, "Role of antioxidant defences in the species-specific response of isolated atria to menadione," *Comparative Biochemistry and Physiology Part C: Toxicology & Pharmacology*, vol. 132, no. 2, pp. 143–151, 2002.

[34] K. Yagi, S. Komura, H. Kojima et al., "Expression of human phospholipid hydroperoxide glutathione peroxidase gene for protection of host cells from lipid hydroperoxide-mediated injury," *Biochemical and Biophysical Research Communications*, vol. 219, no. 2, pp. 486–491, 1996.

[35] B. Mannervik, "The enzymes of glutathione metabolism: an overview," *Biochemical Society Transactions*, vol. 15, no. 4, pp. 717–718, 1987.

[36] A. Meister, "Glutathione metabolism and its selective modification," *The Journal of Biological Chemistry*, vol. 263, no. 33, pp. 17205–17208, 1988.

[37] H. Imai and Y. Nakagawa, "Regulatory and cytoprotective aspects of lipid hydroperoxide metabolism," *Free Radical Biology and Medicine*, vol. 34, no. 2, pp. 145–169, 2003.

[38] D. E. Handy and J. Loscalzo, "Redox regulation of mitochondrial function," *Antioxidants & Redox Signaling*, vol. 16, no. 11, pp. 1323–1367, 2012.

[39] D. Furling, O. Ghribi, A. Lahsaini, M.-E. Mirault, and G. Massicotte, "Impairment of synaptic transmission by transient hypoxia in hippocampal slices: improved recovery in glutathione peroxidase transgenic mice," *Proceedings of the National Academy of Sciences of the United States of America*, vol. 97, no. 8, pp. 4351–4356, 2000.

[40] K. Venardos, G. Harrison, J. Headrick, and A. Perkins, "Effects of dietary selenium on glutathione peroxidase and thioredoxin reductase activity and recovery from cardiac ischemia-reperfusion," *Journal of Trace Elements in Medicine and Biology*, vol. 18, no. 1, pp. 81–88, 2004.

[41] F. D. Suyatna, R. Djohan, A. Nafrialdi, and S. K. Suherman, "The antioxidant effects of curcumin on rat liver mitochondrial dysfunction induced by tert-butylhydroperoxide," *Journal of Ecophysiology and Occupational Health*, vol. 4, pp. 145–151, 2004.

[42] H.-J. Freisleben, "Free radicals and the antioxidant network," in *Free Radical-Related Diseases and Antioxidants in Indonesia*,

H.-J. Freisleben and B. Deisinger, Eds., pp. 1–12, Gardez, Sankt Augustin, Germany, 1999.

[43] V. E. Kagan, E. A. Serbinova, T. Forte, G. Scita, and L. Packer, "Recycling of vitamin E in human low density lipoproteins," *Journal of Lipid Research*, vol. 33, no. 3, pp. 385–397, 1992.

[44] V. E. Kagan, H.-J. Freisleben, M. Tsuchiya, T. Forte, and L. Packer, "Generation of probucol radicals and their reduction by ascorbate and dihydrolipoic acid in human low density lipoproteins," *Free Radical Research Communications*, vol. 15, no. 5, pp. 265–276, 1991.

[45] H.-J. Freisleben and L. Packer, "Free-radical scavenging activities, interactions and recycling of antioxidants," *Biochemical Society Transactions*, vol. 21, no. 2, pp. 325–330, 1993.

[46] M.-H. Pan, T.-M. Huang, and J.-K. Lin, "Biotransformation of curcumin through reduction and glucuronidation in mice," *Drug Metabolism and Disposition*, vol. 27, no. 4, pp. 486–494, 1999.

[47] C. Fiorillo, M. Becatti, A. Pensalfini et al., "Curcumin protects cardiac cells against ischemia-reperfusion injury: effects on oxidative stress, NF-κB, and JNK pathways," *Free Radical Biology and Medicine*, vol. 45, no. 6, pp. 839–846, 2008.

[48] D. Hong, X. Zeng, W. Xu, J. Ma, Y. Tong, and Y. Chen, "Altered profiles of gene expression in curcumin-treated rats with experimentally induced myocardial infarction," *Pharmacological Research*, vol. 61, no. 2, pp. 142–148, 2010.

15

A Review on Potential Mechanisms of *Terminalia chebula* in Alzheimer's Disease

Amir R. Afshari,[1] Hamid R. Sadeghnia,[1,2] and Hamid Mollazadeh[2]

[1]*Pharmacological Research Center of Medicinal Plants, School of Medicine, Mashhad University of Medical Sciences, Mashhad 917794-8564, Iran*
[2]*Neurocognitive Research Center, School of Medicine, Mashhad University of Medical Sciences, Mashhad 917794-8564, Iran*

Correspondence should be addressed to Hamid Mollazadeh; mollazadehh901@mums.ac.ir

Academic Editor: Berend Olivier

The current management of Alzheimer's disease (AD) focuses on acetylcholinesterase inhibitors (AChEIs) and NMDA receptor antagonists, although outcomes are not completely favorable. Hence, novel agents found in herbal plants are gaining attention as possible therapeutic alternatives. The *Terminalia chebula* (Family: Combretaceae) is a medicinal plant with a wide spectrum of medicinal properties and is reported to contain various biochemicals such as hydrolysable tannins, phenolic compounds, and flavonoids, so it may prove to be a good therapeutic alternative. In this research, we reviewed published scientific literature found in various databases: PubMed, Science Direct, Scopus, Web of Science, Scirus, and Google Scholar, with the keywords: *T. chebula*, AD, neuroprotection, medicinal plant, antioxidant, ellagitannin, gallotannin, gallic acid, chebulagic acid, and chebulinic acid. This review shows that *T. chebula* extracts and its constituents have AChEI and antioxidant and anti-inflammatory effects, all of which are currently relevant to the treatment of Alzheimer's disease.

1. Introduction

Alzheimer's disease (AD) is the leading cause of neurodegenerative disease in the geriatric population, accounting for approximately 5 million cases of dementia in the USA according to estimates from the Alzheimer's Association in 2015. Since the disease incidence increases with the progression of age, the risk of developing AD doubles every 5 years, beginning at age 65. Given the growing elderly population in developed countries, projections of future AD prevalence show a fourfold increase through 2050. Consequently, AD has become a major economic health burden because of accrued high healthcare costs, morbidity, and mortality, not to mention the financial burden it has on family members and caregivers due to lost wages and productivity [1].

The pathogenesis of AD is very complicated, but typically cerebral atrophy is clearly evident in postmortem and imaging studies. Combined cortical, limbic, and subcortical pathology leads to dementia typical of AD. Classic microscopic features include neurofibrillary tangles and senile plaques. Also, the clinical features of AD are commonly characterized by psychopathological signs such as language deterioration, memory loss, visuospatial impairment, and poor judgment [2]. Additionally, in AD there is a gradual loss of various neurotransmitters particularly in the basal forebrain. Cholinergic transmission is the earliest and most conspicuously affected in AD. The nucleus basalis in the basal forebrain is affected comparatively early in the process and acetylcholine levels inside the spinal fluid and brain of AD patients quickly reduce with the progression of the disease. This fact supports the cholinergic hypothesis that acetylcholine diminution results in the cognitive decline observed in AD patients finally go to the first symptomatic treatment of AD [3].

Most of the drugs presently available to treat AD are acetylcholinesterase inhibitors (AChEIs): tacrine [4], rivastigmine [5], donepezil [6], and galantamine [7]; but unfortunately all of these drugs have limited effectiveness and side effects [4]. On the other hand, medicinal plants are starting to take an important role in disease treatment, in particular to treat psychiatric and neurological disorders. One reason is because of the discontentment with conventional

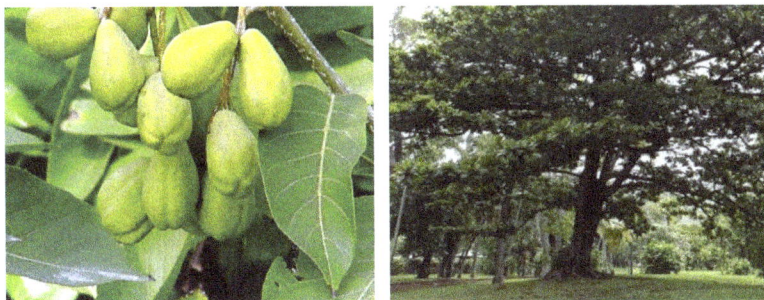

FIGURE 1: *T. chebula* tree and fruits.

treatments and another is because patients are seeking greater self-control over their healthcare decisions [8].

It seems that due to the indiscriminate and excessive use of drugs, their costs, side effects, and interactions, herbal medicines can be a suitable alternative to treat diseases because of their low costs, availability, and fewer drug interactions [9]. Therefore, the search for a new pharmacotherapy from medicinal plants to treat neurodegenerative disorders has remarkably advanced and there are several studies and documents that indicate a significant role of herbal medicines in the treatment of AD [10–12]. One particular herbal remedy is *Terminalia chebula* Retz. (Combretaceae) because of its numerous and different types of phytoconstituents such as polyphenols, terpenes, anthocyanins, flavonoids, alkaloids, and glycosides. In traditional medicine, the fruits of the *T. chebula*, which hold various chemically active compounds responsible for its medicinal properties, have been used in Unani, Ayurveda, and homeopathic medicine since antiquity to treat geriatric diseases and improve memory and brain function [13, 14]. It is also commonly used to treat numerous diseases such as cancer, cardiovascular diseases, paralysis, leprosy, ulcers, gout, arthritis, epilepsy, cough, fever, diarrhea, gastroenteritis, skin disorders, urinary tract infection, and wound infections [15, 16]. Recent studies show that *T. chebula* is effective in the treatment of diabetes [17], bacterial and fungal infections [18, 19], immunodeficiency diseases [20, 21], hyperlipidemia [22], liver diseases [15, 23], stomach ulcer [24], and wounds [25]. Other pharmacological properties and beneficial effects of *T. chebula* are summarized in Table 1.

Hence, this review article aims to sum up the published literature on the pharmacology and phytochemistry of *T. chebula* and its effects on the progression and treatment of AD in order to call attention to this plant as a novel alternative in the treatment of Alzheimer's disease.

2. *Terminalia chebula* Retzius

Terminalia chebula Retzius (Family: Combretaceae), as a shade and ornamental tree with 250 species, is a medicinal plant that grows in the Middle East and tropical regions such as India, China, and Thailand. It can grow to be 25 meters tall and has a variable appearance and spreading branches. The color of the bark is dark brown and is usually cracked. Leaves are thin, elliptic-oblong, cordiform at the base, elliptical, and 7–12 cm long and 4–6.5 cm in width and have a leathery

form with entire margins. The upper surface of the leaves is glabrous opposite of the surface beneath. The flowers are futile with a white to yellowish color and unsightly odor. Flowers have 5–7 cm long spikes, simple or branched, about 4 mm across. The ovary is inferior with 10 stamens. Fruits are yellow to orange-brown when ripe and 2.5–5 cm long and unruffled with an ovate-drupe shape [15, 61].

Moreover, it is called by various names by the local people. For example, in the Thai language the plant's common name is "Kot Phung Pla," and in Indian it is called "Kadukkaai"; and its other names are Black Myrobalan, Ink Tree, or Chebulic Myrobalan (Figure 1) [15].

2.1. Scientific Classification. Its classification is Kingdom: Plantae, Division: Magnoliophyta, Class: Magnoliopsida, Order: Myrtales, Family: Combretaceae, Genus: *Terminalia*, and Species: *Chebula* [15].

2.2. Phytochemical Compositions of T. chebula

2.2.1. Hydrolysable Tannins. Tannins, as a part of the phenolic compounds, are oligomeric and have multiple structural units with free phenolic groups and their molecular weight ranges from 500 to 3000 D. The fruit pulp and dried pericarp of the seeds contain the highest amount of tannins [62]. Tannins consist of hydrolysable and nonhydrolysable tannins and hydrolysable tannins (i.e., gallotannins and ellagitannins) are the main compounds in *T. chebula*.

Gallotannins and ellagitannins are polymers found in the fruits of *T. chebula* [63]. Gallotannins contain gallic acid that has esterified and bonded with the hydroxyl group of a polyol carbohydrate such as glucose [64]. Ellagitannins are formed when oxidative linkage occurs in the galloyl groups in 1,2,3,4,6-pentagalloyl glucose. Ellagitannins differ from gallotannins in that their galloyl groups are linked through C–C bonds, whereas the galloyl groups in gallotannins are linked by depside bonds [65, 66].

Chebulagic acid, a benzopyran tannin, is widely distributed in several plant families: the Combretaceae [67], Euphorbiaceae, Leguminosae, Anacardiaceae, and Fabaceae [31]. Also, in the Combretaceae Family, chebulagic acid is the main constitute of the fruits *T. bellerica, T. chebula,* and *Emblica officinalis* [68].

Chebulinic acid, also known as 1,3,6-tri-*O*-galloyl-2,4-chebuloyl-β-D-glucopyranoside, is an ellagitannin found in

TABLE 1: Structure and pharmacological properties of *T. chebula* active ingredients.

Compound	Category	Chemical structure	Pharmacological properties
Gallotannins	Hydrolysable tannin		Antimicrobial [26], antioxidant [27]
Ellagitannins	Hydrolysable tannin		Anti-inflammatory, anticancer, cardiovascular protection [28], antioxidant, chemopreventive, antiapoptotic, anti-hepatocellular carcinoma (Anti-HCC) [29]
Gallic acid	Phenolic compound		Anti-inflammatory [30], antimutagenic [31], cardioprotective [32], antioxidant [33], anticancer [34], antimicrobial [35], neuroprotective [36], immunosuppressive [37], improved cognition [38]

TABLE 1: Continued.

Compound	Category	Chemical structure	Pharmacological properties
Chebulic acid	Phenolic compound		Anti-HCV [39], antidiabetic [40], hepatoprotective [41], immunosuppressive [37]
Chebulagic acid	Hydrolysable tannin		Hepatoprotective [41], antiviral [42], immunosuppressive [43], antidiabetic [44, 45], neuroprotective [46], antiangiogenesis [47], antiproliferative [48], anti-inflammatory [44]
Chebulinic acid	Hydrolysable tannin		Antisecretory, cytoprotective [49], antiangiogenesis [50], antitumor [51]

TABLE 1: Continued.

Compound	Category	Chemical structure	Pharmacological properties
Ellagic acid	Phenolic compound		Antioxidant [52], anti-inflammatory [53], anti-diabetes-induced sexual dysfunction [54], hepatoprotective [55], antiarrhythmic [56], cognitive enhancer [57, 58]
Anthraquinone glycosides	Phenolic compound		Neuroprotective [59], antidiabetic [60]

the fruits of *T. chebula* or in the leaves of *T. macroptera* [31, 68].

2.2.2. Phenolic Compounds. Phenolic compounds include ellagic acid, a natural potent phenolic antioxidant found in the fruits of *T. chebula* [13]; gallic acid, a trihydroxybenzoic acid found as a part of hydrolysable tannins [69]; tannic acid, a polymer of gallic acid molecules and glucose [70]; and chebulic acid, another phenolic compound in the ripe fruits of *T. chebula and* a component of transformed ellagitannins such as chebulagic acid or chebulinic acid [41].

Glycosides are other phenolic compounds that are widely present in the *Terminalia*, rhubarb, *Senna*, and *Aloe* species. The pericarp of the *T. chebula* fruit contains anthraquinone glycosides [71]. Table 1 shows the main ingredients of *T. chebula* and their chemical structures.

2.2.3. Miscellaneous Compounds. In addition to the above, there are some other compounds that are also present and contribute towards the activity of the plant such as palmitic [72], stearic [73], oleic [74], linoleic [75], and arachidic acids [76], which are present in the fruit kernels.

2.2.4. Methods of Search. This research included articles from 1960 to 2015 that were found in various electronic databases: PubMed, Science Direct, Scopus, Web of Science, Scirus, and Google Scholar by using the search words: *T. chebula*, AD, neuroprotection, medicinal plant, antioxidant, ellagitannin, gallotannin, gallic acid, chebulagic acid, and chebulinic acid. Only current articles that reported the effects of *T. chebula* on AD were included in our study. Then, a comparison of the related mechanisms and evaluation of pharmacology effects in the treatment and progression of AD was done.

2.3. T. chebula and Alzheimer's Disease

2.3.1. Acetyl Cholinesterase (AChE). One of the hypotheses about AD is acetylcholine (ACh) deficiency in the synaptic cleft of the cerebral cortex that causes memory disturbance. Acetyl cholinesterase, also known as AChE or acetylhydrolase, is a hydrolase that hydrolyzes the neurotransmitter acetylcholine. AChE is found at mainly neuromuscular junctions and cholinergic brain synapses where its activity serves to terminate synaptic transmission. It is the primary target of inhibition by organophosphorus compounds such as nerve agents and pesticides. AChE has a very high catalytic activity; each molecule of AChE degrades about 25000 molecules of ACh per second, approaching the limit allowed by diffusion of the substrate [77]. During neurotransmission, ACh is released from the nerve into the synaptic cleft and binds to ACh receptors on the postsynaptic membrane, relaying the signal from the nerve. AChE, also located on the postsynaptic membrane, terminates the signal transmission by hydrolyzing Ach [78]. AChE is found in many types of conducting tissue: central and peripheral tissues, motor and sensory fibers, nerve and muscle, and cholinergic and noncholinergic fibers. The activity of AChE is higher in motor neurons than in sensory neurons [79]. AChE is also found on the red blood cell membranes [80]. Traditionally, necrosis is the pathway that had been thought to cause cell death in AD; however, now it is thought that ACh containing neurons are the most important pathway of neuronal death in AD. The cell death mechanisms in AD are deposition of Aβ, reduced energy metabolism and/or mitochondrial dysfunction, excitotoxicity, and oxidative stress and free radical production. These four mechanisms contribute to necrosis in various diseases such as stroke and AD. Inflammatory responses and their effects on trophic factor function have also been proposed as a main factor for cell death in AD. AChE induces an apoptotic and necrotic cell death by inducing membrane depolarization and NMDA receptor activation with consequent Ca^{2+} influx and modulation of the $\alpha7$ nicotinic acetylcholine receptor in hippocampal cultures. Therefore, AChE has a main role in neurodegeneration and AChEIs could be effective in neuroprotection [81–83]. Increasing expression of splice variants of AChE (R and S) as neuroprotective forms of AChE, with AChEIs, has been effective in preventing the progression of AD. In a study, expression of AChE-R and AChE-S decreased over a period of 12 months in untreated patients. In contrast, treatment with tacrine causes an upregulation in both variants (up to 117%) [84].

Inhibition of AChE leads to accumulation of ACh in the synaptic cleft and results in impeded neurotransmission [78]. The acetyl cholinesterase inhibitors (AChEIs) attenuate the cholinergic deficit underlying the cognitive and neuropsychiatric dysfunctions in patients with neurodegenerative disorders. So, inhibition of brain AChE has been the major therapeutic target of treatment strategies for AD, Parkinson's disease, senile dementia, ataxia, and myasthenia gravis [85]. There are a few synthetic medicines with this mechanism, for example, tacrine, donepezil, and the natural product-based rivastigmine, to treat cognitive dysfunction and memory loss associated with AD [86]. However, these compounds have been reported to have their adverse effects including gastrointestinal disturbances and problems associated with bioavailability, which necessitates the interest in finding better AChE inhibitors from natural sources [87].

In this section we discuss the effectiveness of T. chebula and its constituents on brain functions.

2.3.2. Anticholinesterase Properties. Anticholinesterase properties of T. chebula have been reported in many studies [3, 88–95]. In Sancheti et al.'s study, the inhibitory effects of T. chebula on AChE and butyrylcholinesterase (BChE) were reported. In the in vitro study, methanolic crude extract of the fruits of T. chebula with a concentration of 5 mg/mL inhibited AChE and BChE about 89% and 95%, respectively. Sancheti et al. extracted 1,2,3,4,6-penta-O-galloyl-β-D-glucose (PGG) with a gallotannin structure from T. chebula by chromatographic methods, and they showed it to be the most potent AChE and BChE inhibitor. Bioassay of PGG exhibited its concentration-dependent inhibitory activity on AChE and BChE with IC_{50} values of $29.9 \pm 0.3\,\mu M$ and $27.6 \pm 0.2\,\mu M$, respectively. Then, for deducing the inhibitory activity of PGG, a TLC assay was done with tacrine as a positive control, and the AChE inhibitory effect was visualized clearly in the assay [88]. In addition to the inhibitory effect of methanolic fruit extracts of T. chebula on AChE, the ethyl acetate fraction shows relatively remarkable AChE inhibitory activity. Sulaiman et al. showed that ethyl acetate fraction with doses of 1, 5, 15, and 25 mg/mL inhibited AChE by 29.36%, 32.44%, 45.82%, and 62.32%, respectively. This fraction was more potent than the chloroform and methanolic fraction in AChE inhibition [91]. In a similar in vitro study, Vinutha et al. used the methanolic and aqueous extracts of the fruit of T. chebula and the data showed that IC_{50} values of the aqueous extract of T. chebula (minimum inhibition: 12.45%) are more

potent than the methanolic extract (minimum inhibition: 1.21%) [3].

In addition to the effects of gallotannins on AChE inhibition, tannic acid as an active component of T. chebula has a potential inhibition effect on AChE. Upadhyay and Singh showed the competitive inhibition of AChE by tannic acid in vivo and in vitro. This study focused on the effects of tannic acid from the T. chebula fruit. In vivo treatment with 80% of LC_{50} of tannic acid during 96 h caused a remarkable inhibition in AChE activity in the nervous tissue of *Lymnaea acuminate*. Furthermore, maximum inhibition of AChE activity was detected when the tissue was exposed to 80% of LC_{50} of tannic acid for 96 h, so inhibition of AChE was time- and dose-dependent in the 96 h process. In vitro treatment showed that tannic acid caused dose-dependent AChE inhibition significantly, such that 0.04 mM of tannic acid reduced the AChE activity to 37% of the control in the nervous tissue of *L. acuminata* [92]. In addition, another in vivo research on AChE activity showed that tannic acid completely neutralized the AChE activity in *Naja kaouthia* venom [96].

Parle and Vasudevan in their in vivo study showed that *Abana* (a mixture of medicinal plants containing T. chebula) with doses of 50, 100, and 200 mg/kg administered orally for 15 days can reduce the brain AChE activity in young and aged mice. Passive avoidance apparatus and maze tests were performed on day 16 and the results showed a remarkable dose-dependent reduction in transfer latency and a significant increase in step-down latency tests, indicating significant improvement in memory [93].

Another similar study was done by Dhivya et al. In this in vitro study, AChE inhibitory activity of various plant species containing T. chebula was reported to have AChE inhibition of $41.06 \pm 5.6\%$ (0.1 mg/mL) as well [95].

In a similar study, AChE inhibition of the methanolic extract of T. chebula showed a moderate inhibition with an extract with IC_{50} value of $180 \pm 14.6\,\mu g/mL$ and the percentage of AChE inhibition was 41.06 ± 5.6 at 0.1 mg/mL [97]. In addition, the percentage of AChE inhibition in the extract of T. chebula was 13% (IC_{50} not detected) [14]. Furthermore, in another research, T. chebula could inhibit 89% of AChE activity (5 mg/mL) and 95% of BChE activity (5 mg/mL) [88].

Gallic acid and ellagic acid, as phenolic compounds in the fruits of T. chebula, could also inhibit AChE. Nag and De in their study showed that the inhibitory effect of the methanolic extract of T. chebula (gallic acid: $0.25\,\mu g$, ellagic acid: $0.08\,\mu g$) has a linear relationship with increasing dosage (IC_{50}: 10.96) [89].

2.3.3. Anti-Inflammatory Properties. Cyclooxygenase (COX) and 5-lipoxygenase (5-LOX) are the key enzymes that are involved in inflammation. Reddy et al. investigated chebulagic acid, as a COX-LOX dual inhibitor, from the ethanolic extract of fruits of T. chebula. The results showed that chebulagic acid has a potent COX-LOX dual inhibition activity with IC_{50} values of 15 ± 0.288, 0.92 ± 0.011, and $2.1 \pm 0.057\,\mu M$ for COX-1, COX-2, and 5-LOX, respectively [76].

The water soluble fraction of T. chebula (WFTC) was effective against systemic and local anaphylaxis. Shin et al. showed that the injection of WFTC with doses of

0.01–1.0 g/kg inhibited anaphylactic shock 100%. When WFTC was pretreated at concentrations ranging from 0.005 to 1.0 g/kg, the serum histamine levels were reduced dose-dependently. In addition, this study showed that WFTC increased anti-dinitrophenol and IgE-induced tumor necrosis factor- (TNF-) α production [98].

Lee et al. in their study showed that gallic acid (25 μg) suppressed nuclear factor kappa B (NF-κB) activity and cytokine release. It also remarkably reduced the cyclic AMP response element binding protein/p300 (CBP/p300, a NF-κB coactivator) gene expression, acetylation levels, and CBP/p300 histone acetyltransferase activity. Therefore, gallic acid derived from the extracts of several plants especially *T. chebula* was shown to exert anti-inflammatory activity via the downregulation of the NF-κB pathway in the development of inflammatory diseases, both in vitro and in vivo [30, 99–101].

Kim et al. showed that the inhibition of NF-κB acetylation with gallic acid resulted in reduced cytokine production in microglia cells and the protection of neuronal cells from amyloid β- (Aβ-) induced neurotoxicity. In addition, this research showed a restorative effect of gallic acid on Aβ-induced cognitive dysfunction in mice in Y-maze and passive avoidance tests. Therefore, gallic acid has several roles in neuroinflammatory diseases including (1) preventing Aβ-induced neuronal cell death by inhibiting RelA (as a gene encoding NF-κB) acetylation and cytokine production; (2) protecting neuronal cells from primary microglia-mediated Aβ neurotoxicity; (3) restoring Aβ-induced memory deficits in mice; and (4) suppressing in vivo cytokine production by inhibiting RelA acetylation in brain [101]. Another similar study showed that polyphenolic extracts (containing gallic acid) of medicinal plants such as *T. chebula* are able to inhibit Aβ aggregation, reduce Aβ production, and protect against Aβ neurotoxicity, in vitro [102]. Kim et al. reported the inhibitory effects of gallic acid on inflammatory responses via NF- κB and p38 mitogen-activated protein kinase pathways [103].

In another study, chebulagic acid showed a potent anti-inflammatory effect in lipopolysaccharide- (LPS) stimulated RAW 264.7 (mouse macrophage cell line). Reddy and Reddanna showed the effectiveness of chebulagic acid against inflammatory diseases by different mechanisms such as inhibition of nitric oxide (NO) and prostaglandin E$_2$ production, downregulation of iNOS (inducible nitric oxide synthases), COX-2, 5-LOX, TNF-α, interleukin 6, and inhibitory effects on NF-κB, and decreases in nuclear p50 and p65 protein levels. In addition, the generation of reactive oxygen species (ROS) and phosphorylation of p38, ERK 1/2, and JNK in LPS-stimulated RAW 264.7 cells was suppressed by chebulagic acid in a concentration-dependent manner [44]. In another research, chebulagic acid from the immature seeds of *T. chebula* significantly suppressed the onset and progression of collagen induced arthritis in mice [104]. In a similar study, the aqueous extract of the dried fruit of *T. chebula* showed an anti-inflammatory effect by inhibiting iNOS [105]. Patil et al. in their study showed that administrating the fruit of *T. chebula* (500 mg/kg) via inhibition of iNOS expression can be significantly effective in the progression of inflammation [106]. In vivo anti-inflammatory activity

of *T. chebula* fruit extract at different doses (range: 50 to 500 mg/kg) was evaluated against carrageenan-induced inflammation in rats. In this study, Bag et al. reported that 250 mg/kg (administered orally) caused a 69.96% reduction in carrageenan-induced rat paw edema. This finding suggests that free radical quenching may be one of the mechanisms for its anti-inflammatory activity [107]. Triphala, an Indian Ayurvedic herbal formulation containing *T. chebula*, at a dosage of 1 g/kg, showed an anti-inflammatory effect. Sabina and Rasool in their research showed that the mechanisms of anti-inflammatory properties of this plant include (a) inhibition of lysosomal enzyme release, (b) a significant decrease of inflammatory mediator TNF-α, and (c) a decrease of beta-glucuronidase and lactate dehydrogenase enzymes release. The anti-inflammatory effect of Triphala might be due to the presence of phenolic components and flavonoids [108]. In another study, Ramani and Pradhan showed that the acetone extract of *T. chebula* fruits had a significant effect on controlling Complete Freund's Adjuvant-induced arthritis. This effect leads to a good reduction in paw edema and joint thickness (reduction of ESR values and RF values) in comparison with dexamethasone [109].

2.3.4. Antioxidant Properties. Decreases in antioxidant defense or increases in oxidant status in the body tend to lead to the condition called oxidative stress, which plays a major role in neurological degeneration such as AD [110]. Reactive oxygen species and oxidative stress increase the formation of amyloid-β and senile plaques in the brain are the hallmark of AD [111]. High lipid content, deficient antioxidant values, and high oxygen consumption in the brain are the reasons the central nervous system is vulnerable to oxidative stress. Increased lipid peroxidation, decreased glutathione levels, increased dopamine turnover, and elevated iron and aluminum levels in the brain support the role of oxidative stress in Parkinson's, Amyotrophic Lateral Sclerosis, and AD [112].

In Table 2, we have summarized the roles of oxidative stress in the pathogenesis and progression of AD. Thus, reducing oxidative stress by enhancing antioxidant defense or decreasing the production of reactive oxygen species may be effective in treating AD.

Antioxidant effects of *T. chebula* extract (100 μg/mL) were compared with reference radical scavengers such as quercetin, gallic acid, and t-butylhydroquinone, and *T. chebula* extract showed 95% activity with IC$_{50}$ 2.2 μg/mL [14]. *Terminalia* species such as *T. chebula* and *T. arjuna* with a high content of phenolic constituents showed strong antioxidant and antiaging properties [88]. Oral administration of aqueous extracts of *T. arjuna* causes significant elevation in the activities of antioxidant enzymes such as superoxide dismutase, catalase, and glutathione S-transferase. The strong antioxidant action of the aqueous extract of the *Terminalia* species may play a role in treating age-related diseases such as AD [127]. A similar study done by Mathew and Subramanian showed that the antioxidant activity of the methanolic extract of *T. chebula* (0.1 mg/mL) and IC$_{50}$ was 86.3% and 0.5 μg/mL, respectively. In this study the highest amount of antioxidant activity among 20 plants was found in *T. chebula* due to the presence of gallic acid and ellagic acid. All 20 plants used in

TABLE 2: Major effects of oxidative stress in the pathogenesis of Alzheimer's disease.

Effects of ROS	Result	Biological evidence(s)
Protein oxidation	Increased protein carbonyl content	Increased protein oxidation in frontal pole and occipital pole [113] Decreased ratio of (MAL-6)/(W/S) in AD hippocampus and inferior parietal lobule, decreased the W/S ratio in in vitro models of human synaptosomes oxidation by ROS [114]
DNA oxidation	Direct damage to DNA structure	3-fold increase in mitochondrial DNA oxidation in parietal cortex in AD [115] Increase in oxidative damage to nuclear DNA in AD compared with age-matched control subjects [116] 8-hydroxy-2-deoxyguanosine as a marker of DNA oxidation increases in AD [117]
Lipid peroxidation	Brain phospholipid damage	Increased TBARS levels in AD in hippocampus, piriform cortex, and amygdala [118] Increased lipid peroxidation of AD brain homogenates in vitro due to Fe-H_2O_2 [119] Increased apoptosis in cultured DS and AD neurons inhibited by antioxidant enzymes [112, 120] Decrease in PC, PE, phospholipid precursors, choline, and ethanolamine in hippocampus and inferior parietal lobule in AD [121] Increased aldehydes as a cytotoxic agent in the brain of AD patients [122]
Antioxidant enzymes	Changes in enzymes contents	Elevated GSH-Px, GSSG-R, and CAT activity in hippocampus and amygdala in AD [118] Many studies showed no elevation in enzyme activity [123, 124] or decrease in activity [125]
AGE formation	Pathological changes in protein structure and action	Accelerates aggregation of soluble nonfibrillar Aβ and tau [126]

MAL-6: weakly immobilized protein bound spin label; W/S: strongly immobilized protein bound spin label; TBARS: thiobarbituric acid reactive substances; DS: Down syndrome; PC: phosphatidylcholine; PE: phosphatidylethanolamine; GSH-Px: glutathione peroxidase; GSSG-R: glutathione reductase; CAT: catalase; AGE: advanced glycation end products.

this study were traditional neuroprotective plants that have been used for many years and among them T. chebula was the most potent antioxidant and moderate inhibition of AchE [97]. In the evaluation of antioxidant, anti-inflammatory, membrane-stabilizing, and antilipid peroxidative effects of the hydroalcoholic extract of T. chebula fruits in arthritic disorders, Bag et al. showed that the fruit extract of T. chebula (10 to 100 μg/mL) in carrageenan-induced inflammation in rats reduced the formation of thiobarbituric acid reactive substances in the liver with IC$_{50}$ 94.96 mg/kg. The IC$_{50}$ of the extract in DPPH radical-scavenging activity was 42.14 μg/mL [107]. Antilipid peroxidative capacity of T. chebula was attributed to higher phenolic content, reducing ability, Fe(II) chelating ability, and free radical-scavenging activity. In Khan et al.'s study, the aqueous extracts of yellow T. chebula and black T. chebula showed IC$_{50}$ values of 20.24 $\pm$ 0.9 μg/mL and 17.33 $\pm$ 1.1 μg/mL in the scavenging of the DPPH radical in mice brains, respectively [128]. In an in vitro study done to investigate the biological activities of phenolic compounds and triterpenoid constituents of T. chebula, 9 phenolic compounds and 8 triterpenoids were extracted. Radical-scavenging activities of the phenolic compounds were higher

than the triterpenoids compounds and had potent inhibitory activities against melanogenesis at a concentration of 10 μM and the IC$_{50}$ was 1.4–10.9 μM. These results showed that T. chebula with a high content of polyphenolic ingredients was a potent antioxidant [16]. The extract of the dried fruit pulp of T. chebula (600 mg/kg) could diminish acetic acid-induced colitis in rats with antioxidant effects (free radical-scavenging, antioxidant enzymes enhancing activity and decreasing lipid peroxidation) [129].

In the evaluation of neuroprotective effects, the inhibition of H_2O_2-induced PC12 cell death by T. chebula was investigated. H_2O_2 at 40 μM for 12 h decreased cell viability to 59%. Also, all of the methanol, water, and 95% ethanol extracts of T. chebula increased cell viability at 0.5–5.0 μg/mL, dose-dependently; and among them the water extract was more potent. Antioxidant effects of the extracts were compared and the results showed that methanol extract had good antioxidant activity based on the luminol-H_2O_2-horseradish peroxidase assay and the water extract was shown to have good antioxidant activities in cupric sulfate phenanthroline-H_2O_2 and luminol-H_2O_2 assays. Also, 95% ethanol extract showed good antioxidant activity in the pyrogallol-luminol assay [130]. Effects of *T. chebula* seed extracts on brain-derived neurotrophic factor (BDNF), Cu, Zn-superoxide dismutase (SOD1), and Mn-superoxide dismutase (SOD2) were evaluated by Park et al. Extract with a dose of 100 mg/kg once a day was administrated to gerbils for 7 days before induction of transient cerebral ischemia and the neuroprotective effect of the extract was evaluated in the CA1 hippocampal region on the fourth day after ischemia-reperfusion induction. The results showed that astrocytes and microglia remarkably decreased in the ischemic group compared with the vehicle-treated group and neuron nucleus (as the positive neuron) was distinctively abundant (62%) compared to the vehicle-treated ischemia group (62% versus 12.2%). Protein levels and activity of SOD1, SOD2, and BDNF were much higher in the treated group. These results confirmed the neuroprotective effects of *T. chebula* extracts against neuronal damage in hippocampus [131]. Recently, we have found that the alcoholic extract of *T. chebula* fruits significantly protects against quinolinic acid-induced neurotoxicity by alleviating the oxidative stress parameters (unpublished data).

Many studies used *T. chebula* to modulate the oxidative stress adverse effects in various models of oxidation damage and aging [132–134]. *T. chebula* could enhance the antioxidant defense and modulate oxidative stress due to aging in the liver and kidney of aged rats compared to young albino rats [133] and could protect hepatocytes from damage due to oxidative stress and enhanced total thiol content [41]. Many studies have shown the antioxidant activity of *T. chebula* in various in vivo and in vitro models [16, 135, 136]. In addition, most of the researchers agree with this hypothesis that "pharmacophore, which contains large numbers of –OH group (such as polyphenols), has greater anti-aging properties than those with less numbers of –OH groups." Therefore, two constituents that are potent phenolic compounds are ellagic acid and 4-O-xyloside of ellagic acid. These active ingredients were investigated for their activities on free radical-scavenging, elastase inhibition, expression of matrix metalloproteinase-1 (MMP-1), and type I collagen synthesis in normal human fibroblast cells. Thus, ellagic acid may be useful for the geriatric population [137, 138].

According to the points mentioned above regarding the antioxidant activity of *T. chebula* and the important role of oxidative stress in the pathogenesis of AD, we can conclude that the use of this plant may be effective against the progression of AD.

3. Conclusion

Alzheimer's disease is a debilitating dementia, and only a limited number of therapeutic options are currently available to modify the manifestations of the disease. *T. chebula* has pharmacological activities relevant to dementia therapy (Figure 2). Different extracts from *T. chebula* have exhibited concentration-dependent inhibitory activities on AChE and BChE. Such AChE activities are also described for its active ingredients such as PGG, gallic acid, ellagic acid, and tannic acid. Anti-inflammatory properties of *T. chebula* have been well documented in different experimental systems that could be attributed to chebulagic or gallic acid. *T. chebula* with a

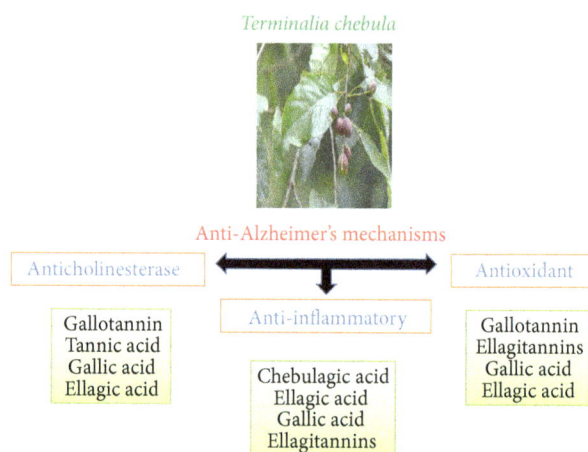

FIGURE 2: Anticholinesterase, anti-inflammatory, and antioxidant properties of *T. chebula* relevant to anti-Alzheimer's therapy.

high content of phenolic constituents exhibits strong antioxidant and neuroprotective properties in vitro and in vivo. The efficacy of *T. chebula* in treating AD should be compared with the current standard pharmacological treatment in animal and clinical testing and researches. Such studies should include the identification of the active principle(s) in order to improve the validation of the clinical trials. Until then, this review provides some evidences on the benefits of *T. chebula* in the treatment of Alzheimer's disease.

Conflict of Interests

The authors confirm that there is no conflict of interests.

References

[1] Y. Stern, "Cognitive reserve and Alzheimer disease," *Alzheimer Disease & Associated Disorders*, vol. 20, no. 2, pp. 112–117, 2006.

[2] H.-R. Adhami, H. Farsam, and L. Krenn, "Screening of medicinal plants from Iranian traditional medicine for acetylcholinesterase inhibition," *Phytotherapy Research*, vol. 25, no. 8, pp. 1148–1152, 2011.

[3] B. Vinutha, D. Prashanth, K. Salma et al., "Screening of selected Indian medicinal plants for acetylcholinesterase inhibitory activity," *Journal of Ethnopharmacology*, vol. 109, no. 2, pp. 359–363, 2007.

[4] K. Chopra, S. Misra, and A. Kuhad, "Current perspectives on pharmacotherapy of Alzheimer's disease," *Expert Opinion on Pharmacotherapy*, vol. 12, no. 3, pp. 335–350, 2011.

[5] S. López, J. Bastida, F. Viladomat, and C. Codina, "Acetylcholinesterase inhibitory activity of some Amaryllidaceae alkaloids and *Narcissus* extracts," *Life Sciences*, vol. 71, no. 21, pp. 2521–2529, 2002.

[6] G. L. Ellman, K. D. Courtney, V. Andres Jr., and R. M. Featherstone, "A new and rapid colorimetric determination of acetylcholinesterase activity," *Biochemical Pharmacology*, vol. 7, no. 2, pp. 88–95, 1961.

[7] I. K. Rhee, M. van de Meent, K. Ingkaninan, and R. Verpoorte, "Screening for acetylcholinesterase inhibitors from Amaryllidaceae using silica gel thin-layer chromatography in combination with bioactivity staining," *Journal of Chromatography A*, vol. 915, no. 1-2, pp. 217–223, 2001.

[8] P. Anand and B. Singh, "A review on cholinesterase inhibitors for Alzheimer's disease," *Archives of Pharmacal Research*, vol. 36, no. 4, pp. 375–399, 2013.

[9] M. M. Dirin, S. Mousavi, A. R. Afshari, K. Tabrizian, and M. H. Ashrafi, "Potential drug-drug interactions in prescriptions dispensed in community and hospital pharmacies in East of Iran," *Journal of Research in Pharmacy Practice*, vol. 3, no. 3, pp. 104–107, 2014.

[10] B. H. May, M. Lit, C. C. L. Xue et al., "Herbal medicine for dementia: a systematic review," *Phytotherapy Research*, vol. 23, no. 4, pp. 447–459, 2009.

[11] S. Akhondzadeh and S. H. Abbasi, "Herbal medicine in the treatment of Alzhelmer's disease," *American Journal of Alzheimer's Disease and other Dementias*, vol. 21, no. 2, pp. 113–118, 2006.

[12] L. L. D. Santos-Neto, M. A. de Vilhena Toledo, P. Medeiros-Souza, and G. A. de Souza, "The use of herbal medicine in Alzheimer's disease—a systematic review," *Evidence-Based Complementary and Alternative Medicine*, vol. 3, no. 4, pp. 441–445, 2006.

[13] A. Saleem, M. Husheem, P. Härkönen, and K. Pihlaja, "Inhibition of cancer cell growth by crude extract and the phenolics of *Terminalia chebula* retz. fruit," *Journal of Ethnopharmacology*, vol. 81, no. 3, pp. 327–336, 2002.

[14] S. K. Ali, A. R. Hamed, M. M. Soltan et al., "In-vitro evaluation of selected Egyptian traditional herbal medicines for treatment of Alzheimer disease," *BMC Complementary and Alternative Medicine*, vol. 13, no. 1, p. 121, 2013.

[15] R. Rathinamoorthy and G. Thilagavathi, "*Terminalia chebula*—review on pharmacological and biochemical studies," *International Journal of PharmTech Research*, vol. 6, no. 1, pp. 97–116, 2014.

[16] A. Manosroi, P. Jantrawut, E. Ogihara et al., "Biological activities of phenolic compounds and triterpenoids from the Galls of *Terminalia chebula*," *Chemistry & Biodiversity*, vol. 10, no. 8, pp. 1448–1463, 2013.

[17] N. K. Rao and S. Nammi, "Antidiabetic and renoprotective effects of the chloroform extract of *Terminalia* chebula Retz. seeds in streptozotocin-induced diabetic rats," *BMC Complementary and Alternative Medicine*, vol. 6, no. 1, article 17, 2006.

[18] K. Aneja and R. Joshi, "Evaluation of antimicrobial properties of fruit extracts of *Terminalia chebula* against dental caries pathogens," *Jundishapur Journal of Microbiology*, vol. 2, no. 3, pp. 105–111, 2009.

[19] B. Dutta, I. Rahman, and T. Das, "Antifungal activity of Indian plant extracts: antimyzetische Aktivität indischer Pflanzenextrakte," *Mycoses*, vol. 41, no. 11-12, pp. 535–536, 1998.

[20] V. Aher and A. Wahi, "Immunomodulatory activity of alcohol extract of *Terminalia chebula* retz combretaceae," *Tropical Journal of Pharmaceutical Research*, vol. 10, no. 5, pp. 567–575, 2011.

[21] M.-J. Ahn, C. Y. Kim, J. S. Lee et al., "Inhibition of HIV-1 integrase by galloyl glucoses from *Terminalia chebula* and flavonol glycoside gallates from *Euphorbia pekinensis*," *Planta Medica*, vol. 68, no. 5, pp. 457–459, 2002.

[22] V. Maruthappan and K. S. Shree, "Hypolipidemic activity of Haritaki (*Terminalia chebula*) in atherogenic diet induced hyperlipidemic rats," *Journal of Advanced Pharmaceutical Technology and Research*, vol. 1, no. 2, pp. 229–235, 2010.

[23] S. Srigopalram and I. A. Jayraaj, "Effect of *Terminalia chebula* retz on den induced hepatocellular carcinogenesis in experimental rats," *International Journal of Pharmacy and Pharmaceutical Sciences*, vol. 4, no. 2, pp. 440–445, 2012.

[24] P. Sharma, T. Prakash, D. Kotresha et al., "Antiulcerogenic activity of *Terminalia chebula* fruit in experimentally induced ulcer in rats," *Pharmaceutical Biology*, vol. 49, no. 3, pp. 262–268, 2011.

[25] M. P. Singh and C. S. Sharma, "Wound healing activity of *Terminalia chebula* in experimentally induced diabetic rats," *International Journal of PharmTech Research*, vol. 1, no. 4, pp. 1267–1270, 2009.

[26] C. Engels, M. Knödler, Y.-Y. Zhao, R. Carle, M. G. Gänzle, and A. Schieber, "Antimicrobial activity of gallotannins isolated from mango (*Mangifera indica* L.) kernels," *Journal of Agricultural and Food Chemistry*, vol. 57, no. 17, pp. 7712–7718, 2009.

[27] X. Zhao, H. Sun, A. Hou, Q. Zhao, T. Wei, and W. Xin, "Antioxidant properties of two gallotannins isolated from the leaves of *Pistacia weinmannifolia*," *Biochimica et Biophysica Acta (BBA)—General Subjects*, vol. 1725, no. 1, pp. 103–110, 2005.

[28] E. Sangiovanni, U. Vrhovsek, G. Rossoni et al., "Ellagitannins from Rubus berries for the control of gastric inflammation: in vitro and in vivo studies," *PLoS ONE*, vol. 8, no. 8, Article ID e71762, 2013.

[29] R. H. Hussein and F. K. Khalifa, "The protective role of ellagitannins flavonoids pretreatment against *N*-nitrosodiethylamine induced-hepatocellular carcinoma," *Saudi Journal of Biological Sciences*, vol. 21, no. 6, pp. 589–596, 2014.

[30] W. Lee, S. Y. Lee, Y. Son, and J. Yun, "Gallic acid decreases inflammatory cytokine secretion through histone acetyltransferase/histone deacetylase regulation in high glucose-induced human monocytes," *Journal of Medicinal Food*, vol. 18, no. 7, pp. 793–801, 2015.

[31] H. Walia and S. Arora, "*Terminalia chebula*—a pharmacognistic account," *Journal of Medicinal Plants Research*, vol. 7, no. 20, pp. 1351–1361, 2013.

[32] D. H. Priscilla and P. S. M. Prince, "Cardioprotective effect of gallic acid on cardiac troponin-T, cardiac marker enzymes, lipid peroxidation products and antioxidants in experimentally induced myocardial infarction in Wistar rats," *Chemico-Biological Interactions*, vol. 179, no. 2-3, pp. 118–124, 2009.

[33] L. D. Reynolds and N. G. Wilson, *Scribes and Scholars*, Cambridge University Press, Cambridge, UK, 1974.

[34] H.-H. Ho, C.-S. Chang, W.-C. Ho, S.-Y. Liao, C.-H. Wu, and C.-J. Wang, "Anti-metastasis effects of gallic acid on gastric cancer cells involves inhibition of NF-κB activity and downregulation of PI3K/AKT/small GTPase signals," *Food and Chemical Toxicology*, vol. 48, no. 8-9, pp. 2508–2516, 2010.

[35] M. A. Farag, D. A. Al-Mahdy, R. Salah El Dine et al., "Structure—activity relationships of antimicrobial gallic acid derivatives from pomegranate and acacia fruit extracts against potato bacterial wilt pathogen," *Chemistry & Biodiversity*, vol. 12, no. 6, pp. 955–962, 2015.

[36] A. Ibrahim, R. El Kareem, and M. Sheir, "Elucidation of acrylamide genotoxicity and neurotoxicity and the protective role of gallic acid and green tea," *Journal of Forensic Toxicology & Pharmacology*, vol. 4, no. 1, article 1, 2015.

[37] S.-I. Hamada, K. Kataoka, J.-T. Woo et al., "Immunosuppressive effects of gallic acid and chebulagic acid on CTL-mediated cytotoxicity," *Biological and Pharmaceutical Bulletin*, vol. 20, no. 9, pp. 1017–1019, 1997.

[38] A. Sarkaki, H. Fathimoghaddam, S. M. T. Mansouri, M. S. Korrani, G. Saki, and Y. Farbood, "Gallic acid improves cognitive, hippocampal long-term potentiation deficits and brain damage induced by chronic cerebral hypoperfusion in rats," *Pakistan Journal of Biological Sciences*, vol. 17, no. 8, pp. 978–990, 2014.

[39] O. S. Ajala, A. Jukov, and C.-M. Ma, "Hepatitis C virus inhibitory hydrolysable tannins from the fruits of *Terminalia chebula*," *Fitoterapia*, vol. 99, pp. 117–123, 2014.

[40] A. T. Pham, K. E. Malterud, B. S. Paulsen, D. Diallo, and H. Wangensteen, "α-Glucosidase inhibition, 15-lipoxygenase inhibition, and brine shrimp toxicity of extracts and isolated compounds from *Terminalia macroptera* leaves," *Pharmaceutical Biology*, vol. 52, no. 9, pp. 1166–1169, 2014.

[41] H.-S. Lee, S.-H. Jung, B.-S. Yun, and K.-W. Lee, "Isolation of chebulic acid from *Terminalia chebula* Retz. and its antioxidant effect in isolated rat hepatocytes," *Archives of Toxicology*, vol. 81, no. 3, pp. 211–218, 2007.

[42] Y. Yang, J. Xiu, J. Liu et al., "Chebulagic acid, a hydrolyzable tannin, exhibited antiviral activity in vitro and in vivo against human enterovirus 71," *International Journal of Molecular Sciences*, vol. 14, no. 5, pp. 9618–9627, 2013.

[43] R. Banerjee, G. Mukherjee, and K. C. Patra, "Microbial transformation of tannin-rich substrate to gallic acid through co-culture method," *Bioresource Technology*, vol. 96, no. 8, pp. 949–953, 2005.

[44] D. B. Reddy and P. Reddanna, "Chebulagic acid (CA) attenuates LPS-induced inflammation by suppressing NF-κB and MAPK activation in RAW 264.7 macrophages," *Biochemical and Biophysical Research Communications*, vol. 381, no. 1, pp. 112–117, 2009.

[45] Y.-N. Huang, D.-D. Zhao, B. Gao et al., "Anti-hyperglycemic effect of chebulagic acid from the fruits of *Terminalia chebula* Retz.," *International Journal of Molecular Sciences*, vol. 13, no. 5, pp. 6320–6333, 2012.

[46] H. J. Kim, J. Kim, K. S. Kang, K. T. Lee, and H. O. Yang, "Neuroprotective effect of chebulagic acid via autophagy induction in SH-SY5Y cells," *Biomolecules and Therapeutics*, vol. 22, no. 4, pp. 275–281, 2014.

[47] A. P. Athira, A. Helen, K. Saja, P. Reddanna, and P. R. Sudhakaran, "Inhibition of angiogenesis *in vitro* by chebulagic acid: a COX-LOX dual inhibitor," *International Journal of Vascular Medicine*, vol. 2013, Article ID 843897, 8 pages, 2013.

[48] N. Kumar, D. Gangappa, G. Gupta, and R. Karnati, "Chebulagic acid from *Terminalia chebula* causes G1 arrest, inhibits NFκB and induces apoptosis in retinoblastoma cells," *BMC Complementary and Alternative Medicine*, vol. 14, article 319, 2014.

[49] V. Mishra, M. Agrawal, S. A. Onasanwo et al., "Anti-secretory and cyto-protective effects of chebulinic acid isolated from the fruits of *Terminalia chebula* on gastric ulcers," *Phytomedicine*, vol. 20, no. 6, pp. 506–511, 2013.

[50] K. Lu, D. Chakraborty, C. Sarkar et al., "Triphala and its active constituent chebulinic acid are natural inhibitors of vascular endothelial growth factor-a mediated angiogenesis," *PLoS ONE*, vol. 7, no. 8, Article ID e43934, 2012.

[51] Z.-C. Yi, Z. Wang, H.-X. Li, M.-J. Liu, R.-C. Wu, and X.-H. Wang, "Effects of chebulinic acid on differentiation of human leukemia K562 cells," *Acta Pharmacologica Sinica*, vol. 25, no. 2, pp. 231–238, 2004.

[52] T. Tanaka, I. Kouno, and G.-I. Nonaka, "Glutathione-mediated conversion of the ellagitannin geraniin into chebulagic acid," *Chemical and Pharmaceutical Bulletin*, vol. 44, no. 1, pp. 34–40, 1996.

[53] M. Mansouri, A. Hemmati, B. Naghizadeh, S. Mard, A. Rezaie, and B. Ghorbanzadeh, "A study of the mechanisms underlying the anti-inflammatory effect of ellagic acid in carrageenan-induced paw edema in rats," *Indian Journal of Pharmacology*, vol. 47, no. 3, pp. 292–298, 2015.

[54] S. Goswami, M. Vishwanath, S. Gangadarappa, R. Razdan, and M. Inamdar, "Efficacy of ellagic acid and sildenafil in diabetes-induced sexual dysfunction," *Pharmacognosy Magazine*, vol. 10, supplement 3, pp. 581–587, 2014.

[55] W. R. García-Niño and C. Zazueta, "Ellagic acid: pharmacological activities and molecular mechanisms involved in liver protection," *Pharmacological Research*, vol. 97, pp. 84–103, 2015.

[56] M. Dianat, N. Amini, M. Badavi, and Y. Farbood, "Ellagic acid improved arrhythmias induced by CaCL2 in the rat stress model," *Avicenna Journal of Phytomedicine*, vol. 5, no. 2, pp. 120–127, 2015.

[57] M. Dolatshahi, Y. Farbood, A. Sarkaki, S. M. T. Mansouri, and A. Khodadadi, "Ellagic acid improves hyperalgesia and cognitive deficiency in 6-hydroxidopamine induced rat model of Parkinson's disease," *Iranian Journal of Basic Medical Sciences*, vol. 18, no. 1, pp. 38–46, 2015.

[58] Y. Farbood, A. Sarkaki, M. Dianat, A. Khodadadi, M. K. Haddad, and S. Mashhadizadeh, "Ellagic acid prevents cognitive and hippocampal long-term potentiation deficits and brain inflammation in rat with traumatic brain injury," *Life Sciences*, vol. 124, pp. 120–127, 2015.

[59] C. Wang, D. Zhang, H. Ma, and J. Liu, "Neuroprotective effects of emodin-8-O-β-d-glucoside in vivo and in vitro," *European Journal of Pharmacology*, vol. 577, no. 1–3, pp. 58–63, 2007.

[60] Y.-L. Xu, L.-Y. Tang, X.-D. Zhou, G.-H. Zhou, and Z.-J. Wang, "Five new anthraquinones from the seed of *Cassia obtusifolia*," *Archives of Pharmacal Research*, vol. 38, no. 6, pp. 1054–1058, 2015.

[61] P. C. Gupta, "Biological and pharmacological properties of *Terminalia chebula* retz. (haritaki)- an overview," *International Journal of Pharmacy and Pharmaceutical Sciences*, vol. 4, supplement 3, pp. 62–68, 2012.

[62] A. Bag, S. K. Bhattacharyya, and R. R. Chattopadhyay, "The development of *Terminalia chebula* Retz. (Combretaceae) in clinical research," *Asian Pacific Journal of Tropical Biomedicine*, vol. 3, no. 3, pp. 244–252, 2013.

[63] I. Mueller-Harvey, "Analysis of hydrolysable tannins," *Animal Feed Science and Technology*, vol. 91, no. 1-2, pp. 3–20, 2001.

[64] N. Lokeswari and K. J. Raju, "Optimization of gallic acid production from terminalia chebula by *Aspergillus niger*," *E-Journal of Chemistry*, vol. 4, no. 2, pp. 287–293, 2007.

[65] R. Niemetz and G. G. Gross, "Enzymology of gallotannin and ellagitannin biosynthesis," *Phytochemistry*, vol. 66, no. 17, pp. 2001–2011, 2005.

[66] T. Yoshida, Y. Amakura, and M. Yoshimura, "Structural features and biological properties of ellagitannins in some plant families of the order myrtales," *International Journal of Molecular Sciences*, vol. 11, no. 1, pp. 79–106, 2010.

[67] P.-S. Chen and J.-H. Li, "Chemopreventive effect of punicalagin, a novel tannin component isolated from *Terminalia catappa*, on H-ras-transformed NIH3T3 cells," *Toxicology Letters*, vol. 163, no. 1, pp. 44–53, 2006.

[68] Q. Han, J. Song, C. Qiao, L. Wong, and H. Xu, "Preparative isolation of hydrolysable tannins chebulagic acid and chebulinic acid from *Terminalia chebula* by high-speed counter-current chromatography," *Journal of Separation Science*, vol. 29, no. 11, pp. 1653–1657, 2006.

[69] H. K. Sharma, S. Soni, P. Kaushal, and C. Singh, "Effect of process parameters on the antioxidant activities of bioactive compounds from Harad (*Terminalia chebula* retz.) Shilpa Soni, H.K. Sharma, Pragati Kaushal and C. Singh Food Engineering &

Technology Department, Sant Longowal Institute of Engineeri," *Agricultural Engineering International: CIGR Journal*, vol. 17, no. 2, 2015.

[70] G. K. B. Lopes, H. M. Schulman, and M. Hermes-Lima, "Polyphenol tannic acid inhibits hydroxyl radical formation from Fenton reaction by complexing ferrous ions," *Biochimica et Biophysica Acta (BBA)—General Subjects*, vol. 1472, no. 1-2, pp. 142–152, 1999.

[71] S. Surveswaran, Y.-Z. Cai, H. Corke, and M. Sun, "Systematic evaluation of natural phenolic antioxidants from 133 Indian medicinal plants," *Food Chemistry*, vol. 102, no. 3, pp. 938–953, 2007.

[72] P. Onial, R. Dayal, M. Rawat, and R. Kumar, "Utilization of *Terminalia chebula* Retz. fruits pericarp as a source of natural dye for textile applications," *Indian Journal of Natural Products and Resources (IJNPR)*, vol. 6, no. 2, pp. 114–121, 2015.

[73] H. G. Kim, J. H. Cho, E. Y. Jeong, J. H. Lim, S. H. Lee, and H. S. Lee, "Growth-inhibiting activity of active component isolated from *Terminalia chebula* fruits against intestinal bacteria," *Journal of Food Protection*, vol. 69, no. 9, pp. 2205–2209, 2006.

[74] P. Onial, M. Rawat, and R. Dayal, "Chemical studies of fatty oil of *Terminalia chebula* seeds kernels," *Analytical Chemistry Letters*, vol. 4, no. 5-6, pp. 359–363, 2014.

[75] X. Zhang, C. Chen, S. He, and F. Ge, "Supercritical-CO_2 fluid extraction of the fatty oil in *Terminalia chebula* and GC-MS analysis," *Journal of Chinese Medicinal Materials*, vol. 20, no. 9, pp. 463–464, 1997.

[76] D. B. Reddy, T. C. M. Reddy, G. Jyotsna et al., "Chebulagic acid, a COX–LOX dual inhibitor isolated from the fruits of *Terminalia chebula* Retz., induces apoptosis in COLO-205 cell line," *Journal of Ethnopharmacology*, vol. 124, no. 3, pp. 506–512, 2009.

[77] P. Anand, B. Singh, and N. Singh, "A review on coumarins as acetylcholinesterase inhibitors for Alzheimer's disease," *Bioorganic and Medicinal Chemistry*, vol. 20, no. 3, pp. 1175–1180, 2012.

[78] M. Pohanka, "Alpha7 nicotinic acetylcholine receptor is a target in pharmacology and toxicology," *International Journal of Molecular Sciences*, vol. 13, no. 2, pp. 2219–2238, 2012.

[79] J. R. Suarez-Lopez, J. H. Himes, D. R. Jacobs Jr., B. H. Alexander, and M. R. Gunnar, "Acetylcholinesterase activity and neurodevelopment in boys and girls," *Pediatrics*, vol. 132, no. 6, pp. e1649–e1658, 2013.

[80] C. F. Bartels, T. Zelinski, and O. Lockridge, "Mutation at codon 322 in the human acetylcholinesterase (ACHE) gene accounts for YT blood group polymorphism," *The American Journal of Human Genetics*, vol. 52, no. 5, pp. 928–936, 1993.

[81] S. Greenfield and D. J. Vaux, "Parkinson's disease, Alzheimer's disease and motor neurone disease: identifying a common mechanism," *Neuroscience*, vol. 113, no. 3, pp. 485–492, 2002.

[82] T. Day and S. A. Greenfield, "A peptide derived from acetylcholinesterase induces neuronal cell death: characterisation of possible mechanisms," *Experimental Brain Research*, vol. 153, no. 3, pp. 334–342, 2003.

[83] P. T. Francis, A. Nordberg, and S. E. Arnold, "A preclinical view of cholinesterase inhibitors in neuroprotection: do they provide more than symptomatic benefits in Alzheimer's disease?" *Trends in Pharmacological Sciences*, vol. 26, no. 2, pp. 104–111, 2005.

[84] T. Darreh-Shori, E. Hellström-Lindahl, C. Flores-Flores, Z. Z. Guan, H. Soreq, and A. Nordberg, "Long-lasting acetylcholinesterase splice variations in anticholinesterase-treated Alzheimer's disease patients," *Journal of Neurochemistry*, vol. 88, no. 5, pp. 1102–1113, 2004.

[85] A. Borisovskaya, M. Pascualy, and S. Borson, "Cognitive and neuropsychiatric impairments in Alzheimer's disease: current treatment strategies," *Current Psychiatry Reports*, vol. 16, no. 9, pp. 1–9, 2014.

[86] M. H. Oh, P. J. Houghton, W. K. Whang, and J. H. Cho, "Screening of Korean herbal medicines used to improve cognitive function for anti-cholinesterase activity," *Phytomedicine*, vol. 11, no. 6, pp. 544–548, 2004.

[87] V. Schulz, "Ginkgo extract or cholinesterase inhibitors in patients with dementia: what clinical trials and guidelines fail to consider," *Phytomedicine*, vol. 10, no. 4, pp. 74–79, 2003.

[88] S. Sancheti, S. Sancheti, B.-H. Um, and S.-Y. Seo, "1,2,3,4,6-penta-O-galloyl-β-D-glucose: a cholinesterase inhibitor from *Terminalia chebula*," *South African Journal of Botany*, vol. 76, no. 2, pp. 285–288, 2010.

[89] G. Nag and B. De, "Acetylcholinesterase inhibitory activity of *Terminalia chebula*, *Terminalia bellerica* and *Emblica officinalis* and some phenolic compounds," *International Journal of Pharmacy and Pharmaceutical Sciences*, vol. 3, no. 3, pp. 121–124, 2011.

[90] A. P. Murray, M. B. Faraoni, M. J. Castro, N. P. Alza, and V. Cavallaro, "Natural AChE inhibitors from plants and their contribution to Alzheimer's disease therapy," *Current Neuropharmacology*, vol. 11, no. 4, pp. 388–413, 2013.

[91] C. Sulaiman, C. Sadashiva, S. George, and I. Balachandran, "Acetylcholinestrase inhibition and antioxidant activity of *Terminalia chebula*, Retz," *Journal of Tropical Medicinal Plants*, vol. 13, no. 2, pp. 125–127, 2012.

[92] A. Upadhyay and D. K. Singh, "Inhibition kinetics of certain enzymes in the nervous tissue of vector snail *Lymnaea acuminata* by active molluscicidal components of *Sapindus mukorossi* and *Terminalia chebula*," *Chemosphere*, vol. 85, no. 6, pp. 1095–1100, 2011.

[93] M. Parle and M. Vasudevan, "Memory enhancing activity of Abana: an indian ayurvedic poly-herbal formulation," *Journal of Health Science*, vol. 53, no. 1, pp. 43–52, 2007.

[94] H. Walia, J. Kaur, and S. Arora, "Antioxidant efficacy of fruit extracts of *Terminalia chebula* prepared by sequential method using TA-102 strain of *Salmonella typhimurium*," *Spatula DD*, vol. 2, no. 2, pp. 165–171, 2012.

[95] P. Dhivya, M. Sobiya, P. Selvamani, and S. Latha, "An approach to Alzheimer's disease treatment with cholinesterase inhibitory activity from various plant species," *International Journal of PharmTech Research*, vol. 6, no. 5, pp. 1450–1467, 2014.

[96] P. Pithayanukul, P. Ruenraroengsak, R. Bavovada, N. Pakmanee, and R. Suttisri, "In vitro. Investigation of the protective effects of tannic acid against the activities of *Naja kaouthia*. Venom," *Pharmaceutical Biology*, vol. 45, no. 2, pp. 94–97, 2007.

[97] M. Mathew and S. Subramanian, "In vitro screening for anti-cholinesterase and antioxidant activity of methanolic extracts of ayurvedic medicinal plants used for cognitive disorders," *PLoS ONE*, vol. 9, no. 1, Article ID e86804, 2014.

[98] T. Y. Shin, H. J. Jeong, D. K. Kim et al., "Inhibitory action of water soluble fraction of *Terminalia chebula* on systemic and local anaphylaxis," *Journal of Ethnopharmacology*, vol. 74, no. 2, pp. 133–140, 2001.

[99] K.-C. Choi, Y.-H. Lee, M. G. Jung et al., "Gallic acid suppresses lipopolysaccharide-induced nuclear factor-κB signaling by preventing RelA acetylation in A549 lung cancer cells," *Molecular Cancer Research*, vol. 7, no. 12, pp. 2011–2021, 2009.

[100] N. D. Das, K. H. Jung, J. H. Park et al., "*Terminalia chebula* extract acts as a potential NF-κB inhibitor in human lymphoblastic T cells," *Phytotherapy Research*, vol. 25, no. 6, pp. 927–934, 2011.

[101] M.-J. Kim, A.-R. Seong, J.-Y. Yoo et al., "Gallic acid, a histone acetyltransferase inhibitor, suppresses β-amyloid neurotoxicity by inhibiting microglial-mediated neuroinflammation," *Molecular Nutrition & Food Research*, vol. 55, no. 12, pp. 1798–1808, 2011.

[102] Y.-J. Wang, P. Thomas, J.-H. Zhong et al., "Consumption of grape seed extract prevents amyloid-β deposition and attenuates inflammation in brain of an alzheimer's disease mouse," *Neurotoxicity Research*, vol. 15, no. 1, pp. 3–14, 2009.

[103] S.-H. Kim, C.-D. Jun, K. Suk et al., "Gallic acid inhibits histamine release and pro-inflammatory cytokine production in mast cells," *Toxicological Sciences*, vol. 91, no. 1, pp. 123–131, 2006.

[104] V. Nair, S. Singh, and Y. K. Gupta, "Anti-arthritic and disease modifying activity of *Terminalia chebula* Retz. in experimental models," *Journal of Pharmacy and Pharmacology*, vol. 62, no. 12, pp. 1801–1806, 2010.

[105] T. Moeslinger, R. Friedl, I. Volf, M. Brunner, E. Koller, and P. G. Spieckermann, "Inhibition of inducible nitric oxide synthesis by the herbal preparation Padma 28 in macrophage cell line," *Canadian Journal of Physiology and Pharmacology*, vol. 78, no. 11, pp. 861–866, 2000.

[106] R. Patil, B. Nanjwade, and F. Manvi, "Evaluation of anti-inflammatory and antiarthritic effect of sesbania grandiflora bark and fruit of *Terminalia chebula* in rats," *International Journal of Pharmacology and Biological Sciences*, vol. 5, no. 1, pp. 37–46, 2011.

[107] A. Bag, S. Kumar Bhattacharyya, N. Kumar Pal, and R. R. Chattopadhyay, "Anti-inflammatory, anti-lipid peroxidative, antioxidant and membrane stabilizing activities of hydroalcoholic extract of *Terminalia chebula* fruits," *Pharmaceutical Biology*, vol. 51, no. 12, pp. 1515–1520, 2013.

[108] E. P. Sabina and M. Rasool, "An in vivo and in vitro potential of Indian ayurvedic herbal formulation Triphala on experimental gouty arthritis in mice," *Vascular Pharmacology*, vol. 48, no. 1, pp. 14–20, 2008.

[109] Y. R. Ramani and S. Pradhan, "Antiarthritic activity of acetone extract of *Terminalia chebula*," *WebmedCentral Pharmacology*, vol. 3, no. 2, Article ID WMC003057, pp. 1–9, 2012.

[110] P. Srivastava, H. N. Raut, R. S. Wagh, H. M. Puntambekar, and M. J. Kulkarni, "Purification and characterization of an antioxidant protein (~16 kDa) from *Terminalia chebula* fruit," *Food Chemistry*, vol. 131, no. 1, pp. 141–148, 2012.

[111] C. S. Atwood, M. E. Obrenovich, T. Liu et al., "Amyloid-β: a chameleon walking in two worlds: a review of the trophic and toxic properties of amyloid-β," *Brain Research Reviews*, vol. 43, no. 1, pp. 1–16, 2003.

[112] B. Uttara, A. V. Singh, P. Zamboni, and R. T. Mahajan, "Oxidative stress and neurodegenerative diseases: a review of upstream and downstream antioxidant therapeutic options," *Current Neuropharmacology*, vol. 7, no. 1, pp. 65–74, 2009.

[113] K. Hensley, N. Hall, R. Subramaniam et al., "Brain regional correspondence between Alzheimer's disease histopathology and biomarkers of protein oxidation," *Journal of Neurochemistry*, vol. 65, no. 5, pp. 2146–2156, 1995.

[114] K. Hensley, J. Carney, N. Hall, W. Shaw, and D. A. Butterfield, "Electron paramagnetic resonance investigations of free radical-induced alterations in neocortical synaptosomal membrane protein infrastructure," *Free Radical Biology and Medicine*, vol. 17, no. 4, pp. 321–331, 1994.

[115] R. X. Santos, S. C. Correia, X. Zhu et al., "Mitochondrial DNA oxidative damage and repair in aging and Alzheimer's disease," *Antioxidants & Redox Signaling*, vol. 18, no. 18, pp. 2444–2457, 2013.

[116] P. Mecocci, U. MacGarvey, and M. F. Beal, "Oxidative damage to mitochondrial DNA is increased in Alzheimer's disease," *Annals of Neurology*, vol. 36, no. 5, pp. 747–751, 1994.

[117] H.-T. Lee, C.-S. Lin, C.-S. Lee, C.-Y. Tsai, and Y.-H. Wei, "Increased 8-hydroxy-2′-deoxyguanosine in plasma and decreased mRNA expression of human 8-oxoguanine DNA glycosylase 1, anti-oxidant enzymes, mitochondrial biogenesis-related proteins and glycolytic enzymes in leucocytes in patients with systemic lupus erythematosus," *Clinical & Experimental Immunology*, vol. 176, no. 1, pp. 66–77, 2014.

[118] M. A. Lovell, W. D. Ehmann, S. M. Butler, and W. R. Markesbery, "Elevated thiobarbituric acid-reactive substances and antioxidant enzyme activity in the brain in Alzheimer's disease," *Neurology*, vol. 45, no. 8, pp. 1594–1601, 1995.

[119] K. V. Subbarao, J. S. Richardson, and L. C. Ang, "Autopsy samples of Alzheimer's cortex show increased peroxidation in vitro," *Journal of Neurochemistry*, vol. 55, no. 1, pp. 342–345, 1990.

[120] I. T. Lott, "Antioxidants in Down syndrome," *Biochimica et Biophysica Acta (BBA)—Molecular Basis of Disease*, vol. 1822, no. 5, pp. 657–663, 2012.

[121] L. Whiley, A. Sen, J. Heaton et al., "Evidence of altered phosphatidylcholine metabolism in Alzheimer's disease," *Neurobiology of Aging*, vol. 35, no. 2, pp. 271–278, 2014.

[122] R. J. Mark, M. A. Lovell, W. R. Markesbery, K. Uchida, and M. P. Mattson, "A role for 4-hydroxynonenal, an aldehydic product of lipid peroxidation, in disruption of ion homeostasis and neuronal death induced by amyloid β-peptide," *Journal of Neurochemistry*, vol. 68, no. 1, pp. 255–264, 1997.

[123] A. Klugman, D. P. Naughton, M. Isaac, I. Shah, A. Petroczi, and N. Tabet, "Antioxidant enzymatic activities in alzheimer's disease: the relationship to acetylcholinesterase inhibitors," *Journal of Alzheimer's Disease*, vol. 30, no. 3, pp. 467–474, 2012.

[124] L. Balazs and M. Leon, "Evidence of an oxidative challenge in the Alzheimer's brain," *Neurochemical Research*, vol. 19, no. 9, pp. 1131–1137, 1994.

[125] R. A. Omar, Y.-J. Chyan, A. C. Andorn, B. Poeggeler, N. K. Robakis, and M. A. Pappolla, "Increased expression but reduced activity of antioxidant enzymes in Alzheimer's disease," *Journal of Alzheimer's Disease*, vol. 1, no. 3, pp. 139–145, 1999.

[126] N. Sasaki, S. Toki, H. Chowei et al., "Immunohistochemical distribution of the receptor for advanced glycation end products in neurons and astrocytes in Alzheimer's disease," *Brain Research*, vol. 888, no. 2, pp. 256–262, 2001.

[127] N. Verma and M. Vinayak, "Effect of *Terminalia arjuna* on antioxidant defense system in cancer," *Molecular Biology Reports*, vol. 36, no. 1, pp. 159–164, 2009.

[128] A. Khan, H. Nazar, S. M. Sabir et al., "Antioxidant activity and inhibitory effect of some commonly used medicinal plants against lipid per-oxidation in mice brain," *African Journal of Traditional, Complementary and Alternative Medicines*, vol. 11, no. 5, pp. 83–90, 2014.

[129] M. K. Gautam, S. Goel, R. R. Ghatule, A. Singh, G. Nath, and R. K. Goel, "Curative effect of *Terminalia chebula* extract on acetic

acid-induced experimental colitis: role of antioxidants, free radicals and acute inflammatory marker," *Inflammopharmacology*, vol. 21, no. 5, pp. 377–383, 2013.

[130] C. L. Chang and C. S. Lin, "Phytochemical composition, antioxidant activity, and neuroprotective effect of *Terminalia chebula* Retzius extracts," *Evidence-Based Complementary and Alternative Medicine*, vol. 2012, Article ID 125247, 7 pages, 2012.

[131] J. H. Park, H. S. Joo, K.-Y. Yoo et al., "Extract from *Terminalia chebula* seeds protect against experimental ischemic neuronal damage via maintaining SODs and BDNF levels," *Neurochemical Research*, vol. 36, no. 11, pp. 2043–2050, 2011.

[132] M. Na, K. Bae, S. Sik Kang et al., "Cytoprotective effect on oxidative stress and inhibitory effect on cellular aging of *Terminalia chebula* fruit," *Phytotherapy Research*, vol. 18, no. 9, pp. 737–741, 2004.

[133] R. Mahesh, S. Bhuvana, and V. M. H. Begum, "Effect of *Terminalia chebula* aqueous extract on oxidative stress and antioxidant status in the liver and kidney of young and aged rats," *Cell Biochemistry and Function*, vol. 27, no. 6, pp. 358–363, 2009.

[134] H.-Y. Cheng, T.-C. Lin, K.-H. Yu, C.-M. Yang, and C.-C. Lin, "Antioxidant and free radical scavenging activities of *Terminalia chebula*," *Biological and Pharmaceutical Bulletin*, vol. 26, no. 9, pp. 1331–1335, 2003.

[135] R. Sarkar and N. Mandal, "Hydroalcoholic extracts of Indian medicinal plants can help in amelioration from oxidative stress through antioxidant properties," *Journal of Complementary and Integrative Medicine*, vol. 9, no. 1, pp. 1–9, 2012.

[136] A. Manosroi, P. Jantrawut, T. Akihisa, W. Manosroi, and J. Manosroi, "In vitro anti-aging activities of *Terminalia chebula* gall extract," *Pharmaceutical Biology*, vol. 48, no. 4, pp. 469–481, 2010.

[137] K. W. Lee, Y. J. Kim, D.-O. Kim, H. J. Lee, and C. Y. Lee, "Major phenolics in apple and their contribution to the total antioxidant capacity," *Journal of Agricultural and Food Chemistry*, vol. 51, no. 22, pp. 6516–6520, 2003.

[138] S. C. Mondal, P. Singh, B. Kumar, S. K. Singh, S. K. Gupta, and A. Verma, "Ageing and potential anti-aging phytochemicals: an overview," *World Journal of Pharmacy and Pharmaceutical Sciences*, vol. 4, no. 1, pp. 426–454, 2014.

16

Pharmacological Evaluation of Antidepressant-Like Effect of Genistein and Its Combination with Amitriptyline: An Acute and Chronic Study

Gaurav Gupta,[1,2] Tay Jia Jia,[1] Lim Yee Woon,[1] Dinesh Kumar Chellappan,[1] Mayuren Candasamy,[1] and Kamal Dua[3]

[1]*Department of Life Science, School of Pharmacy, International Medical University, Bukit Jalil, Kuala Lumpur 57000, Malaysia*
[2]*School of Medicine and Public Health, University of Newcastle, Newcastle, NSW 2308, Australia*
[3]*School of Biomedical Science, University of Newcastle, Newcastle, NSW 2308, Australia*

Correspondence should be addressed to Gaurav Gupta; gauravpharma25@gmail.com

Academic Editor: Berend Olivier

The present study was designed to evaluate the acute and chronic antidepressant effect of genistein in combination with amitriptyline in mice. Animals were divided into six groups ($n = 6$) for treatment with water, genistein, or amitriptyline, either alone or in combination for ten days. Animals were subjected to locomotor activity testing; tail suspension test (TST); and forced swim test (FST) and immobility time was recorded on day one and day ten. Acute treatment of all treatment groups did not significantly reduce the immobility time ($p > 0.05$). Chronic treatment of combination of genistein (10 mg/kg) and amitriptyline (5 mg/kg and 10 mg/kg) significantly reduced the immobility time as compared to control group ($p < 0.001$) and was comparable to amitriptyline alone (10 mg/kg). However, no changes in anti-immobility activity in combination of subeffective doses of genistein (5 mg/kg) and amitriptyline (5 mg/kg) were observed. Genistein at its standard dose (10 mg/kg) rendered synergistic effects in combination with subeffective dose of amitriptyline (5 mg/kg) and additive effects in combination with therapeutic dose of amitriptyline (10 mg/kg).

1. Introduction

Depression is the most common affective disorders (defined as disorders of mood rather than disturbances of thought or cognition); it may range from very mild conditions, bordering on normality, to severe (psychotic) depression accompanied by hallucinations and delusions. The emotional symptoms of depression described by Diagnostic and Statistical Manual of Mental Disorders are lack of interest, sadness, guiltiness, and suicidal thoughts while lack of sleep, headaches, pain, sleep disorders, changes in appetite, gastrointestinal disorders, and changes in psychomotor function are the physical symptoms of depression. Around 6.3 to 15.7% of the world's population is estimated to suffer depression once in life according to World Health Organization International Consortium of Psychiatric Epidemiology (WHO-ICPE). Additionally, 7 to 12% in men and 20 to 25% in woman are the estimation of lifetime prevalence of major depression in adults [1, 2].

Tricyclic antidepressant like amitriptyline is chemically heterocyclic compounds used effectively for treating depression since it acts as a serotonin-norepinephrine reuptake inhibitor, thereby increasing the concentration of these transmitters in the synapse. Since many side effects due to chronic administration limit the therapeutic treatment, so it is necessary to unveil new targeted drugs with the claim of a more favourable tolerability and efficacy profile [3].

Natural compounds including genistein, a soy isoflavone, have been suggested in treatment of depression. It is a potential molecule as legumes are part of traditional diets in many regions of the world. However, studies conducted in patients with depression are limited. A randomised controlled trial has demonstrated that depression scores decrease significantly after 1 and 2 years of genistein treatment in postmenopausal women [4]. Animal models are also useful to study the antidepressant-like activity. Treatment of genistein 10 mg/kg for 14 days in ovariectomised rats has been shown to reduce the immobility time, the marker of depression in forced swim test [5]. Beside that, consumption of dietary genistein renders a wide range of potential health benefits including alleviation of menopausal symptoms, chemoprevention of breast and prostate cancers, and cardioprotective effect [6, 7].

In the present study, we aimed to investigate the effect of genistein in combination with amitriptyline administered acutely and chronically on animal behaviour in tail suspension test (TST) and forced swim test (FST) and locomotor activity testing in mice. We hypothesised that genistein would potentiate the antidepressant effect of amitriptyline. Ultimately, the combined therapy allows lower dose of amitriptyline to be employed and hence reduces its magnitude of side effects and may be effective in cases of treatment-resistant depression.

2. Materials and Methods

2.1. Animals. Adult male albino mice (BALB/c strain) weighing 20–30 g were used in this study. They were housed in group of 6 at a controlled temperature ($25 \pm 1°C$) and humidity ($50 \pm 10\%$) with 12 h light/dark cycle (lights on at 7:00 am) with free access to standard pellet and water. Animals were used only once in each test. The experimental protocol was approved by the Laboratory Animal Care and Use Committee, International Medical University, Kuala Lumpur, Malaysia.

2.2. Drugs and Treatment. Amitriptyline (Sigma-Aldrich) and genistein (Sigma-Aldrich) were purchased from CHEMO-LAB Supplies (Malaysia). All drugs were dissolved in reverse osmosis (RO) water and administered 1 hour before test. All test solutions were freshly prepared and administered orally in a volume of 10 mL/kg body weight for 10 days. Animals were randomly divided into 6 groups ($n = 6$) as follows. The doses were selected based on those reported in the literature.

All the mice were administered orally one hour before the locomotor activity testing; TST and FST were carried out on day one and day ten as follows:

Group 1: [control]: RO water (0.5 mL),

Group 2: [standard]: amitriptyline 10 mg/kg,

Group 3: [standard]: genistein 10 mg/kg,

Group 4: [test]: genistein 5 mg/kg + amitriptyline 5 mg/kg,

Group 5: [test]: genistein 10 mg/kg + amitriptyline 5 mg/kg,

Group 6: [test]: genistein 10 mg/kg + amitriptyline 10 mg/kg.

2.3. Locomotor Activity Testing. The locomotor activity was measured on innate pretreated mice by an actophotometer. Actophotometer functioned on photoelectric cells that were attached in circuit with a counter. When the ray of light dropping on the photocell was cut off by the animal, a count

was noted. These cutoffs were calculated for a period of 10 min and the number was used as a degree of the locomotor activity of the animal [8].

2.4. Tail Suspension Test (TST). The TST was conducted according to the method of Steru et al. [9]. Mice both acoustically and visually isolated were suspended by their tail in the TST apparatus (50 height × 45 width × 12 cm depths) on the first day and tenth day of drug administration. The duration of immobility was recorded for test period of 5 minutes. Mice were considered immobile when they hung passively and completely motionless.

2.5. Forced Swim Test (FST). According to the FST method described by Porsolt et al., the mice were placed individually into 5 L glass beakers filled with 15 cm height of water. The water was changed frequently to eliminate fur, urine, and excrement after each test was done. When the mice remained floating in the water without struggling, making only minimum movements of its limbs necessary to keep its head above the water surface, they were considered to be immobile. This was classified as induced depression. The total duration of immobility was recorded during 5-minute test. The immobility period was calculated by subtracting total time (5 minutes) from time spent in escaping behaviour such as swimming and climbing. Swimming was defined as movements throughout the glass beaker and climbing was considered as upward-directed movements of forepaws by the side of glass beaker. Antidepressant drug treatment reduced the length of time the animals remain immobile and increased the escaping behaviour [10–12].

2.6. Statistical Analysis. All results were presented as mean ± SEM and $^{***}p < 0.001$, $^{**}p < 0.01$, and $^{*}p < 0.05$ were considered significant. Data were analyzed by one-way ANOVA, followed by Dunnett's post hoc test using Graph Pad Prism version 5.0.

3. Results

Body weight was evaluated before and after 10 days of treatment and weight gain is shown in Figure 1. Although weight loss was observed in the combination of genistein (10 mg/kg) and amitriptyline (10 mg/kg), there was no significant differences in body weight gain among all the treatment groups ($p > 0.05$).

In locomotor activity, as per Table 1, amitriptyline (10 mg/kg) shows a nonsignificant increase, whereas genistein significantly increases a locomotor activity alone and in combination with different doses of amitriptyline, respectively ($p < 0.05$; $p < 0.01$; and $p < 0.001$).

In TST, as shown in Figure 2, all treatment groups did not alter the total immobility time as compared to control group on the first day of experiment.

The behavioural effects after 10-day treatment are shown in Figure 3. On 10th day, individual treatments of amitriptyline (10 mg/kg) and genistein (10 mg/kg) produced significant decrease in immobility time as compared to control group ($p < 0.05$). The decrease in immobility time of genistein

TABLE 1: Effects of the standard drugs and their combined treatments on locomotor activity.

Treatment (dose, mg/kg, p.o.)	Activity counts (s)
Normal control	165.36 ± 9.05
Amitriptyline 10 mg/kg	67.03 ± 5.38
Genistein 10 mg/kg	226.4 ± 12.35[c]
Genistein 5 mg/kg + amitriptyline 5 mg/kg	153.7 ± 13.27[b]
Genistein 10 mg/kg + amitriptyline 5 mg/kg	189.3 ± 10.14[c]
Genistein 10 mg/kg + amitriptyline 10 mg/kg	102.35 ± 14.12[a]

Values are expressed in mean ± SEM, where $n = 6$.
[a] $p < 0.05$, compared with normal control group.
[b] $p < 0.01$, compared with normal control group.
[c] $p < 0.001$, compared with normal control group.

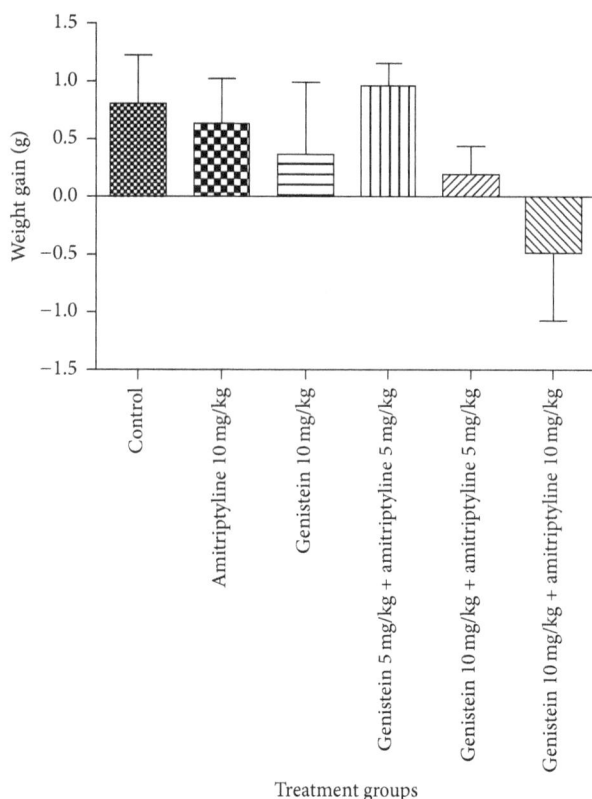

FIGURE 1: Effects of the standard drugs and their combined treatments on body weight gain in mice after 10 days. Values represent the mean ± SEM ($n = 6$). Data were analyzed with one-way ANOVA followed by Dunnett's post hoc test.

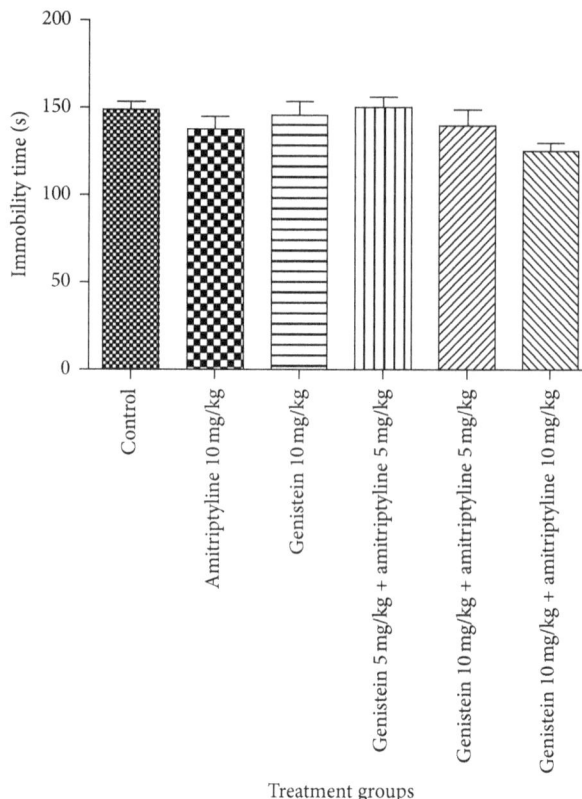

FIGURE 2: Effects of the standard drugs and their combined treatments on immobility time on 1st day. Values represent the mean ± SEM ($n = 6$). Data were analyzed with one-way ANOVA followed by Dunnett's post hoc test.

was comparable to amitriptyline. Coadministration of genistein (10 mg/kg) with amitriptyline (5 mg/kg and 10 mg/kg) significantly decreased the immobility time as compared to control group ($p < 0.001$) and were comparable to standard amitriptyline (10 mg/kg) and genistein (10 mg/kg) alone. However, the combination of genistein and amitriptyline at subeffective doses (5 mg/kg) did not significantly reduce the immobility time as compared to control group ($p > 0.05$).

In FST, on day one, mean immobility period was reduced in animals treated with amitriptyline 10 mg/kg alone, genistein 10 mg/kg alone, and combined use of genistein 5 mg/kg with amitriptyline 5 mg/kg and genistein 10 mg/kg with amitriptyline 5 mg/kg and genistein 10 mg/kg with amitriptyline 10 mg/kg compared to control group but there was no statistically significant difference in duration of immobility in all groups of animals compared to animals in control group on first day, Figure 4. After ten days of administration, decrease in mean duration of immobility in all groups of animals was found to be statistically significant comparable to that of control groups, Figure 5. Genistein with dose of 10 mg/kg and amitriptyline with dose of 5 mg/kg in combination group showed most significant decrease in immobility period in FST as compared to control group on day ten ($p < 0.001$).

4. Discussion

Acute treatment of amitriptyline does not produce antidepressant effect similar to previous findings [13]. This may be due to delayed onset of action of antidepressant drugs observed in clinical settings. However, some studies have demonstrated that amitriptyline reduces the immobility time in rodents on the first day of behavioural test [14, 15]. Nonetheless, amitriptyline administered chronically exerts antidepressant activity. It is widely accepted that monoamines

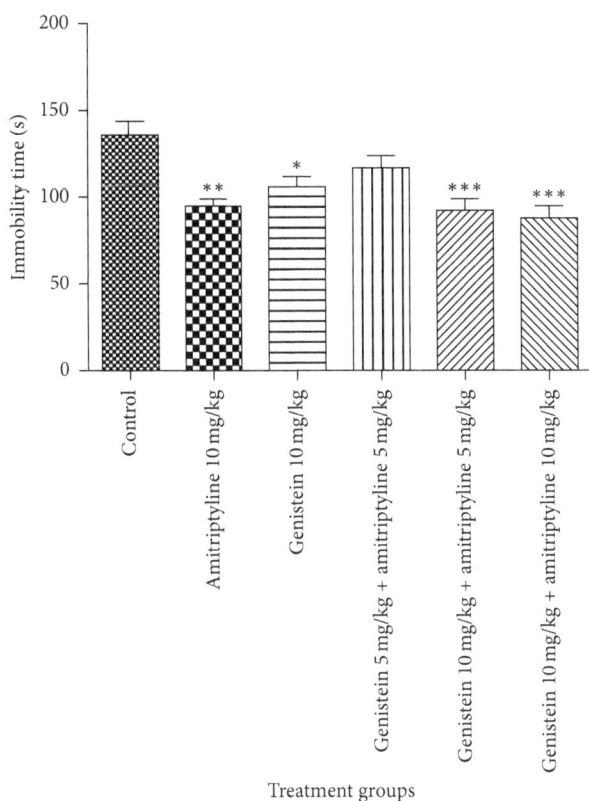

FIGURE 3: Effects of the standard drugs and their combined treatments on immobility time on 10th day. Values represent the mean $\pm$ SEM (n = 6). $^{***}p < 0.001$, $^{**}p < 0.01$, and $^*p < 0.05$ were considered significant as compared to control group. Data were analyzed with one-way ANOVA followed by Dunnett's post hoc test.

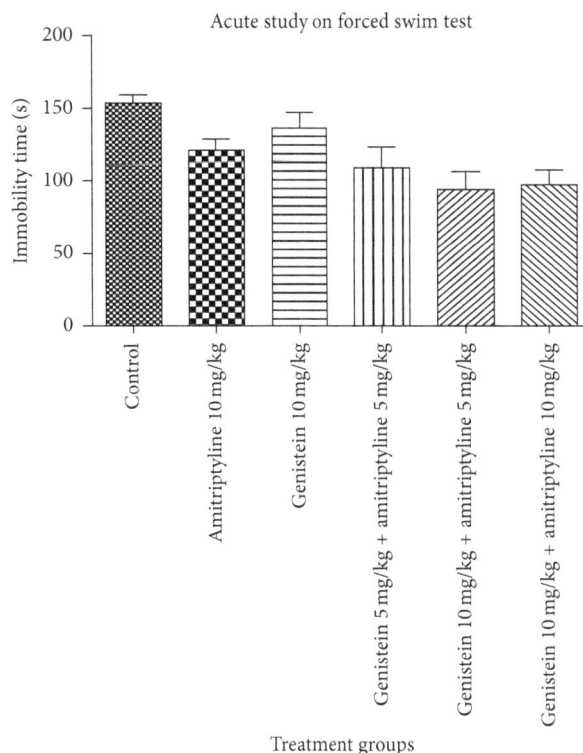

FIGURE 4: Immobility time (sec) in mice in forced swim test. Values represent the mean $\pm$ SEM (n = 6). All groups were compared with vehicle control (one-way ANOVA followed by Dunnett's test).

reuptake inhibition is crucial for its action. By blocking the serotonin and noradrenaline transporters, amitriptyline increases the neurotransmitters in the synapse and hence enhances neurotransmission [16]. Recent studies have reported that it activates fibroblast growth factor receptor signalling in glial cells which contribute to its antidepressant action [17]. Several mechanisms involved in the mediation of the antidepressant action after repeated treatment have been proposed. It is suggested that chronic treatment may enhance dopamine transmission in nucleus accumbens and also produce peptide of luteinizing hormone releasing hormone that modulates affective disorder [18–20].

Consistent with previous findings [5, 21], acute treatment of genistein does not exert antidepressant-like activity but repeated treatment shows antidepressant effect which is comparable to amitriptyline. Genistein has poor oral bioavailability. It is rapidly eliminated from plasma and excreted in the urine within 24 hours after single dose [6, 22, 23]. Hence, daily administration of genistein might increase plasma concentration of genistein but should not expect a dramatic increase in plasma level after 2-3 doses of treatment. A six-month randomised controlled trial has shown that plasma levels of genistein increase in first and sixth month with daily soy isoflavone administration [24].

Chronic genistein (10 mg/kg) in combination with therapeutic doses of amitriptyline (10 mg/kg) has significant antidepressant activity as compared to control group and is comparable to individual treatments. This suggests an additive effect at antidepressant dose of amitriptyline. On the other hand, genistein (10 mg/kg) in combination with subeffective doses of amitriptyline (5 mg/kg) administered chronically exerts antidepressant effect which is comparable to individual treatments, suggesting synergistic effect at subeffective dose of amitriptyline. Nevertheless, subeffective dose of genistein (5 mg/kg) fails to augment antidepressant effect of amitriptyline.

One of the side effects of tricyclic antidepressants is weight gain. In this study, we failed to demonstrate body weight gain in mice treated with amitriptyline. Studies in rats have revealed that there is no linkage between weight gain and amitriptyline treatment [25, 26]. From here, we cannot model the body weight changes of combination therapy in clinical setting. Additionally, genistein in agreement with previous report does not increase body weight in rats [5].

Genistein presents mainly in leguminous plants where 1 gram of soy protein contains $250\,\mu g$ of genistein [7]. Moreover, 10 mg/kg body weight of genistein for rats corresponds with 600 mg for a human [27]. The underlying mechanism of genistein in depression remains unclear. Genistein shares structural features with oestrogen-oestradiol-17β [7]. It can penetrate the blood-brain barrier after administration and bind differentially to α or β oestrogen receptors (OR) in

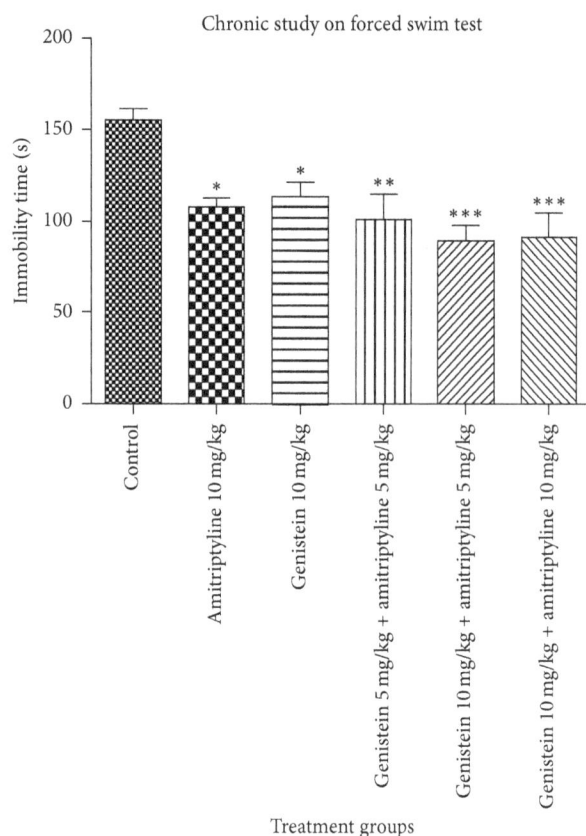

FIGURE 5: Immobility time (sec) in mice in forced swim test. Values represent the mean ± SEM ($n = 6$). $^{*}p < 0.05$, $^{**}p < 0.01$, and $^{***}p < 0.001$ were considered significant; all groups were compared with vehicle control (one-way ANOVA followed by Dunnett's test).

To our knowledge, the current study first time demonstrates the additive and synergistic effect of genistein in combination with antidepressant drug. Genistein (10 mg/kg) can be an adjunctive treatment with amitriptyline (10 mg/kg) for patients resistant to the conventional treatments. Additionally, genistein (10 mg/kg) in combination with subeffective dose of amitriptyline (5 mg/kg) may reduce the dose and thus the side effects of antidepressant drugs. This is important in cases of childhood depression or postnatal depression where safety of medication is being questioned.

Our results constitute further studies concerning the locomotor activity. Although previous studies have demonstrated that amitriptyline and genistein do not affect locomotor activity in rodents, locomotor activity shall be assessed to distinguish antidepressants from psychostimulants to prevent false positive results [34]. Further investigations, for instance, measurement of corticosterone, pharmacokinetic studies, and toxicology assessments, are recommended for better understanding of the observed phenomenon.

5. Conclusions

In summary, the present study supports the hypothesis that genistein enhanced the antidepressant effect of amitriptyline in tail suspension test. These findings might be important in the development of new treatment strategies and in the medical practice. The synergistic effect could mean a higher response for those with treatment-resistant depression and reduces the magnitude of side effects with low dose of antidepressant drugs.

Conflict of Interests

The authors declare no competing interests.

References

[1] American Psychiatric Association, *Diagnostic and Statistical Manual of Mental Disorders, (DSM-IV-R)*, American Psychiatric Association, Washington, DC, USA, 4th edition, 1994.

[2] Z. Rihmer and J. Angst, "Mood disorders: epidemiology," in *Kaplan & Sadock's Comprehensive Textbook of Psychiatric*, B. J. Sadock and V. A. Sadocl, Eds., pp. 1576–1582, Lippincott Williams & Wilkins, Philadelphia, Pa, USA, 8th edition, 2005.

[3] M. J. Owens, W. N. Morgan, S. J. Plott, and C. B. Nemeroff, "Neurotransmitter receptor and transporter binding profile of antidepressants and their metabolites," *Journal of Pharmacology and Experimental Therapeutics*, vol. 283, no. 3, pp. 1305–1322, 1997.

[4] M. Atteritano, S. Mazzaferro, A. Bitto et al., "Genistein effects on quality of life and depression symptoms in osteopenic postmenopausal women: a 2-year randomized, double-blind, controlled study," *Osteoporosis International*, vol. 25, no. 3, pp. 1123–1129, 2014.

[5] A. Kageyama, H. Sakakibara, W. Zhou et al., "Genistein regulated serotonergic activity in the hippocampus of ovariectomized rats under forced swimming stress," *Bioscience, Biotechnology, and Biochemistry*, vol. 74, no. 10, pp. 2005–2010, 2010.

the hippocampus [28]. Studies have concluded that antidepressant effect may involve OR β rather than OR α [29]. Furthermore, genistein may regulate serotonergic pathway under stressful conditions. In their study, genistein decreased serotonin turnover ratio (5-HIAA/5-HT), indicating serotonin level increased in hippocampus. Monoamine-oxidase A (MAO-A) is a mitochondrial enzyme involved in metabolism of monoamines such as dopamine and serotonin. MAO-A inhibitors are effective in treatment of depression. Hence genistein may regulate activity of MAO-A in brain [30]. Oxidative stresses are correlated with the pathophysiology of depression [31]. Therefore it suggests that antioxidant property of genistein may contribute to its antidepressant-like activity.

Importantly, genistein in moderation is well tolerated [32, 33]. Larger doses of genistein have been demonstrated to increase apoptosis and may be contraindicated in cancer regimens. In clinical trials, gastrointestinal adverse effects are the most common reason for treatment discontinuation. In addition, there is no change in endometrial thickness and breast density with daily administration of 54 mg of genistein for 3 years in postmenopausal women [32].

[6] V. Kalaiselvan, M. Kalaivani, A. Vijayakumar, K. Sureshkumar, and K. Venkateskumar, "Current knowledge and future direction of research on soy isoflavones as a therapeutic agents," *Pharmacognosy Reviews*, vol. 4, no. 8, pp. 111–117, 2010.

[7] R. A. Dixon and D. Ferreira, "Genistein," *Phytochemistry*, vol. 60, no. 3, pp. 205–211, 2002.

[8] S. K. Kulkarni, *Handbook of Experimental Pharmacology*, Vallabh Prakashan, New Delhi, India, 3rd edition, 2005.

[9] L. Steru, R. Chermat, B. Thierry, and P. Simon, "The tail suspension test: a new method for screening antidepressants in mice," *Psychopharmacology*, vol. 85, no. 3, pp. 367–370, 1985.

[10] R. D. Porsolt, A. Bertin, and M. Jalfre, "Behavioral despair in mice: a primary screening test for antidepressants," *Archives Internationales de Pharmacodynamie et de Therapie*, vol. 229, no. 2, pp. 327–336, 1977.

[11] M. J. Detke, M. Rickels, and I. Lucki, "Active behaviors in the rat forced swimming test differentially produced by serotonergic and noradrenergic antidepressants," *Psychopharmacology*, vol. 121, no. 1, pp. 66–72, 1995.

[12] F. Borsini and A. Meli, "Is the forced swimming test a suitable model for revealing antidepressant activity?" *Psychopharmacology*, vol. 94, no. 2, pp. 147–160, 1988.

[13] J. F. Cryan, C. Mombereau, and A. Vassout, "The tail suspension test as a model for assessing antidepressant activity: review of pharmacological and genetic studies in mice," *Neuroscience and Biobehavioral Reviews*, vol. 29, no. 4-5, pp. 571–625, 2005.

[14] A. Enríquez-Castillo, J. Alamilla, J. Barral et al., "Differential effects of caffeine on the antidepressant-like effect of amitriptyline in female rat subpopulations with low and high immobility in the forced swimming test," *Physiology and Behavior*, vol. 94, no. 3, pp. 501–509, 2008.

[15] S. Aithal, T. V. Hooli, R. Patil, H. V. Varun, and E. S. Swetha, "Evaluation of antidepressant activity of topiramate in mice," *Asian Journal of Pharmaceutical and Clinical Research*, vol. 7, no. 1, pp. 174–176, 2014.

[16] C. Leucht, M. Huhn, and S. Leucht, "Amitriptyline versus placebo for major depressive disorder," *Cochrane Database of Systematic Reviews*, vol. 12, Article ID CD009138, 2012.

[17] K. Hisaoka, M. Tsuchioka, R. Yano et al., "Tricyclic antidepressant amitriptyline activates fibroblast growth factor receptor signaling in glial cells: involvement in glial cell line-derived neurotrophic factor production," *The Journal of Biological Chemistry*, vol. 286, no. 24, pp. 21118–21128, 2011.

[18] F. Borsini, E. Nowakowska, L. Pulvirenti, and R. Samanin, "Repeated treatment with amitriptyline reduces immobility in the behavioural 'despair' test in rats by activating dopaminergic and β-adrenergic mechanisms," *Journal of Pharmacy and Pharmacology*, vol. 37, no. 2, pp. 137–138, 1985.

[19] L. Cervo and R. Samanin, "Repeated treatment with imipramine and amitriptyline reduced the immobility of rats in the swimming test by enhancing dopamine mechanisms in the nucleus accumbens," *Journal of Pharmacy and Pharmacology*, vol. 40, no. 2, pp. 155–156, 1988.

[20] M. R. Jain and N. K. Subhedar, "Increase in number of LHRH neurones in septal-preoptic area of rats following chronic amitriptyline treatment: implication in antidepressant effect," *Brain Research*, vol. 604, no. 1-2, pp. 7–15, 1993.

[21] N. S. Sapronov and S. B. Kasakova, "Effects of synthetic and plant-derived selective modulators of estrogen receptors on depression-like behavior of female rats," *Bulletin of Experimental Biology and Medicine*, vol. 146, no. 1, pp. 73–76, 2008.

[22] S. H. Kwon, M. J. Kang, J. S. Huh et al., "Comparison of oral bioavailability of genistein and genistin in rats," *International Journal of Pharmaceutics*, vol. 337, no. 1-2, pp. 148–154, 2007.

[23] M. G. Busby, A. R. Jeffcoat, L. T. Bloedon et al., "Clinical characteristics and pharmacokinetics of purified soy isoflavones: single-dose administration to healthy men," *American Journal of Clinical Nutrition*, vol. 75, no. 1, pp. 126–136, 2002.

[24] C. E. Gleason, C. M. Carlsson, J. H. Barnet et al., "A preliminary study of the safety, feasibility and cognitive efficacy of soy isoflavone supplements in older men and women," *Age and Ageing*, vol. 38, no. 1, pp. 86–93, 2009.

[25] J. Nobrega and D. V. Coscina, "Effects of chronic amitriptyline and desipramine on food intake and body weight in rats," *Pharmacology Biochemistry and Behavior*, vol. 27, no. 1, pp. 105–112, 1987.

[26] S. Ranjbar, N. B. Pai, and C. Deng, "The association of antidepressant medication and body weight gain," *Online Journal of Health and Allied Sciences*, vol. 12, no. 1, pp. 1–9, 2013.

[27] H. Sakakibara, Y. Honda, S. Nakagawa, H. Ashida, and K. Kanazawa, "Simultaneous determination of all polyphenols in vegetables, fruits, and teas," *Journal of Agricultural and Food Chemistry*, vol. 51, no. 3, pp. 571–581, 2003.

[28] T.-H. Tsai, "Concurrent measurement of unbound genistein in the blood, brain and bile of anesthetized rats using microdialysis and its pharmacokinetic application," *Journal of Chromatography A*, vol. 1073, no. 1-2, pp. 317–322, 2005.

[29] A. A. Walf and C. A. Frye, "Rapid and estrogen receptor beta mediated actions in the hippocampus mediate some functional effects of estrogen," *Steroids*, vol. 73, no. 9-10, pp. 997–1007, 2008.

[30] T. Hatano, T. Fukuda, T. Miyase, T. Noro, and T. Okuda, "Phenolic constituents of licorice. III. Structures of glicoricone and licofuranone, and inhibitory effects of licorice constituents of monoamine oxidase," *Chemical and Pharmaceutical Bulletin*, vol. 39, no. 5, pp. 1238–1243, 1991.

[31] H. Herken, A. Gurel, S. Selek et al., "Adenosine deaminase, nitric oxide, superoxide dismutase, and xanthine oxidase in patients with major depression: impact of antidepressant treatment," *Archives of Medical Research*, vol. 38, no. 2, pp. 247–252, 2007.

[32] H. Marini, A. Bitto, D. Altavilla et al., "Breast safety and efficacy of genistein aglycone for postmenopausal bone loss: a follow-up study," *Journal of Clinical Endocrinology and Metabolism*, vol. 93, no. 12, pp. 4787–4796, 2008.

[33] M. Evans, J. G. Elliott, P. Sharma, R. Berman, and N. Guthrie, "The effect of synthetic genistein on menopause symptom management in healthy postmenopausal women: a multi-center, randomized, placebo-controlled study," *Maturitas*, vol. 68, no. 2, pp. 189–196, 2011.

[34] K. Socała, D. Nieoczym, E. Wyska, E. Poleszak, and P. Wlaź, "Sildenafil, a phosphodiesterase type 5 inhibitor, enhances the antidepressant activity of amitriptyline but not desipramine, in the forced swim test in mice," *Journal of Neural Transmission*, vol. 119, no. 6, pp. 645–652, 2012.

17

Targeting AGEs Signaling Ameliorates Central Nervous System Diabetic Complications in Rats

Mohamed Naguib Zakaria,[1] Hany M. El-Bassossy,[1,2] and Waleed Barakat[1,3]

[1]*Department of Pharmacology and Toxicology, Faculty of Pharmacy, Zagazig University, Zagazig 44519, Egypt*
[2]*Department of Pharmacology, Faculty of Pharmacy, King Abdulaziz University, Jeddah 80200, Saudi Arabia*
[3]*Department of Pharmacology, Faculty of Pharmacy, University of Tabuk, Tabuk 71491, Saudi Arabia*

Correspondence should be addressed to Waleed Barakat; waled055@yahoo.com

Academic Editor: Berend Olivier

Diabetes is a chronic endocrine disorder associated with several complications as hypertension, advanced brain aging, and cognitive decline. Accumulation of advanced glycation end products (AGEs) is an important mechanism that mediates diabetic complications. Upon binding to their receptor (RAGE), AGEs mediate oxidative stress and/or cause cross-linking with proteins in blood vessels and brain tissues. The current investigation was designed to investigate the effect of agents that decrease AGEs signaling, perindopril which increases soluble RAGE (sRAGE) and alagebrium which cleaves AGEs cross-links, compared to the standard antidiabetic drug, gliclazide, on the vascular and *central nervous system* (CNS) complications in STZ-induced (50 mg/kg, IP) diabetes in rats. Perindopril ameliorated the elevation in blood pressure seen in diabetic animals. In addition, both perindopril and alagebrium significantly inhibited memory decline (performance in the Y-maze), neuronal degeneration (Fluoro-Jade staining), AGEs accumulation in serum and brain, and brain oxidative stress (level of reduced glutathione and activities of catalase and malondialdehyde). These results suggest that blockade of AGEs signaling after diabetes induction in rats is effective in reducing diabetic CNS complications.

1. Introduction

Diabetes mellitus is an endocrine disorder resulting from inadequate insulin release or insulin insensitivity [1]. The prevalence of diabetes worldwide was estimated to be 2.8% in 2000 and 4.4% in 2030 [2]. The prevalence of diabetes in Egypt was 3.9% in 2000 and is expected to rise to 6.8% by the year 2030 which would make Egypt one of the highest 10 countries with diabetes in 2030 [2].

Diabetes often results in microvascular and macrovascular complications such as retinopathy, peripheral neuropathy, stroke, and coronary heart disease [1]. Hypertension is very frequently associated with diabetic subjects, irrespective of whether they are type 1 or type 2 [3]. Diabetes induces advanced brain aging and may ultimately result in deficits in cognitive performance [4] and increased risk of developing clinical manifestations of Alzheimer's disease [5].

Although several drugs are available to control elevated blood glucose level in diabetic patients, many diabetic patients still suffer from diabetic complications and so new treatment strategies are required to manipulate these chronic widely spreading complications.

Poor glycemic control increases the accumulation of advanced glycation end products (AGEs) [6] and oxidative stress, which may lead to cellular and molecular damage [7] that contributes to diabetes-induced brain aging [8]. AGEs have been associated with increased oxidative stress [9] and inhibition of reactive oxygen species (ROS) was shown to interfere with the formation of AGEs [10]. AGEs activate the receptor for advanced glycation end products (RAGE) [11] which is implicated in the pathogenesis and progression of chronic diseases such as diabetes and immune/inflammatory disorders [12]. In addition, RAGE expression was increased in human diabetic kidney [13].

The AGE/RAGE interaction promotes reactive oxygen species (ROS) production [14] and activates protein kinase C (PKC) and nuclear factor-kappa B (NF-κB) [15]. In addition, ROS themselves may fuel further generation of AGEs [16]. Soluble RAGE (sRAGE) is the extracellular ligand-binding domain of RAGE that binds ligands and blocks their interaction with, and activation of, cell surface receptors [11]. Chronic administration of sRAGE protects against macro- and microvascular complications in the great vessels, heart, kidney, retina, and peripheral nerve [12].

Among other actions of AGEs are effects on extracellular matrix proteins and basement membrane components and formation of protein cross-links which can cause or facilitate vascular complications [17, 18]. The AGE cross-link breaker alagebrium (ALT-711) has been shown to cleave preformed AGE cross-links and reduce tissue levels of AGEs [19] resulting in improved total arterial compliance in aged humans with vascular stiffening [18].

Previous studies have demonstrated a relationship between the renin-angiotensin system (RAS) and the accumulation of AGEs in experimental diabetes [20]. ACE inhibition was shown to reduce the accumulation of serum AGEs in diabetes, possibly via effects on oxidative pathways [20] and by increasing the production and secretion of sRAGE into plasma as shown with perindopril which caused an increase in plasma sRAGE in patients [21].

The present study was designed to investigate the possible effect of agents that decrease AGEs signaling (perindopril which increases sRAGE level or alagebrium which cleaves AGEs-induced protein cross-links) on the impact of diabetes on blood pressure and CNS functions in STZ diabetic rats.

2. Material and Methods

2.1. Animals. Adult male Wistar rats weighing 170 ± 20 g were obtained from the National Research Institute (Cairo, Egypt). All experimental procedures were approved by the Ethical Committee for Animal Handling at Zagazig University (ECAHZU).

2.2. Drugs and Chemicals. STZ was purchased from Sigma-Aldrich (Germany), and perindopril (Coversyl tablets) and gliclazide (Diamicron tablets) were purchased from Servier Egypt Industries, while alagebrium was purchased from Chemos (Germany).

2.3. Study Protocol. Diabetes was induced by streptozotocin (STZ, 50 mg/kg, IP) [22] and rats with stable hyperglycemia (300–400 mg/dL) after 8 weeks of STZ injection were randomly distributed among four groups ($n = 6$) and received alagebrium (10 mg/kg) [23, 24], perindopril (4 mg/kg) [25, 26], or gliclazide (10 mg/kg) [27] daily as oral suspension in 0.5% carboxymethyl cellulose (CMC) for another 6 weeks. In addition, 6 nondiabetic rats received similar volume of CMC daily for the same duration and served as control. Eight weeks after diabetes induction was previously shown to be necessary for development of significant vascular complications as shown in our previous studies [28].

2.4. Behavior Changes. Behavior changes were assessed in Y-maze as a score: 0, no entrance to target arm; 1, entrance to target arm only and staying in it; 2, entrance to nontarget arm first and then target arm; 3, entrance to target arm first and passing three arms in more than four minutes; 4, entrance to target arm first and passing three arms within four minutes; 5, entrance to target arm first and passing three arms in less than one minute [29, 30].

2.5. Blood Glucose and Blood Pressure Measurement. Twelve hours after the last injection, body weight and blood glucose were measured (Glucometer Bionime GM100 Blood Glucose Meter) and blood pressure was recorded (Power Lab 26T, LTS) in a conscious and slightly restrained rat by tail cuff method as previously described [31].

2.6. Blood and Tissue Sampling. Blood was collected from the retroorbital plexus under topical ophthalmic anesthetic, centrifuged at 3000 ×g, 4°C for 20 min (Hermle Z326K), and serum was stored at −20°C for later determination of serum AGEs level.

Animals were sacrificed and brain was carefully isolated and frozen at −80°C and 20 μm sections were prepared using cryostat (Slee, Mainz, Germany) and used for the detection of neuronal degeneration by Fluoro-Jade B staining [32].

The whole brain was cut from olfactory bulb to the cerebellum. The distance between sections was 400 μm and the trimmed portion of the brain was homogenated and used for detection of AGEs or oxidative stress biomarkers.

2.7. Determination of Neuronal Degeneration by Fluoro-Jade B Staining (FJ-B). Fluoro-Jade staining was performed using the method described previously [33]. Fluoro-Jade stained slides were visualized under fluorescent microscope (Leica DM500, Leica, Germany). At least ten different fields were photographed from each section and the images were analyzed by ImageJ software.

2.8. Detection of AGEs Level in Serum and Brain. Advanced glycation end products (AGEs) level was detected in serum and brain homogenates (extracted with PBS) fluorometrically [34, 35] at excitation wavelength 370 nm and emission at 445 nm by LS45 fluorescence spectrophotometer (PerkinElmer).

2.9. Determination of Oxidative Stress Biomarkers in the Brain. Brain catalase (CAT) activity [36], reduced glutathione (GSH) [37], and malondialdehyde (MDA) [38] content in the brain were determined colorimetrically.

2.10. Statistical Analysis. Data are expressed as mean ± SEM. Statistical analysis was performed using one-way analysis of variance (ANOVA) followed by Tukey's post hoc test at $P < 0.05$ using Graphpad Prism software.

TABLE 1: Effects of alagebrium (10 mg/kg), perindopril (4 mg/kg), or gliclazide (10 mg/kg) on body weight, blood glucose level, blood pressure (diastolic and systolic), and serum AGEs level in STZ-induced diabetes in rats. Data are presented as mean ± SEM (n = 6).

Parameter	Control	Diabetic	Alagebrium	Perindopril	Gliclazide
Body weight (gm)	301.6 ± 9.1	238.9 ± 8.8*	241.8 ± 8.6*	230.5 ± 7.2*	220.5 ± 7.5*
Blood glucose level (mg/dL)	122.7 ± 5.3	552.3 ± 27.7*	562 ± 19.3*	555.8 ± 18.8*	487.8 ± 63.5*
Diastolic blood pressure (mmHg)	77.5 ± 2.8	110.3 ± 6.4*	111.5 ± 7.6*	81.4 ± 3.9#	93.8 ± 8.5
Systolic blood pressure (mmHg)	105.1 ± 3.1	125.6 ± 4.1*	133.8 ± 3.9*	108.7 ± 3.4	115 ± 5.3
Serum AGEs (fluorescent units)	46.8 ± 1.7	128.5 ± 5.3*	103.5 ± 4.5*#	106.2 ± 3.7*#	120.8 ± 2.9*

*Significantly different from control group. #Significantly different from diabetic group at $P < 0.05$ using ANOVA followed by Tukey's post hoc test.

3. Results

3.1. Body Weight.
In the current study, diabetes caused a significant decrease in body weight in comparison to control rats (239 versus 302 gm). Meanwhile, treatment with alagebrium, perindopril, and gliclazide did not cause any significant change in body weight compared to diabetic rats as shown in Table 1.

3.2. Blood Glucose.
Blood glucose level was significantly increased after STZ injection in comparison to control rats (552 versus 123 mg/dL). However, treatment with alagebrium, perindopril, and gliclazide did not cause any significant change in blood glucose level compared to diabetic rats (Table 1).

3.3. Blood Pressure

3.3.1. Diastolic Blood Pressure.
The present study has demonstrated a significant increase in diastolic blood pressure in diabetic rats compared to control rats (110 versus 77 mmHg). On the other hand, treatment with perindopril caused a significant decrease in diastolic blood pressure compared to diabetic rats (81 versus 110 mmHg) as shown in Table 1.

3.3.2. Systolic Blood Pressure.
In addition, diabetes caused a significant increase in systolic blood pressure in comparison to control rats (126 versus 105 mmHg), while treatment with alagebrium, perindopril, and gliclazide did not cause any significant change in systolic blood pressure compared to diabetic rats as shown in Table 1.

3.4. Serum Advanced Glycation End Products (AGEs).
Diabetes was associated with a significant increase in serum AGEs level in comparison to control rats (128 versus 47 units). Meanwhile, treatment with alagebrium, perindopril, and gliclazide caused a significant decrease in serum AGEs level compared to diabetic rats (103, 106, and 121 versus 128 units, resp.) as shown in Table 1.

3.5. Brain Advanced Glycation End Products (AGEs).
The elevation in serum AGEs was also associated with an increase in brain AGEs level in diabetic rats in comparison to control rats (7.8 versus 3.4 units). Similarly, treatment with alagebrium, perindopril, and gliclazide caused a significant decrease in

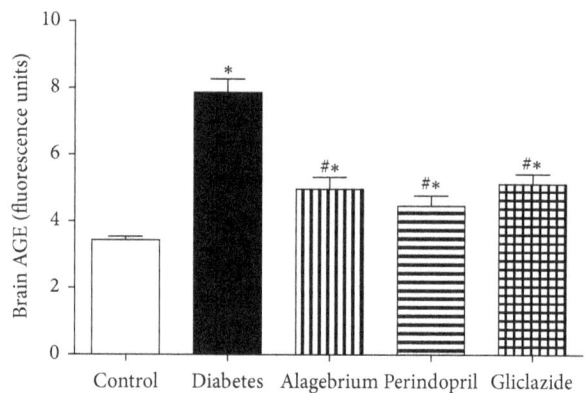

FIGURE 1: Effects of alagebrium (10 mg/kg), perindopril (4 mg/kg), or gliclazide (10 mg/kg) on brain AGEs level in STZ-induced diabetes in rats. Data are presented as mean ± SEM (n = 6). *Significantly different from control group. #Significantly different from diabetic group at $P < 0.05$ using ANOVA followed by Tukey's post hoc test.

serum AGEs level compared to diabetic rats (5, 4.5, and 5.1 versus 7.8 units, resp.) as shown in Figure 1.

3.6. Neuronal Degeneration.
In the current study, diabetes caused a significant increase in neuronal degeneration as evidenced by the increase in Fluoro-Jade (FJ) fluorescence in comparison to control rats (2.9 versus 1.9 units). Meanwhile, only treatment with perindopril caused a significant decrease in FJ fluorescence as compared to diabetic rats (2.3 versus 2.9 units) as shown in Figure 2.

3.7. Behavioural Change in Y-Maze.
The present study has shown that diabetes caused a significant decrease in Y-maze score in comparison to control rats (1.6 versus 4.7 units). On the other hand, treatment with alagebrium, perindopril, and gliclazide caused a significant increase in Y-maze score compared to diabetic rats (3.5, 3.5, and 4.2 versus 1.6, resp.) as shown in Figure 3.

3.8. Brain Oxidative Stress

3.8.1. Catalase.
Administration of STZ caused a significant decrease in brain catalase activity in comparison to

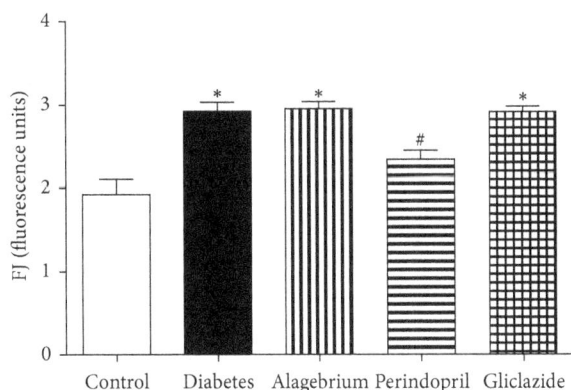

FIGURE 2: Effects of alagebrium (10 mg/kg), perindopril (4 mg/kg), or gliclazide (10 mg/kg) on neuronal degeneration (Fluoro-Jade fluorescence) in STZ-induced diabetes in rats. Data are presented as mean ± SEM (n = 6). *Significantly different from control group. #Significantly different from diabetic group at $P < 0.05$ using ANOVA followed by Tukey's post hoc test.

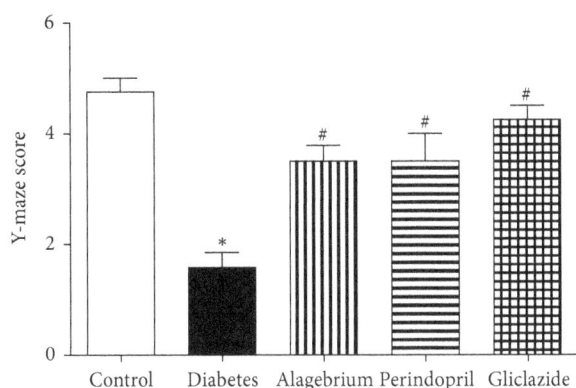

FIGURE 3: Effects of alagebrium (10 mg/kg), perindopril (4 mg/kg), or gliclazide (10 mg/kg) on Y-maze score in STZ-induced diabetes in rats. Data are presented as mean ± SEM (n = 6). *Significantly different from control group. #Significantly different from diabetic group at $P < 0.05$ using ANOVA followed by Tukey's post hoc test.

control rats (0.21 versus 0.32 μmoles/min/mg). Brain catalase activity was significantly increased following treatment with gliclazide in comparison to diabetic rats (0.34 versus 0.21 μmoles/min/mg) as shown in Figure 4(a).

3.8.2. GSH. Similarly, diabetes caused a significant decrease in brain GSH content in comparison to control rats (1 versus 1.4 units). However, treatment with alagebrium, perindopril, and gliclazide did not cause any change in brain GSH content compared to diabetic rats as shown in Figure 4(b).

3.8.3. MDA. In the current study, diabetes caused a significant increase in brain MDA content in comparison to control rats (4 versus 3 μmoles/g). In addition, treatment with alagebrium, perindopril, and gliclazide caused a significant decrease in brain MDA content in comparison to diabetic rats (3.1, 3, and 3.1 versus 4 μmoles/g, resp.) as shown in Figure 4(c).

4. Discussion

The present study was designed to investigate the impact of diabetes on blood pressure and some central nervous system (CNS) functions. Also, this study investigated the possible beneficial effects of alagebrium, a highly potent AGE-cross-link breaker that has the ability to reverse already-formed AGE cross-links [39–42], and perindopril, a brain-penetrating angiotensin-converting enzyme (ACE) inhibitor [43] known to increase plasma sRAGE level [21], against these diabetic complications.

In the current study, diabetes was associated with a decrease in body weight which was not altered by treatment with alagebrium, perindopril, and gliclazide. These findings keep pace with previous studies in diabetic rats [44, 45].

In addition, STZ administration caused a significant increase in blood glucose level as previously described [46–48]. The elevation in blood glucose level following STZ injection was not altered by treatment with alagebrium, perindopril, and gliclazide at the tested doses and timepoint.

The present investigation has shown that diabetes caused a significant increase in diastolic blood pressure, which was decreased by treatment with perindopril only confirming its hypotensive effect [25]. Similarly, diabetes caused a significant increase in systolic blood pressure which was not altered by any of the treatments used. Elevation of blood pressure was previously reported following induction of diabetes [3, 49, 50] and STZ-induced hypertension was prevented by perindopril treatment [3].

AGEs are the end product of a nonenzymatic reaction with sugar derivatives which leads to irreversible protein-protein cross-links [51]. When AGEs link to long-lived proteins, such as collagen in the arterial wall, they contribute to arterial stiffening [52]. Furthermore, AGEs bind to specific AGE-binding receptors on endothelial cells and quench nitric oxide, thereby leading to endothelial dysfunction [25]. The increased formation of advanced glycation end products (AGEs) constitutes a potential mechanism of hyperglycaemia-induced micro- and macrovascular disease in diabetes [53].

Diabetes was associated with an increase in serum AGEs level after STZ administration, which was decreased by treatment with alagebrium and perindopril. Several studies have demonstrated the involvement of AGEs in micro- and macrovascular complications of diabetes [54] and similar elevation in AGEs was previously reported following induction of diabetes [44, 55].

Alagebrium breaks established AGE cross-links between proteins [56]. Alagebrium therapy was previously shown to be associated with reduced AGEs accumulation and RAGE expression in diabetic rats [19]. Previous animal studies and initial phase I and II patient studies demonstrated reduced vascular stiffness and improved endothelial function by alagebrium [57]. Several studies have also shown that ACE inhibition reduced the accumulation of serum AGEs in diabetes, possibly via effects on oxidative pathways [20, 58].

In the current study, diabetes caused a significant increase in brain AGEs which was prevented by treatment with alagebrium, perindopril, and gliclazide.

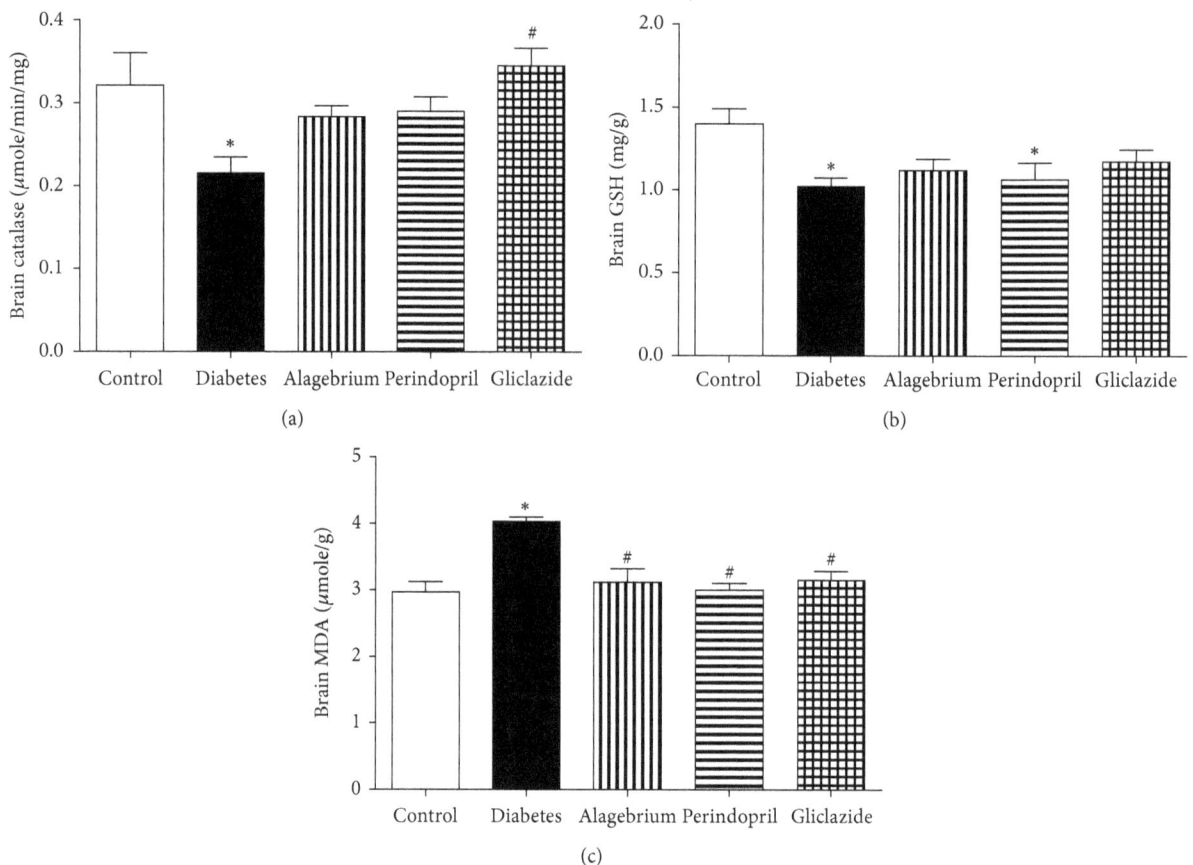

FIGURE 4: Effects of alagebrium (10 mg/kg), perindopril (4 mg/kg), or gliclazide (10 mg/kg) on (a) brain catalase activity, (b) brain GSH content, and (c) brain MDA content in STZ-induced diabetes in rats. Data are presented as mean ± SEM ($n = 6$). *Significantly different from control group. #Significantly different from diabetic group at $P < 0.05$ using ANOVA followed by Tukey's post hoc test.

AGEs were reported to be directly neurotoxic to cultured neurons [59] promoting neuronal cell death and contributing to neurodegenerative disorders such as Alzheimer's disease (AD) [60]. This explains why diabetes caused a significant increase in neuronal degeneration as evidenced by Fluoro-Jade (FJ) fluorescence, which was prevented only by treatment with perindopril.

The ability of perindopril to abolish the enhanced neuronal degeneration might be partly mediated by its ability to reduce AGEs level, increase the production of sRAGE [21], and reduce elevated blood pressure [3] as previously demonstrated.

The changes in neuronal degeneration were accompanied by parallel changes in behavior as diabetes caused a significant decrease in Y-maze score. Similar alterations in memory were previously reported following induction of diabetes [61, 62].

Rats treated with perindopril had near-normal performance in the Y-maze. Perindopril was previously reported to prevent cognitive impairment in AD mouse model through the suppression of microglia/astrocyte activation and the attenuation of oxidative stress [43]. In addition, antihypertensive treatment based on perindopril was demonstrated

to reduce cognitive decline in patients with cerebrovascular disease [63].

Surprisingly, alagebrium and gliclazide also improved rat performance in the Y-maze although they had no influence on neuronal degeneration measured by Fluoro-Jade fluorescence. Alagebrium was shown to ameliorate Aβ-induced neuronal death in rat brains [60] which is linked to Alzheimer's disease and associated memory defects [64]. However, in the present study, alagebrium had no effect on neuronal degeneration which indicates that this effect might be attributed to another action and needs further investigation. Gliclazide was shown to stimulate peroxisome proliferator activated receptor gamma (PPAR-γ) and exert antiamyloidogenic and anti-inflammatory effects, which may play a role in delaying and reducing the risk of neurodegeneration as previously demonstrated [65]. This could explain the effectiveness of gliclazide in improving rat performance in the Y-maze without alteration in neuronal degeneration.

This research has shown that diabetes caused a state of brain oxidative stress as evidenced by the decrease in brain catalase activity, decrease in brain GSH content, and increase in brain MDA content. Treatment with gliclazide caused a significant increase in brain catalase activity and a decrease in brain MDA activity, while treatment with alagebrium and perindopril caused a decrease in brain MDA activity suggesting antioxidant action.

STZ is known to increase production of ROS [66] and MDA [3], while reducing antioxidant capacity [67] as GSH level [3] in diabetic animals.

In addition to the ligation of RAGE, AGEs may increase generation of ROS by decreasing activities of superoxide dismutase (SOD) and catalase and diminishing glutathione stores [68].

Diabetes-associated increase in superoxide production was prevented by alagebrium [19] which also increased the availability of GSH [40], glutathione peroxidase, and superoxide dismutase activities in aging rats and reduced oxidative stress [41]. This antioxidant action of alagebrium might partly explain its neuroprotective effect that caused improvement in the performance in Y-maze without alteration in neuronal degeneration and further studies are required to explain this phenomenon.

Treatment with perindopril was shown to prevent STZ-induced oxidative stress in rats by increasing GSH and decreasing MDA levels [3]. In addition, it reduced oxidative stress and increased plasma antioxidant capacity in hypertensive patients [69].

Gliclazide has antioxidant effect [70] acting as a general free radical scavenger [71, 72], which was shown to prevent the increase of MDA and SOD during diabetes [73].

Although the results from experimental studies concerning alagebrium [74, 75] were promising, safety and/or efficacy in clinical studies seems to be a concern [53, 76]. Alagebrium showed beneficial effects on a range of cardiovascular variables in hypertensive individuals [56, 57], whereas other clinical trials in heart failure patients did not show any beneficial effects [77, 78]. In addition, the cardioprotective effects of 1-year exercise training in previously sedentary older subjects were not potentiated by alagebrium [51].

5. Conclusion

Diabetes is associated with vascular and behavioral complications including hypertension and dementia which might be mediated by brain oxidative stress and neuronal degeneration. Although perindopril was effective in reducing the elevated blood pressure induced by diabetes, this effect could not be fully attributed to amelioration of AGEs signaling since perindopril is a known ACEI and alagebrium was not effective against elevated blood pressure.

Blockade of AGEs signaling by alagebrium and perindopril in rats as late as 8 weeks after diabetes induction was effective in reducing CNS complications only which suggests the possible use of these drugs to manage diabetic central complications together with conventional antidiabetic therapies. Whether similar effects would be observed in human diabetic patients is the main question and needs further investigation.

Conflict of Interests

The authors confirm that there is no known conflict of interests associated with the publication of this paper.

Acknowledgment

This work was funded by Zagazig University (8K2/M3, 2009).

References

[1] S. A. Wrighten, G. G. Piroli, C. A. Grillo, and L. P. Reagan, "A look inside the diabetic brain: contributors to diabetes-induced brain aging," *Biochimica et Biophysica Acta—Molecular Basis of Disease*, vol. 1792, no. 5, pp. 444–453, 2009.

[2] S. Wild, G. Roglic, A. Green, R. Sicree, and H. King, "Global prevalence of diabetes: estimates for the year 2000 and projections for 2030," *Diabetes Care*, vol. 27, no. 5, pp. 1047–1053, 2004.

[3] B. M. Patel, S. S. Agarwal, and S. V. Bhadada, "Perindopril protects against streptozotocin-induced hyperglycemic myocardial damage/alterations," *Human & Experimental Toxicology*, vol. 31, no. 11, pp. 1132–1143, 2012.

[4] W. H. Gispen and G.-J. Biessels, "Cognition and synaptic plasticity in diabetes mellitus," *Trends in Neurosciences*, vol. 23, no. 11, pp. 542–549, 2000.

[5] G. J. Biessels, L. P. Van der Heide, A. Kamal, R. L. A. W. Bleys, and W. H. Gispen, "Ageing and diabetes: implications for brain function," *European Journal of Pharmacology*, vol. 441, no. 1-2, pp. 1–14, 2002.

[6] S.-Y. Goh and M. E. Cooper, "The role of advanced glycation end products in progression and complications of diabetes," *The Journal of Clinical Endocrinology & Metabolism*, vol. 93, no. 4, pp. 1143–1152, 2008.

[7] C. Dominguez, E. Ruiz, M. Gussinye, and A. Carrascosa, "Oxidative stress at onset and in early stages of type 1 diabetes in children and adolescents," *Diabetes Care*, vol. 21, no. 10, pp. 1736–1742, 1998.

[8] L. P. Reagan, "Glucose, stress, and hippocampal neuronal vulnerability," *International Review of Neurobiology*, vol. 51, pp. 289–324, 2002.

[9] D. Suzuki, T. Miyata, N. Saotome et al., "Immunohistochemical evidence for an increased oxidative stress and carbonyl modification of proteins in diabetic glomerular lesions," *Journal of the American Society of Nephrology*, vol. 10, no. 4, pp. 822–832, 1999.

[10] T. Nishikawa, D. Edelstein, X. L. Du et al., "Normalizing mitochondrial superoxide production blocks three pathways of hyperglycaemic damage," *Nature*, vol. 404, no. 6779, pp. 787–790, 2000.

[11] R. Ramasamy, S. J. Vannucci, S. S. D. Yan, K. Herold, S. F. Yan, and A. M. Schmidt, "Advanced glycation end products and RAGE: a common thread in aging, diabetes, neurodegeneration, and inflammation," *Glycobiology*, vol. 15, no. 7, pp. 16R–28R, 2005.

[12] S. F. Yan, R. Ramasamy, and A. M. Schmidt, "Soluble RAGE: therapy and biomarker in unraveling the RAGE axis in chronic disease and aging," *Biochemical Pharmacology*, vol. 79, no. 10, pp. 1379–1386, 2010.

[13] N. Tanji, G. S. Markowitz, C. Fu et al., "Expression of advanced glycation end products and their cellular receptor RAGE diabetic nephropathy and nondiabetic renal disease," *Journal of the*

American Society of Nephrology, vol. 11, no. 9, pp. 1656–1666, 2000.

[14] M.-P. Wautier, O. Chappey, S. Corda, D. M. Stern, A. M. Schmidt, and J.-L. Wautier, "Activation of NADPH oxidase by AGE links oxidant stress to altered gene expression via RAGE," *American Journal of Physiology—Endocrinology and Metabolism*, vol. 280, no. 5, pp. E685–E694, 2001.

[15] T. Wendt, N. Tanji, J. Guo et al., "Glucose, glycation, and RAGE: implications for amplification of cellular dysfunction in diabetic nephropathy," *Journal of the American Society of Nephrology*, vol. 14, no. 5, pp. 1383–1395, 2003.

[16] M. B. Yim, H.-S. Yim, C. Lee, S.-O. Kang, and P. B. Chock, "Protein glycation: creation of catalytic sites for free radical generation," *Annals of the New York Academy of Sciences*, vol. 928, pp. 48–53, 2001.

[17] D. C. Perantie, A. Lim, J. Wu et al., "Effects of prior hypoglycemia and hyperglycemia on cognition in children with type 1 diabetes mellitus," *Pediatric Diabetes*, vol. 9, no. 2, pp. 87–95, 2008.

[18] D. Susic, J. Varagic, J. Ahn, and E. D. Frohlich, "Crosslink breakers: a new approach to cardiovascular therapy," *Current Opinion in Cardiology*, vol. 19, no. 4, pp. 336–340, 2004.

[19] M. T. Coughlan, J. M. Forbes, and M. E. Cooper, "Role of the AGE crosslink breaker, alagebrium, as a renoprotective agent in diabetes," *Kidney International*, vol. 72, pp. S54–S60, 2007.

[20] J. M. Forbes, M. E. Cooper, V. Thallas et al., "Reduction of the accumulation of advanced glycation end products by ACE inhibition in experimental diabetic nephropathy," *Diabetes*, vol. 51, no. 11, pp. 3274–3282, 2002.

[21] J. M. Forbes, S. R. Thorpe, V. Thallas-Bonke et al., "Modulation of soluble receptor for advanced glycation end products by angiotensin-converting enzyme-1 inhibition in diabetic nephropathy," *Journal of the American Society of Nephrology*, vol. 16, no. 8, pp. 2363–2372, 2005.

[22] M. Ramanathan, A. K. Jaiswal, and S. K. Bhattacharya, "Differential effects of diazepam on anxiety in streptozotocin induced diabetic and non-diabetic rats," *Psychopharmacology*, vol. 135, no. 4, pp. 361–367, 1998.

[23] M. T. Coughlan, V. Thallas-Bonke, J. Pete et al., "Combination therapy with the advanced glycation end product crosslink breaker, alagebrium, and angiotensin converting enzyme inhibitors in diabetes: synergy or redundancy?" *Endocrinology*, vol. 148, no. 2, pp. 886–895, 2007.

[24] J.-B. Kim, B.-W. Song, S. Park et al., "Alagebrium chloride, a novel advanced glycation end-product cross linkage breaker, inhibits neointimal proliferation in a diabetic rat carotid balloon injury model," *Korean Circulation Journal*, vol. 40, no. 10, pp. 520–526, 2010.

[25] T. Mashhoody, K. Rastegar, and F. Zal, "Perindopril may improve the hippocampal reduced glutathione content in rats," *Advanced Pharmaceutical Bulletin*, vol. 4, no. 2, pp. 155–159, 2014.

[26] H. Sun, N. Ge, M. Shao et al., "Lumbrokinase attenuates diabetic nephropathy through regulating extracellular matrix degradation in Streptozotocin-induced diabetic rats," *Diabetes Research and Clinical Practice*, vol. 100, no. 1, pp. 85–95, 2013.

[27] H. M. El-Bassossy, A. Fahmy, and D. Badawy, "Cinnamaldehyde protects from the hypertension associated with diabetes," *Food and Chemical Toxicology*, vol. 49, no. 11, pp. 3007–3012, 2011.

[28] N. Hassan, H. M. El-Bassossy, and M. N. M. Zakaria, "Heme oxygenase-1 induction protects against hypertension associated

with diabetes: effect on exaggerated vascular contractility," *Naunyn-Schmiedeberg's Archives of Pharmacology*, vol. 386, no. 3, pp. 217–226, 2013.

[29] T. Baluchnejadmojarad and M. Roghani, "Chronic epigallocatechin-3-gallate ameliorates learning and memory deficits in diabetic rats via modulation of nitric oxide and oxidative stress," *Behavioural Brain Research*, vol. 224, no. 2, pp. 305–310, 2011.

[30] S. Nasri, M. Roghani, T. Baluchnejadmojarad, M. Balvardi, and T. Rabani, "Chronic cyanidin-3-glucoside administration improves short-term spatial recognition memory but not passive avoidance learning and memory in streptozotocin-diabetic rats," *Phytotherapy Research*, vol. 26, no. 8, pp. 1205–1210, 2012.

[31] H. M. El-Bassossy, R. El-Fawal, and A. Fahmy, "Arginase inhibition alleviates hypertension associated with diabetes: effect on endothelial dependent relaxation and NO production," *Vascular Pharmacology*, vol. 57, no. 5-6, pp. 194–200, 2012.

[32] W. Barakat, N. Safwet, N. N. El-Maraghy, and M. N. M. Zakaria, "Candesartan and glycyrrhizin ameliorate ischemic brain damage through downregulation of the TLR signaling cascade," *European Journal of Pharmacology*, vol. 724, no. 1, pp. 43–50, 2014.

[33] Y. Li, P. J. Lein, C. Liu et al., "Spatiotemporal pattern of neuronal injury induced by DFP in rats: a model for delayed neuronal cell death following acute OP intoxication," *Toxicology and Applied Pharmacology*, vol. 253, no. 3, pp. 261–269, 2011.

[34] G. Munch, R. Keis, A. Wessels et al., "Determination of advanced glycation end products in serum by fluorescence spectroscopy and competitive ELISA," *European Journal of Clinical Chemistry and Clinical Biochemistry*, vol. 35, no. 9, pp. 669–677, 1997.

[35] R. Sampathkumar, M. Balasubramanyam, M. Rema, C. Premanand, and V. Mohan, "A novel advanced glycation index and its association with diabetes and microangiopathy," *Metabolism: Clinical and Experimental*, vol. 54, no. 8, pp. 1002–1007, 2005.

[36] A. K. Sinha, "Colorimetric assay of catalase," *Analytical Biochemistry*, vol. 47, no. 2, pp. 389–394, 1972.

[37] E. Beutler, O. Duron, and B. M. Kelly, "Improved method for the determination of blood glutathione," *The Journal of Laboratory and Clinical Medicine*, vol. 61, pp. 882–888, 1963.

[38] T. Yoshioka, K. Kawada, T. Shimada, and M. Mori, "Lipid peroxidation in maternal and cord blood and protective mechanism against activated-oxygen toxicity in the blood," *American Journal of Obstetrics and Gynecology*, vol. 135, no. 3, pp. 372–376, 1979.

[39] M. T. Coughlan, J. M. Forbes, and M. E. Cooper, "Role of the AGE crosslink breaker, alagebrium, as a renoprotective agent in diabetes," *Kidney International Supplements*, vol. 72, pp. S54–S60, 2007.

[40] A. Dhar, K. M. Desai, and L. Wu, "Alagebrium attenuates acute methylglyoxal-induced glucose intolerance in Sprague-Dawley rats," *British Journal of Pharmacology*, vol. 159, no. 1, pp. 166–175, 2010.

[41] Y. Guo, M. Lu, J. Qian, and Y.-L. Cheng, "Alagebrium chloride protects the heart against oxidative stress in aging rats," *Journals of Gerontology—Series A: Biological Sciences and Medical Sciences*, vol. 64, no. 6, pp. 629–635, 2009.

[42] S. Vasan, P. Foiles, and H. Founds, "Therapeutic potential of breakers of advanced glycation end product-protein crosslinks," *Archives of Biochemistry and Biophysics*, vol. 419, no. 1, pp. 89–96, 2003.

[43] Y.-F. Dong, K. Kataoka, Y. Tokutomi et al., "Perindopril, a centrally active angiotensin-converting enzyme inhibitor, prevents

cognitive impairment in mouse models of Alzheimer's disease," *The FASEB Journal*, vol. 25, no. 9, pp. 2911–2920, 2011.

[44] M. Guglielmotto, M. Aragno, E. Tamagno et al., "AGEs/RAGE complex upregulates BACE1 via NF-κB pathway activation," *Neurobiology of Aging*, vol. 33, no. 1, pp. 196.e13–196.e27, 2012.

[45] L. Michea, V. Irribarra, I. A. Goecke, and E. T. Marusic, "Reduced Na-K pump but increased Na-K-2Cl cotransporter in aorta of streptozotocin-induced diabetic rat," *The American Journal of Physiology: Heart and Circulatory Physiology*, vol. 280, no. 2, pp. H851–H858, 2001.

[46] C. Di Filippo, R. Marfella, S. Cuzzocrea et al., "Hyperglycemia in streptozotocin-induced diabetic rat increases infarct size associated with low levels of myocardial HO-1 during ischemia/reperfusion," *Diabetes*, vol. 54, no. 3, pp. 803–810, 2005.

[47] M. Elsner, B. Guldbakke, M. Tiedge, R. Munday, and S. Lenzen, "Relative importance of transport and alkylation for pancreatic beta-cell toxicity of streptozotocin," *Diabetologia*, vol. 43, no. 12, pp. 1528–1533, 2000.

[48] L. P. Reagan, A. M. Magariños, D. K. Yee et al., "Oxidative stress and HNE conjugation of GLUT3 are increased in the hippocampus of diabetic rats subjected to stress," *Brain Research*, vol. 862, no. 1-2, pp. 292–300, 2000.

[49] S. Funakawa, T. Okahara, M. Imanishi, T. Komori, K. Yamamoto, and Y. Tochino, "Renin-angiotensin system and prostacyclin biosynthesis in streptozotocin diabetic rats," *European Journal of Pharmacology*, vol. 94, no. 1-2, pp. 27–33, 1983.

[50] Y.-J. Liu, Y. Nakagawa, and T. Ohzeki, "Gene expression of 11β-hydroxysteroid dehydrogenase type 1 and type 2 in the kidneys of insulin-dependent diabetic rats," *Hypertension*, vol. 31, no. 3, pp. 885–889, 1998.

[51] M. H. Oudegeest-Sander, M. G. M. O. Rikkert, P. Smits et al., "The effect of an advanced glycation end-product crosslink breaker and exercise training on vascular function in older individuals: a randomized factorial design trial," *Experimental Gerontology*, vol. 48, no. 12, pp. 1509–1517, 2013.

[52] G. L. Bakris, A. J. Bank, D. A. Kass, J. M. Neutel, R. A. Preston, and S. Oparil, "Advanced glycation end-product crosslink breakers: a novel approach to cardiovascular pathologies related to the aging process," *American Journal of Hypertension*, vol. 17, supplement 3, pp. 23S–30S, 2004.

[53] L. Engelen, C. D. A. Stehouwer, and C. G. Schalkwijk, "Current therapeutic interventions in the glycation pathway: evidence from clinical studies," *Diabetes, Obesity and Metabolism*, vol. 15, no. 8, pp. 677–689, 2013.

[54] V. Radoi, D. Lixandru, M. Mohora, and B. Virgolici, "Advanced glycation end products in diabetes mellitus: mechanism of action and focused treatment," *Proceedings of the Romanian Academy, Series B*, vol. 1, pp. 9–19, 2012.

[55] S. Cardoso, R. X. Santos, S. C. Correia et al., "Insulin-induced recurrent hypoglycemia exacerbates diabetic brain mitochondrial dysfunction and oxidative imbalance," *Neurobiology of Disease*, vol. 49, no. 1, pp. 1–12, 2013.

[56] D. A. Kass, E. P. Shapiro, M. Kawaguchi et al., "Improved arterial compliance by a novel advanced glycation end-product crosslink breaker," *Circulation*, vol. 104, no. 13, pp. 1464–1470, 2001.

[57] S. J. Zieman, V. Melenovsky, L. Clattenburg et al., "Advanced glycation endproduct crosslink breaker (alagebrium) improves endothelial function in patients with isolated systolic hypertension," *Journal of Hypertension*, vol. 25, no. 3, pp. 577–583, 2007.

[58] K. Šebeková, R. Schinzel, G. Münch, Z. Krivošíková, R. Dzúrik, and A. Heidland, "Advanced glycation end-product levels in subtotally nephrectomized rats: beneficial effects of angiotensin II receptor 1 antagonist losartan," *Mineral and Electrolyte Metabolism*, vol. 25, no. 4–6, pp. 380–383, 1999.

[59] M. Takeuchi, R. Bucala, T. Suzuki et al., "Neurotoxicity of advanced glycation end-products for cultured cortical neurons," *Journal of Neuropathology and Experimental Neurology*, vol. 59, no. 12, pp. 1094–1105, 2000.

[60] K. Byun, E. Bayarsaikhan, D. Kim et al., "Induction of neuronal death by microglial AGE-albumin: implications for Alzheimer's disease," *PLoS ONE*, vol. 7, no. 5, Article ID e37917, 2012.

[61] P. T. Kumar, S. Antony, M. S. Nandhu, J. Sadanandan, G. Naijil, and C. S. Paulose, "Vitamin D3 restores altered cholinergic and insulin receptor expression in the cerebral cortex and muscarinic M3 receptor expression in pancreatic islets of streptozotocin induced diabetic rats," *The Journal of Nutritional Biochemistry*, vol. 22, no. 5, pp. 418–425, 2011.

[62] A. Nitta, R. Murai, N. Suzuki et al., "Diabetic neuropathies in brain are induced by deficiency of BDNF," *Neurotoxicology and Teratology*, vol. 24, no. 5, pp. 695–701, 2002.

[63] C. Tzourio, C. Anderson, N. Chapman et al., "Effects of blood pressure lowering with perindopril and indapamide therapy on dementia and cognitive decline in patients with cerebrovascular disease," *Archives of Internal Medicine*, vol. 163, no. 9, pp. 1069–1075, 2003.

[64] J. W. Wright and J. W. Harding, "The brain RAS and Alzheimer's disease," *Experimental Neurology*, vol. 223, no. 2, pp. 326–333, 2010.

[65] K. Alagiakrishnan and P. Senior, "Antidiabetic drugs and their potential role in treating mild cognitive impairment and Alzheimer's disease," *Discovery Medicine*, vol. 16, no. 90, pp. 277–286, 2013.

[66] P. A. Low and K. K. Nickander, "Oxygen free radical effects in sciatic nerve in experimental diabetes," *Diabetes*, vol. 40, no. 7, pp. 873–877, 1991.

[67] C. Hermenegildo, A. Raya, J. Roma, and F. J. Romero, "Decreased glutathione peroxidase activity in sciatic nerve of alloxan-induced diabetic mice and its correlation with blood glucose levels," *Neurochemical Research*, vol. 18, no. 8, pp. 893–896, 1993.

[68] J.-M. Jiang, Z. Wang, and D.-D. Li, "Effects of AGEs on oxidation stress and antioxidation abilities in cultured astrocytes," *Biomedical and Environmental Sciences*, vol. 17, no. 1, pp. 79–86, 2004.

[69] L. Ghiadoni, A. Magagna, D. Versari et al., "Different effect of antihypertensive drugs on conduit artery endothelial function," *Hypertension*, vol. 41, no. 6, pp. 1281–1286, 2003.

[70] X. Qiang, J. Satoh, M. Sagara et al., "Gliclazide inhibits diabetic neuropathy irrespective of blood glucose levels in streptozotocin-induced diabetic rats," *Metabolism: Clinical and Experimental*, vol. 47, no. 8, pp. 977–981, 1998.

[71] I. M. Salman and M. N. Inamdar, "Effect of gliclazide on cardiovascular risk factors involved in split-dose streptozotocin induced neonatal rat model: a chronic study," *International Journal of Basic & Clinical Pharmacology*, vol. 1, no. 3, pp. 196–201, 2012.

[72] C. M. Sena, T. Louro, P. Matafome, E. Nunes, P. Monteiro, and R. Seiça, "Antioxidant and vascular effects of gliclazide in type 2 diabetic rats fed high-fat diet," *Physiological Research*, vol. 58, no. 2, pp. 203–209, 2009.

[73] Y.-B. Wu, L.-L. Shi, Y.-J. Wu, W.-H. Xu, L. Wang, and M.-S. Ren, "Protective effect of gliclazide on diabetic peripheral neuropathy through Drp-1 mediated-oxidative stress and apoptosis," *Neuroscience Letters*, vol. 523, no. 1, pp. 45–49, 2012.

[74] R. Candido, J. M. Forbes, M. C. Thomas et al., "A breaker of advanced glycation end products attenuates diabetes-induced myocardial structural changes," *Circulation Research*, vol. 92, no. 7, pp. 785–792, 2003.

[75] M. Lassila, K. K. Seah, T. J. Allen et al., "Accelerated nephropathy in diabetic apolipoprotein E-knockout mouse: role of advanced glycation end products," *Journal of the American Society of Nephrology*, vol. 15, no. 8, pp. 2125–2138, 2004.

[76] N. Fujimoto, J. L. Hastings, G. Carrick-Ranson et al., "Cardiovascular effects of 1 year of alagebrium and endurance exercise training in healthy older individuals," *Circulation: Heart Failure*, vol. 6, no. 6, pp. 1155–1164, 2013.

[77] J. W. L. Hartog, S. Willemsen, D. J. van Veldhuisen et al., "Effects of alagebrium, an advanced glycation endproduct breaker, on exercise tolerance and cardiac function in patients with chronic heart failure," *European Journal of Heart Failure*, vol. 13, no. 8, pp. 899–908, 2011.

[78] W. C. Little, M. R. Zile, D. W. Kitzman, W. G. Hundley, T. X. O'Brien, and R. C. Degroof, "The effect of alagebrium chloride (ALT-711), a novel glucose cross-link breaker, in the treatment of elderly patients with diastolic heart failure," *Journal of Cardiac Failure*, vol. 11, no. 3, pp. 191–195, 2005.

18

Enzyme Inhibitory Properties, Antioxidant Activities, and Phytochemical Profile of Three Medicinal Plants from Turkey

Gokhan Zengin,[1] Gokalp Ozmen Guler,[2] Abdurrahman Aktumsek,[1] Ramazan Ceylan,[1] Carene Marie Nancy Picot,[3] and M. Fawzi Mahomoodally[3]

[1]Department of Biology, Science Faculty, Selçuk University Campus, 42250 Konya, Turkey
[2]Department of Biological Education, Ahmet Keleşoğlu Education Faculty, Necmettin Erbakan University, 42090 Konya, Turkey
[3]Department of Health Sciences, Faculty of Science, University of Mauritius, 230 Réduit, Mauritius

Correspondence should be addressed to Gokhan Zengin; gokhanzengin@selcuk.edu.tr
and M. Fawzi Mahomoodally; f.mahomoodally@uom.ac.mu

Academic Editor: Berend Olivier

We aimed to investigate the inhibitory potential of three medicinal plants (*Hedysarum varium*, *Onobrychis hypargyrea*, and *Vicia truncatula*) from Turkey against key enzymes involved in human pathologies, namely, diabetes (α-amylase and α-glucosidase), neurodegenerative disorders (tyrosinase, acetylcholinesterase, and butyrylcholinesterase), and hyperpigmentation (tyrosinase). The antioxidant potential, phenolic and flavonoid content of ethyl acetate, and methanolic and aqueous extracts were investigated using *in vitro* assays. The total antioxidant capacity (TAC), β-carotene/linoleic acid bleaching activity, 1,1-diphenyl-2-picrylhydrazyl free radical (DPPH$^\bullet$), 2,2-azino-bis(3-ethylbenzothiazoline-6-sulfonic acid) (ABTS$^{\bullet+}$), cupric ion reducing antioxidant capacity (CUPRAC), ferric reducing antioxidant power (FRAP), and metal chelating activity on ferrous ions were used to evaluate the antioxidant capabilities of the extracts. The half-maximal inhibitory concentrations (IC_{50}) of the extracts on cholinesterase, tyrosinase, and α-amylase were significantly higher than the references, galantamine, kojic acid, and acarbose, respectively. The half-maximal effective concentrations (EC_{50}) of the extracts on TAC, CUPRAC, and FRAP were significantly higher than trolox. The phenol and flavonoid contents of the plant extracts were in the range 20.90 ± 0.190–83.25 ± 0.914 mg gallic acid equivalent/g extract and 1.45 ± 0.200–39.71 ± 0.092 mg rutin equivalent/g extract, respectively. The plants were found to possess moderate antioxidant capacities and interesting inhibitory action against key enzymes.

1. Introduction

Turkey has been described as one of the countries which has the richest floral biodiversity worldwide [1]. Indeed, this is due to its unique geographical location, climatic conditions, and geomorphological characteristics [2, 3]. Approximately, 10,500 species have been identified in Turkey and 30% were found to be endemic [2]. The relatively high rate of endemism in Turkey provides an indication of the richest biodiversity in this area [1].

Herbal medicinal systems, knowledge, and practices have been transmitted through the ages. For centuries, medicinal plants were the only resources available for the treatment of several diseases which plagued humanity. In fact, many of today's drugs have been derived from medicinal plants [1].

Additionally, the World Health Organisation has reported that 80% of the world's population relies on herbal medicine for primary health care [2]. Recently, several ethnobotanical studies have reported the widespread usage of plants for curative purposes among the local Turkish people [2, 4, 5]. However, to the best of our knowledge, several medicinal plants used as folk Turkish medicine have not received scientific attention yet.

In Turkey, the Fabaceae family is the second largest family after Asteraceae and the most economically important family after Poaceae [6, 7]. Ethnobotanical studies have reported that important taxa from Fabaceae family have been used in folk medicine. For instance, *Onobrychis gracilis* is commonly used for cold and flu [8]; *Vicia faba* is used to treat gastrovascular disorders [9]; *Vicia cracca* subsp. *stenophylla* is used as an anticough agent [10]; *Vicia ervilia* is used to treat diabetes [11]. In the present investigation, 3 Fabaceae species, namely, *Hedysarum varium*, *Onobrychis hypargyrea*, and *Vicia truncatula*, were evaluated for their possible antioxidant activities and inhibitory action on cholinesterase, tyrosinase, α-amylase, and α-glucosidase.

2. Materials and Methods

2.1. Plant Material and Extraction.

Hedysarum varium (Hv) (38°1′49.25″N, 32°30′10.91″S) was collected from Konya, and *Onobrychis hypargyrea* (Oh) (40°18′30.00″N, 32°58′39.00″S) and *Vicia truncatula* (Vt) (40°27′17.00″N, 32°37′27.00″S) were collected from Ankara. The plants were identified by Dr. Murad Aydin Sanda, the senior taxonomist of the Department of Biology, Selçuk University, Konya, Turkey, and voucher specimens were deposited at the herbarium of the laboratory. The aerial parts of the plants were dried at room temperature. Air-dried samples (10 g) were macerated in 200 mL solvent (ethyl acetate (EA), methanol (MeOH), or water (Aq)) at room temperature for 24 h. The extracts were concentrated under reduced pressure and organic extracts were dissolved in methanol while the aqueous extract was dissolved in water.

2.2. Quantification of Phenolic Compounds

2.2.1. Determination of Total Phenol Content. The total phenol content was determined as described by Slinkard and Singleton [12] with slight modifications. Briefly, 0.25 mL plant extract was mixed with a tenfold diluted Folin-Ciocalteu reagent solution and the mixture was shaken vigorously. After 3 min, 0.75 mL sodium carbonate solution (1%) was added to the mixture and was allowed to react for 2 h at room temperature. The absorbance was then read at 760 nm. The total phenol content was expressed as mg gallic acid equivalents (GAE) per g crude extract using a gallic acid standard curve.

2.2.2. Determination of Total Flavonoid Content. The total flavonoid content was determined following the method described by Berk et al. [13]. Briefly, 1 mL aluminium trichloride (2%) solution in methanol was added to 1 mL plant extract. The absorbance of the mixture was read at 415 nm after 10 min incubation at room temperature. The total flavonoid content was expressed as mg rutin equivalents (RE) per g crude extract using a rutin standard curve.

2.3. Determination of Antioxidant Activities

2.3.1. Total Antioxidant Capacity (TAC). The reduction of molybdenum(VI) to molybdenum(V) by the plant extracts was used to assess the total antioxidant capacity following the method described by Berk et al. [13] with slight modifications. An aliquot of plant extract (0.3 mL) was combined with 3 mL of reagent solution (0.6 M sulfuric acid, 28 mM sodium phosphate, and 4 mM ammonium molybdate). The absorbance was read at 695 nm after 90 min incubation at 95°C. EC_{50}, that is, the effective concentration at which the absorbance was 0.5, was calculated for the plant extracts and trolox.

2.3.2. β-Carotene/Linoleic Acid Bleaching Activity. The antilipid peroxidation capacities of the plant extracts were measured by β-carotene/linoleic acid bleaching [14]. A stock solution of β-carotene and linoleic acid was prepared from 0.5 mg β-carotene dissolved in 1 mL chloroform, 25 μL linoleic acid, and 200 mg Tween 40. The chloroform was completely evaporated using a vacuum evaporator and 100 mL of oxygenated distilled water was added to the residual mixture. The mixture was shaken vigorously and 1.5 mL of this mixture was added to 0.5 mL plant extract and the absorbance at time 0 was measured at 490 nm. The absorbance was monitored at regular intervals, that is, at 30, 60, 90, and 120 min. The bleaching rate (R) of β-carotene was calculated according to

$$R = \left[\frac{\ln (a/b)}{t} \right], \quad (1)$$

where ln represents natural log, a is the absorbance at time 0, and b is the absorbance at time t (30, 60, 90, and 120 min). The antioxidant activity (AA) was calculated in terms of percentage inhibition relative to the control from

$$AA = \left[\frac{\left(R_{\text{Control}} - R_{\text{Sample}} \right)}{R_{\text{Control}}} \right] \times 100. \quad (2)$$

IC_{50}, that is, the concentration of plant extract/trolox required to scavenge 50% of linoleate, was then determined.

2.3.3. 1,1-Diphenyl-2-picrylhydrazyl (DPPH) Free Radical Scavenging Assay. The effect of the plant extracts on DPPH radical was assessed according to the method described by Sarikurkcu [15]. Briefly, 1 mL of plant extract was added to 4 mL DPPH solution (0.004%) in methanol. The absorbance was measured at 517 nm after 30 min incubation at room temperature in the dark. The radical scavenging activity was calculated as follows: % inhibition = [(Abs_{blank} − Abs_{sample})/Abs_{blank}] × 100, where Abs_{blank} is absorbance of the blank and Abs_{sample} is absorbance of the sample. Trolox is used as a positive control and IC_{50} was then determined.

2.3.4. 2,2-Azino-bis(3-ethylbenzothiazoline-6-sulfonic acid) (ABTS) Radical Cation Scavenging Activity. The scavenging activity of the plant extracts on ABTS$^{\bullet+}$ radical was measured according to the method of Re et al. [16] with slight modifications. ABTS$^{\bullet+}$ radical was produced by reacting 7 mM ABTS solution with 2.45 mM potassium persulfate. The mixture was allowed to stand for 12 to 16 h in the dark at room temperature. The resulting ABTS solution was diluted with methanol and adjusted to absorbance of 0.700 ± 0.02 at 734 nm. Plant extract (1 mL) was added to ABTS solution (2 mL) and after 30 min incubation at room temperature the absorbance was measured at 734 nm. The radical scavenging activity was calculated as follows: % inhibition = [(Abs_{blank} − Abs_{sample})/Abs_{blank}] × 100, where Abs_{blank} is absorbance of the blank and Abs_{sample} is absorbance of the sample. Trolox is used as a positive control and IC_{50} was then calculated.

2.3.5. Cupric Ion Reducing Antioxidant Capacity (CUPRAC) Assay. The cupric ion reducing antioxidant capacity

(CUPRAC) was determined according to the method described by Apak et al. [17]. Plant extract (0.5 mL) was added to the reaction mixture containing 10 mM copper chloride (1 mL), 7.5 mM neocuproine (1 mL), and 1 M ammonium acetate buffer at pH 7 (1 mL). The absorbance was read at 450 nm after 30 min incubation at room temperature. EC_{50} was determined for each plant extract.

2.3.6. Ferric Reducing Antioxidant Power (FRAP) Assay. The FRAP assay was carried out as described by Aktumsek et al. [18] with slight modifications. Plant extract (0.1 mL) was added to FRAP reagent solution (2 mL) containing 0.3 M acetate buffer, pH 3.6, 10 mM 2,4,6-tris(2-pyridyl)-s-triazine (TPTZ) in 40 mM HCl, and 20 mM ferric chloride in a ratio of 10 : 1 : 1 (v/v/v). The absorbance was then measured at 593 nm after 30 min incubation at room temperature. EC_{50} of the plant extract was then determined.

2.3.7. Metal Chelating Activity on Ferrous Ions. The metal chelating activities of the plant extracts on ferrous ions were determined by the method described by Aktumsek et al. [18]. Briefly, 2 mL of plant extract was added to 0.05 mL 2 mM iron chloride. The reaction was initiated by the addition of 0.2 mL 5 mM ferrozine. The absorbance was read at 562 nm after 10 min incubation at room temperature. The chelating activity was calculated as follows: % inhibition = [(Abs_{blank} − Abs_{sample})/Abs_{blank}]×100, where Abs_{blank} is absorbance of the blank and Abs_{sample} is absorbance of the sample. EDTA is used as a positive control and IC_{50} was calculated.

2.4. Determination of Cholinesterase, Tyrosinase, α-Amylase, and α-Glucosidase Activity

2.4.1. Cholinesterase Inhibition Assay. Cholinesterase inhibitory activity was measured using Ellman's method as previously reported by Aktumsek et al. [18] with slight modifications. The plant extract (50 μL) was mixed with dithiobisnitro-benzoate (DTNB) (125 μL) and cholinesterase solution (25 μL) in Tris-HCl buffer (pH 8.0) in a 96-well microplate. The reaction was initiated by the addition of 25 μL of acetylthiocholine iodide or butyrylthiocholine chloride. The absorbance was read at 405 nm after 10 min incubation at room temperature. The anticholinesterase activity was calculated as follows: % inhibition = [(Abs_{blank} − Abs_{sample})/Abs_{blank}]×100, where Abs_{blank} is absorbance of the blank and Abs_{sample} is absorbance of the sample. Galantamine is used as a positive control and IC_{50} value was determined.

2.4.2. Tyrosinase Inhibition Assay. Tyrosinase inhibitory activity was measured using the modified dopachrome method previously described by Orhan et al. [19] with slight modifications. Plant extract (25 μL) was mixed with tyrosinase solution (40 μL) and phosphate buffer (pH 6.8) (100 μL) in a 96-well microplate and incubated for 15 min at 37°C. L-DOPA (40 μL) was then added to the mixture to initiate the reaction. The absorbance was read at 492 nm after 10 min incubation at 37°C. The percentage inhibition of tyrosinase was calculated as follows: % inhibition = [(Abs_{blank} − Abs_{sample})/Abs_{blank}] × 100, where Abs_{blank} is

absorbance of the blank and Abs_{sample} is absorbance of the sample. Kojic acid is used as a positive control and IC_{50} was calculated.

2.4.3. α-Amylase Inhibition Assay. α-Amylase inhibitory activity was performed using the Caraway-Somogyi iodine-potassium iodide method [20] with some modifications. Briefly, plant extract (25 μL) was mixed with α-amylase solution (50 μL) in phosphate buffer (pH 6.9) with 6 mM sodium chloride in a 96-well microplate and incubated for 10 min at 37°C. The reaction was initiated by the addition of 0.05% starch solution (50 μL). The reaction mixture was incubated for 10 min at 37°C. The reaction was then stopped by the addition of 1 M HCl (25 μL), followed by addition of the iodine-potassium iodide solution (100 μL). The absorbance was measured at 630 nm. The percentage inhibition of α-amylase was calculated as follows: % inhibition = [(Abs_{blank} − Abs_{sample})/Abs_{blank}]×100, where Abs_{blank} is absorbance of the blank and Abs_{sample} is absorbance of the sample. Acarbose is used as a positive control and IC_{50} was determined.

2.4.4. α-Glucosidase Inhibition Assay. α-Glucosidase inhibitory activity was performed following the previous method described by Palanisamy et al. [21] with some modifications. Plant extract (50 μL) was mixed with glutathione (50 μL), α-glucosidase solution (50 μL) in phosphate buffer (pH 6.8), and PNPG (50 μL) in a 96-well microplate and incubated for 15 min at 37°C. The reaction was stopped by the addition of 0.2 M sodium carbonate (50 μL) and the absorbance was read at 400 nm. The percentage inhibition of α-glucosidase was calculated as follows: % inhibition = [(Abs_{blank} − Abs_{sample})/Abs_{blank}]×100, where Abs_{blank} is absorbance of the blank and Abs_{sample} is absorbance of the sample. Acarbose is used as a positive control and IC_{50} was determined.

2.5. Statistical Analysis. The experiments were carried out in triplicate. The results are expressed as mean ± standard deviation (SD). The differences between the different extracts were analyzed using one-way analysis of variance (ANOVA) followed by Tukey's honestly significant difference post hoc test with α = 0.05 using SPSS v. 14.0.

3. Results

3.1. Quantification of Phenolic Compounds. The total phenol and flavonoid content of the plant extracts are summarised in Table 1. Oh extracts yielded higher phenol content in the following order: OhEA > OhMeOH > OhAq. On the other hand, it was observed that the flavonoid content of the plant extracts varied in the following order: MeOH > Aq > EA. The methanolic and aqueous extracts of Hv showed the highest flavonoid content.

3.2. Determination of Antioxidant Activities. Table 2 summarises the reducing power and radical scavenging and metal chelating capacities of Hv, Oh, and Vt extracts. It was found that the plant extracts showed variable radical scavenging capabilities on DPPH• and ABTS•+. Methanolic extracts of Hv and Oh and aqueous extract of Oh (IC_{50}: 0.30 ± 0.005,

TABLE 1: Total phenol and flavonoid content of the plant extracts.

Plant extracts	Total phenol content (mg GAE/g extract)	Total flavonoid content (mg RE/g extract)
HvEA	20.96 ± 1.291	2.41 ± 0.205
HvMeOH	45.11 ± 1.399	39.71 ± 0.092
HvAq	37.97 ± 1.033	34.53 ± 2.001
OhEA	83.25 ± 0.914	9.92 ± 0.030
OhMeOH	73.20 ± 0.756	27.00 ± 0.544
OhAq	69.38 ± 0.992	25.20 ± 0.088
VtEA	27.19 ± 1.283	1.45 ± 0.200
VtMeOH	20.90 ± 0.190	22.45 ± 0.325
VtAq	25.86 ± 0.085	8.67 ± 0.109

Hv: *Hedysarum varium*; Oh: *Onobrychis hypargyrea*; Vt: *Vicia truncatula*; EA: ethyl acetate extract; MeOH: methanolic extract; Aq: aqueous extract.

0.29 ± 0.002, and 0.27 ± 0.001 mg/mL, resp.) significantly ($P < 0.05$) scavenged DPPH$^\bullet$ as compared to the positive control trolox (IC$_{50}$: 0.31 ± 0.003 mg/mL). On the other hand, it was observed that the plant extracts scavenged ABTS$^{\bullet+}$ but were significantly ($P < 0.05$) less active than trolox (IC$_{50}$: 0.18 ± 0.004 mg/mL). Likewise, the plant extracts showed low chelating activity on ferrous ions. Ethyl acetate extracts of Hv and Vt (IC$_{50}$: 1.07 ± 0.006 and 1.05 ± 0.001 mg/mL, resp.) showed potent β-carotene bleaching capacities as compared to trolox (IC$_{50}$: 1.10 ± 0.004 mg/mL). Additionally, it was noted that the plant extracts exhibited variable reducing potential. However, as shown in Table 2, none of the plant extracts exhibited reducing activity which was significantly ($P < 0.05$) lower than trolox.

It was observed that the plant extracts exhibited variable inhibitory effects on cholinesterases (acetyl cholinesterase and butyryl cholinesterase), tyrosinase, α-amylase, and α-glucosidase (Table 3). The plant extracts were significantly ($P < 0.05$) less active than the positive controls galantamine, kojic acid, and acarbose against cholinesterases, tyrosinase, and α-amylase, respectively. However, Hv extracts (IC$_{50}$: 3.77 ± 0.016, 2.88 ± 0.051, and 5.18 ± 0.078 mg/mL for ethyl acetate, methanolic, and aqueous extract, resp.), methanolic and aqueous extracts of Oh (IC$_{50}$: 3.89 ± 0.097 and 5.86 ± 0.050 mg/mL, resp.), and ethyl acetate extract of Vt (IC$_{50}$: 2.74 ± 0.044 mg/mL) significantly ($P < 0.05$) inhibited α-glucosidase as compared to acarbose (IC$_{50}$: 6.67 ± 0.200 mg/mL).

4. Discussion

The use of plant-based products for the management and treatment of diseases is gaining much momentum from both scientific and consumer perspectives. Indeed, herbal therapies have been used for curative purposes since the dawn of civilisation. The relentless efforts for wellbeing and to combat diseases have guided scientists as well as health care providers towards safer and natural alternatives such as medicinal plants. Currently, there is a renewed interest in natural inhibitors from plant-based medicines to modulate physiological effects of enzymes linked to several pathologies such

as diabetes, obesity, neurodegenerative diseases, and inflammation, amongst others. The present study has endeavoured to investigate the possible inhibitory effects of three medicinal plants to modulate key enzymes involved in diabetes (α-amylase and α-glucosidase), neurodegenerative disorders (tyrosinase, acetylcholinesterase, and butyrylcholinesterase), and melanogenesis (tyrosinase).

Diabetes is a chronic disease characterised by elevated blood sugar level which leads to the onset of serious health complications such as cardiovascular problems, nephropathy, and neuropathy [22]. The inhibition of α-amylase and α-glucosidase which are involved in the hydrolysis of sugars *in vivo* has been an important strategy for the management of diabetes thereby lowering postprandial glucose level. Inhibitors of α-glucosidase delay the breaking down of carbohydrate in the gut and decrease postprandial blood glucose peak in diabetic patients. Synthetic oral hypoglycaemic agents such as acarbose, miglitol, and voglibose are currently used for the treatment of diabetes [23]. However, their side effects, such as abdominal discomforts and flatulence, have guided research towards safer and more effective alternatives notably from natural sources [24]. In the present study, the plant extracts showed inhibition against both α-amylase and α-glucosidase. Additionally, it was noted that the plant extracts were potent inhibitors of α-glucosidase and the methanolic and aqueous extracts of Hv and Oh showed significantly lower IC$_{50}$ values than acarbose and therefore can be potentially useful as an effective therapy for postprandial hyperglycemia with minimal side effects. This is in line with report of Picot et al. [25] who reported natural α-glucosidase inhibitors from plants to have strong inhibition towards the activity of the enzyme compared to acarbose.

Plant extracts from the present study were found to inhibit acetylcholinesterase although their inhibitory action was less potent than the known inhibitor galantamine. It was also found that some of the plant extracts showed inhibition against another cholinesterase enzyme, butyrylcholinesterase. Inhibition of cholinesterases, the key enzymes in the breakdown of acetylcholine, is considered one of the treatment strategies against several neurological disorders. The inhibition of cholinesterases leads to an increase in the concentration of acetylcholine in the brain which subsequently results in an increase in communication between the brain nerve cells [22, 26]. Indeed, both acetylcholinesterase and butyrylcholinesterase inhibitors have been key targets for the treatment of neurodegenerative disorders such as Alzheimer's disease [27, 28]. Cholinesterase inhibitors constitute, to date, the most effective approach to treat the cognitive symptoms of neurological disorders. Hence, plants studied in the present study can be of therapeutic utility both on cognitive performances and on the quality of life in these patients.

Tyrosinase is a key enzyme responsible for the hydroxylation of tyrosine to L-DOPA and its subsequent oxidation to dopaquinone [29]. Dopaquinone and its derivatives produced via the biosynthesis of melanin by tyrosinase are thought to play a pivotal role in the degeneration of nigrostriatal dopaminergic neurons in Parkinson's disease [30]. Tyrosinase inhibitors have attracted much interest due

TABLE 2: Reducing power, metal chelation activity, and radical scavenging potential of the plant extracts.

| Plant extracts/positive controls | IC$_{50}$ (mg/mL) | | | | TAC | EC$_{50}$ (mg/mL) | |
	DPPH•	ABTS•+	Metal chelating	β-Carotene/linoleic acid bleaching activity		CUPRAC	FRAP
HvEA	6.27 ± 1.523**	11.81 ± 0.682**	NA	1.07 ± 0.006*	1.18 ± 0.013**	3.01 ± 0.279**	1.98 ± 0.107**
HvMeOH	0.30 ± 0.005*	2.75 ± 0.004**	51.54 ± 4.795**	1.10 ± 0.009**	1.54 ± 0.045**	0.69 ± 0.031**	0.44 ± 0.007**
HvAq	0.35 ± 0.014**	1.50 ± 0.039**	1.40 ± 0.010**	1.10 ± 0.006**	2.85 ± 0.001**	0.80 ± 0.008**	0.43 ± 0.007**
OhEA	0.31 ± 0.003**	1.20 ± 0.007**	NA	1.14 ± 0.008**	0.90 ± 0.014**	0.81 ± 0.021**	0.34 ± 0.005**
OhMeOH	0.29 ± 0.002*	1.27 ± 0.007**	47.27 ± 1.255**	1.12 ± 0.070**	1.09 ± 0.021**	0.89 ± 0.056**	0.39 ± 0.003**
OhAq	0.27 ± 0.001*	1.22 ± 0.014**	16.79 ± 0.456**	1.06 ± 0.007**	1.44 ± 0.101**	0.80 ± 0.011**	0.37 ± 0.004**
VtEA	1.15 ± 0.002**	5.91 ± 0.083**	10.80 ± 1.453**	1.05 ± 0.001*	1.13 ± 0.004**	1.58 ± 0.276**	1.33 ± 0.061**
VtMeOH	0.84 ± 0.060**	6.23 ± 0.035**	32.35 ± 2.493**	1.12 ± 0.008**	2.48 ± 0.035**	1.44 ± 0.098**	1.16 ± 0.026**
VtAq	0.47 ± 0.004**	5.50 ± 0.252**	20.62 ± 0.060**	1.12 ± 0.003**	3.35 ± 0.008**	1.13 ± 0.015**	0.65 ± 0.009**
Trolox	0.31 ± 0.003	0.18 ± 0.004	ND	1.10 ± 0.004	0.59 ± 0.006	0.11 ± 0.008	0.05 ± 0.003
EDTA	ND	ND	0.04 ± 0.001	ND	ND	ND	ND

Hv: *Hedysarum varium*; Oh: *Onobrychis hypargyrea*; Vt: *Vicia truncatula*; EA: ethyl acetate extract; MeOH: methanolic extract; Aq: aqueous extract. *Values significantly ($P < 0.05$) lower than the positive control. **Values significantly ($P < 0.05$) higher than the positive control. NA: not active; ND: not determined.

TABLE 3: Inhibition concentration of the plant extracts on cholinesterases, tyrosinase, α-amylase, and α-glucosidase.

| Plant extracts/positive controls | IC_{50} (mg/mL) | | | | |
| | Cholinesterases | | Tyrosinase | α-Amylase | α-Glucosidase |
	Acetylcholinesterase	Butyrylcholinesterase			
HvEA	$1.44 \pm 0.001^{**}$	$3.29 \pm 0.018^{**}$	$2.63 \pm 0.035^{**}$	$3.65 \pm 0.188^{**}$	$3.77 \pm 0.016^{*}$
HvMeOH	$1.50 \pm 0.044^{**}$	NA	$2.50 \pm 0.014^{**}$	$5.59 \pm 0.191^{**}$	$2.88 \pm 0.051^{*}$
HvAq	$9.22 \pm 0.527^{**}$	NA	$3.46 \pm 0.012^{**}$	$13.39 \pm 0.219^{**}$	$5.18 \pm 0.078^{*}$
OhEA	$1.46 \pm 0.016^{**}$	$3.81 \pm 0.252^{**}$	$4.30 \pm 0.057^{**}$	$4.92 \pm 0.335^{**}$	$20.95 \pm 0.581^{**}$
OhMeOH	$1.63 \pm 0.018^{**}$	NA	$3.50 \pm 0.069^{**}$	$5.51 \pm 0.141^{**}$	$3.89 \pm 0.097^{*}$
OhAq	$4.46 \pm 0.024^{**}$	NA	$21.76 \pm 1.357^{**}$	$11.84 \pm 0.465^{**}$	$5.86 \pm 0.050^{*}$
VtEA	$1.57 \pm 0.003^{**}$	$3.15 \pm 0.052^{**}$	$3.21 \pm 0.012^{**}$	$2.07 \pm 0.095^{**}$	$2.74 \pm 0.044^{*}$
VtMEOH	$1.60 \pm 0.008^{**}$	NA	$2.26 \pm 0.010^{**}$	$4.21 \pm 0.180^{**}$	$8.68 \pm 0.214^{**}$
VtAq	$5.55 \pm 0.080^{**}$	NA	$4.41 \pm 0.145^{**}$	$13.74 \pm 0.514^{**}$	$8.31 \pm 0.355^{**}$
Galantamine	0.002 ± 0.000	0.002 ± 0.001	ND	ND	ND
Kojic acid	ND	ND	0.14 ± 0.001	ND	ND
Acarbose	ND	ND	ND	1.00 ± 0.023	6.67 ± 0.200

Hv: *Hedysarum varium*; Oh: *Onobrychis hypargyrea*; Vt: *Vicia truncatula*; EA: ethyl acetate extract; MeOH: methanolic extract; Aq: aqueous extract. *Values significantly ($P < 0.05$) lower than the positive control. **Values significantly ($P < 0.05$) higher than the positive control.

to the key role of tyrosinase in mammalian melanogenesis [31]. Inhibitors of the tyrosinase enzyme, such as kojic acid (by-product in the fermentation of malting rice, produced naturally by several species of fungi such as *Aspergillus oryzae*), azelaic acid (isolated from wheat, rye, and barley and produced naturally by *Malassezia furfur*), and arbutin (extracted from bearberry plants), have been utilised in the pharmaceutical and cosmetic industry for their potential of thwarting the excessive production of melanin. However, controversies still persist in the literature concerning their safety and efficacy [31, 32]. Interestingly, plant extracts evaluated in the present study were found to inhibit tyrosinase activity but at higher concentration than the known inhibitor kojic acid.

The variation in activity of the plant extracts against these enzymes might be explained based on the complex composition and potential synergistic effect(s) of individual phytochemicals present in each sample. Interestingly, we found varying concentration of phenolics and flavonoids in extracts of these plants. Previously, it has been reported that inhibitory activity of plant extracts might be due to the presence of several phytochemicals such as flavonoids, saponins, and tannins. Additionally, studies on α-amylase and α-glucosidase inhibitors isolated from medicinal plants suggest that several potential inhibitors belong to flavonoid class which has features of inhibiting metabolic enzymes. Recently, it has been shown that phenolics play a role in mediating amylase inhibition and therefore have potential to contribute to the management of type 2 diabetes [33].

Free radicals are known to play a pivotal role in the onset and exacerbation of several pathologies [34]. By counteracting these free radicals, antioxidants help in preserving good health. Indeed, phytochemicals have received much interest owing to their molecular structure which consists of hydroxyl groups on aromatic rings and this has been associated with their functionality as oxidant scavengers [35]. Phytochemicals act by inhibiting oxidative chain reactions

at cellular level thereby increasing their therapeutic efficacy [36]. In the present study, the phenolic content of the plant extracts was estimated using the Folin-Ciocalteau method. This method is rapid and simple but also measures various interfering nonphenolic compounds such as ascorbic acid, thiol, and nitrogen containing compounds [37]. Flavonoids are the major class of phenolic compounds and are known to exhibit strong antioxidant activities [38, 39]. Interestingly, in the present study, it was observed that Oh extract showed high phenolic and flavonoid content.

Various assays were employed to study the antioxidant potential of the extracts of Hv, Oh, and Vt. The gross antioxidant capacities of the plant extracts were determined using two methods, namely, the TAC and β-carotene bleaching assays. The TAC assay is based on the reduction of Mo(IV) to Mo(V) by antioxidants and the formation of green phosphate/Mo(V) compound [36]. On the other hand, the ability of the plant extracts to scavenge linoleate-derived free radicals and thus prevent β-carotene bleaching was also investigated [40]. It was observed that Oh extracts actively reduced Mo(IV) to Mo(V) but their EC_{50} values were significantly higher than the standard trolox. It was also noted that ethyl acetate extracts showed IC_{50} significantly lower than trolox for the β-carotene bleaching assay. This was associated with the "polar paradox theory" which suggests that nonpolar antioxidants are more effective in relatively nonpolar systems [24]. The high phenolic and flavonoid content of Oh were linked to the observed gross antioxidant capacity.

The reducing power of plant extracts is regarded as an indication of their antioxidant capacities [41]. FRAP and CUPRAC were used to assess the reductive potentials of the plant extracts. The plant extracts exerted variable reducing potentials thereby suggesting that phenolic compounds acted as reductones. Reductones are thought to exert antioxidant action by donating a hydrogen atom thus breaking the chain reaction [42]. Additionally, it was reported that reductones react with peroxide precursors thereby preventing peroxide formation [43].

The free radical quenching potential of the plant extracts was determined using two nitrogen-centered radicals, namely, DPPH$^\bullet$ and ABTS$^{\bullet+}$. DPPH$^\bullet$ is a stable dark purple free radical which turns into a yellow stable diamagnetic molecule upon reaction with antioxidants [44]. On the other hand, ABTS$^{\bullet+}$ is a blue radical cation which is converted into a colourless form in the presence of a hydrogen donor [42]. Results from the present study have demonstrated that the plant extracts showed good abilities to quench both DPPH$^\bullet$ and ABTS$^{\bullet+}$. The ability of the plant extracts to quench DPPH$^\bullet$ and ABTS$^{\bullet+}$ was related to the observed high phenol content.

One of the most important mechanisms of action of antioxidants involves the chelation of prooxidant metals such as iron. Iron promotes oxidation by acting as catalyst of free radical chain reactions [45]. The chelation of iron by phytochemicals decreases its prooxidant effect through the stabilisation of its oxidised form [40]. Indeed, the plant extracts were found to chelate iron but were less potent than EDTA.

5. Conclusion

Data gathered from the present investigation demonstrated that Hv, Oh, and Vt possessed antioxidant capabilities and also exhibited inhibitory potential against cholinesterase, tyrosinase, α-amylase, and α-glucosidase *in vitro*. Furthermore, to date, no such scientific information on these plants has been gathered. However, it was observed that the antioxidant capacities and α-amylase, cholinesterase, and tyrosinase inhibitory activities of the plant extracts were less potent than the controls. Thus, it might be argued that the plants possessed moderate antioxidant and enzyme inhibitory properties. Further studies are needed for the identification of bioactive constituents for the determination of molecular mechanisms involved in antioxidant and enzymatic activities of these plant extracts.

Conflict of Interests

The authors declare that there is no conflict of interests regarding the publication of this paper.

Acknowledgment

This research was supported by the Scientific and Technological Research Council of Turkey (TUBITAK) (Project no. 113Z892).

References

[1] E. Özdemir and K. Alpınar, "An ethnobotanical survey of medicinal plants in western part of central Taurus Mountains: Aladaglar (Nigde-Turkey)," *Journal of Ethnopharmacology*, vol. 166, pp. 53–65, 2015.

[2] B. Güler, E. Manav, and E. Uğurlu, "Medicinal plants used by traditional healers in Bozüyük (Bilecik–Turkey)," *Journal of Ethnopharmacology*, vol. 173, pp. 39–47, 2015.

[3] M. Mükemre, L. Behçet, and U. Çakılcıoğlu, "Ethnobotanical study on medicinal plants in villages of Çatak (Van-Turkey)," *Journal of Ethnopharmacology*, vol. 166, pp. 361–374, 2015.

[4] S. A. Sargin, "Ethnobotanical survey of medicinal plants in Bozyazı district of Mersin, Turkey," *Journal of Ethnopharmacology*, vol. 173, pp. 105–126, 2015.

[5] M. Y. Paksoy, S. Selvi, and A. Savran, "Ethnopharmacological survey of medicinal plants in Ulukışla (Niğde-Turkey)," *Journal of Herbal Medicine*, 2015.

[6] D. F. Chamberlain, "Glycyrrhiza," in *Flora of Turkey and the East Aegean 364 Islands*, P. H. Davis, Ed., pp. 260–263, Edinburgh University Press, Edinburgh, UK, 1970.

[7] P. H. Davis, R. R. Mill, and K. Tan, *Flora of Turkey and the East Aegean Islands*, vol. 10, supplement 1, Edinburgh University Press, Edinburgh, UK, 1988.

[8] S. Demirci and N. Özhatay, "An ethnobotanical study in Kahramanmaraş (Turkey); wild plants used for medicinal purpose in Andirin, Kahramanmaraş," *Turkish Journal of Pharmaceutical Sciences*, vol. 9, no. 1, pp. 75–92, 2012.

[9] S. A. Sargin, E. Akçicek, and S. Selvi, "An ethnobotanical study of medicinal plants used by the local people of Alaşehir (Manisa) in Turkey," *Journal of Ethnopharmacology*, vol. 150, no. 3, pp. 860–874, 2013.

[10] S. Hayta, R. Polat, and S. Selvi, "Traditional uses of medicinal plants in ElazIğ (Turkey)," *Journal of Ethnopharmacology*, vol. 154, no. 3, pp. 613–623, 2014.

[11] E. Yeşilada, G. Honda, E. Sezik et al., "Traditional medicine in Turkey. V. Folk medicine in the inner Taurus Mountains," *Journal of Ethnopharmacology*, vol. 46, no. 3, pp. 133–152, 1995.

[12] K. Slinkard and V. L. Singleton, "Total phenol analyses: automation and comparison with manual methods," *American Journal of Enology and Viticulture*, vol. 28, pp. 49–55, 1977.

[13] S. Berk, B. Tepe, S. Arslan, and C. Sarikurkcu, "Screening of the antioxidant, antimicrobial and DNA damage protection potentials of the aqueous extract of *Asplenium ceterach* DC," *African Journal of Biotechnology*, vol. 10, no. 44, pp. 8902–8908, 2011.

[14] C. Sarikurkcu, F. Eryigit, M. Cengiz, B. Tepe, A. Cakir, and E. Mete, "Screening of the antioxidant activity of the essential oil and methanol extract of *Mentha pulegium* L. from Turkey," *Spectroscopy Letters*, vol. 45, no. 5, pp. 352–358, 2012.

[15] C. Sarikurkcu, "Antioxidant activities of solvent extracts from endemic *Cyclamen mirabile* Hildebr. tubers and leaves," *African Journal of Biotechnology*, vol. 10, no. 5, pp. 831–839, 2011.

[16] R. Re, N. Pellegrini, A. Proteggente, A. Pannala, M. Yang, and C. Rice-Evans, "Antioxidant activity applying an improved ABTS radical cation decolorization assay," *Free Radical Biology and Medicine*, vol. 26, no. 9-10, pp. 1231–1237, 1999.

[17] R. Apak, K. Güçlü, M. Özyürek, S. Esin Karademir, and E. Erçağ, "The cupric ion reducing antioxidant capacity and polyphenolic content of some herbal teas," *International Journal of Food Sciences and Nutrition*, vol. 57, no. 5-6, pp. 292–304, 2006.

[18] A. Aktumsek, G. Zengin, G. O. Guler, Y. S. Cakmak, and A. Duran, "Antioxidant potentials and anticholinesterase activities of methanolic and aqueous extracts of three endemic *Centaurea* L. species," *Food and Chemical Toxicology*, vol. 55, pp. 290–296, 2013.

[19] I. E. Orhan, F. S. Senol, A. R. Gulpinar, N. Sekeroglu, M. Kartal, and B. Sener, "Neuroprotective potential of some terebinth coffee brands and the unprocessed fruits of *Pistacia terebinthus* L. and their fatty and essential oil analyses," *Food Chemistry*, vol. 130, no. 4, pp. 882–888, 2012.

[20] X.-W. Yang, M.-Z. Huang, Y.-S. Jin, L.-N. Sun, Y. Song, and H.-S. Chen, "Phenolics from *Bidens bipinnata* and their amylase inhibitory properties," *Fitoterapia*, vol. 83, no. 7, pp. 1169–1175, 2012.

[21] U. D. Palanisamy, L. T. Ling, T. Manaharan, and D. Appleton, "Rapid isolation of geraniin from *Nephelium lappaceum* rind waste and its anti-hyperglycemic activity," *Food Chemistry*, vol. 127, no. 1, pp. 21–27, 2011.

[22] A. Abirami, G. Nagarani, and P. Siddhuraju, "In vitro antioxidant, anti-diabetic, cholinesterase and tyrosinase inhibitory potential of fresh juice from *Citrus hystrix* and *C. maxima* fruits," *Food Science and Human Wellness*, vol. 3, no. 1, pp. 16–25, 2014.

[23] S. Gurudeeban, K. Satyavani, and T. Ramanathan, "Alpha glucosidase inhibitory effect and enzyme kinetics of coastal medicinal plants," *Bangladesh Journal of Pharmacology*, vol. 7, no. 3, pp. 186–191, 2012.

[24] G. Zengin, C. Sarikurkcu, A. Aktumsek, and R. Ceylan, "*Sideritis galatica* Bornm.: a source of multifunctional agents for the management of oxidative damage, Alzheimer's's and diabetes mellitus," *Journal of Functional Foods*, vol. 11, pp. 538–547, 2014.

[25] C. M. N. Picot, A. H. Subratty, and M. F. Mahomoodally, "Inhibitory potential of five traditionally used native antidiabetic medicinal plants on α-amylase, α-glucosidase, glucose entrapment, and amylolysis kinetics in vitro," *Advances in Pharmacological Sciences*, vol. 2014, Article ID 739834, 7 pages, 2014.

[26] J. S. Choi, M. N. Islam, M. Y. Ali, E. J. Kim, Y. M. Kim, and H. A. Jung, "Effects of C-glycosylation on anti-diabetic, anti-Alzheimer's disease and anti-inflammatory potential of apigenin," *Food and Chemical Toxicology*, vol. 64, pp. 27–33, 2014.

[27] J. K. R. da Silva, L. C. Pinto, R. M. R. Burbano et al., "Essential oils of Amazon *Piper* species and their cytotoxic, antifungal, antioxidant and anti-cholinesterase activities," *Industrial Crops and Products*, vol. 58, pp. 55–60, 2014.

[28] F. S. Senol, I. E. Orhan, and O. Ustun, "In vitro cholinesterase inhibitory and antioxidant effect of selected coniferous tree species," *Asian Pacific Journal of Tropical Medicine*, vol. 8, no. 4, pp. 269–275, 2015.

[29] D. D. Orhan, F. S. Senol, S. Hosbas, and I. E. Orhan, "Assessment of cholinesterase and tyrosinase inhibitory and antioxidant properties of *Viscum album* L. samples collected from different host plants and its two principal substances," *Industrial Crops and Products*, vol. 62, pp. 341–349, 2014.

[30] T. Hasegawa, "Tyrosinase-expressing neuronal cell line as in vitro model of Parkinson's disease," *International Journal of Molecular Sciences*, vol. 11, no. 3, pp. 1082–1089, 2010.

[31] T.-S. Chang, "An updated review of tyrosinase inhibitors," *International Journal of Molecular Sciences*, vol. 10, no. 6, pp. 2440–2475, 2009.

[32] S. Parvez, M. Kang, H.-S. Chung et al., "Survey and mechanism of skin depigmenting and lightening agents," *Phytotherapy Research*, vol. 20, no. 11, pp. 921–934, 2006.

[33] M. I. Kazeem, J. O. Adamson, and I. A. Ogunwande, "Modes of inhibition of α-amylase and α-glucosidase by aqueous extract of morinda lucida benth leaf," *BioMed Research International*, vol. 2013, Article ID 527570, 6 pages, 2013.

[34] N. Demir, O. Yildiz, M. Alpaslan, and A. A. Hayaloglu, "Evaluation of volatiles, phenolic compounds and antioxidant activities of rose hip (*Rosa* L.) fruits in Turkey," *LWT—Food Science and Technology*, vol. 57, no. 1, pp. 126–133, 2014.

[35] A. B. Tukun, N. Shaheen, C. P. Banu, M. Mohiduzzaman, S. Islam, and M. Begum, "Antioxidant capacity and total phenolic contents in hydrophilic extracts of selected Bangladeshi medicinal plants," *Asian Pacific Journal of Tropical Medicine*, vol. 7, no. 1, pp. S568–S573, 2014.

[36] N. Akhtar, Ihsan-ul-Haq, and B. Mirza, "Phytochemical analysis and comprehensive evaluation of antimicrobial and antioxidant properties of 61 medicinal plant species," *Arabian Journal of Chemistry*, 2015.

[37] H. H. Doğan, "Evaluation of phenolic compounds, antioxidant activities and fatty acid composition of *Amanita ovoidea* (Bull.) Link. in Turkey," *Journal of Food Composition and Analysis*, vol. 31, no. 1, pp. 87–93, 2013.

[38] K. Robards, P. D. Prenzler, G. Tucker, P. Swatsitang, and W. Glover, "Phenolic compounds and their role in oxidative processes in fruits," *Food Chemistry*, vol. 66, no. 4, pp. 401–436, 1999.

[39] J.-H. Xie, C.-J. Dong, S.-P. Nie et al., "Extraction, chemical composition and antioxidant activity of flavonoids from *Cyclocarya paliurus* (Batal.) Iljinskaja leaves," *Food Chemistry*, vol. 186, pp. 97–105, 2015.

[40] M. Z. Končić, M. Barbarić, I. Perković, and B. Zorc, "Antiradical, chelating and antioxidant activities of hydroxamic acids and hydroxyureas," *Molecules*, vol. 16, no. 8, pp. 6232–6242, 2011.

[41] M. B. Gholivand, M. Piryaei, and S. M. Maassoumi, "Antioxidant activity of *Ziziphora tenuoir* methanolic extracts and comparison of the essential oil in two stages of growth," *Chinese Journal of Natural Medicines*, vol. 12, no. 7, pp. 505–511, 2014.

[42] R. S. Kumar, B. Rajkapoor, and P. Perumal, "Antioxidant activities of *Indigofera cassioides* Rottl. Ex. DC. using various in vitro assay models," *Asian Pacific Journal of Tropical Biomedicine*, vol. 2, no. 4, pp. 256–261, 2012.

[43] I. Geckil, B. Ates, G. Durmaz, S. Erdogan, and I. Yilmaz, "Antioxidant, free radicalscavenging and metal characteristics of propolis," *American Journal of Biochemistry and Biotechnology*, vol. 1, pp. 27–31, 2005.

[44] U. I. Alhaji, N. U. Samuel, M. Aminu et al., "In vitro antitrypanosomal activity, antioxidant property and phytochemical constituents of aqueous extracts of nine Nigerian medicinal plants," *Asian Pacific Journal of Tropical Disease*, vol. 4, no. 5, pp. 348–355, 2014.

[45] T. M. Chaouche, F. Haddouchi, R. Ksouri, and F. Atik-Bekkara, "Evaluation of antioxidant activity of hydromethanolic extracts of some medicinal species from South Algeria," *Journal of the Chinese Medical Association*, vol. 77, no. 6, pp. 302–307, 2014.

19

High-Dose Estradiol-Replacement Therapy Enhances the Renal Vascular Response to Angiotensin II via an AT_2-Receptor Dependent Mechanism

Tahereh Safari,[1] Mehdi Nematbakhsh,[2,3,4] Roger G. Evans,[5] and Kate M. Denton[5]

[1]Department of Physiology, Zahedan University of Medical Sciences, Isfahan, Iran
[2]Water & Electrolytes Research Center, Isfahan University of Medical Sciences, Isfahan, Iran
[3]Department of Physiology, Isfahan University of Medical Sciences, Isfahan, Iran
[4]Isfahan MN Institute of Basic & Applied Sciences Research, Isfahan, Iran
[5]Department of Physiology, Monash University, Clayton, VIC, Australia

Correspondence should be addressed to Mehdi Nematbakhsh; nematbakhsh@med.mui.ac.ir

Academic Editor: Todd C. Skaar

Physiological levels of estrogen appear to enhance angiotensin type 2 receptor- (AT_2R-) mediated vasodilatation. However, the effects of supraphysiological levels of estrogen, analogous to those achieved with high-dose estrogen replacement therapy in postmenopausal women, remain unknown. Therefore, we pretreated ovariectomized rats with a relatively high dose of estrogen (0.5 mg/kg/week) for two weeks. Subsequently, renal hemodynamic responses to intravenous angiotensin II (Ang II, 30–300 ng/kg/min) were tested under anesthesia, while renal perfusion pressure was held constant. The role of AT_2R was examined by pretreating groups of rats with PD123319 or its vehicle. Renal blood flow (RBF) decreased in a dose-related manner in response to Ang II. Responses to Ang II were enhanced by pretreatment with estradiol. For example, at $300 \, \text{ng} \, \text{kg}^{-1} \, \text{min}^{-1}$, Ang II reduced RBF by 45.7 ± 1.9% in estradiol-treated rats but only by 27.3 ± 5.1% in vehicle-treated rats. Pretreatment with PD123319 blunted the response of RBF to Ang II in estradiol-treated rats, so that reductions in RBF were similar to those in rats not treated with estradiol. We conclude that supraphysiological levels of estrogen promote AT_2R-mediated renal vasoconstriction. This mechanism could potentially contribute to the increased risk of cardiovascular disease associated with hormone replacement therapy using high-dose estrogen.

1. Introduction

Women have a lower prevalence of renal and cardiovascular disease than men, at least before menopause [1–5]. The mechanistic basis of sexual dimorphism in the susceptibility to cardiovascular and renal disease remains incompletely understood. However, there is evidence that the renin angiotensin system (RAS) [6, 7] and sex hormones, especially estradiol [1], are critical players.

Angiotensin II (Ang II), the main component of RAS, is of major importance in the regulation of blood pressure, body fluid volume, and electrolyte balance [8]. Even small increases in the plasma concentration of this peptide increase arterial pressure and renal vascular resistance [9]. Ang II

also plays an important role in the progression of renal diseases [10, 11]. Activation of the Ang II receptor type 1 (AT_1R) induces vasoconstriction [7, 12, 13]. For the most part, activation of Ang II receptor type 2 (AT_2R) has been shown to induce vasodilation [7, 12]. However, there are reports that its activation can induce vasoconstriction, at least in specific vascular beds such as the renal medulla [14, 15].

There is now compelling evidence that estrogen can upregulate AT_2R function in the systemic and renal vasculature [12]. This action is thought to underlie some of the protection from cardiovascular disease afforded to premenopausal women [16–18]. But such a conclusion is at odds with the observed increase in the incidence of renal [19] and cardiovascular [20] diseases in women taking oral contraceptives. One possible explanation for this paradox relates to the dose of estrogen. That is, while physiological levels of estrogen may blunt Ang II-induced vasoconstriction by upregulating AT_2R signaling cascades, high-dose estrogen might have the opposite effect or even transform the normal vasodilator influence of AT_2R activation into a vasoconstrictor action, as has been observed in the renal medulla [14, 15]. To test this hypothesis, in the current study we examined the effects of ovariectomy and hormone "replacement" with a high dose beyond the physiological range, on responses of the renal vasculature of the rat to Ang II *in vivo*. To determine the role of the AT_2R, rats were studied during treatment with the AT_2R antagonist PD123319 or its vehicle.

2. Methods

2.1. Animals. Female Wistar rats (10 to 15 weeks of age) were used in this study (n = 28). The rats were housed individually at a temperature of 23–25°C with a 12 h light/dark cycle, with the dark period between 19:00 and 07:00 hours. The rats had free access to water and food. The rats were acclimatized to this diet for at least one week prior to surgery. The experimental procedures were approved in advance by the Isfahan University of Medical Sciences Ethics Committee.

2.2. Ovariectomy. The animals were anesthetized with ketamine (75 mg/kg, i.p.). An incision measuring 2 cm in length was made in the subabdominal area. The abdominal muscles were opened and the intestine was retracted. The ureteric tube and the vascular base of ovaries were ligated, and the ovaries were removed. The muscle and skin incisions were closed with sutures and the animals were allowed to recover under a heat lamp. After recovery, the animals were allowed to acclimatize to the regular diet for one week. Then, they were randomly divided into four experimental groups. Two groups (n = 5 each) received 0.5 mg/kg/week estradiol valerate (Aburaihan Co., Tehran, Iran) in sesame oil via intramuscular injections for two weeks. Two groups (n = 5 each) received the sesame oil only. At the end of the two-week run-in period, a terminal experiment was performed under general anesthesia, during which groups of estradiol and vehicle-treated rats were treated with the AT_2R antagonist PD123319 or its vehicle, and renal vascular responses to Ang II were examined (see below). A fifth group (n = 8) was sham operated. These animals were not subjected to the terminal experiment, but body weight and uterine weight were determined two weeks after surgery to allow comparison with the other experimental groups.

2.3. Terminal Procedures. Rats were anesthetized (Inactin; thiobutabarbital, 175 mg kg^{-1} i.p.; Sigma, St. Louis, MO, USA) and the trachea was isolated and cannulated to facilitate ventilation. Catheters were implanted into the jugular vein and the carotid and femoral arteries. Mean arterial pressure (MAP) was measured from the carotid artery. Femoral arterial pressure was considered as the renal perfusion pressure (RPP). In order to maintain this pressure at control levels (to avoid the direct effect of RPP elevation induced by Ang II administration) during infusion of Ang II, an adjustable

clamp was placed around the aorta above the level of the renal arteries. The left kidney was placed in a stable cup. A flow probe (type 2SB; Transonic Systems, Ithaca, NY, USA) was placed around the renal artery, so that left kidney renal blood flow (RBF) could be monitored by transit-time ultrasound flowmetry. Body temperature was continuously monitored throughout the experiment. Experimental manipulations commenced 30–60 minutes after completion of the surgical preparation. MAP, RPP, and RBF were measured continuously throughout the experiment as 2-second averages, via a data acquisition system. Renal vascular resistance was calculated as MAP/RBF.

2.4. Experimental Protocol. Groups of ovariectomized female rats and ovariectomized rats treated with high-dose estradiol received either the AT_2R antagonist PD123319 (1 mg kg^{-1} plus 1 mg kg^{-1} h^{-1} from stock of 0.5 mg/mL) or its vehicle (2 mL kg^{-1} plus 2 mL kg^{-1} h^{-1} 154 mmol L^{-1} NaCl) intravenously. This dose of PD123319 was similar to previous studies [21–23], and it was selected based on Macari et al.'s report that PD123319 is highly selective for AT2R at doses less than 1000 μg/kg/min [24]. The antagonist infusions continued for the whole experiment. Thirty minutes after commencing the infusion of PD123319 or its vehicle, a series of intravenous (via the jugular vein) infusions of Ang II (0, 30, 100, and 300 ng kg^{-1} min^{-1}) commenced in all rats. Each dose was administered until equilibration of arterial blood pressure was achieved (about 10 min), and then the measurements were performed for 3–5 minutes. The rats were killed by overdose of anesthetic at the end of the experiments, and the kidney and uterus were removed and weighted.

2.5. Statistical Analysis. Data are expressed as mean ± SEM. One-way analysis of variance (ANOVA) was applied to baseline data. Between-groups comparisons were then made using Tukey's test. Repeated measures ANOVA was used to determine whether the responses to Ang II were altered by estrogen therapy or PD123319 or an interaction between these two treatments. The Greenhouse-Geisser correction was applied to P values derived from within-subjects factors [25]. Two-tailed P ≤ 0.05 was considered statistically significant.

3. Results

3.1. Baseline Measurements. No significant differences were observed between the groups with respect to body weight, kidney weight, MAP, RPP, RBF, and RVR. However, uterine weight was 5-fold greater in estradiol-treated animals compared to vehicle-treated animals (Table 1 and Figure 1). In addition, the uterine weight of sham operated rats was 2.7-fold greater than that of the vehicle-treated ovariectomized rats but 47% less than in the estradiol-treated rats (Table 1). Collectively, these observations indicate that the dose of estradiol we used was supraphysiological.

3.2. Responses to PD123319 and Its Vehicle. There was little or no change in MAP after treatment with PD123319 or

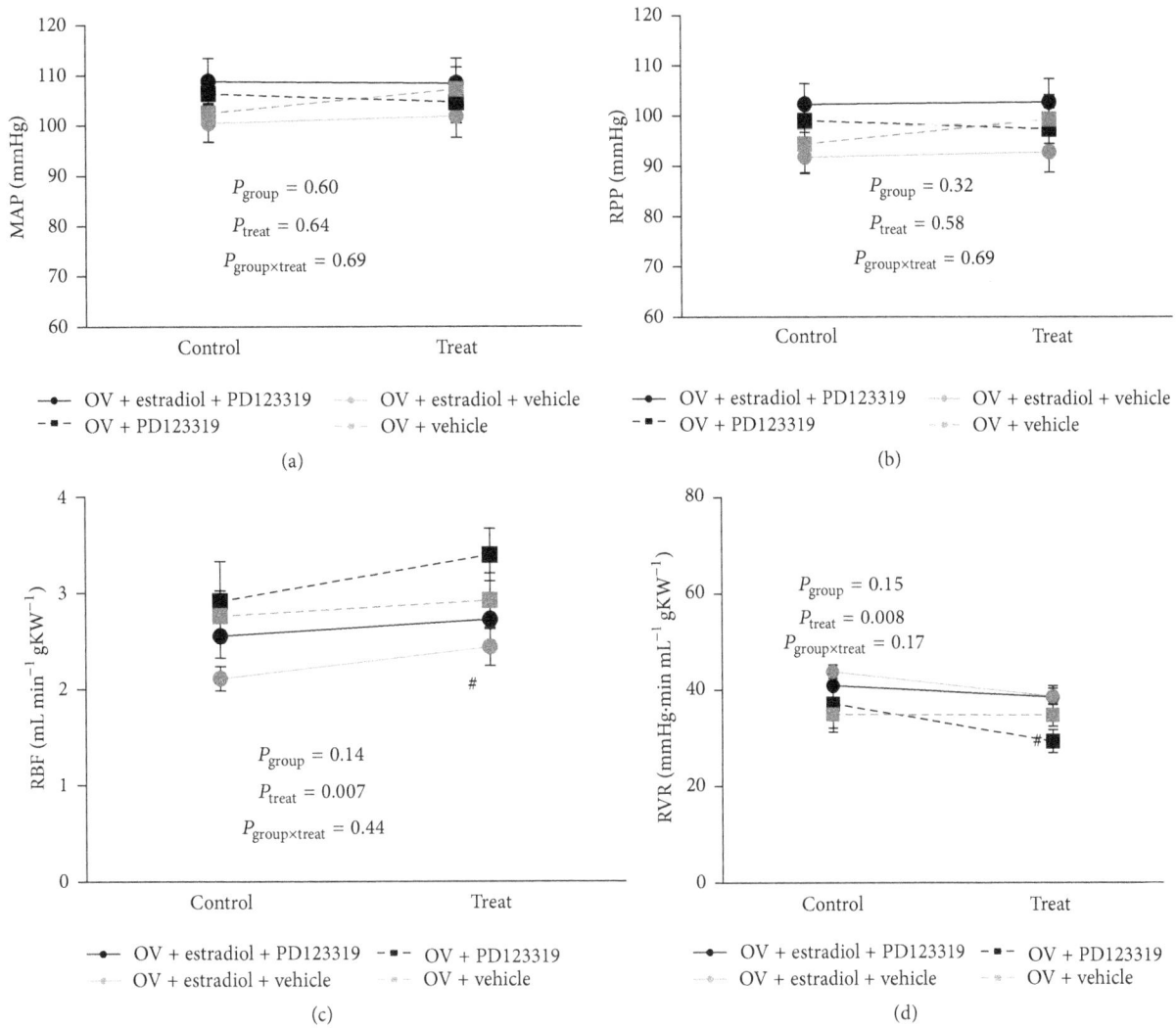

FIGURE 1: Hemodynamic variables before and after administration of vehicle or PD123319. Data are presented as mean ± SEM. The P values were derived from repeated measures ANOVA with factor groups, treatment, and their interaction. $n = 5$ per group. MAP, mean arterial pressure; RPP, renal perfusion pressure; RBF, renal blood flow per gram kidney weight; RVR, renal vascular resistance; OV, ovariectomized group.

TABLE 1: Hemodynamic variables before vehicle or PD123319 administration and body, uterus, and kidney weights at postmortem.

Group	BW g	UW mg	KW g	MAP mmHg	RPP mmHg	RBF mL/min/g KW	RVR mmHg/mL/min/g KW
OV	192 ± 8	35 ± 4	0.66 ± 0.03	103 ± 6	94 ± 6	2.7 ± 0.3	35 ± 3
OV + PD	203 ± 11	45 ± 12	0.70 ± 0.03	106 ± 2	99 ± 2	2.9 ± 0.4	37 ± 6
OV + E	185 ± 9	202 ± 19*	0.62 ± 0.03	100 ± 4	91.7 ± 3	2.1 ± 0.1	44 ± 1
OV + E + PD	183 ± 6	201 ± 26*	0.72 ± 0.04	109 ± 5	102 ± 4	2.5 ± 0.2	44 ± 2
Sham	190 ± 4	107 ± 7#	—	—	—	—	—
P_{ANOVA}	0.4	<0.0001	0.2	0.5	0.3	0.2	0.3

Data are presented as mean ± SEM of $n = 5$. The P values were derived from one-way ANOVA. Specific contrasts were generated by Tukey's *post hoc* comparisons. *$P \leq 0.05$ for comparison with ovariectomized rats treated with the vehicles for estrogen and PD123319. #$P \leq 0.05$ for comparison with all ovariectomized rats. OV: ovariectomized, E: estradiol, PD: PD123319, BW: body weight, UW: uterus weight, KW: kidney weight, MAP: mean arterial pressure, RPP: renal perfusion pressure, RBF: renal blood flow per gram kidney weight, and RVR: renal vascular resistance.

its vehicle commenced (Figure 1). Across all 20 rats, RBF increased by $12.6 \pm 3.5\%$ and RVR reduced by $8.5 \pm 2.8\%$ after administration of either PD123319 or its vehicle. However, these responses were indistinguishable in rats treated with PD123319 relative to those treated with its vehicle. Thus, it appears that renal vasodilatation occurred over time during the experiment, independent of whether rats were treated with PD123319 or its vehicle.

3.3. Responses to Ang II Infusion. Ang II infusion resulted in dose-related increases in MAP in female rats (Figure 2). The increases in MAP in response to graded doses of Ang II infusion were not significantly altered by pretreatment with either estradiol or PD123319. However, in all groups, RPP was kept relatively constant during Ang II infusion by manipulation of the aortic clamp (Figure 2).

RBF decreased and RVR increased in a dose-related fashion in response to infusion of Ang II (Figure 2; $P_{dose} < 0.0001$). In ovariectomized rats pretreated with the vehicle for estradiol, responses to Ang II appeared to be little affected by PD123319. For example, $300 \, \text{ng} \, \text{kg}^{-1} \, \text{min}^{-1}$ Ang II reduced RBF by $27 \pm 5\%$ and increased RVR by $42 \pm 14\%$ in rats pretreated with the vehicle for estradiol and then treated with PD123319 and reduced RBF by $23 \pm 9\%$ and increased RVR by $36 \pm 23\%$ in rats pretreated with the vehicle for estradiol and then treated with the vehicle for PD123319 (Figure 2). The greatest response to Ang II was observed in ovariectomized rats treated with estradiol but not PD123319. For example, $300 \, \text{ng} \, \text{kg}^{-1} \, \text{min}^{-1}$ Ang II reduced RBF by $46 \pm 2\%$ and increased RVR by $101 \pm 7\%$ in this group (Figure 2). In contrast, responses of RBF to Ang II in rats pretreated with estradiol and then treated with PD123319 were similar to those of the two groups that were not treated with estradiol. For example, $300 \, \text{ng} \, \text{kg}^{-1} \, \text{min}^{-1}$ Ang II reduced RBF by $30 \pm 7\%$ and increased RVR by $46 \pm 14\%$ in this group (Figure 2).

4. Discussion

This study was designed to determine the acute RBF response to Ang II infusion in the presence of fixed RPP in ovariectomized rats treated with supraphysiological dose of estradiol. The major new finding of the current study was that the renal vasoconstrictor response to Ang II in ovariectomized rats was enhanced by high-dose estradiol pretreatment. Interestingly, this enhanced response was not observed when AT_2R were acutely blocked with PD123319. Taken together with previous observations in the literature, discussed in detail below, our current observations suggest that the impact of estrogen on AT_2R function may be more complex than previously thought. That is, while physiological levels of estrogen might promote the vasodilator actions of AT_2R activation in the renal vasculature, supraphysiological levels might instead promote vasoconstriction. It is tempting to speculate that such a phenomenon might underlie, at least in part, the apparently deleterious effects of high-dose estrogen therapy on risk of cardiovascular and renal disease in postmenopausal women.

It is generally regarded that AT_2R, located on endothelial cells, predominately mediates vasodilatation via the generation of nitric oxide and as such opposes the vasoconstrictor actions driven by the AT_1R [26, 27]. However, AT_2R-mediated vasoconstriction has been observed under a variety of conditions, including in the mesenteric vasculature of spontaneously hypertensive rats (SHR) *in vitro* [28], the cerebral vasculature during hemorrhage in rats *in vivo* [29], the rat hydronephrotic kidney [30], the kidneys of rats with heart failure [31], and the renal medullary circulation of both normal rats and rabbits [15] and rats with renovascular hypertension [14]. The AT_2R also appears to mediate ~20% of Ang II-induced vasoconstriction in SHR during development of hypertension [32]. It is suggested that AT_2R-mediated vasoconstriction is due to an increase in smooth muscle cell AT_2R expression [26]. Our current findings indicate that supraphysiological levels of estrogen are also able to promote the vasoconstrictor actions of AT_2R activation.

In contrast to our current findings, there is considerable evidence that physiological levels of estrogen promote the vasodilator action of AT_2R. For example, a lower AT_1R/AT_2R ratio was found in female as compared to male SHR and this was associated with a lower arterial pressure in the females [33]. Also, it has been demonstrated that low dose Ang II decreases arterial pressure in females via AT_2R activation [34] and that this effect was abolished by ovariectomy and restored by estrogen replacement [35]. In addition, it has been demonstrated that the attenuated pressor response to chronic Ang II infusion observed in female mice is abolished in estrogen receptor alpha knockout mice [36] and in aged reproductively senescent mice [37]. Evidence also suggests that arterial pressure is kept normal during pregnancy by a decreased vascular responsiveness to Ang II modulated in part by upregulation of AT_2R expression. This was demonstrated in AT_2R null mice in which arterial pressure rose significantly during pregnancy [38]. Finally, Ang II caused dose-dependent forearm vasodilatation in female patients following 3-week candesartan treatment; and PD123319 infusion elevated baseline forearm vascular resistance, suggesting that tonic AT_2R-mediated vasodilatation contributes to the hemodynamic profile of AT_1R blockade [39]. Thus, there appears to be a complex relationship between the bioavailability of estrogen and the regulation of AT_2R function.

A number of limitations of our current study should be acknowledged. Firstly, we did not assess the impact of estrogen therapy on the expression of angiotensin receptors in the kidney. Secondly, we did not investigate the mechanisms underlying AT_2R-mediated renal vasoconstriction, which remain unknown [24]. Thus, the precise mechanisms that underlie the complex dose-response relationship for estrogen, which allow physiological levels to promote AT_2R-mediated renal vasodilation and high levels to promote AT_2R-mediated vasoconstriction, must be the subject of future studies. However, our study also has a number of strengths. Firstly, we can be confident that the dose of estradiol we used was supraphysiological, since it resulted in marked hypertrophy of the uterus. Secondly, we can be confident that the dose of PD123319 used was sufficient to block AT_2R in the kidney, since we have previously shown

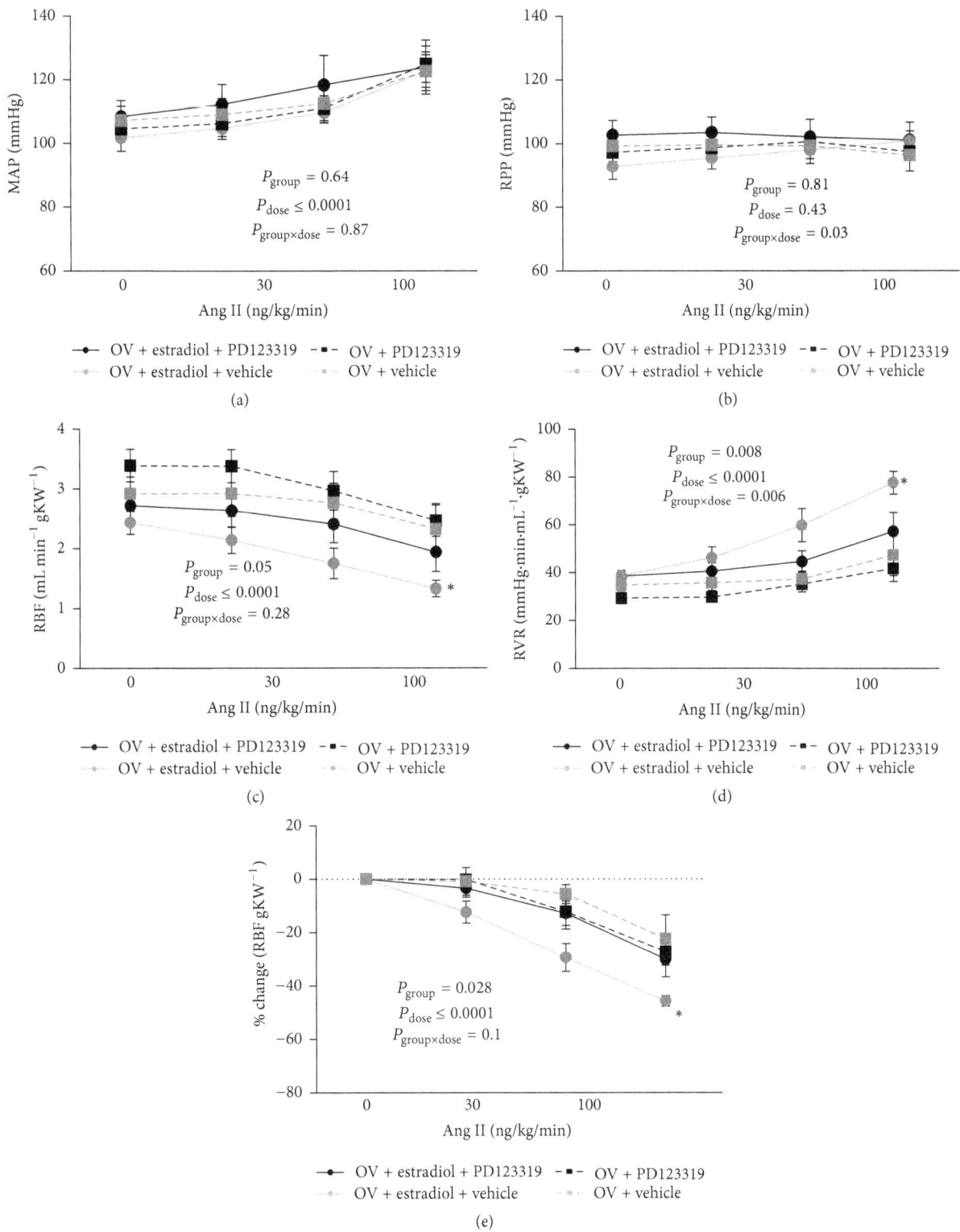

FIGURE 2: Effects of vehicle or PD123319, on responses to Ang II infusion. Data are shown as mean ± SEM. The data for RBF are also presented as percentage change from baseline. P values were derived from repeated measures ANOVA with factors group, dose (of Ang II), and their interaction. ∗ represents $P \leq 0.05$ for comparison of the response to 300 ng/kg/min in ovariectomized rats treated with estradiol and the vehicle for PD123319 compared with all other groups, derived from Tukey's *post hoc* test. $n = 5$ per group. MAP, mean arterial pressure; RPP, renal perfusion pressure; RBF, renal blood flow per gram kidney weight; RVR, renal vascular resistance; OV, ovariectomized group.

this dose to abolish AT_2R-mediated vasoconstriction in the renal medullary circulation of rats [14].

In conclusion, our current findings indicate that supraphysiological levels of estrogen can promote AT_2R-mediated vasoconstriction. This action could potentially underlie some of the detrimental influence of high-dose estrogen replacement therapy on the risk of cardiovascular disease.

Conflict of Interests

The authors declare that they have no conflict of interests.

Acknowledgment

This research was supported by Isfahan University of Medical Sciences (Grant no. 189120).

References

[1] T. Hannedouche, P. Chauveau, E. Kalou, G. Albouze, B. Lacour, and P. Jungers, "Factors affecting progression in advanced chronic renal failure," *Clinical Nephrology*, vol. 39, no. 6, pp. 312–320, 1993.

[2] D.-H. Kang, E. S. Yu, K.-I. Yoon, and R. Johnson, "The impact of gender on progression of renal disease: potential role of estrogen-mediated vascular endothelial growth factor regulation and vascular protection," *The American Journal of Pathology*, vol. 164, no. 2, pp. 679–688, 2004.

[3] J. A. Miller, D. Z. Cherney, J. A. Duncan et al., "Gender differences in the renal response to renin-angiotensin system blockade," *Journal of the American Society of Nephrology*, vol. 17, no. 9, pp. 2554–2560, 2006.

[4] J. F. Reckelhoff, "Gender differences in the regulation of blood pressure," *Hypertension*, vol. 37, no. 5, pp. 1199–1208, 2001.

[5] S. Silbiger and J. Neugarten, "Gender and human chronic renal disease," *Gender Medicine*, vol. 5, supplement 1, pp. S3–S10, 2008.

[6] S. Oparil and A. P. Miller, "Gender and blood pressure," *Journal of Clinical Hypertension*, vol. 7, no. 5, pp. 300–309, 2005.

[7] J. C. Sullivan, "Sex and the renin-angiotensin system: inequality between the sexes in response to RAS stimulation and inhibition," *American Journal of Physiology—Regulatory Integrative and Comparative Physiology*, vol. 294, no. 4, pp. R1220–R1226, 2008.

[8] J. E. Hall, M. W. Brands, and J. R. Henegar, "Angiotensin II and long-term arterial pressure regulation: the overriding dominance of the kidney," *Journal of the American Society of Nephrology*, vol. 10, supplement 12, pp. S258–S265, 1999.

[9] P. B. M. W. M. Timmermans, P. C. Wong, A. T. Chiu et al., "Angiotensin II receptors and angiotensin II receptor antagonists," *Pharmacological Reviews*, vol. 45, no. 2, pp. 205–251, 1993.

[10] G. Remuzzi, N. Perico, M. Macia, and P. Ruggenenti, "The role of renin-angiotensin-aldosterone system in the progression of chronic kidney disease," *Kidney International. Supplement*, vol. 99, pp. S57–S65, 2005.

[11] S. R. Silbiger and J. Neugarten, "The impact of gender on the progression of chronic renal disease," *American Journal of Kidney Diseases*, vol. 25, no. 4, pp. 515–533, 1995.

[12] I. Armando, M. Jezova, A. V. Juorio et al., "Estrogen upregulates renal angiotensin II AT2 receptors," *The American Journal of Physiology—Renal Physiology*, vol. 283, no. 5, pp. F934–F943, 2002.

[13] G. Nickenig, A. T. Bäumer, C. Grohè et al., "Estrogen modulates AT1 receptor gene expression in vitro and in vivo," *Circulation*, vol. 97, no. 22, pp. 2197–2201, 1998.

[14] L. M. Duke, R. E. Widdop, M. M. Kett, and R. G. Evans, "AT2 receptors mediate tonic renal medullary vasoconstriction in renovascular hypertension," *British Journal of Pharmacology*, vol. 144, no. 4, pp. 486–492, 2005.

[15] L. M. Duke, G. A. Eppel, R. E. Widdop, and R. G. Evans, "Disparate roles of AT2 receptors in the renal cortical and medullary circulations of anesthetized rabbits," *Hypertension*, vol. 42, no. 2, pp. 200–205, 2003.

[16] C. J. Pepine, W. W. Nichols, and D. F. Pauly, "Estrogen and different aspects of vascular disease in women and men," *Circulation Research*, vol. 99, no. 5, pp. 459–461, 2006.

[17] V. Regitz-Zagrosek and U. Seeland, "Sex and gender differences in clinical medicine," in *Sex and Gender Differences in Pharmacology*, vol. 214 of *Handbook of Experimental Pharmacology*, pp. 3–22, 2012.

[18] F. Grodstein, J. E. Manson, G. A. Colditz, W. C. Willett, F. E. Speizer, and M. J. Stampfer, "A prospective, observational study of postmenopausal hormone therapy and primary prevention of cardiovascular disease," *Annals of Internal Medicine*, vol. 133, no. 12, pp. 933–941, 2000.

[19] E. Brandle, E. Gottwald, H. Melzer, and H. G. Sieberth, "Influence of oral contraceptive agents on kidney function and protein metabolism," *European Journal of Clinical Pharmacology*, vol. 43, no. 6, pp. 643–646, 1992.

[20] D. H. Friedlander and A. P. Snell, "Acute coronary artery disease and oral contraceptives," *Australian and New Zealand Journal of Medicine*, vol. 5, no. 1, pp. 12–16, 1975.

[21] A. Mansoori, S. Oryan, and M. Nematbakhsh, "Role of mas receptor antagonist (A779) on pressure diuresis and natriuresis and renal blood flow in the absence of angiotensin II receptors type 1 and 2 in female and male rats," *Journal of Physiology and Pharmacology*, vol. 65, no. 5, pp. 633–639, 2014.

[22] T. Safari, M. Nematbakhsh, L. M. Hilliard, R. G. Evans, and K. M. Denton, "Sex differences in the renal vascular response to angiotensin II involves the Mas receptor," *Acta Physiologica*, vol. 206, no. 2, pp. 150–156, 2012.

[23] L. M. Hilliard, M. Nematbakhsh, M. M. Kett et al., "Gender differences in pressure-natriuresis and renal autoregulation: role of the angiotensin type 2 receptor," *Hypertension*, vol. 57, no. 2, pp. 275–282, 2011.

[24] D. Macari, S. Bottari, S. Whitebread, M. De Gasparo, and N. Levens, "Renal actions of the selective angiotensin AT2 receptor ligands CGP 42112B and PD 123319 in the sodium-depleted rat," *European Journal of Pharmacology*, vol. 249, no. 1-2, pp. 85–93, 1993.

[25] J. Ludbrook, "Repeated measurements and multiple comparisons in cardiovascular research," *Cardiovascular Research*, vol. 28, no. 3, pp. 303–311, 1994.

[26] E. S. Jones, A. Vinh, C. A. McCarthy, T. A. Gaspari, and R. E. Widdop, "AT2 receptors: functional relevance in cardiovascular disease," *Pharmacology & Therapeutics*, vol. 120, no. 3, pp. 292–316, 2008.

[27] C. A. McCarthy, R. E. Widdop, K. M. Denton, and E. S. Jones, "Update on the angiotensin AT2 receptor," *Current Hypertension Reports*, vol. 15, no. 1, pp. 25–30, 2013.

[28] R. M. Touyz, D. Endemann, G. He, J.-S. Li, and E. L. Schiffrin, "Role of AT$_2$ receptors in angiotensin II-stimulated contraction of small mesenteric arteries in young SHR," *Hypertension*, vol. 33, no. 1, part 2, pp. 366–372, 1999.

[29] L. Näveri, C. Strömberg, and J. M. Saavedra, "Angiotensin II AT2 receptor stimulation increases cerebrovascular resistance during hemorrhagic hypotension in rats," *Regulatory Peptides*, vol. 52, no. 1, pp. 21–29, 1994.

[30] K. Hayashi, H. Suzuki, and T. Saruta, "Segmental differences in angiotensin receptor subtypes in interlobular artery of hydronephrotic rat kidneys," *American Journal of Physiology*, vol. 265, no. 6, part 2, pp. F881–F885, 1993.

[31] P. F. Mento, M. E. Maita, and B. M. Wilkes, "Renal hemodynamics in rats with myocardial infarction: selective antagonism of angiotensin receptor subtypes," *American Journal of Physiology—Heart and Circulatory Physiology*, vol. 271, part 2, no. 6, pp. H2306–H2312, 1996.

[32] C. Chatziantoniou and W. J. Arendshorst, "Angiotensin receptor sites in renal vasculature of rats developing genetic hypertension," *American Journal of Physiology*, vol. 265, no. 6, article 2, pp. F853–F862, 1993.

[33] M. M. Silva-Antonialli, R. C. A. Tostes, L. Fernandes et al., "A lower ratio of AT1/AT2 receptors of angiotensin II is found in female than in male spontaneously hypertensive rats," *Cardiovascular Research*, vol. 62, no. 3, pp. 587–593, 2004.

[34] A. K. Sampson, K. M. Moritz, E. S. Jones, R. L. Flower, R. E. Widdop, and K. M. Denton, "Enhanced angiotensin II type 2 receptor mechanisms mediate decreases in arterial pressure attributable to chronic low-dose angiotensin II in female rats," *Hypertension*, vol. 52, no. 4, pp. 666–671, 2008.

[35] A. K. Sampson, L. M. Hilliard, K. M. Moritz et al., "The arterial depressor response to chronic low-dose angiotensin II infusion in female rats is estrogen dependent," *American Journal of Physiology—Regulatory Integrative and Comparative Physiology*, vol. 302, no. 1, pp. R159–R165, 2012.

[36] B. Xue, J. Pamidimukkala, D. B. Lubahn, and M. Hay, "Estrogen receptor-α mediates estrogen protection from angiotensin II-induced hypertension in conscious female mice," *The American Journal of Physiology—Heart and Circulatory Physiology*, vol. 292, no. 4, pp. H1770–H1776, 2007.

[37] K. M. Mirabito, L. M. Hilliard, G. A. Head, R. E. Widdop, and K. M. Denton, "Pressor responsiveness to angiotensin II in female mice is enhanced with age: role of the angiotensin type 2 receptor," *Biology of Sex Differences*, vol. 5, no. 1, article 13, 2014.

[38] K. M. Mirabito, L. M. Hilliard, Z. Wei et al., "Role of inflammation and the angiotensin type 2 receptor in the regulation of arterial pressure during pregnancy in mice," *Hypertension*, vol. 64, no. 3, pp. 626–631, 2014.

[39] S. Phoon and L. G. Howes, "Forearm vasodilator response to angiotensin II in elderly women receiving candesartan: role of AT$_2$-receptors," *Journal of Renin-Angiotensin-Aldosterone System*, vol. 3, no. 1, pp. 36–39, 2002.

20

Melatonin and Ischemic Stroke: Mechanistic Roles and Action

Syed Suhail Andrabi,[1] Suhel Parvez,[1] and Heena Tabassum[1,2]

[1]Department of Medical Elementology and Toxicology, Jamia Hamdard (Hamdard University), New Delhi 110062, India
[2]Department of Biochemistry, Jamia Hamdard (Hamdard University), New Delhi 110062, India

Correspondence should be addressed to Heena Tabassum; heenatabassum@jamiahamdard.ac.in

Academic Editor: Ivar von Kugelgen

Stroke is one of the most devastating neurological disabilities and brain's vulnerability towards it proves to be fatal and socio-economic loss of millions of people worldwide. Ischemic stroke remains at the center stage of it, because of its prevalence amongst the several other types attacking the brain. The various cascades of events that have been associated with stroke involve oxidative stress, excitotoxicity, mitochondrial dysfunction, upregulation of Ca^{2+} level, and so forth. Melatonin is a neurohormone secreted by pineal and extra pineal tissues responsible for various physiological processes like sleep and mood behaviour. Melatonin has been implicated in various neurological diseases because of its antioxidative, antiapoptotic, and anti-inflammatory properties. We have previously reviewed the neuroprotective effect of melatonin in various models of brain injury like traumatic brain injury and spinal cord injury. In this review, we have put together the various causes and consequence of stroke and protective role of melatonin in ischemic stroke.

1. Introduction

The brain is a highly active metabolic and complex organ of our body that performs important functions, thus, making it highly susceptible to different assaults. Any disruption in the normal functioning of the brain can lead to loss of homeostasis that can have devastating implication on whole body. Stroke leads to long-term severe disability and death [1]. There are many types of strokes like ischemic stroke, hemorrhagic stroke, and transient ischemic stroke but ischemic stroke constitutes 85% of all stroke cases which is the second leading cause of death worldwide [2, 3]. However, no effective treatment has been found to prevent the brain damage in such cases except tissue plasminogen activator with narrow therapeutic window [4–6] and there is an unmet need to develop therapeutics for neuroprotection from ischemic stroke [7]. Stroke is a broad term that refers to a range of abnormalities that are caused by occlusion or haemorrhage of one of the main arteries supplying blood to brain tissues [8]. One of the major causes of disability in ischemic stroke is the curtailment of cerebral blood flow (CBF) to a critical threshold that propagates brain damage [9]. Focal cerebral ischemia involves reduction in CBF to a specific vascular territory, usually encountered clinically due to thrombotic, hemorrhagic, or embolic strokes [10]. Within minutes of a focal ischemic stroke taking place, the core of brain tissue exposed to the most dramatic blood flow reduction is fatally injured and subsequently undergoes necrotic cell death and is called ischemia core [11]. Deprivation of oxygen by stroke is a major cause of severe neurological disability [12]. This core region is surrounded by a zone of less severely affected tissue which is rendered functionally silent by reduced blood flow but remains metabolically active [13]. This surrounding region known as the ischemic penumbra may comprise as much as half of the total lesion volume during the initial phase of ischemia and represents the region in which there is opportunity for recovery via post-stroke therapy [14]. The majority of strokes are a result of focal ischemia and one of the major blood vessels affected is the middle cerebral artery (MCA) [15]. Another type of stroke, global cerebral ischemia, involves a reduction or absence of CBF to the entire brain, situations usually encountered in severe hypotension or acute cardiac arrest. In all cases, the stroke ultimately involves dysfunction or death of brain cells, giving rise to cerebral infraction. Ischemic stroke leads to neurological deficits, cognitive impairment, and sensory impairment or in severe cases suicidal ideation [16]. This review will explore the role of reactive oxygen species (ROS), excitotoxicity, apoptosis, and current pharmacological interventions by melatonin in ischemic stroke.

2. ROS and Ischemic Stroke

Oxidative reactions are essential biological reactions necessary for producing high energy compounds which fuel cellular metabolic processes [17]. These processes include transfer of electrons and can generate by-products known as free radicals [18]. Brain cells have very low capacity to attenuate the effects of oxidative stress hence highly susceptible to oxidative damage involved in pathogenesis of various neurodegenerative diseases [19]. The brain derives its energy almost exclusively from oxidative metabolism in mitochondria respiratory chain that produces ROS by electron transport chain complexes in mitochondria [20]. ROS formation also takes place by degradation of free fatty acids by phospholipase A2 into arachidonic acid and subsequent oxidation of arachidonic acid by cyclooxygenase and lipoxygenase [21]. As a part of host immune system, NADPH oxidase activity in macrophages, neutrophils, and microglia also contributes to ROS production that is detrimental for the brain cells [22]. This overload of free radicals includes hydroxyl radicals ($^{\bullet}OH$), superoxide ($O_2^{\bullet-}$), hydrogen peroxide (H_2O_2), nitric oxide (NO), and peroxynitrite (OONO-). These free radicals promote macromolecule damage such as DNA, lipids, proteins, and carbohydrates oxidation, blood brain barrier (BBB) breakdown, and microglial infiltration into the ischemic territory [23]. This production of ROS can act as intracellular signalling molecule for various destructive pathways which include apoptotic pathway. Once activated, it leads to release of apoptotic factors such as cytochrome c and apoptosis-inducing factor (AIF), ultimately leading to neuronal death [24]. In ischemia/reperfusion, the production of ROS is particularly significant during reperfusion phase that is the hallmark in the pathogenesis of cerebral ischemia [25].

3. Excitotoxicity

Excitotoxicity, a type of neurotoxicity, occurs when there is excessive release of neurotransmitter like glutamate for prolonged time. Glutamate is the major excitory neurotransmitter responsible for neuronal growth, axon guidance, brain development, maturation, and synaptic plasticity in health and disease [26]. Glutamate acts through three families of receptors, a-amino-3-hydroxy-5-methyl-4-isoxazole-propionic acid (AMPA), N-methyl-D-aspartate (NMDA), and kainate receptors. Out of these three, NMDA receptor is widely implicated in ischemic stroke [27]. The sequence of excitotoxicity starts with the release of excessive glutamate in the extracellular space. Excessive release of glutamate plays a prominent role in various nervous system disorders like brain trauma and ischemic injury and other neurodegenerative diseases [28]. Glutamate excitotoxicity leads to overloading of Ca^{2+} through NMDA receptor leading to activation of poly

(ADP-ribose) polymerase-1 (PARP-1) and formation of poly (ADP-ribose) (PAR) polymer. PAR polymer is highly toxic to cells, killing them by sending death signals through AIF [29]. Glutamate induced overstimulation of NMDA receptor leads to increase in levels of intracellular Ca^{2+} [26]. Calcium is one of the most important signalling molecules in cell biology and maintenance of Ca^{2+} is crucial for the normal functioning of cell. In pathological conditions including ischemia/reperfusion, mitochondria accumulate significant amount of Ca^{2+} via mitochondrial calcium uniporter (MCU) from cytosol [30]. Influx of excessive Ca^{2+} into mitochondrial matrix propagates disruption of normal bioenergetic, mitochondrial ROS and increase in mitochondrial membrane permeability [31]. Excessive release of glutamate induced excitotoxicity leads to progressive neuronal death in cerebral ischemia through mitochondrial impairment and functional collapse [32].

4. Mitochondria and Ischemic Stroke

Mitochondria, a cellular powerhouse, carry out oxidative phosphorylation and generation of energy for cell. Besides being powerhouse of cell, mitochondria act as death centre by releasing several kinds of death factors like cytochrome c and AIF [43]. Once these factors are released from mitochondria, they can induce Caspase dependent (cytochrome c) and Caspase independent (AIF) cell death pathways [44]. This regulation of cell death is an important aspect of cell survival [45]. However, in cell stress, brain injury, trauma, and ischemic cell death become unregulated and lead to neurodegeneration and stroke [46]. Mitochondrial membrane contains a multicomponent protein channel composed of voltage dependent anionic channel (VDAC) in the outer membrane and adenine-nucleotide translocator (ANT) in the inner membrane [47]. Cyclophilin D (CypD), a matrix protein, and other proteins like pro- and antiapoptotic proteins primarily regulate the formation of the channel known as mitochondrial permeability transition pore (mPTP) [48, 49]. Bcl-2 associated proteins contain various antiapoptotic proteins (bcl-2, bcl-xl) and proapoptotic proteins (bax, bak) which are prime regulators of apoptosis and necrotic death [50–52]. These proapoptotic proteins play an essential role in the release of cytochrome c in cytosol through opening of mPTP [53]. During mitochondrial dysfunction, ROS/RNS and elevated Ca^{2+} levels lead to opening of mitochondrial permeability transition pore [54]. Mitochondrial overload of Ca^{2+} concentration induces mPTP opening which leads to inhibition of ATP synthesis, production of ROS, release of cytochrome c, and cell death via both apoptosis and necrosis (Figure 1) [55–57].

4.1. Caspase Dependent Apoptosis. Cascade of reactions lead to the opening of mPTP causing the release of proapoptotic proteins like cytochrome c into the cytosol from intermembrane space of mitochondria [58]. Once this component of electron transport chain is released into cytosol, it forms "apoptosome" by activating Apaf-1 and pro-Caspase-9. Activation of pro-Caspase-9 leads to formation of Caspase-9

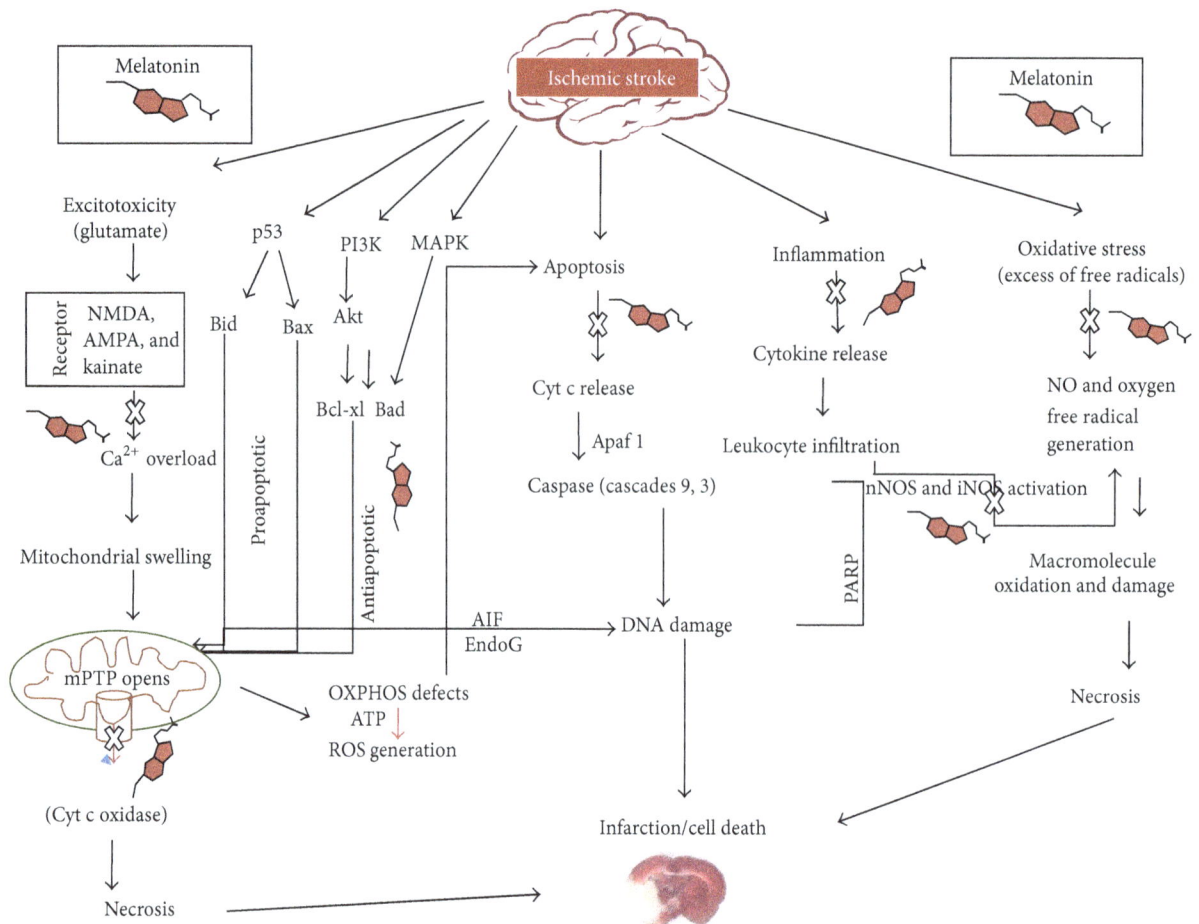

FIGURE 1: The flowchart shows a complex webbed array of events involved in the pathogenesis of cerebral ischemic injury and the role played by melatonin as neuroprotectant. Stroke onset triggers a chain of mechanisms, including activation of glutamate receptors, calcium overload with subsequent activation of apoptosis, and toxic radical release. Induction of mitochondrial permeability transition by opening of the permeability transition pore (mPTP) dissipates the mitochondrial membrane potential. These events result in cessation of electron transport and ATP formation, mitochondrial swelling, and permeabilization of the outer mitochondrial membrane, allowing the efflux of several proapoptotic molecules, including cytochrome c and apoptosis-inducing factor (AIF). In turn, cytochrome c and AIF activate a series of downstream effectors that eventually lead to the fragmentation of nuclear DNA resulting in cellular death. The cell may be also destructed by apoptosis or necrosis in case of mPTP opening and PARP activation. Triggers such as inflammation initiate the "extrinsic" pathway to programmed cell death. Conversely, calcium overload and oxygen free radicals appear to exert their effect predominantly at the mitochondrial level via the "intrinsic" pathway. In addition, crossover activation between the "extrinsic" and "intrinsic" pathway may take place through proapoptotic intermediates such as the BID protein. AIF, ATP, adenosine triphosphate; BAK; BAX, Bcl$_2$-associated × protein; Bcl$_2$, B-cell lymphoma 2 protein family; Bcl-X$_L$, B-cell lymphoma-extra-large; and BID, p53 tumor suppressor protein. The ischemia-induced inflammation then further maintains these processes via cytokine release and iNOS activation leading to oxidative stress and necrosis. Melatonin limits the extent of ischemic brain injury by interacting at multisteps of the ischemic cascade. The cross indicates the interference by melatonin.

which in turn activates Caspase-3 [59]. Caspase-3 has been identified as key mediator for apoptosis in animal models of ischemic stroke [60, 61]. Apoptotic protein Caspase-3 cleaves various substrate proteins such as DNA repair enzyme PARP-1. PARP-1 inactivation leads to DNA damage ultimately resulting in cell death [62].

4.2. Caspase Independent Apoptosis. Mitochondria can also induce apoptosis through Caspase independent pathway by releasing death proteins/factors into the cytosol. One of

the best studied cell death pathways of Caspase independent proteins is release of AIF [63]. In ischemic stroke, permeability of outer mitochondrial membrane leads to the release of AIF in cytosol by proteolysis through calcium dependent calpains and calcium independent cathepsins [64]. In cytosol, AIF interacts with cyclophilin A and their translocation into nucleus leads to DNA degradation and cell death [65]. It has been well established that AIF dependent neuronal death plays a key role in acute brain injury model system of cerebral ischemia, traumatic brain injury, and epileptic seizures [66].

4.3. Parthanatos: A New Form of Cell Death in Stroke. Parthanatos, a new form of death mediated by PARP-1, activated product PAR polymer, known as *Par,* and *Thanatos,* a Greek word meaning "death" [67]. Oxidative stress induced free radical generation causes disruption of macromolecules like proteins, lipids, and DNA. Excessive synthesis of NO reacts to $O_2^{\bullet-}$ forms OONO- which causes DNA damage and leads to activation of DNA repairing enzyme PARP-1 [68]. Overactivation of PARP-1 causes cell death by consumption of excessive NAD^+ or formation of toxic PAR polymer. Depletion of NAD^+ causes ATP depletion and drop in cellular energy subsequently leading to cell demise [69]. PARP-1 also induces release of AIF from mitochondria leading to apoptosis [70]. In cell stress, DNA damage overactivates the nuclear enzyme PARP-1 producing toxic PAR polymer leading to neuronal injury via AIF release from mitochondria [71]. Inhibition of PAR polymer mediated death signalling may offer new therapeutic strategies to prevent cell injury in stroke.

4.4. Inflammation and Stroke. After primary events of stroke induced immunogenic cascade and immune modulatory activated inflammatory signalling contribute to ischemic damage of brain [72, 73]. There is large body evidence that ischemia involves the activation of various immune cells like monocytes, microglia, and astrocytes that exacerbates that long-term brain injury [74–76]. This recruitment of immune cells leads to the activation of various other cascades and secretion of cytokines and chemokines like IL-1, IL-6, IL-8, IL-10, and TNF-α modulates various inflammatory pathways in ischemia [77, 78]. Ischemia-induced BBB disruption causes infiltration of leukocytes into brain resulting in neuronal cell death [79]. Activated microglia release various inflammatory molecules, ROS and nitric oxide, that are detrimental for brain cells [80, 81].

4.5. Endogenous Neuroprotectants in Stroke. Endogenously occurring compounds are being implicated in various diseases like cancer and neurodegenerative diseases for their chemopreventive and neuroprotective properties. Endogenously occurring bioactive compounds such as estrogens [82, 83] and progesterone [84, 85] have been widely studied for their neuroprotective role in stroke. Among these endogenous compounds, melatonin represents one of the extensively studied compounds because of its pleiotropic neuroprotective effect in stroke (Tables 1, 2, and 3).

5. Melatonin

Melatonin (N-acetyl-5-methoxytrptamine) is a natural hormone secreted by pineal gland and extra pineal tissues and others such as retina, gut, bone marrow, kidney, astrocytes, platelets, and glia cells and has been used in therapies from decades in various diseases for its antioxidative and antiapoptotic properties [85–87]. Melatonin is an ideal neuroprotective agent as it readily crosses the BBB and lacks toxicity in comparison to other neuroprotectants and has

been widely used for dietary supplement in various countries [88].

5.1. Biology and Pharmacology of Melatonin. Melatonin is formed from amino acid tryptophan by pinealocytes and rate of its synthesis depends on the activity of two enzymes, serotonin N-acetyltransferase and tryptophan hydroxylase (TPH) [89]. Tryptophan is converted into 5-hydroxytryptophan which in turn forms serotonin with the help of an enzyme aromatic amino acid decarboxylase. Serotonin is then converted into N-acetylserotonin which is the main step in the formation of melatonin. Finally, N-serotonin is converted into melatonin by another enzyme, Hydroxyindole O-methyltransferase. Out of the two, serotonin N-acetyltransferase is the main regulatory enzyme that plays pivotal role in the biosynthetic pathway of melatonin [90, 91]. Metabolism of melatonin usually takes place in liver by cytochrome P_{450} and is converted to 6-hydroxymelatonin. 6-Hydroxymelatonin is then excreted through urine in the conjugated form with sulfate and glucuronic acid [92]. There is evidence supporting the role of melatonin in regulation of various physiological functions like modulation of sleep, mood, behavior, anti-inflammatory activities, radical scavenging, immunomodulatory activities, antiangiogenic activity, and anticarcinogenic properties, and so forth [93–97]. Melatonin receptors are widely distributed in CNS as well as in the peripheral organs which acts as a lipophilic and hydrophilic molecule and able to pass the morphophysiological barriers such as the BBB [98]. Melatonin activity is mediated by the specific receptors in cellular membranes by two high affinity melatonin receptors, MT1 and MT2, which belong to the seven-transmembrane G protein-coupled receptor (GPCR) superfamily, and through nuclear receptors RZR/ROR [99]. These melatonin receptors are primarily found in the endogenous circadian master clock suprachiasmatic nuclei (SCN), located in the hypothalamus of the mammalian cells, being localized primarily to neuronal elements, and in many other organs as well, coordinate the synthesis of melatonin in the pineal gland, and also participate in several neuroendocrine and physiological processes [100].

5.2. Neuroprotective Action of Melatonin. Amphiphilic melatonin being a potent antioxidative and antiapoptotic agent has been used clinically in various CNS disorders [101]. It has been used in various neurodegenerative diseases like Alzheimer's, Parkinson, and stroke due to its property of inhibiting apoptotic pathways and by activating survival pathways due to its protective properties [102]. Melatonin has conferred a cerebral-protective effect, as shown by reduced infarct volume, lowered brain edema, and increased neurological scores by inducing upregulation of SIRT1 which is also associated with an increase in the antiapoptotic factor, Bcl2, and a reduction in the proapoptotic factor, Bax [103]. Melatonin (5 mg/kg) pretreatment *intraperitoneally* has diminished the increased expression of Nox2 and Nox4, reduced ROS levels, and inhibited cell apoptosis which may contribute to its antioxidant and antiapoptotic effects during

TABLE 1: Effect of melatonin on ischemic model of rat.

Dose	Duration	Effect/result	References
5 mg/kg b.w, i.p	30 min before MCAO	↓ROS, ↓NOX2, and ↓NOX4 expression, ↓TUNEL positive cells	[33]
5 mg/kg b.w, i.p	30 min before and 60, 120 min after occlusion	↓nitrite level, ↓MDA, and ↓Ca^{2+}	[34]
5 mg/kg b.w, i.p	At 90 min of reperfusion	↑PSD-95, ↑GAP-45, and ↑MMP-9	[35]
5 mg/kg b.w, i.p	Prior to MCAO	↑parvalbumin and ↑hippocalcin ↓Ca^{2+}	[36]
5 mg/kg b.w, i.p	Prior to MCAO	↓phosphorylation of Raf-1, MEK1/2, ERK 1/2, and ↓TUNEL positive cells	[37]

TABLE 2: Effect of melatonin in mice model of ischemic stroke.

Dose	Duration	Effect/result	References
10 mg/kg b.w, i.p	Twice at ischemia reperfusion	↑SIRT1, ↑BCL-2, and ↓Bax. ↓mitochondrial membrane potential, ↑mitochondrial complex I, ↑mitochondrial cytochrome c, and ↓cytoplasmic cytochrome c level	[38]
5 mg/kg b.w, i.v	Upon reperfusion	↑TIMP expression, ↑PAI activity, ↓uPA activity, and ↓MMP-9	[39]
4 mg/kg b.w, oral	After 24 hr ischemia for 29 days through drinking water	↑neuronal survival, ↑rotarod, ↑grip strength, and ↓anxiety and ↓hyperactivity	[40]

brain ischemia reperfusion [38]. Mitochondrial apoptotic protein cytochrome c release was directly inhibited by melatonin (10 mg/kg b.wt.) in the model of ischemic injury [33]. Melatonin given in chronic dose has shown to redeem both impaired adult neurogenesis and the decreased density of hippocampal granule cells and reduced synaptic inhibition in Ts65Dn mouse (TS) by increasing the density and/or activity of glutamatergic synapses in the hippocampus leading to recovery of hippocampal LTP in trisomic animals. These results show that melatonin possesses cognitive-enhancing effects as seen in adult TS mice that could be mediated by the normalization of their electrophysiological and neuromorphological abnormalities. This evidence point out that melatonin represents an effective treatment in retarding the progression of Down's syndrome neuropathology [104]. Melatonin and its metabolites have been able to modulate the oxidative stress by reducing ROS, MDA, and NO and restored the GSH and SOD level in various ischemic studies [105, 106].

6. Neuroprotective Mechanisms of Melatonin in Ischemic Stroke

6.1. Reduced Oxidative Damage. It has been well documented that oxidative stress is involved in ischemic injury especially after reperfusion. It has shown that melatonin is effective antioxidant in various *in vitro* and *in vivo* models of neurodegenerative diseases not only by scavenging free radicals but also by increasing the gene expression of antioxidative enzymes like GPx, GR, and SOD [107]. Dihydroethidium (DHE) fluorescence study using a live-animal imaging system (IVIS) showed that melatonin attenuated the free radical production via MT2 receptor in mice model of ischemia [108].

6.2. Antiapoptotic Activity of Melatonin. Mitochondria are the prime target for melatonin in neurodegenerative diseases as it maintains mitochondrial homeostasis. Melatonin is known for its ability to inhibit release of cytochrome c from Ca^{2+} mediated mitochondria [109]. Mitochondria membrane potential is crucial factor for the maintenance of cellular bioenergetic homeostasis and its dissipation leads to formation of mPTP in stroke. Melatonin has increased the expression of antiapoptotic proteins like bcl-2 through SIRT1 pathways in mice model of cerebral ischemia. It has also decreased the expression of apoptotic factor Bax [33, 38, 103–110].

6.3. Inhibition of Mitochondrial Permeability Transition Pore (mPTP). Inhibition of mPTP remains one of the prime targets in neurodegenerative diseases to block the release of death factors into cytosol [111]. It has been widely accepted that opening of mPTP takes place in stroke due to multiple stress factors, oxidative stress, and Ca^{2+} stress in mitochondria [112]. Stroke induced infarction has been seen greatly reduced in cyclophilin D deficient mice of MCAO [113]. It has been revealed by patch clamp electrophysiology that minute concentration of melatonin (250 μM) directly inhibits the mPTP by interacting with channel directly [42]. Melatonin seems to maintain the mitochondrial membrane potential in various models of PCNs and PSNs that indirectly inhibits the formation of mPTP [114].

6.4. Regulation of Ca^{2+} Level. Excitotoxicity is one of the major events in stroke mediated via glutamate induced NMDA receptor that leads to elevation of mitochondrial level of Ca^{2+} [115]. Studies have shown that excessive Ca^{2+} leads

TABLE 3: Effect of melatonin on OGD model.

Dose	Duration	Effect/result	References
10 and 100 nM	Before OGD for 24 hrs	$\uparrow$activation of Akt, $\downarrow$phosphorylation of JNK	[41]
$10^{-5}, 10^{-7}, 10^{-9}$	After reperfusion	$\downarrow$mitochondrial membrane potential, $\downarrow$cytoplasmic cytochrome c and $\downarrow$Caspase-3 and $\downarrow$DNA damage	[39]
100 to 250 μM	At time of OGD and oxygen-glucose resupply	$\downarrow$mPTP, $\downarrow$mitochondrial depolarization, $\downarrow$Ca^{2+} level, $\downarrow$Caspase-3 activation, $\downarrow$DNA fragmentation, and $\downarrow$cytochrome c release	[42]

to release of proapoptotic factor by opening of mPTP in pathological conditions [116]. *In vitro* and *in vivo* studies have revealed that melatonin has perpetuated the calcium buffering proteins, parvalbumin and hippocalcin, in hippocampal cells and male Sprague-Dawley rats to attenuate the ischemic injury [117]. Stroke induced Ca^{2+} level was supposed to be reduced through inhibition of acid sensing ion channel 1a (ASIC1a) in MCAO model of stroke by melatonin [36].

6.5. Anti-Inflammatory Role of Melatonin in Stroke.
After ischemic injury, an immune response is initiated that leads to production of proinflammatory cytokines and recruitment of various inflammatory cells like neutrophils, T-cells, macrophage, and monocytes that exacerbate the ischemic injury [118]. Melatonin regulates NO level, proinflammatory cytokines, and various enzymes like COX2 and iNOS in various neurodegenerative diseases [119]. Melatonin attenuates ischemic damage by reducing the infiltration of inflammatory cell leukocytes and microglia through MT2 receptor as shown by gp91^{phos} staining in CI/R model of mice [120]. Melatonin has mediated its anti-inflammatory effect by attenuating the glial fibrillary acidic protein level in rat model of cerebral ischemia. It has been shown that melatonin also reduces the activation of microglia and infiltration of monocytes. [121]. Melatonin successfully reduced the microglia production of NO by decreasing the iNOS level in ischemic model of rat [106].

6.6. Regulation of PI3K/Akt Pathway.
It is well documented that PI3K/Akt pathway plays important role in neuronal death and survival [122]. Melatonin has shown positive modulation through this pathway in various neurodegenerative disorders [123]. PI3K/Akt pathway is the important survival pathway in neurons by targeting antiapoptotic factors like Bcl-2 protein family activated by Akt. These antiapoptotic proteins inhibit apoptosis by subjugating the apoptotic pathways in mitochondria. Studies have shown that activating the Akt leads to neuroprotection by inhibiting apoptosis in various models of stroke [124, 125]. Melatonin has strongly inhibited autophagy and stimulated the PI3K/Akt prosurvival pathway in MCAO model of ischemia [126]. Melatonin can target PI3K/Akt pathway, mTOR, or the forkhead transcription factor pAFX and also restore JNK1/2 and ERK 1/2 phosphorylated levels, thereby preventing the proapoptotic actions of the dephosphorylated proteins [127]. Reports are available on the role of phosphatidyl inositol-3 kinase/Akt

signaling in acute melatonin-induced neuroprotection, while ERK-1/-2 and/or JNK-1/-2 rather appear to be involved in melatonin's long-term effects [128].

6.7. Regulation of MAP Kinase Pathway.
Few others suggest that protection from cerebral ischemic injury was attributed to the maintenance of signalling via the mitogen activated protein kinase pathway, leading to the prevention of Bad dephosphorylation. MAP kinase pathway has been involved in various cellular processes like cell differentiation, growth, death, and cell survival. Bcl-xl, an apoptotic protein, is regulated in mitochondria through phosphorylation of p38 MAPK imparts neuroprotection in MCAO model of mice [128]. Phosphorylation of ERK1/2 via activated Raf and MEK by various growth factors leads to phosphorylation of antiapoptotic protein, Bad, by phosphorylated ribosomal S6 kinase (p90RSK). Melatonin has alleviated the neuronal death in cerebral ischemia by activating signalling cascade of Raf/MEK/ERK/p90RSK in ischemic model [37, 129].

6.8. Regulation of Endothelin-1 Pathway.
Several other mechanisms behind melatonin's neuroprotective action have been proposed. A study shows that melatonin, both when prophylactically administered and when acutely applied, is a powerful endothelin converting enzyme-1 (ECE-1) inhibitor. In humans, endothelin-1 is implicated in the evolution of arterial hypertension, stimulates platelet aggregation, and also reinforces the formation of ROS. Activation of the endothelin-1 pathway is therefore considered to confer an increased risk of stroke and MEL as its inhibitor have been proposed as a treatment for vascular disease [130].

6.8.1. Role of Nrf2.
Investigators have suggested that melatonin as a neuroprotectant in cerebral ischemia may involve mechanisms like reduction in ROS production, and activation of the nuclear factor-erythroid 2-related factor 2 (Nrf2), which is a master regulator of endogenous antioxidant defenses followed by overexpression of phase II enzymes such as heme oxygenase-1, which has a potent antioxidant and anti-inflammatory effect [131].

6.8.2. Receptor Proteins Involved in Melatonin Neuroprotection.
Melatonin acts via high affinity G-protein-coupled melatonin receptors, MT1 and MT2, which have been identified *in vitro* autoradiography and conventional binding

assays, also cloned and characterized in mammals. The specific receptors have been found in human brain regions like medial preoptic area, anterior hypothalamus, paraventricular and anteroventral thalamic nuclei, hippocampus, cerebral and cerebellar cortex, and retina. The available data indicates that the melatonin receptor is associated with membrane and is also linked to secondary messengers such as cAMP, cGMP, diacylglycerol, arachidonic acid, IP3, and inorganic calcium. Melatonin also regulates the third messengers, namely, the phosphorylation of CREB and expression of c-Fos [132]. Data suggest that melatonin exhibits a protective effect against ischemic stroke in mice model which is MT2 melatonin receptor-associated. Studies have indicated that melatonin elicits its neuroprotective effect in ischemic stroke through MT2 receptor as revealed by using MT2 receptor antagonist luzindole [108]. Also, activation of the MT2 melatonin receptor in the hippocampal region with melatonin treatment shown by immunoreactive responses may be involved in its neuroprotective action against transient cerebral ischemic damage [133]. But few studies using knock-out mice show contradictory results that both MT1 and MT2 receptors are not necessary for neuroprotection by MEL against ischemia [134].

7. Future Perspectives of Melatonin

Melatonin, a neurohormone, has been found effective in various animal models of brain injury. Several research studies are being done on assessing protective role of melatonin in humans. Melatonin, a potent antiapoptotic and antioxidative neuroprotectant with no serious toxicity, raises hopes that it might be used for humans for stroke treatment. The bulk of studies published have used pharmacological interventions against ROS production and apoptosis. There is need to explore different mechanisms of melatonin in neuroprotection of different models of brain injury that will be more effective at endogenous levels of body that might be important especially at later stage of age when melatonin level is attenuated. There is need to design more efficient clinical trials to explore the clinical aspect of protective role of melatonin in detail against various neurodegenerative diseases.

Conflict of Interests

The authors declare that there is no conflict of interests.

Acknowledgments

Dr. Heena Tabassum is grateful to Department of Biotechnology, Government of India, for financial grant (DBT BioCARe Program, sanction no. BT/Bio-CARe/01/10219/2013-14). The Grant (no. F. 30-1/2013(SA-II)/RA-2012-14-GE-WES-2400), received as Research Award (2012–14) from the University Grants Commission (UGC), New Delhi, Government of India, to Dr. Suhel Parvez, is thankfully acknowledged. Syed Suhail Andrabi was supported by a Junior Research Fellowship of the UGC-Basic Research Fellowship Program (Grant no. F.25-1/2013-14(BSR)/7-91/2007(BSR)).

References

[1] C. D. Mathers, T. Boerma, and D. Ma Fat, "Global and regional causes of death," *British Medical Bulletin*, vol. 92, no. 1, pp. 7–32, 2009.

[2] R. W. V. Flynn, R. S. M. MacWalter, and A. S. F. Doney, "The cost of cerebral ischaemia," *Neuropharmacology*, vol. 55, no. 3, pp. 250–256, 2008.

[3] R. S. Pandya, L. Mao, H. Zhou et al., "Central nervous system agents for ischemic stroke: neuroprotection mechanisms," *Central Nervous System Agents in Medicinal Chemistry*, vol. 11, no. 2, pp. 81–97, 2011.

[4] Y. Jin, N. Raviv, A. Barnett et al., "The shh signaling pathway is upregulated in multiple cell types in cortical ischemia and influences the outcome of stroke in an animal model," *PLoS ONE*, vol. 10, no. 4, Article ID e0124657, 2015.

[5] B. Wali, T. Ishrat, S. Won, D. G. Stein, and I. Sayeed, "Progesterone in experimental permanent stroke: a dose-response and therapeutic time-window study," *Brain*, vol. 137, no. 2, pp. 486–502, 2013.

[6] A. Canazza, L. Minati, C. Boffano, E. Parati, and S. Binks, "Experimental models of brain ischemia: a review of techniques, magnetic resonance imaging, and investigational cell-based therapies," *Frontiers in Neurology*, vol. 5, article 19, 2014.

[7] R. Jin, X. Zhu, and G. Li, "Embolic middle cerebral artery occlusion (MCAO) for ischemic stroke with homologous blood clots in rats," *Journal of Visualized Experiments*, no. 91, Article ID 51956, 2014.

[8] K.-A. Hossmann, "The two pathophysiologies of focal brain ischemia: implications for translational stroke research," *Journal of Cerebral Blood Flow and Metabolism*, vol. 32, no. 7, pp. 1310–1316, 2012.

[9] W.-D. Heiss, "The ischemic penumbra: how does tissue injury evolve?" *Annals of the New York Academy of Sciences*, vol. 1268, no. 1, pp. 26–34, 2012.

[10] T. M. Woodruff, J. Thundyil, S.-C. Tang, C. G. Sobey, S. M. Taylor, and T. V. Arumugam, "Pathophysiology, treatment, and animal and cellular models of human ischemic stroke," *Molecular Neurodegeneration*, vol. 6, no. 1, article 11, 2011.

[11] A. Purushotham, B. C. V. Campbell, M. Straka et al., "Apparent diffusion coefficient threshold for delineation of ischemic core," *International Journal of Stroke*, vol. 10, no. 3, pp. 348–353, 2015.

[12] M. Fisher and B. Bastan, "Identifying and utilizing the ischemic penumbra," *Neurology*, vol. 79, no. 13, pp. S79–S85, 2012.

[13] M. Fisher and B. Bastan, "Identifying and utilizing the ischemic penumbra," *Neurology*, vol. 79, no. 13, supplement 1, pp. S79–S85, 2012.

[14] H. Li, N. Zhang, H.-Y. Lin et al., "Histological, cellular and behavioral assessments of stroke outcomes after photo-thrombosis-induced ischemia in adult mice," *BMC Neuroscience*, vol. 15, article 58, 2014.

[15] T. Chiang, R. O. Messing, and W. H. Chou, "Mouse model of middle cerebral artery occlusion," *Journal of Visualized Experiments*, vol. 13, no. 48, p. 2761, 2011.

[16] M. Pompili, P. Venturini, D. A. Lamis et al., "Suicide in stroke survivors: epidemiology and prevention," *Drugs and Aging*, vol. 32, no. 1, pp. 21–29, 2014.

[17] H. Sies, "Oxidative stress: a concept in redox biology and medicine," *Redox Biology*, vol. 4, pp. 180–183, 2015.

[18] B. Halliwell, "Free radicals and antioxidants—quo vadis?" *Trends in Pharmacological Sciences*, vol. 32, no. 3, pp. 125–130, 2011.

[19] M. L. Dallas, J. P. Boyle, C. J. Milligan et al., "Carbon monoxide protects against oxidant-induced apoptosis *via* inhibition of $K_v2.1$," *The FASEB Journal*, vol. 25, no. 5, pp. 1519–1530, 2011.

[20] J. W. Thompson, S. V. Narayanan, and M. A. Perez-Pinzon, "Redox signaling pathways involved in neuronal ischemic preconditioning," *Current Neuropharmacology*, vol. 10, no. 4, pp. 354–369, 2012.

[21] R. M. Adibhatla and J. F. Hatcher, "Phospholipase A(2), reactive oxygen species, and lipid peroxidation in CNS pathologies," *Journal of Biochemistry and Molecular Biology*, vol. 41, no. 8, pp. 560–567, 2008.

[22] H.-M. Gao, H. Zhou, and J.-S. Hong, "NADPH oxidases: novel therapeutic targets for neurodegenerative diseases," *Trends in Pharmacological Sciences*, vol. 33, no. 6, pp. 295–303, 2012.

[23] J. C. Lee and M. H. Won, "Neuroprotection of antioxidant enzymes against transient global cerebral ischemia in gerbils," *Anatomy & Cell Biology*, vol. 47, no. 3, pp. 149–156, 2014.

[24] K. Niizuma, H. Yoshioka, H. Chen et al., "Mitochondrial and apoptotic neuronal death signaling pathways in cerebral ischemia," *Biochimica et Biophysica Acta—Molecular Basis of Disease*, vol. 1802, no. 1, pp. 92–99, 2010.

[25] T. H. Sanderson, C. A. Reynolds, R. Kumar, K. Przyklenk, and M. Hüttemann, "Molecular mechanisms of ischemia-reperfusion injury in brain: pivotal role of the mitochondrial membrane potential in reactive oxygen species generation," *Molecular Neurobiology*, vol. 47, no. 1, pp. 9–23, 2013.

[26] T. W. Lai, S. Zhang, and Y. T. Wang, "Excitotoxicity and stroke: identifying novel targets for neuroprotection," *Progress in Neurobiology*, vol. 115, pp. 157–188, 2014.

[27] A. Lau and M. Tymianski, "Glutamate receptors, neurotoxicity and neurodegeneration," *Pflügers Archiv*, vol. 460, no. 2, pp. 525–542, 2010.

[28] A. M. Dolga, N. Terpolilli, F. Kepura et al., "$K_{Ca}2$ channels activation prevents $[Ca^{2+}]i$ deregulation and reduces neuronal death following glutamate toxicity and cerebral ischemia," *Cell Death and Disease*, vol. 2, no. 4, article e147, 2011.

[29] S. A. Andrabi, H. C. Kang, J.-F. Haince et al., "Iduna protects the brain from glutamate excitotoxicity and stroke by interfering with poly(ADP-ribose) polymer-induced cell death," *Nature Medicine*, vol. 17, no. 6, pp. 692–699, 2011.

[30] Q. Zhao, S. Wang, Y. Li et al., "The role of the mitochondrial calcium uniporter in cerebral ischemia/reperfusion injury in rats involves regulation of mitochondrial energy metabolism," *Molecular Medicine Reports*, vol. 7, no. 4, pp. 1073–1080, 2013.

[31] L. C. Constantino, C. I. Tasca, and C. R. Boeck, "The role of NMDA receptors in the development of brain resistance through pre- and postconditioning," *Aging and Disease*, vol. 5, no. 6, pp. 430–441, 2014.

[32] M. M. Harraz, S. M. Eacker, X. Wang, T. M. Dawson, and V. L. Dawson, "MicroRNA-223 is neuroprotective by targeting glutamate receptors," *Proceedings of the National Academy of Sciences of the United States of America*, vol. 109, no. 46, pp. 18962–18967, 2012.

[33] X. Wang, B. E. Figueroa, I. G. Stavrovskaya et al., "Metha-zolamide and melatonin inhibit mitochondrial cytochrome C release and are neuroprotective in experimental models of ischemic injury," *Stroke*, vol. 40, no. 5, pp. 1877–1885, 2009.

[34] P. Bhattacharya, A. K. Pandey, S. Paul, and R. Patnaik, "Mela-tonin renders neuroprotection by protein kinase C mediated aquaporin-4 inhibition in animal model of focal cerebral ischemia," *Life Sciences*, vol. 100, no. 2, pp. 97–109, 2014.

[35] S.-H. Tai, H.-Y. Chen, E.-J. Lee et al., "Melatonin inhibits postischemic matrix metalloproteinase-9 (MMP-9) activation via dual modulation of plasminogen/plasmin system and endogenous MMP inhibitor in mice subjected to transient focal cerebral ischemia," *Journal of Pineal Research*, vol. 49, no. 4, pp. 332–341, 2010.

[36] X. Hu, P. Li, Y. Guo et al., "Microglia/macrophage polarization dynamics reveal novel mechanism of injury expansion after focal cerebral ischemia," *Stroke*, vol. 43, no. 11, pp. 3063–3070, 2012.

[37] W.-S. Juan, S.-Y. Huang, C.-C. Chang et al., "Melatonin improves neuroplasticity by upregulating the growth-associated protein-43 (GAP-43) and NMDAR postsynaptic density-95 (PSD-95) proteins in cultured neurons exposed to glutamate excitotoxicity and in rats subjected to transient focal cerebral ischemia even during a long-term recovery period," *Journal of Pineal Research*, vol. 56, no. 2, pp. 213–223, 2014.

[38] H. Li, Y. Wang, D. Feng et al., "Alterations in the time course of expression of the Nox family in the brain in a rat experimental cerebral ischemia and reperfusion model: effects of melatonin," *Journal of Pineal Research*, vol. 57, no. 1, pp. 110–119, 2014.

[39] Y.-X. Han, S.-H. Zhang, X.-M. Wang, and J.-B. Wu, "Inhibition of mitochondria responsible for the anti-apoptotic effects of melatonin during ischemia-reperfusion," *Journal of Zhejiang University Science B*, vol. 7, no. 2, pp. 142–147, 2006.

[40] E. Kilic, Ü. Kilic, M. Bacigaluppi et al., "Delayed melatonin administration promotes neuronal survival, neurogenesis and motor recovery, and attenuates hyperactivity and anxiety after mild focal cerebral ischemia in mice," *Journal of Pineal Research*, vol. 45, no. 2, pp. 142–148, 2008.

[41] J. Song, S. M. Kang, W. T. Lee, K. A. Park, K. M. Lee, and J. E. Lee, "The beneficial effect of melatonin in brain endothelial cells against oxygen-glucose deprivation followed by reperfusion-induced injury," *Oxidative Medicine and Cellular Longevity*, vol. 2014, Article ID 639531, 14 pages, 2014.

[42] S. A. Andrabi, I. Sayeed, D. Siemen, G. Wolf, and T. F. W. Horn, "Direct inhibition of the mitochondrial permeability transition pore: a possible mechanism responsible for anti-apoptotic effects of melatonin," *The FASEB Journal*, vol. 18, no. 7, pp. 869–871, 2004.

[43] C. Thornton and H. Hagberg, "Role of mitochondria in apop-totic and necroptotic cell death in the developing brain," *Clinica Chimica Acta*, 2015.

[44] M. H. Singh, S. M. Brooke, I. Zemlyak, and R. M. Sapolsky, "Evidence for caspase effects on release of cytochrome c and AIF in a model of ischemia in cortical neurons," *Neuroscience Letters*, vol. 469, no. 2, pp. 179–183, 2010.

[45] L. Portt, G. Norman, C. Clapp, M. Greenwood, and M. T. Green-wood, "Anti-apoptosis and cell survival: a review," *Biochimica et Biophysica Acta—Molecular Cell Research*, vol. 1813, no. 1, pp. 238–259, 2011.

[46] S. Fulda, A. M. Gorman, O. Hori, and A. Samali, "Cellular stress responses: cell survival and cell death," *International Journal of Cell Biology*, vol. 2010, Article ID 214074, 23 pages, 2010.

[47] E. A. Jonas, G. A. Porter Jr., G. Beutner, N. Mnatsakanyan, and K. N. Alavian, "Cell death disguised: the mitochondrial permeability transition pore as the c-subunit of the F_1F_O ATP synthase," *Pharmacological Research*, 2015.

[48] V. Giorgio, S. S. von Stockum, M. Antoniel et al., "Dimers of mitochondrial ATP synthase form the permeability transition pore," *Proceedings of the National Academy of Sciences of the United States of America*, vol. 110, no. 15, pp. 5887–5892, 2013.

[49] H. Huang, X. Hu, C. O. Eno, G. Zhao, C. Li, and C. White, "An interaction between Bcl-x$_L$ and the voltage-dependent anion channel (VDAC) promotes mitochondrial Ca^{2+} uptake," *Journal of Biological Chemistry*, vol. 288, no. 27, pp. 19870–19881, 2013.

[50] J. Karch, J. Q. Kwong, and A. R. Burr, "Bax and Bak function as the outer membrane component of the mitochondrial permeability pore in regulating necrotic cell death in mice," *Elife*, vol. 27, no. 2, Article ID e00772, 2013.

[51] S.-Y. Ryu, P. M. Peixoto, O. Teijido, L. M. Dejean, and K. W. Kinnally, "Role of mitochondrial ion channels in cell death," *BioFactors*, vol. 36, no. 4, pp. 255–263, 2010.

[52] Q. Chen, H. Xu, A. Xu et al., "Inhibition of Bcl-2 sensitizes mitochondrial permeability transition pore (MPTP) opening in ischemia-damaged mitochondria," *PLOS ONE*, vol. 10, no. 3, Article ID e0118834, 2015.

[53] L. M. Dejean, S.-Y. Ryu, S. Martinez-Caballero, O. Teijido, P. M. Peixoto, and K. W. Kinnally, "MAC and Bcl-2 family proteins conspire in a deadly plot," *Biochimica et Biophysica Acta—Bioenergetics*, vol. 1797, no. 6-7, pp. 1231–1238, 2010.

[54] C. Brenner and M. Moulin, "Physiological roles of the permeability transition pore," *Circulation Research*, vol. 111, no. 9, pp. 1237–1247, 2012.

[55] R. Abeti and A. Y. Abramo, "Mitochondrial Ca^{2+} in neurodegenerative disorders," *Pharmacological Research*, vol. 6618, no. 15, pp. 91–92, 2015.

[56] J. Yuan, "Neuroprotective strategies targeting apoptotic and necrotic cell death for stroke," *Apoptosis*, vol. 14, no. 4, pp. 469–477, 2009.

[57] M. A. Moskowitz, E. H. Lo, and C. Iadecola, "The science of stroke: mechanisms in search of treatments," *Neuron*, vol. 67, no. 2, pp. 181–198, 2010.

[58] N. R. Sims and H. Muyderman, "Mitochondria, oxidative metabolism and cell death in stroke," *Biochimica et Biophysica Acta*, vol. 1802, no. 1, pp. 80–91, 2010.

[59] H. Zhang, Y.-W. Zhang, Y. Chen et al., "Appoptosin is a novel pro-apoptotic protein and mediates cell death in neurodegeneration," *Journal of Neuroscience*, vol. 32, no. 44, pp. 15565–15576, 2012.

[60] B. R. S. Broughton, D. C. Reutens, and C. G. Sobey, "Apoptotic mechanisms after cerebral ischemia," *Stroke*, vol. 40, no. 5, pp. e331–e339, 2009.

[61] L. Jie, C. Yuqin, D. Yao, H. Shuai, and W. Yuanyuan, "Occlusion of middle cerebral artery induces apoptosis of cerebellar cortex neural cells via caspase-3 in rats," *Turkish Neurosurgery*, vol. 21, no. 4, pp. 567–574, 2011.

[62] S. Nowsheen and E. S. Yang, "The intersection between DNA damage response and cell death pathways," *Experimental Oncology*, vol. 34, no. 3, pp. 243–254, 2012.

[63] E. Norberg, S. Orrenius, and B. Zhivotovsky, "Mitochondrial regulation of cell death: processing of apoptosis-inducing factor (AIF)," *Biochemical and Biophysical Research Communications*, vol. 396, no. 1, pp. 95–100, 2010.

[64] E.-M. Öxler, A. Dolga, and C. Culmsee, "AIF depletion provides neuroprotection through a preconditioning effect," *Apoptosis*, vol. 17, no. 10, pp. 1027–1038, 2012.

[65] B. M. Polster, "AIF, reactive oxygen species, and neurodegeneration: a 'complex' problem," *Neurochemistry International*, vol. 62, no. 5, pp. 695–702, 2013.

[66] N. Doti, C. Reuther, P. L. Scognamiglio et al., "Inhibition of the AIF/CypA complex protects against intrinsic death pathways induced by oxidative stress," *Cell Death & Disease*, vol. 16, no. 5, article e993, 2014.

[67] S. A. Andrabi, T. M. Dawson, and V. L. Dawson, "Mitochondrial and nuclear cross talk in cell death: parthanatos," *Annals of the New York Academy of Sciences*, vol. 1147, pp. 233–241, 2008.

[68] E. Batnasan, R. Wang, J. Wen et al., "17-Beta estradiol inhibits oxidative stress-induced accumulation of AIF into nucleolus and PARP1-dependent cell death via estrogen receptor alpha," *Toxicology Letters*, vol. 232, no. 1, pp. 1–9, 2015.

[69] K. K. David, S. A. Andrabi, T. M. Dawson, and V. L. Dawson, "Parthanatos, a messenger of death," *Frontiers in Bioscience*, vol. 14, no. 3, pp. 1116–1128, 2009.

[70] Y. Wang, N. S. Kim, X. Li et al., "Calpain activation is not required for AIF translocation in PARP-1-dependent cell death (parthanatos)," *Journal of Neurochemistry*, vol. 110, no. 2, pp. 687–696, 2009.

[71] S.-H. Baek, O.-N. Bae, E.-K. Kim, and S.-W. Yu, "Induction of mitochondrial dysfunction by poly(ADP-ribose) polymer: implication for neuronal cell death," *Molecules and Cells*, vol. 36, no. 3, pp. 258–266, 2013.

[72] J. Pei, X. You, and Q. Fu, "Inflammation in the pathogenesis of ischemic stroke," *Frontiers in Bioscience*, vol. 20, no. 4, pp. 772–783, 2015.

[73] C. Iadecola and J. Anrather, "The immunology of stroke: from mechanisms to translation," *Nature Medicine*, vol. 17, no. 7, pp. 796–808, 2011.

[74] M. Kawabori and M. A. Yenari, "Inflammatory responses in brain ischemia," *Current Medicinal Chemistry*, vol. 22, no. 10, pp. 1258–1277, 2015.

[75] G. Yilmaz and D. N. Granger, "Leukocyte recruitment and ischemic brain injury," *NeuroMolecular Medicine*, vol. 12, no. 2, pp. 193–204, 2010.

[76] Á. Chamorro, A. Meisel, A. M. Planas, X. Urra, D. Van de Beek, and R. Veltkamp, "The immunology of acute stroke," *Nature Reviews Neurology*, vol. 8, no. 7, pp. 401–410, 2012.

[77] B. M. Famakin, "The immune response to acute focal cerebral ischemia and associated post-stroke immunodepression: a focused review," *Aging and Disease*, vol. 5, no. 5, pp. 307–326, 2014.

[78] L. Wu, K. Zhang, G. Hu, H. Yang, C. Xie, and X. Wu, "Inflammatory response and neuronal necrosis in rats with cerebral ischemia," *Neural Regeneration Research*, vol. 9, no. 19, pp. 1753–1762, 2014.

[79] T. Dziedzic, "Systemic inflammation as a therapeutic target in acute ischemic stroke," *Expert Review of Neurotherapeutics*, vol. 15, no. 5, pp. 523–531, 2015.

[80] D. N. Doll, T. L. Barr, and J. W. Simpkins, "Cytokines: their role in stroke and potential use as biomarkers and therapeutic targets," *Aging and Disease*, vol. 5, no. 5, pp. 294–306, 2014.

[81] H. C. Pan, C. N. Yang, Y. W. Hung et al., "Reciprocal modulation of C/EBP-α and C/EBP-β by IL-13 in activated microglia prevents neuronal death," *European Journal of Immunology*, vol. 43, no. 11, pp. 2854–2865, 2013.

[82] E. C. Koellhoffer and L. D. McCullough, "The effects of estrogen in ischemic stroke," *Translational Stroke Research*, vol. 4, no. 4, pp. 390–401, 2013.

[83] D. A. Schreihofer and Y. Ma, "Estrogen receptors and ischemic neuroprotection: who, what, where, and when?" *Brain Research*, vol. 1514, pp. 107–122, 2013.

[84] I. Sayeed and D. G. Stein, "Progesterone as a neuroprotective factor in traumatic and ischemic brain injury," *Progress in Brain Research*, vol. 175, pp. 219–237, 2009.

[85] H.-M. Zhang and Y. Zhang, "Melatonin: a well-documented antioxidant with conditional pro-oxidant actions," *Journal of Pineal Research*, vol. 57, no. 2, pp. 131–146, 2014.

[86] A. Galano, D. X. Tan, and R. J. Reiter, "Melatonin as a natural ally against oxidative stress: a physicochemical examination," *Journal of Pineal Research*, vol. 51, no. 1, pp. 1–16, 2011.

[87] J. J. García, L. López-Pingarrón, P. Almeida-Souza et al., "Protective effects of melatonin in reducing oxidative stress and in preserving the fluidity of biological membranes: a review," *Journal of Pineal Research*, vol. 56, no. 3, pp. 225–237, 2014.

[88] E. Miller, A. Morel, L. Saso, and J. Saluk, "Melatonin redox activity. Its potential clinical applications in neurodegenerative disorders," *Current Topics in Medicinal Chemistry*, vol. 15, no. 2, pp. 163–169, 2015.

[89] A. Chattoraj, T. Liu, L. S. Zhang, Z. Huang, and J. Borjigin, "Melatonin formation in mammals: *in vivo* perspectives," *Reviews in Endocrine and Metabolic Disorders*, vol. 10, no. 4, pp. 237–243, 2009.

[90] J. B. Zawilska, D. J. Skene, and J. Arendt, "Physiology and pharmacology of melatonin in relation to biological rhythms," *Pharmacological Reports*, vol. 61, no. 3, pp. 383–410, 2009.

[91] P. M. Iuvone, G. Tosini, N. Pozdeyev, R. Haque, D. C. Klein, and S. S. Chaurasia, "Circadian clocks, clock networks, arylalkylamine *N*-acetyltransferase, and melatonin in the retina," *Progress in Retinal and Eye Research*, vol. 24, no. 4, pp. 433–456, 2005.

[92] I. Semak, E. Korik, M. Antonova, J. Wortsman, and A. Slominski, "Metabolism of melatonin by cytochrome P450s in rat liver mitochondria and microsomes," *Journal of Pineal Research*, vol. 45, no. 4, pp. 515–523, 2008.

[93] B. Claustrat and J. Leston, "Melatonin: physiological effects in humans," *Neurochirurgie*, vol. 61, no. 2-3, pp. 77–84, 2015.

[94] R. Hardeland and B. Poeggeler, "Melatonin and synthetic melatonergic agonists: actions and metabolism in the central nervous system," *Central Nervous System Agents in Medicinal Chemistry*, vol. 12, no. 3, pp. 189–216, 2012.

[95] B. P. Lucke-Wold, K. E. Smith, L. Nguyen et al., "Sleep disruption and the sequelae associated with traumatic brain injury," *Neuroscience & Biobehavioral Reviews*, vol. 55, pp. 68–77, 2015.

[96] B. V. Jardim, L. C. Ferreira, T. F. Borin et al., "Evaluation of the anti-angiogenic action of melatonin in breast cancer," *BMC Proceedings*, vol. 7, supplement 2, article P11, 2003.

[97] A. Korkmaz, T. Topal, D.-X. Tan, and R. J. Reiter, "Role of melatonin in metabolic regulation," *Reviews in Endocrine and Metabolic Disorders*, vol. 10, no. 4, pp. 261–270, 2009.

[98] B. Lacoste, D. Angeloni, S. Dominguez-Lopez et al., "Anatomical and cellular localization of melatonin MT_1 and MT_2 receptors in the adult rat brain," *Journal of Pineal Research*, vol. 58, no. 4, pp. 397–417, 2015.

[99] E. R. V. Rios, E. T. Venncio, N. F. M. Rocha et al., "Melatonin: pharmacological aspects and clinical trends," *International Journal of Neuroscience*, vol. 120, no. 9, pp. 583–590, 2010.

[100] Y.-H. Wu, J. Ursinus, J.-N. Zhou et al., "Alterations of melatonin receptors MT1 and MT2 in the hypothalamic suprachiasmatic nucleus during depression," *Journal of Affective Disorders*, vol. 148, no. 2-3, pp. 357–367, 2013.

[101] B. M. Escribano, A. Colín-González, A. Santamaría, and I. Túnez, "The role of melatonin in multiple sclerosis, Huntington's disease and cerebral ischemia," *CNS & Neurological Disorders—Drug Targets*, vol. 13, no. 6, pp. 1096–1119, 2014.

[102] G. Sarlak, A. Jenwitheesuk, B. Chetsawang, and P. Govitrapong, "Effects of melatonin on nervous system aging: neurogenesis and neurodegeneration," *Journal of Pharmacological Sciences*, vol. 123, no. 1, pp. 9–24, 2013.

[103] Y. Yang, S. Jiang, Y. Dong et al., "Melatonin prevents cell death and mitochondrial dysfunction via a SIRT1-dependent mechanism during ischemic-stroke in mice," *Journal of Pineal Research*, vol. 58, no. 1, pp. 61–70, 2015.

[104] A. Corrales, R. Vidal, S. García et al., "Chronic melatonin treatment rescues electrophysiological and neuromorphological deficits in a mouse model of Down syndrome," *Journal of Pineal Research*, vol. 56, no. 1, pp. 51–61, 2014.

[105] V. H. Ozacmak, F. Barut, and H. S. Ozacmak, "Melatonin provides neuroprotection by reducing oxidative stress and HSP70 expression during chronic cerebral hypoperfusion in ovariectomized rats," *Journal of Pineal Research*, vol. 47, no. 2, pp. 156–163, 2009.

[106] S. R. Pandi-Perumal, A. S. Bahammam, G. M. Brown et al., "Melatonin antioxidative defense: therapeutic implications for aging and neurodegenerative processes," *Neurotoxicity Research*, vol. 23, no. 3, pp. 267–300, 2013.

[107] X. Wang, "The antiapoptotic activity of melatonin in neurodegenerative diseases," *CNS Neuroscience and Therapeutics*, vol. 15, no. 4, pp. 345–357, 2009.

[108] C.-M. Chern, J.-F. Liao, Y.-H. Wang, and Y.-C. Shen, "Melatonin ameliorates neural function by promoting endogenous neurogenesis through the MT2 melatonin receptor in ischemic-stroke mice," *Free Radical Biology and Medicine*, vol. 52, no. 9, pp. 1634–1647, 2012.

[109] V. K. Rao, E. A. Carlson, and S. S. Yan, "Mitochondrial permeability transition pore is a potential drug target for neurodegeneration," *Biochimica et Biophysica Acta—Molecular Basis of Disease*, vol. 1842, no. 8, pp. 1267–1272, 2014.

[110] N. R. Sims and H. Muyderman, "Mitochondria, oxidative metabolism and cell death in stroke," *Biochimica et Biophysica Acta—Molecular Basis of Disease*, vol. 1802, no. 1, pp. 80–91, 2010.

[111] M. K. E. Schäfer, A. Pfeiffer, M. Jaeckel, A. Pouya, A. M. Dolga, and A. Methner, "Regulators of mitochondrial Ca^{2+} homeostasis in cerebral ischemia," *Cell and Tissue Research*, vol. 357, no. 2, pp. 395–405, 2014.

[112] G. Yu, F. Wu, and E.-S. Wang, "BQ-869, a novel NMDA receptor antagonist, protects against excitotoxicity and attenuates cerebral ischemic injury in stroke," *International Journal of Clinical and Experimental Pathology*, vol. 8, no. 2, pp. 1213–1225, 2015.

[113] X. Wang, "The antiapoptotic activity of melatonin in neurodegenerative diseases," *CNS Neuroscience & Therapeutics*, vol. 15, no. 4, pp. 345–357, 2009.

[114] Y. Gouriou, P. Bijlenga, and N. Demaurex, "Mitochondrial Ca^{2+} uptake from plasma membrane Cav3.2 protein channels contributes to ischemic toxicity in PC12 cells," *The Journal of Biological Chemistry*, vol. 288, no. 18, pp. 12459–12468, 2013.

[115] P.-O. Koh, "Melatonin regulates the calcium-buffering proteins, parvalbumin and hippocalcin, in ischemic brain injury," *Journal of Pineal Research*, vol. 53, no. 4, pp. 358–365, 2012.

[116] P. Bhattacharya, A. K. Pandey, S. Paul, and R. Patnaik, "Melatonin renders neuroprotection by protein kinase C mediated

aquaporin-4 inhibition in animal model of focal cerebral ischemia," *Life Sciences*, vol. 100, no. 2, pp. 97–109, 2014.

[117] H. Alluri, C. A. Shaji, M. L. Davis, and B. Tharakan, "Oxygen-glucose deprivation and reoxygenation as an in vitro ischemia-reperfusion injury model for studying blood-brain barrier dysfunction," *Journal of Visualized Experiments*, no. 99, Article ID e52699, 2015.

[118] E. Esposito and S. Cuzzocrea, "Antiinflammatory activity of melatonin in central nervous system," *Current Neuropharmacology*, vol. 8, no. 3, pp. 228–242, 2010.

[119] W. Balduini, S. Carloni, S. Perrone et al., "The use of melatonin in hypoxic-ischemic brain damage: an experimental study," *Journal of Maternal-Fetal and Neonatal Medicine*, vol. 25, no. 1, pp. 119–124, 2012.

[120] K. Liang, Y. Ye, Y. Wang, J. Zhang, and C. Li, "Formononetin mediates neuroprotection against cerebral ischemia/reperfusion in rats via downregulation of the Bax/Bcl-2 ratio and upregulation PI3K/Akt signaling pathway," *Journal of the Neurological Sciences*, vol. 344, no. 1-2, pp. 100–104, 2014.

[121] Z. Pei and R. T. Cheung, "Pretreatment with melatonin exerts anti-inflammatory effects against ischemia/reperfusion injury in a rat middle cerebral artery occlusion stroke model," *Journal of Pineal Research*, vol. 37, no. 2, pp. 85–91, 2004.

[122] Y. Feng, S. Lu, J. Wang, P. Kumar, L. Zhang, and A. J. Bhatt, "Dexamethasone-induced neuroprotection in hypoxic-ischemic brain injury in newborn rats is partly mediated via Akt activation," *Brain Research*, vol. 1589, pp. 68–77, 2014.

[123] A. Hafeez, O. Elmadhoun, C. Peng et al., "Reduced apoptosis by ethanol and its association with PKC-δ and Akt signaling in ischemic stroke," *Aging and Disease*, vol. 5, no. 6, pp. 366–372, 2014.

[124] Y. Zheng, J. Hou, J. Liu et al., "Inhibition of autophagy contributes to melatonin-mediated neuroprotection against transient focal cerebral ischemia in rats," *Journal of Pharmacological Sciences*, vol. 124, no. 3, pp. 354–364, 2014.

[125] L. Zhao, X. Liu, J. Liang et al., "Phosphorylation of p38 MAPK mediates hypoxic preconditioning-induced neuroprotection against cerebral ischemic injury via mitochondria translocation of Bcl-xL in mice," *Brain Research*, vol. 1503, pp. 78–88, 2013.

[126] P.-O. Koh, "Melatonin attenuates the cerebral ischemic injury via the MEK/ERK/p90RSK/Bad signaling cascade," *Journal of Veterinary Medical Science*, vol. 70, no. 11, pp. 1219–1223, 2008.

[127] F. Luchetti, B. Canonico, M. Betti et al., "Melatonin signaling and cell protection function," *The FASEB Journal*, vol. 24, no. 10, pp. 3603–3624, 2010.

[128] Ü. Kilic, E. Kilic, R. J. Reiter, C. L. Bassetti, and D. M. Hermann, "Signal transduction pathways involved in melatonin-induced neuroprotection after focal cerebral ischemia in mice," *Journal of Pineal Research*, vol. 38, no. 1, pp. 67–71, 2005.

[129] P.-O. Koh, "Melatonin prevents ischemic brain injury through activation of the mTOR/p70S6 kinase signaling pathway," *Neuroscience Letters*, vol. 444, no. 1, pp. 74–78, 2008.

[130] E. Kilic, Ü. Kilic, R. J. Reiter, C. L. Bassetti, and D. M. Hermann, "Prophylactic use of melatonin protects against focal cerebral ischemia in mice: role of endothelin converting enzyme-1," *Journal of Pineal Research*, vol. 37, no. 4, pp. 247–251, 2004.

[131] E. Parada, I. Buendia, R. León et al., "Neuroprotective effect of melatonin against ischemia is partially mediated by alpha-7 nicotinic receptor modulation and HO-1 overexpression," *Journal of Pineal Research*, vol. 56, no. 2, pp. 204–212, 2014.

[132] J. Vanecek, "Cellular mechanisms of melatonin action," *Physiological Reviews*, vol. 78, no. 3, pp. 687–721, 1998.

[133] C. H. Lee, K.-Y. Yoo, J. H. Choi et al., "Melatonin's protective action against ischemic neuronal damage is associated with up-regulation of the MT2 melatonin receptor," *Journal of Neuroscience Research*, vol. 88, no. 12, pp. 2630–2640, 2010.

[134] U. Kilic, B. Yilmaz, M. Ugur et al., "Evidence that membrane-bound G protein-coupled melatonin receptors MT1 and MT2 are not involved in the neuroprotective effects of melatonin in focal cerebral ischemia," *Journal of Pineal Research*, vol. 52, no. 2, pp. 228–235, 2012.

21

Protective Effect of *Diospyros kaki* against Glucose-Oxygen-Serum Deprivation-Induced PC12 Cells Injury

Fatemeh Forouzanfar,[1] **Shaghayegh Torabi,**[2] **Vahid R. Askari,**[3] **Elham Asadpour,**[4] **and Hamid R. Sadeghnia**[1,2,3]

[1]*Neurocognitive Research Center, School of Medicine, Mashhad University of Medical Sciences, Mashhad 917794-8564, Iran*
[2]*Pharmacological Research Center of Medicinal Plants, School of Medicine, Mashhad University of Medical Sciences, Mashhad 917794-8564, Iran*
[3]*Department of Pharmacology, School of Medicine, Mashhad University of Medical Sciences, Mashhad 917794-8564, Iran*
[4]*Anesthesiology and Critical Care Research Center, Shiraz University of Medical Sciences, Shiraz, Iran*

Correspondence should be addressed to Hamid R. Sadeghnia; sadeghniahr@mums.ac.ir

Academic Editor: Masahiro Oike

Ischemic cerebrovascular disease is one of the most common causes of death in the world. Recent interests have been focused on natural antioxidants and anti-inflammatory agents as potentially useful neuroprotective agents. *Diospyros kaki* (persimmon) has been shown to exert anti-inflammatory, antioxidant, and antineoplastic effects. However, its effects on ischemic damage have not been evaluated. Here, we used an *in vitro* model of cerebral ischemia and studied the effects of hydroalcoholic extract of peel (PeHE) and fruit pulp (PuHE) of persimmon on cell viability and markers of oxidative damage mainly intracellular reactive oxygen species (ROS) induced by glucose-oxygen-serum deprivation (GOSD) in PC12 cells. GOSD for 6 h produced significant cell death which was accompanied by increased levels of ROS. Pretreatment with different concentrations of PeHE and PuHE (0–500 μg/mL) for 2 and 24 h markedly restored these changes only at high concentrations. However, no significant differences were seen in the protection against ischemic insult between different extracts and the time of exposure. The experimental results suggest that persimmon protects the PC12 cells from GOSD-induced injury via antioxidant mechanisms. Our findings might raise the possibility of potential therapeutic application of persimmon for managing cerebral ischemic and other neurodegenerative disorders.

1. Introduction

Oxidative stress plays an important role in nerve cell damage and is closely related to the pathogenesis of many central nervous system diseases such as cerebral ischemia, Alzheimer's disease, and Parkinson's disease. During neuropathological states, excessive reactive oxygen species (ROS) generation caused significant damage to cellular macromolecules (i.e., cellular lipids, proteins, or DNA), leading to cellular death [1]. Deprivation of neurons from glucose-oxygen-serum deprivation (GOSD) is a reliable *in vitro* model for understanding of the molecular mechanisms of ischemia-induced neuronal damage and also for the discovery and development of novel compounds for better treatment of cerebral ischemia [2].

Recently, there are intensive interests towards neuroprotective properties of herbal products in ischemic brain injury because of relatively high therapeutic value and less serious side effects [3]. Persimmon (*Diospyros kaki*), which belongs to the Ebenaceae family, is a deciduous small tree native to Eastern Asia and has also been cultivated in Northeastern India, Middle East, Spain, and many other regions. The dry residue of persimmon fruit is known to have many bioactive compounds such as flavonoids, polyphenol (especially tannins), carotenoids, dietary fibers, and minerals [4, 5]. In many traditional medicinal systems, the extract of persimmon fruit is used as antitussive, carminative, and sedative agent and to heal bronchial complaints and hypertension [4, 5]. Recently, it has been shown that persimmon possesses several pharmacological activities such as strong radical scavenging and antioxidant properties [6] and antigenotoxic [6] and anticarcinogenic [7, 8] and anti-inflammatory [9] and anti-hypertensive [10] and antidiabetic [11] effects.

To our knowledge, no study has previously investigated the effect of persimmon fruit against cerebral ischemia, *in vitro* or *in vivo*. Considering that persimmon has antioxidant and anti-inflammatory properties, the aim of the present study was to investigate the effects of hydroalcoholic extracts of persimmon fruit peel and pulp on GOSD-induced PC12 cells injury. Role of intracellular ROS was also investigated.

2. Material and Methods

2.1. Cell Line and Reagents. A PC12 cell line was obtained from Pasteur Institute (Tehran, Iran). High glucose Dulbecco's Modified Eagles Medium (DMEM, 4.5 g/L) and fetal calf serum (FCS) were purchased from Gibco (Carlsbad, CA). Glucose-free DMEM, 3-(4,5-dimethylthiazol-2-yl)-2,5-diphenyl tetrazolium (MTT), $2',7'$-dichlorodihydrofluorescein diacetate (H$_2$DCF-DA), and other cell culture materials were purchased from Sigma (St. Louis, MO).

2.2. Preparation of PuHE (Pulp Hydroalcoholic Extract) and PeHE (Peel Hydroalcoholic Extract). Fresh fruits of a commercial cultivar in Khorasan province (Iran) were harvested and authenticated by herbarium of Ferdowsi University of Mashhad (Mashhad, Iran, voucher specimen number 11-0203-1).

The pulps and peels of whole seedless fruits were separated, washed, and then shaken with ethanol (70%) and water for 2 days. The resulting extracts were then filtered and concentrated under reduced pressure to get pulp hydroalcoholic extract (PuHE) and peel hydroalcoholic extract (PeHE), respectively. The yields were found to be about 27% w/w.

Stock solutions of PuHE and PeHE were prepared in deionized water and desired working concentrations were made from the stock using complete medium.

2.3. Cell Culture. PC12 cells were cultured in DMEM supplemented with 10% FCS and 100 units/mL of penicillin/streptomycin. All cells were maintained in a humidified atmosphere containing 5% CO$_2$ at 37°C [12].

2.4. Induction of Cell Injury by GOSD. To mimic the ischemic condition, PC12 cells were placed into in an incubation chamber containing "37°C, 5% CO$_2$, and 95% N$_2$" and cultured in glucose- and serum-free DMEM supplemented with 100 U/mL penicillin and 100 U/mL streptomycin for 6 h [2].

2.5. Cell Proliferation (MTT) Assay. MTT was used to identify viable cells which reduce it to a violet formazan dye [13]. PC12 cells (5000/well) were seeded out in 96-well tissue culture plates and, after 24 h, the cells were pretreated with PuHE and PeHE (0–500 μg/mL) for 2 and 24 h and then subjected to GOSD insult for 6 h, respectively. The concentrations and times were chosen based on earlier experiments. Controls were treated identically. At 6 h after GOSD insult, MTT was added to each well to achieve a final concentration

of 0.5 mg/mL. After incubation at 37°C for 4 h, the medium was removed and 100 μL of dimethyl sulfoxide was added to each well and kept for 10 min and the absorbance at 570 and 620 nm (background) was measured using StatFAX303 plate reader. All experiments were carried out in triplicate; the percentage of viable cells was calculated as the mean ± SEM with controls set to 100%.

2.6. Measurement of Intracellular Reactive Oxygen Species (ROS). The determination of intracellular ROS levels was accomplished with a fluorescent probe, H$_2$DCF-DA, as described previously with minor modifications [12]. H$_2$DCF-DA readily diffuses through the cell membrane and is enzymatically hydrolyzed by intracellular esterases to nonfluorescent H$_2$DCF, which is then rapidly oxidized to highly fluorescent DCF ($2',7'$-dichlorofluorescin) in the presence of ROS. The DCF fluorescence intensity is believed to parallel the amount of intracellular ROS [14]. In brief, PC12 cells (10^4 cells/well) were pretreated with different concentrations of PuHE and PeHE (0–500 μg/mL) for 2 h and then subjected to GOSD for 6 h in which the same treatments were applied. At 6 h after ischemic insult, the cells were incubated with 20 μM H$_2$DCF-DA at 37°C for 30 min in the dark. The DCF fluorescence intensity was detected using a FLUO-star galaxy fluorescence plate reader (Perkin Elmer 2030, Multilabel reader, Finland) with excitation wavelength set at 485 nm and emission wavelength set at 530 nm.

2.7. Statistical Analysis. The results are presented as the mean ± standard error (SEM). The values were compared using the one-way analysis of variance (ANOVA) followed by Tukey's post hoc test for multiple comparisons. The p values less than 0.05 were considered to be statistically significant.

3. Results

3.1. Effects of PeHE and PuHE on Cell Viability following GOSD Insult in PC12 Cells. Exposure to GOSD for 6 h significantly decreased cell viability as compared with control cells. The average survival rate of cells under the GOSD condition was about 36%.

Pretreatment with PeHE for 2 h significantly attenuated GOSD-induced damage to PC12 cells only at high concentration (500 μg/mL; 110.5 ± 4.2; $p < 0.001$) as compared to GOSD group (37.0 ± 4.0) (Figure 1(a)). Also, pretreatment with PeHE for 24 h significantly attenuated GOSD-induced PC12 cells death at concentration of 500 μg/mL (27.3 ± 10.0; $p < 0.01$) (Figure 1(b)).

In the same way, pretreatment with PuHE for 2 h significantly attenuated cell death induced by GOSD at concentration of 500 μg/mL (105.0 ± 5.3; $p < 0.001$) as compared to GOSD group (35.0 ± 2.0) (Figure 1(c)). Again, pretreatment with PuHE for 24 h significantly increased cell survival following ischemic insult at concentration of 500 μg/mL (57.5 ± 9.5; $p < 0.001$) and at concentration of 400 μg/mL (29.0 ± 13.0; $p < 0.05$) (Figure 1(d)).

3.2. Effects of PeHE and PuHE on ROS Production following GOSD Insult in PC12 Cells. GOSD significantly increased the

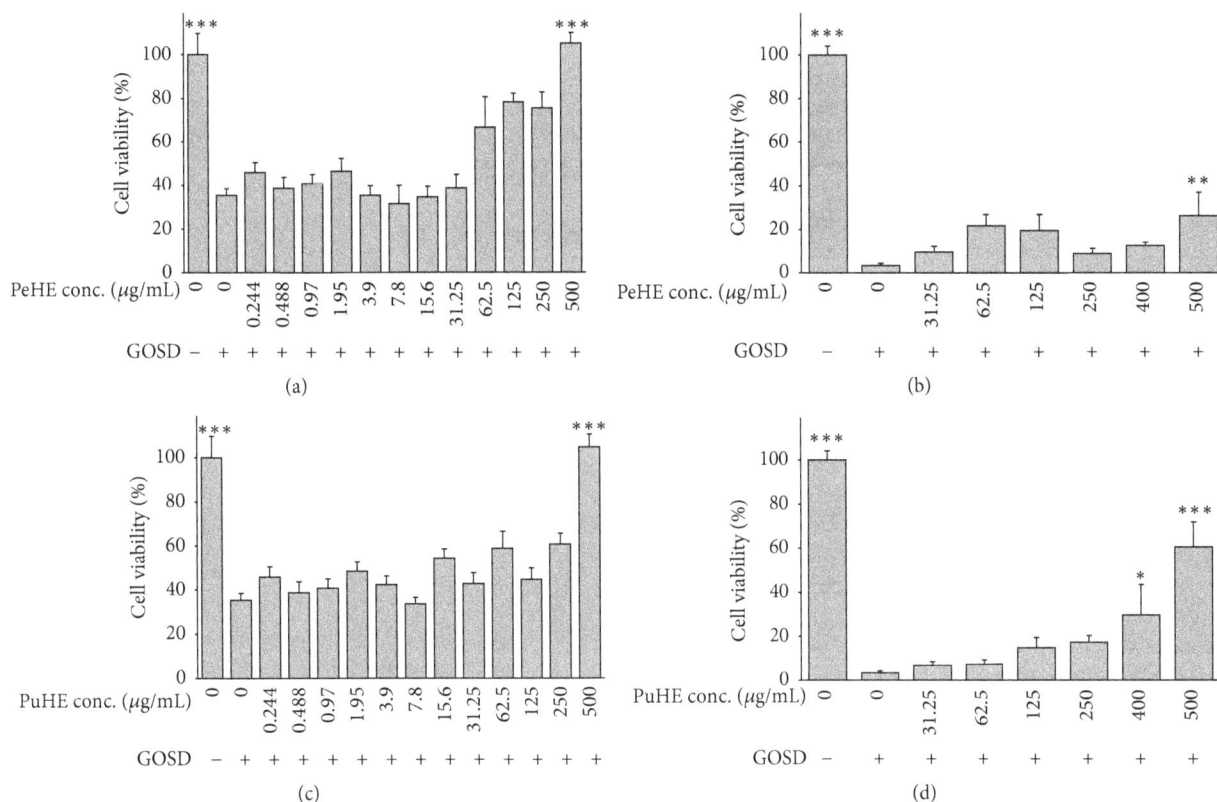

FIGURE 1: Effects of hydroalcoholic extracts of fruit peel (PeHE) and pulp (PuHE) of *Diospyros kaki* on PC12 cells death induced by glucose-oxygen-serum deprivation (GOSD). PC12 cells were treated with PeHE for 2 h (a) and 24 h (b) or PuHE for 2 h (c) and 24 h (d) and then subjected to GOSD for 6 h. the data are presented as mean ± SD from independent experiments performed in triplicate. $^*p < 0.05$, $^{**}p < 0.01$, and $^{***}p < 0.001$ as compared to ischemic group.

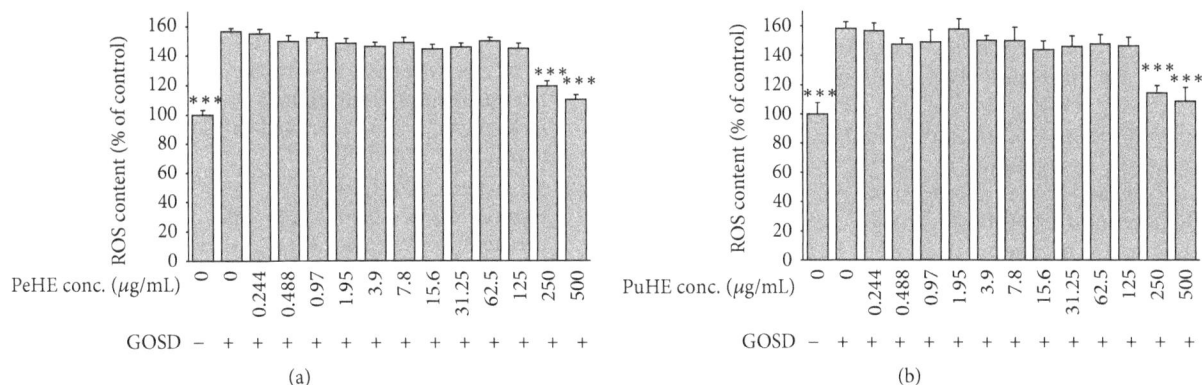

FIGURE 2: Effects of hydroalcoholic extracts of fruit peel (PeHE) and pulp (PuHE) of *Diospyros kaki* on ROS production in glucose-oxygen-serum deprivation- (GOSD-) treated PC12 cells. PC12 cells were preincubated with PeHE (a) or PuHE (b) for 2 h prior to GOSD insult. Then, PC12 cells were loaded with DCF-DA, and intracellular ROS were detected by fluorimetry. The data are represented as mean ± SD from independent experiments performed in triplicate. $^{***}p < 0.001$ as compared to ischemic group.

number of DCF-positive cells illustrating an elevation of ROS production to 156%. As shown in Figure 2(a), pretreatment with PeHE for 2 h resulted in a significant ($p < 0.001$) reduction in ROS production following GOSD (121.4 ± 2.0 and 110.4±2.0 at concentrations of 250 and 500 μg/mL, resp.).

As illustrated in Figure 2(b), pretreatment with PuHE for 2 h caused a significant reduction of ROS production

following GOSD (114.3 ± 4.2; $p < 0.01$ and 108.4 ± 9; $p < 0.001$ at concentrations of 250 and 500 μg/mL, resp.).

4. Discussion

According to our knowledge, this is the first report of the neuroprotective effect of *D. kaki* fruit extract. In the present study, we demonstrated that pretreatment with peel and pulp fruit extracts of *D. kaki* was able to promote cell survival and depress ROS increase upon GOSD stress in PC12 cells. Recently, substantial efforts have been invested for identifying optimal drugs that can reduce ischemic brain damage [2].

It is well known that ischemia increases the formation of ROS in brain tissues and antioxidants and ROS scavengers can decrease tissue damage following ischemic injury [15–17]. Excessive production of ROS will act as damaging molecule causing cell death either directly, through interacting and destroying cellular proteins, lipids, and DNA, or indirectly, by affecting normal cellular signaling pathways and gene regulation [15, 18].

One possible mechanism underlying the attenuation of ROS generation following ischemic insult is due to antioxidant and free radical scavenger properties of persimmon. Previous studies have shown that flavonoids from persimmon peel and leaf could protect against hydrogen proxide-induced oxidative damage, *in vitro* [19, 20]. High molecular weight persimmon tannin also ameliorates oxidative damage and cognition deficits in D-galactose-induced senescent mice [21]. Tian et al. showed that administration of high molecular weight persimmon condensed tannin (HMWPT) significantly protected serum and liver antioxidant enzymes from damage and prevented lipid peroxidation in bromobenzene-treated mice [22]. In addition, several studies suggest that persimmon leaves extract and its flavonoids exhibit neuroprotective effects and protect rats from both focal and global cerebral ischemic injury, *in vivo*, as well as cortical neurons from hypoxia-induced injury, *in vitro* [23, 24]. High-performance liquid chromatography (HPLC) analysis also revealed that gallic acid and quercetin were the major phenolic components in the fruit extracts of persimmon [25].

Also, antiaging and memory enhancing effects of oligomeric proanthocyanidins isolated from persimmon fruits have also been described in a senescence-accelerated mouse prone model [26–28]. A recent study showed that ethanol extract of *Diospyros kaki* leaves significantly attenuated the upregulation of vascular endothelial growth factor, fibroblast growth factor, interleukin-6, and matrix metalloproteinase-2 (MMP-2) protein levels, in alkali burn-induced corneal neovascularization in rats [29]. Kim et al. also showed that ethanol extract of *Diospyros kaki* leaves prevented degenerative retinal diseases in N-methyl-N-nitrosourea- (MNU-) induced retinal degeneration in mice [30].

5. Conclusions

In summary, the results of the current study suggest that persimmon is able to protect cultured PC12 cells against damage induced by GOSD. These effects of persimmon are, at least in part, attributable to its antioxidant property. This study on the neuroprotective effects of persimmon may suggest the possible application of persimmon in clinical setting to prevent and treat the common neurological insults.

Conflict of Interests

The authors declare that they have no conflict of interests.

Acknowledgment

This work was supported by the Office of the Vice Chancellor for Research and Technology of Mashhad University of Medical Sciences under Grant no. 901050. The authors are gratefully acknowledging this financial support.

References

[1] V. Shukla, S. K. Mishra, and H. C. Pant, "Oxidative stress in neurodegeneration," *Advances in Pharmacological Sciences*, vol. 2011, Article ID 572634, 13 pages, 2011.

[2] C.-H. Wang, W.-J. Lee, V. K. Ghanta, W.-T. Wang, S.-Y. Cheng, and C.-M. Hsueh, "Molecules involve in the self-protection of neurons against glucose-oxygen-serum deprivation (GOSD)-induced cell damage," *Brain Research Bulletin*, vol. 79, no. 3-4, pp. 169–176, 2009.

[3] K. Suk, "Regulation of neuroinflammation by herbal medicine and its implications for neurodegenerative diseases: a focus on traditional medicines and flavonoids," *NeuroSignals*, vol. 14, no. 1-2, pp. 23–33, 2005.

[4] U. V. Mallavadhani, A. K. Panda, and Y. R. Rao, "Pharmacology and chemotaxonomy of Diospyros," *Phytochemistry*, vol. 49, no. 4, pp. 901–951, 1998.

[5] S. Singh and H. Joshi, "Diospyros kaki (Ebenaceae): a review," *Asian Journal of Research in Pharmaceutical Sciences*, vol. 1, no. 3, pp. 55–58, 2011.

[6] I.-C. Jang, E.-K. Jo, M.-S. Bae et al., "Antioxidant and antigenotoxic activities of different parts of persimmon (*Diospyros kaki* cv. Fuyu) fruit," *Journal of Medicinal Plants Research*, vol. 4, no. 2, pp. 155–160, 2010.

[7] M. Kawase, N. Motohashi, K. Satoh et al., "Biological activity of persimmon (*Diospyros kaki*) peel extracts," *Phytotherapy Research*, vol. 17, no. 5, pp. 495–500, 2003.

[8] Y. Achiwa, H. Hibasami, H. Katsuzaki, K. Imai, and T. Komiya, "Inhibitory effects of persimmon (*Diospyros kaki*) extract and related polyphenol compounds on growth of human lymphoid leukemia cells," *Bioscience, Biotechnology and Biochemistry*, vol. 61, no. 7, pp. 1099–1101, 1997.

[9] M. Del Carmen Recio, R. M. Giner, S. Manez et al., "Investigations on the steroidal anti-inflammatory activity of triterpenoids from *Diospyros leucomelas*," *Planta Medica*, vol. 61, no. 1, pp. 9–12, 1995.

[10] K. Kawakami, S. Aketa, H. Sakai, Y. Watanabe, H. Nishida, and M. Hirayama, "Antihypertensive and vasorelaxant effects of water-soluble proanthocyanidins from persimmon leaf tea in spontaneously hypertensive rats," *Bioscience, Biotechnology and Biochemistry*, vol. 75, no. 8, pp. 1435–1439, 2011.

[11] C. Li, W. Bei, Y. Li, and J. Lou, "Ethylacetate extract of *Diospyros kaki* leaf for preventing and treating hyperglycemic, diabetes and metabolic syndromes," *Faming Zhuanli Shenqing Gongkai Shuomingshu*, vol. 32, pp. 21–23, 2007.

[12] F. Forouzanfar, A. Afkhami Goli, E. Asadpour, A. Ghorbani, and H. R. Sadeghnia, "Protective effect of *Punica granatum* L. against serum/glucose deprivation-induced PC12 cells injury," *Evidence-Based Complementary and Alternative Medicine*, vol. 2013, Article ID 716730, 9 pages, 2013.

[13] T. Mosmann, "Rapid colorimetric assay for cellular growth and survival: application to proliferation and cytotoxicity assays," *Journal of Immunological Methods*, vol. 65, no. 1-2, pp. 55–63, 1983.

[14] H. Wang and J. A. Joseph, "Quantifying cellular oxidative stress by dichlorofluorescein assay using microplate reader," *Free Radical Biology and Medicine*, vol. 27, no. 5-6, pp. 612–616, 1999.

[15] Y. Li, Y. Bao, B. Jiang et al., "Catalpol protects primary cultured astrocytes from in vitro ischemia-induced damage," *International Journal of Developmental Neuroscience*, vol. 26, no. 3-4, pp. 309–317, 2008.

[16] J. Yamada, S. Yoshimura, H. Yamakawa et al., "Cell permeable ROS scavengers, Tiron and Tempol, rescue PC12 cell death caused by pyrogallol or hypoxia/reoxygenation," *Neuroscience Research*, vol. 45, no. 1, pp. 1–8, 2003.

[17] M. Tagami, K. Yamagata, K. Ikeda et al., "Vitamin E prevents apoptosis in cortical neurons during hypoxia and oxygen reperfusion," *Laboratory Investigation*, vol. 78, no. 11, pp. 1415–1429, 1998.

[18] P. H. Chan, "Reactive oxygen radicals in signaling and damage in the ischemic brain," *Journal of Cerebral Blood Flow & Metabolism*, vol. 21, no. 1, pp. 2–14, 2001.

[19] Y. A. Lee, E. J. Cho, and T. Yokozawa, "Protective effect of persimmon (*Diospyros kaki*) peel proanthocyanidin against oxidative damage under H_2O_2-induced cellular senescence," *Biological and Pharmaceutical Bulletin*, vol. 31, no. 6, pp. 1265–1269, 2008.

[20] W. Bei, W. Peng, Y. Ma, and A. Xu, "Flavonoids from the leaves of *Diospyros kaki* reduce hydrogen peroxide-induced injury of NG108-15 cells," *Life Sciences*, vol. 76, no. 17, pp. 1975–1988, 2005.

[21] Y. Tian, B. Zou, L. Yang et al., "High molecular weight persimmon tannin ameliorates cognition deficits and attenuates oxidative damage in senescent mice induced by D-galactose," *Food and Chemical Toxicology*, vol. 49, no. 8, pp. 1728–1736, 2011.

[22] Y. Tian, B. Zou, C.-M. Li, J. Yang, S.-F. Xu, and A. E. Hagerman, "High molecular weight persimmon tannin is a potent antioxidant both ex vivo and in vivo," *Food Research International*, vol. 45, no. 1, pp. 26–30, 2012.

[23] W. Bei, W. Peng, L. Zang, Z. Xie, D. Hu, and A. Xu, "Neuroprotective effects of a standardized extract of *Diospyros kaki* leaves on MCAO transient focal cerebral ischemic rats and cultured neurons injured by glutamate or hypoxia," *Planta Medica*, vol. 73, no. 7, pp. 636–643, 2007.

[24] W. Bei, L. Zang, J. Guo et al., "Neuroprotective effects of a standardized flavonoid extract from *Diospyros kaki* leaves," *Journal of Ethnopharmacology*, vol. 126, no. 1, pp. 134–142, 2009.

[25] F. Pu, X.-L. Ren, and X.-P. Zhang, "Phenolic compounds and antioxidant activity in fruits of six *Diospyros kaki* genotypes," *European Food Research and Technology*, vol. 237, no. 6, pp. 923–932, 2013.

[26] Y. A. Lee, E. J. Cho, and T. Yokozawa, "Oligomeric proanthocyanidins improve memory and enhance phosphorylation of vascular endothelial growth factor receptor-2 in senescence-accelerated mouse prone/8," *British Journal of Nutrition*, vol. 103, no. 4, pp. 479–489, 2010.

[27] T. Yokozawa, Y. A. Lee, E. J. Cho, K. Matsumoto, C. H. Park, and N. Shibahara, "Anti-aging effects of oligomeric proanthocyanidins isolated from persimmon fruits," *Drug Discoveries & Therapeutics*, vol. 5, no. 3, pp. 109–118, 2011.

[28] T. Yokozawa, Y. A. Lee, Q. Zhao, K. Matsumoto, and E. J. Cho, "Persimmon oligomeric proanthocyanidins extend life span of senescence-accelerated mice," *Journal of Medicinal Food*, vol. 12, no. 6, pp. 1199–1205, 2009.

[29] S. J. Yang, H. Jo, K.-A. Kim, H. R. Ahn, S. W. Kang, and S. H. Jung, "Diospyros kaki extract inhibits alkali burn-induced corneal neovascularization," *Journal of Medicinal Food*, vol. 19, no. 1, pp. 106–109, 2016.

[30] K.-A. Kim, S. W. Kang, H. R. Ahn, Y. Song, S. J. Yang, and S. H. Jung, "The leaves of persimmon (*Diospyros kaki* Thunb.) ameliorate N-methyl-N-nitrosourea (MNU)-induced retinal degeneration in mice," *Journal of Agricultural and Food Chemistry*, vol. 63, no. 35, pp. 7750–7759, 2015.

22

In Vitro Study on Glucose Utilization Capacity of Bioactive Fractions of *Houttuynia cordata* in Isolated Rat Hemidiaphragm and Its Major Phytoconstituent

Manish Kumar,[1] **Satyendra K. Prasad,**[1,2] **and Siva Hemalatha**[1]

[1]*Pharmacognosy Research Laboratory, Department of Pharmaceutics, Indian Institute of Technology (Banaras Hindu University), Varanasi 221005, India*
[2]*Department of Pharmaceutical Sciences, R. T. M. Nagpur University, Nagpur 440033, India*

Correspondence should be addressed to Siva Hemalatha; shemalatha.phe@itbhu.ac.in

Academic Editor: Thérèse Di Paolo-Chênevert

Objective. The whole plant of *Houttuynia cordata* has been reported to have potent antihyperglycemic activity. Therefore, the present study was undertaken to investigate the glucose utilization capacity of bioactive fractions of ethanol extract of *Houttuynia cordata* (HC) in isolated rat hemidiaphragm. *Methods.* All the fractions, that is, aqueous (AQ), hexane (HEX), chloroform (CHL), and ethyl acetate (EA), obtained from ethanol extract of *H. cordata* were subjected to phytochemical standardization use in quercetin as a marker with the help of HPTLC. Further, glucose utilization capacity by rat hemidiaphragm was evaluated in 12 different sets of *in vitro* experiments. In the study, different fractions from *H. cordata* as mentioned above were evaluated, where insulin was used as standard and quercetin as a biological standard. *Results.* Among all the tested fractions, AQ and EA significantly increased glucose uptake by isolated rat hemidiaphragm compared to negative control. Moreover, AQ fractions enhanced the uptake of glucose significantly ($p < 0.05$) and was found to be more effective than insulin. *Conclusions.* The augmentation in glucose uptake by hemidiaphragm in presence of AQ and EA fractions may be attributed to the presence of quercetin, which was found to be 7.1 and 3.2% w/w, respectively, in both the fractions.

1. Introduction

Diabetes mellitus is a group of metabolic disorders, characterized by hyperglycemia resulting from the defects in insulin secretion, insulin action, or both [1]. Numbers of therapies have been used to improve the status of diabetes by different mechanisms such as inhibition of carbohydrate metabolizing enzymes, manipulation of glucose transporters, β-cell regeneration, and enhancing the insulin releasing activity [2]. Although oral hypoglycemic agents and insulin are the cornerstones of treatment of diabetes and are effective in controlling hyperglycemia, they have prominent side effects and many limitations exist in their use [3]. Therefore, the management of diabetes without any side effect is still a challenge to the medical system. Many efforts have been made to identify new hypoglycemic agents obtained from different sources especially from medicinal plants because of their effectiveness, fewer side effects, and relatively low cost. Several medicinal plants have been investigated for their beneficial use in different types of diabetes in the traditional system of medicine; however, studies related to their biologically active components are still lacking and require a great encouragement [4].

Houttuynia cordata Thunb. (Saururaceae) is a single species of its genus and is native to Japan, South-East Asia, and Himalayas. The whole plant of *H. cordata* is being widely used as a medicinal salad in North-East region of India for lowering the blood glucose level and is commonly known by the name Jamyrdoh [5]. Traditionally it is used to cure various human ailments throughout South-East Asia, namely, cancer, coughs, dysentery, enteritis, fever, snake bites, and skin disorders. Pharmacologically this plant has been validated for antioxidant, antihypertension, antiedema, anti-inflammatory, antipyretic, antipurulent, antihyperglycemic, and aldose reductase inhibitory activities [6–9]. The major active constituents of *H. cordata* include quercetin, chlorogenic acid, caffeic acid, hyperin, and rutin which have exhibited antioxidant, antihyperglycmic, anticancer, and neuroprotective effects in various experimental models [10–15]. With these reports, it was suggested that flavonoids are molecules capable to interact with more than one target and therefore termed as privileged structures in accordance with Patchett's definition [16]. Conventional antidiabetic agents can affect several pathways of glucose metabolism such as insulin secretion, glucose uptake by target organs, and nutrient absorption. As the plant has been reported for its antihyperglycaemic potential; therefore, estimation of glucose content in rat hemidiaphragm may act as a reliable method for determining the efficiency of the plant in *in vitro* peripheral uptake of glucose. Therefore, on the basis of above background the present study was undertaken for the first time to assess the potential role of different fraction of *H. cordata* on the peripheral utilization of glucose.

2. Material and Methods

2.1. Plant Material. Whole plant of *H. cordata* was collected during the months of June–September (2012) from various areas of the West and East Jaintia Hills district (namely, Jowai, Mihmyntdu, Khliehriat, and Ladrymbai) of Meghalaya, North-East, India. Voucher herbarium specimen (COG/HC/011-2012) was prepared and preserved along with sample of crude drug in the Pharmacognosy research laboratory of Department of Pharmaceutics, Indian Institute of Technology, Banaras Hindu University, Varanasi (UP), India. The plant material was identified and authenticated by Dr. B. K. Sinha (Scientist In-charge), Botanical Survey of India, Shillong, Meghalaya.

2.2. Preparation and Standardization of Extract and Its Fractions. Whole plant of *H. cordata* was washed with water, shade dried, and ground in a mill and was passed through sieve #40 to obtain a homogenous powder. The coarsely powdered plant material (1 Kg) of *H. cordata* was exhaustively extracted for 24 h by soxhlation using 95% ethanol (3 L v/v) as solvent for extraction. The resulting extract was filtered and concentrated under reduced pressure to obtain the crude ethanol extract of *H. cordata* (EHC) (yield: 13.2% w/w). The ethanol extract was then subjected to successive fractionation by suspending in aqueous media and then partitioning with solvents of varying polarity such as hexane, chloroform, and ethyl acetate in order of their ascending polarity.

Further, all the fractions, that is, aqueous (AQ), hexane (HEX), chloroform (CHL), and ethyl acetate (EA), from *H. cordata* were standardized with quercetin (QC) using high performance thin layer chromatography (HPTLC). Mobile phase for developing the chromatogram was composed of chloroform : methanol and formic acid mixture in the ratio 7.5 : 1.5 : 1 (v/v/v). The concentration of quercetin was taken as 0.5 mg/mL, while that of the fractions was taken as 5 mg/mL in methanol. The study was carried out using Camag-HPTLC instrumentation (Camag, Mutten, Switzerland) equipped with Linomat V sample applicator, Camag TLC scanner 3, Camag TLC visualizer, and WINCATS 4 software for data interpretation. The R_f values were recorded and the developed plate was screened and photodocumented at ultra violet range with wavelength (λ_{max}) of 254 nm (details in Supplementary data; see Supplementary Material available online at http://dx.doi.org/10.1155/2016/2573604).

2.3. Study of Glucose Utilization by Isolated Rat Hemidiaphragm Technique. Glucose uptake by rat hemidiaphragm was estimated by the method described by Hemalatha et al. [17], using regular insulin (Biocon Ltd.) as a positive control group and rat's hemidiaphragm for the assay. Glucose uptake per gram of tissue was calculated as the difference between the initial and final glucose content in the incubated medium [18].

2.4. Animals. Albino rats of Charles foster strain with body weights of 160–200 g were obtained from the Central Animal House (Reg. number 542/02/ab/CPCSEA), Institute of Medical Science (IMS), Banaras Hindu University (BHU), Varanasi, India. Rats were fed with normal laboratory pellet diet (Hindustan lever Ltd., India) with water *ad libitum* and were housed in polypropylene cages under standard laboratory condition [12 h light/12 h darkness, (21±2°C)]. The experimental protocol has been approved by the institutional animal ethics committee (Reference number Dean/10-11/58 dated 07.03.2011).

2.5. Assessment of Glucose Utilization by Rat Hemidiaphragm Method. For the estimation of glucose utilization by rat hemidiaphragm, twelve sets containing three numbers of graduated test tubes (n = 3) each were taken. Group I was served as a control which contained 2 mL of Tyrode's solution with 2% glucose and group II contained 2 mL Tyrode's solution with 2% glucose and regular insulin (Biocon Ltd.), that is, 1 mL of 0.25 IU/mL of solution. Group III contained 2 mL of Tyrode's solution with 2% glucose and 1 mL of (1 mg/mL) solution of quercetin, used as biological standard. Group IV contained 2 mL of Tyrode's solution with 2% glucose and regular insulin (1 mL of 0.25 IU/mL solution) and 1 mL of (1 mg/mL) solution of quercetin. Group V contained 2 mL of Tyrode's solution with 2% glucose and 1 mL of (25 mg/mL) of AQ fraction. Group VI contained 2 mL of Tyrode's solution with 2% glucose and 1 mL of (25 mg/mL) of AQ fraction and regular insulin (1 mL of 0.25 IU/mL solution). Group VII contained 2 mL of Tyrode's solution with 2% glucose and 1 mL of (25 mg/mL) of EA fraction. Group VIII contained 2 mL of Tyrode's solution with 2% glucose and 1 mL of (25 mg/mL) of EA fraction and regular insulin (1 mL of 0.25 IU/mL solution). Group IX contained 2 mL of Tyrode's solution with 2% glucose and 1 mL of (25 mg/mL) of CHL fraction. Group X contained 2 mL of Tyrode's solution with 2% glucose and 1 mL of (25 mg/mL) of CHL fraction and regular insulin (1 mL of 0.25 IU/mL solution). Group XI contained 2 mL of Tyrode's solution with 2% glucose and 1 mL of (25 mg/mL) of HEX fraction. Group XII contained 2 mL of Tyrode's solution with 2% glucose and 1 mL of (25 mg/mL) of HEX fraction and regular insulin (1 mL of 0.25 IU/mL solution).

TABLE 1: Effect of different fractions of *H. cordata* on glucose utilization by isolated rat hemidiaphragm.

Group	Incubation medium	Glucose uptake (mg/g/30 min)
Control	Tyrode solution with glucose (2%)	15.74 ± 0.38
Insulin	Tyrode solution with glucose (2%) + insulin (0.25 IU/mL)	29.65 ± 0.54^a
QC	Tyrode solution with glucose (2%) + quercetin (1 mg/mL)	31.42 ± 1.87^a
Insulin + QC	Tyrode solution with glucose (2%) + insulin (0.25 IU/mL) + quercetin (1 mg/mL)	34.10 ± 1.03^a
AQ	Tyrode solution with glucose (2%) + aqueous fraction (25 mg/mL)	$35.26 \pm 0.52^{a,b}$
Insulin + AQ	Tyrode solution with glucose (2%) + insulin (0.25 IU/mL) + aqueous fraction (25 mg/mL)	$36.21 \pm 1.63^{a,b}$
EA	Tyrode solution with glucose (2%) + ethyl acetate fraction (25 mg/mL)	24.58 ± 0.56^a
Insulin + EA	Tyrode solution with glucose (2%) + insulin (0.25 IU/mL) + ethyl acetate fraction (25 mg/mL)	28.60 ± 0.33^a
CHL	Tyrode solution with glucose (2%) + chloroform fraction (25 mg/mL)	19.32 ± 0.84
Insulin + CHL	Tyrode solution with glucose (2%) + insulin (0.25 IU/mL) + chloroform fraction (25 mg/mL)	23.33 ± 0.54^a
HEX	Tyrode solution with glucose (2%) + hexane fraction (25 mg/mL)	17.41 ± 0.81
Insulin + HEX	Tyrode solution with glucose (2%) + insulin (0.25 IU/mL) + hexane fraction (25 mg/mL)	22.32 ± 0.36^a

All results are expressed as mean ± SEM. Statistical comparison was determined by one-way ANOVA followed by Tukey's multiple comparison test. $^a p < 0.05$, statistically significant compared to control group; $^b p < 0.05$ compared to insulin.
AQ: aqueous fraction, EA: ethyl acetate fraction, CHL: chloroform fraction, and HEX: hexane fraction of *H. cordata*.

The final volume of all the test tubes was made up to 4 mL with distilled water to match the volume of the test tubes of group IV. Albino rats were sacrificed by cervical dislocation after overnight fasting. The diaphragms were dissected out quickly with minimal strain and divided into two equal halves. Two diaphragms from the same animal were not used for the same set of experiment. The hemidiaphragms were placed in test tubes and incubated for 30 min at 37°C in an atmosphere of 95% oxygen and 5% CO_2 with shaking at 140 cycles/min. Glucose uptake per gram of tissue was calculated as the difference between the initial and final glucose content in the incubated medium.

2.6. Statistical Analysis. The data were analyzed with Graph-Pad Prism version 5 (San Diego, CA). Statistical analysis was done by one-way ANOVA, followed by Tukey's multiple comparison test. Data are expressed as mean ± SEM. A level of $p < 0.05$ was accepted as statistically significant.

3. Result

Different concentrations of fractions and quercetin were subjected to HPTLC analyses using mobile phase as chloroform : methanol and formic acid in the ratio 7.5 : 1.5 : 1 (v/v/v). R_f value of quercetin was reported to be 0.48 and the quercetin content was found to be 7.1% and 3.2% w/w in AQ and EA fractions, respectively, whereas CHL and HEX fractions did not show any measurable quercetin content (Figures 1(a), 1(b), and 1(c)).

In the present study different fractions from *H. cordata*, namely, aqueous, ethyl acetate, chloroform, and hexane fraction, were estimated for glucose utilization capacity by isolated rat hemidiaphragm. Among all the tested fractions, AQ fractions enhanced the uptake of glucose by isolated rat hemidiaphragm significantly ($p < 0.05$), which was found to be more effective than insulin (Table 1). Moreover, quercetin which was used as biological marker also showed significant glucose uptake ($p < 0.05$) when compared to glucose uptake

by rat hemidiaphragm of control group (Tyrode's solution with 2% glucose + rat hemidiaphragm) only (Table 1).

4. Discussion

Several investigations have demonstrated the beneficial effects of *H. cordata*. In our previous studies ethanol extract of *H. cordata* has been shown to possess antihyperglycemic activity, increase the antioxidant status of pancreatic β-cells, and promote the insulin secretion in rodents [8]. In the present study, we have made an attempt to investigate the plausible mechanism of action for the above proposed activity. From the literature search it was found that many herbs and plant products have been shown to have antidiabetic action due to high flavonoids contents, which are known to be bioactive antidiabetic principles. The positive results of the *in vivo* study that was undertaken previously by us in rodents for antidiabetic potential of *H. cordata* may be due the presence of flavonoid compounds.

The estimation of glucose content in rat hemidiaphragm was employed for *in vitro* study of peripheral uptake of glucose. The results showed that the AQ and EA fractions significantly increased glucose uptake by isolated rat hemidiaphragm as compared to normal control (Table 1). Furthermore, the AQ fractions enhanced the uptake of glucose significantly ($p < 0.05$) and were found to be more effective than insulin. Administration of QC significantly ($p < 0.05$) enhanced the uptake of glucose compared to control group as observed in insulin treated group. However, there was no significant difference observed when AQ fractions and insulin administered groups were together compared to AQ fraction alone. It is reported that insulin stimulates glucose transport in the isolated rat diaphragm primarily through a translocation of functional glucose transport units from an intracellular membrane pool to the plasma membrane [19]. As we have discussed earlier *H. cordata* enhances the insulin secretion; therefore it may be one of the rationale for glucose utilization by rat hemidiaphragm.

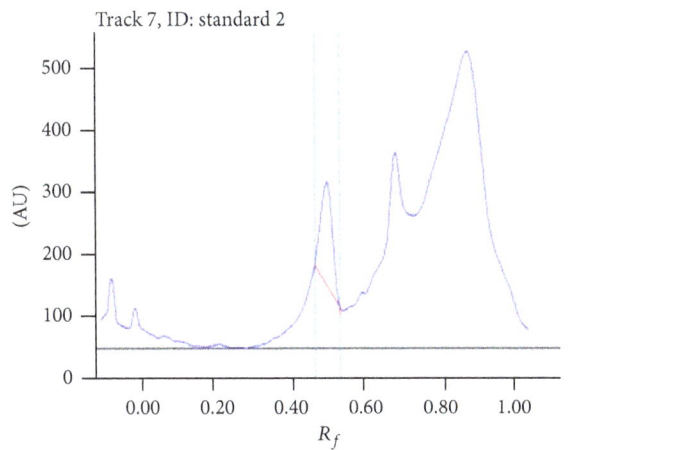

Peak	Start R_f	Start height	Max R_f	Max height	Max %	End R_f	End height	Area	Area %
1	0.47	3.5	0.52	186.5	100.00	0.54	14.1	4952.5	100.00

(a)

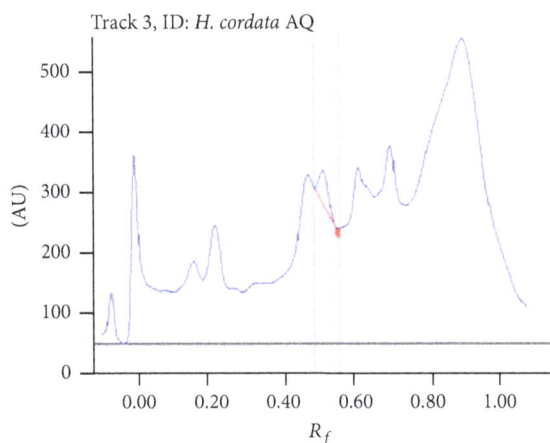

Peak	Start R_f	Start height	Max R_f	Max height	Max %	End R_f	End height	Area	Area %
1	0.48	0.1	0.51	103.7	100	0.54	0.9	2143.0	100.00

(b)

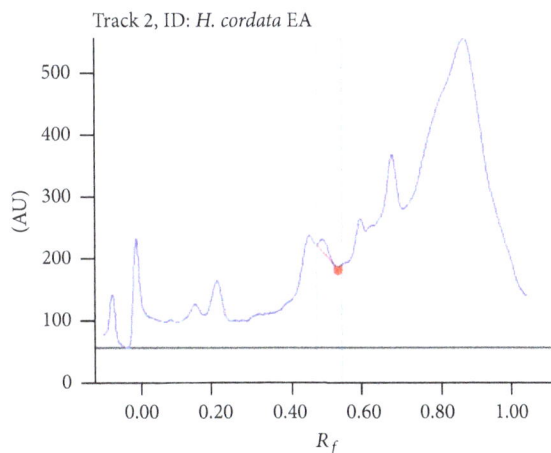

Peak	Start R_f	Start height	Max R_f	Max height	Max %	End R_f	End height	Area	Area %
1	0.49	0.4	0.51	57.3	100.00	0.54	0.4	1118.9	100.00

(c)

FIGURE 1: HPTLC chromatograms of quercetin (a); HPTLC chromatograms of quercetin in AQ fraction of *H. cordata* (b); HPTLC chromatograms of quercetin in EA fraction of *H. cordata* (c).

It is interesting to note that the quercetin content in AQ and EA fractions was significant as compared to CL and HEX (Figures 1(a), 1(b), and 1(c)), where it was not detected. *H. cordata* has been previously reported for the presence of a number of phenolic compounds such as quercitrin, afzelin, hyperin, rutin, quercetin, chlorogenic acid, and caffeic acid. However, amongst them, quercetin and rutin have been reported to possess action towards increase in glucose uptake by rat hemidiaphragm [20]. The results from the present study revealed that the augmentation in glucose utilization by hemidiaphragm in presence of AQ fractions may be attributed to the presence of quercetin, as it represents the major component of these fractions. However, the role of other phytoconstituents cannot be discounted unless verified by further experiments.

5. Conclusion

In the present study, glucose utilization capacity of different fractions of *H. cordata* was carried out on isolated rat hemidiaphragm. Among the tested fractions, aqueous fraction showed increased utilization of the glucose by hemidiaphragm, which may be attributed to the presence of high water soluble flavonoid contents. These results suggest that *H. cordata* had some extra pancreatic mechanism like glucose uptake by peripheral tissues.

Conflict of Interests

The authors report no conflict of interests. The authors alone are responsible for the content and writing of the paper.

Acknowledgments

Financial assistance provided by Rajiv Gandhi National Fellowship Scheme (RGNFS) to Mr. Manish Kumar is greatly acknowledged. The authors also wished to acknowledge Dr. B. K. Sinha, Botanical Survey of India, Shillong, Meghalaya, for identification and authentication of the plant.

References

[1] WHO Definition, "Diagnosis and classification of diabetes mellitus and its complications, part 1: diagnosis and classification of diabetes mellitus," Report of WHO Consultation, World Health Organization, Geneva, Switzerland, 1999.

[2] A. K. Tiwari and J. M. Rao, "Diabetes mellitus and multiple therapeutic approaches of phytochemicals: present status and future prospects," *Current Science*, vol. 83, no. 1, pp. 30–38, 2002.

[3] J. K. Grover, S. Yadav, and V. Vats, "Medicinal plants of India with anti-diabetic potential," *Journal of Ethnopharmacology*, vol. 81, no. 1, pp. 81–100, 2002.

[4] M. Modak, P. Dixit, J. Londhe, S. Ghaskadbi, and T. P. A. Devasagayam, "Indian herbs and herbal drugs used for the treatment of diabetes," *Journal of Clinical Biochemistry and Nutrition*, vol. 40, no. 3, pp. 163–173, 2007.

[5] M. Kumar, S. K. Prasad, and S. Hemalatha, "A current update on the phytopharmacological aspects of *Houttuynia cordata* Thunb," *Pharmacognosy Reviews*, vol. 8, no. 15, pp. 22–35, 2014.

[6] H. M. Lu, Y. Z. Liang, L. Z. Yi, and X. J. Wu, "Anti-inflammatory effect of *Houttuynia cordata* injection," *Journal of Ethnopharmacology*, vol. 104, no. 1-2, pp. 245–249, 2006.

[7] A. Probstle and R. Bauer, "Aristolactams and a 4,5-dioxoaporphine derivative from *Houttuynia cordata*," *Planta Medica*, vol. 58, no. 6, pp. 568–569, 1992.

[8] M. Kumar, S. K. Prasad, S. Krishnamurthy, and S. Hemalatha, "Antihyperglycemic activity of *Houttuynia cordata* Thunb. in streptozotocin-induced diabetic rats," *Advances in Pharmacological Sciences*, vol. 2014, Article ID 809438, 12 pages, 2014.

[9] M. Kumar, D. Laloo, S. K. Prasad, and S. Hemalatha, "Aldose reductase inhibitory potential of different fractions of *Houttuynia cordata* Thunb," *Journal of Acute Disease*, vol. 3, no. 1, pp. 64–68, 2014.

[10] M. A. Ansari, H. M. Abdul, G. Joshi, W. O. Opii, and D. A. Butterfield, "Protective effect of quercetin in primary neurons against Aβ(1–42): relevance to Alzheimer's disease," *Journal of Nutritional Biochemistry*, vol. 20, no. 4, pp. 269–275, 2009.

[11] H.-Y. Chen, J.-H. Wang, Z.-X. Ren, and X.-B. Yang, "Protective effect of hyperin on focal cerebral ischemia reperfusion injury in rat," *Zhong Xi Yi Jie He Xue Bao*, vol. 4, no. 5, pp. 526–529, 2006.

[12] S.-M. Huang, H.-C. Chuang, C.-H. Wu, and G.-C. Yen, "Cytoprotective effects of phenolic acids on methylglyoxal-induced apoptosis in Neuro-2A cells," *Molecular Nutrition and Food Research*, vol. 52, no. 8, pp. 940–949, 2008.

[13] M. M. Khan, A. Ahmad, T. Ishrat et al., "Rutin protects the neural damage induced by transient focal ischemia in rats," *Brain Research*, vol. 1292, pp. 123–135, 2009.

[14] C. Shi, L. Zhao, B. Zhu et al., "Protective effects of *Ginkgo biloba* extract (EGb761) and its constituents quercetin and ginkgolide B against beta-amyloid peptide-induced toxicity in SH-SY5Y cells," *Chemico-Biological Interactions*, vol. 181, pp. 115–123, 2009.

[15] L. Zhang, W.-P. Zhang, K.-D. Chen, X.-D. Qian, S.-H. Fang, and E.-Q. Wei, "Caffeic acid attenuates neuronal damage, astrogliosis and glial scar formation in mouse brain with cryoinjury," *Life Sciences*, vol. 80, no. 6, pp. 530–537, 2007.

[16] A. A. Patchett and R. P. Nargund, "Privileged structures—An update," in *Annual Reports in Medicinal Chemistry*, vol. 35, chapter 26, pp. 289–298, Elsevier, Philadelphia, Pa, USA, 2000.

[17] S. Hemalatha, N. Sachdeva, A. K. Wahi, P. N. Singh, and J. P. N. Chansouria, "Effect of aqueous extract of fruits of *Withania coagulans* on glucose utilization by rat hemidiaphragm," *Indian Journal of Natural products*, vol. 21, no. 2, pp. 20–21, 2005.

[18] D. K. Patel, K. Sairam, and S. Hemalatha, "Evaluation of glucose utilization capacity of bioactivity guided fractions of *Hybanthus enneaspermus* and *Pedalium murex* in isolated rat hemidiaphragm," *Journal of Acute Disease*, vol. 2, pp. 33–36, 2013.

[19] L. J. Wardzala and B. Jeanrenaud, "Potential mechanism of insulin action on glucose transport in the isolated rat diaphragm. Apparent translocation of intracellular transport units to the plasma membrane," *The Journal of Biological Chemistry*, vol. 256, no. 14, pp. 7090–7093, 1981.

[20] J. Ramulu and P. Goverdhan, "Hypoglycemic and antidiabetic activity of flavonoids: boswellic acid, ellagic acid, quercetin, rutin on streptozotocin-nicotinamide induced type 2 diabetic rats," *International Journal of Pharmacy and Pharmaceutical Sciences*, vol. 4, no. 2, pp. 251–256, 2012.

23

Role of Mas Receptor Antagonist A799 in Renal Blood Flow Response to Ang 1-7 after Bradykinin Administration in Ovariectomized Estradiol-Treated Rats

Aghdas Dehghani,[1,2] **Shadan Saberi,**[1,2] **and Mehdi Nematbakhsh**[1,2,3]

[1]*Water & Electrolytes Research Center, Isfahan University of Medical Sciences, Isfahan 81745, Iran*
[2]*Department of Physiology, Isfahan University of Medical Sciences, Isfahan 81745, Iran*
[3]*Isfahan*[MN] *Institute of Basic & Applied Sciences Research, Isfahan 81546, Iran*

Correspondence should be addressed to Mehdi Nematbakhsh; nematbakhsh@med.mui.ac.ir

Academic Editor: Thérèse Di Paolo-Chênevert

Background. The accompanied role of Mas receptor (MasR), bradykinin (BK), and female sex hormone on renal blood flow (RBF) response to angiotensin 1-7 is not well defined. We investigated the role of MasR antagonist (A779) and BK on RBF response to Ang 1-7 infusion in ovariectomized estradiol-treated rats. *Methods.* Ovariectomized Wistar rats received estradiol (OVE) or vehicle (OV) for two weeks. Catheterized animals were subjected to BK and A799 infusion and mean arterial pressure (MAP), RBF, and renal vascular resistance (RVR) responses to Ang 1-7 (0, 100, and 300 ng kg^{-1} min^{-1}) were determined. *Results.* Percentage change of RBF (%RBF) in response to Ang1-7 infusion increased in a dose-dependent manner. In the presence of BK, when MasR was not blocked, %RBF response to Ang 1-7 in OVE group was greater than OV group significantly ($P < 0.05$). Infusion of 300 ng kg^{-1} min^{-1} Ang 1-7 increased RBF by 6.9 ± 1.9% in OVE group versus 0.9 ± 1.8% in OV group. However when MasR was blocked, %RBF response to Ang 1-7 in OV group was greater than OVE group insignificantly. *Conclusion.* Coadministration of BK and A779 compared to BK alone increased RBF response to Ang 1-7 in vehicle treated rats. Such observation was not seen in estradiol treated rats.

1. Introduction

Women are shown to be protected against cardiovascular and renal diseases before menopause, suggesting that estrogen has beneficial roles in this respect [1–3]. Estrogen affects renin-angiotensin system (RAS) by stimulating the depressor pathway of this system [4–6], while this sex hormone enhances the kallikrein-kinin system (KKS), leading to the renoprotective effect [7, 8].

The heptapeptide angiotensin 1-7 (Ang 1-7) is a biologically active peptide of RAS, especially in the kidney [9, 10] via G-protein coupled Mas receptor (MasR) [11]. Ang 1-7 induces vasodilator response to attenuate the actions of angiotensin II (Ang II) [12] and therefore plays pivotal role in cardiovascular and renal systems [13, 14]. Endogenous levels of Ang 1-7 are increased by angiotensin converting enzyme (ACE) or Ang II type 1 receptor (AT1R) inhibitors

indicating that the protective effects of ACE or AT1R blockers are exerted by augmenting of this peptide [15, 16]. Ang 1-7 formation is different in the circulation and kidney [17, 18]. In circulation, neutral endopeptidase (NEP) is the main enzyme that produces Ang 1-7 [19], while the major enzyme that contributes to renal Ang 1-7 synthesis is ACE2 as ACE homologue [17, 18]. In general, the ACE2/Ang 1-7/Mas axis has a key role in renal hemodynamics.

KKS is also involved in the control of renal hemodynamics and function [20]. This system forms active peptides called kinins that have two distinct receptors, namely, B1 and B2 receptors [21]. Bradykinin (BK) is a main component of the KKS generated from kininogens by the kallikreins [21] and is expressed within the kidney [22]. In the kidney, the local infusion of BK enhances sodium and water excretion [23], while it mediates some functions via B2 receptor, including vasodilatation, natriuresis, and dieresis [23, 24]. It is well known that ACE participates in degradation of BK, and ACE inhibitor elevates the BK level. Therefore, the positive effects of ACE inhibitor in the kidney can be exerted by enhancing and prolonging the effects of BK [25, 26]. Ang 1-7 increases BK-induced vasodilator effects by activation of mediated factors, nitric oxide (NO) and prostaglandin release [21, 27]. It is demonstrated that cooperation between Ang 1-7 and BK potentiates vasodilatory response, mediated by endothelium-dependent release of NO [27], and coadministration of Ang 1-7 and BK causes hypotension [28]. In addition, B2 receptor antagonist, HOE-140, abolishes the vasodepressor effects of Ang 1-7 [28]. On the other hand, inhibition of MasR by A779 leads to blockade of BK and potentiating activity of Ang 1-7, indicating that MasR is involved in mediating the vasodilation effect [29].

Renal diseases usually are influenced by RBF disturbance [30–32] hormone dependently [3], and MasR, BK, and NO are abundant in the kidney too [33–36]. On the other hand, female sex hormone, estrogen, plays an important role in regulation of RAS and KKS [5–7]. This complex data raises the question about the role of estrogen and BK in renal Ang 1-7-Mas axis function.

Therefore, it is hypothesized that BK and estradiol may influence RBF response to Ang 1-7 via MasR. To examine this hypothesis, MasR was inhibited by A779 and in the presence of BK, the response of RBF to Ang 1-7 was measured in ovariectomized rats treated with estradiol, and the results were compared with those obtained from the control group.

2. Methods and Materials

2.1. Animals. Female rats were housed in the animal room with controlled temperature of 23–25°C and 12 h light/dark cycle. The rats were kept in cages with free access to water and chow. All experimental procedures were in advance confirmed by Isfahan University of Medical Sciences Ethics Committee.

Female Wistar rats (200 ± 20 g) were anesthetized (0.06 g/kg of ketamine 10% and xylazine 2% solution) and ovariectomized as described before [37]. After one week of recovery, the animals were randomly assigned into two groups named OVE as the treated group and OV as the control group. The animals in OVE group received estradiol valerate (500 g/kg/twice weekly, im) dissolved in sesame oil, while OV group received vehicle (sesame oil) for estradiol for two weeks. The animals were then subjected to surgical procedure.

2.2. Surgical Procedure. The rats were anesthetized by urethane (1.7 g/kg^{-1} i.p.; Merck, Germany). The trachea was cannulated for air ventilation and polyethylene catheters were inserted into the carotid and femoral arteries and jugular vein for direct mean arterial pressure (MAP) and renal perfusion pressure (RPP) measurements and drug administration, respectively. Arterial catheters were connected to a pressure transducer and bridge amplifier (Scientific Concepts, Melbourne, VIC, Australia) and attached to a data acquisition system. The bladder also was catheterized to collect urine output. Body temperature was monitored continuously through

the experiment. An adjustable clamp was put around the aorta above the renal artery to maintain RPP at the control level during Ang 1-7 infusion. With midline incision, the kidney was exposed and placed in a kidney cup. A transit-time ultrasound flow probe (Type 2BS; Transonic Systems, Ithaca, NY, USA) was placed around the renal artery to measure RBF. Then, 30–60 minutes after the equilibration period, basal MAP, RPP, and RBF were recorded and RVR was calculated as RPP/RBF.

2.3. Experimental Protocol. Both groups of OV and OVE underwent the experimental protocol according to the following procedure. After measurement of MAP, RPP, and RBF in the equilibration time, A779 or combination of BK and A779 was infused via the vein catheter. Therefore, in each group, we assigned two subgroups. Subgroup 1 and subgroup 2 from OV group received BK and BK + A779, respectively. Such treatments were applied in subgroups 1 and 2 from OVE group. A779 is a selective MasR antagonist and also has negligible affinity for Ang II receptors [38]. It was administrated at bolus doses of 50 μg/kg followed by continuous infusion at 50 μg/kg/h. BK as B2 agonist was infused at 150 μg/kg/h. Both BK and A779 were infused for the entire duration of experiment until the experiment was finished (end of Ang 1-7 infusion).

Thirty minutes after administration of agonist and antagonist, intravenous infusion of Ang 1-7 at graded doses of 0, 100, and 300 ng kg^{-1} min^{-1} was performed using a microsyringe pump (New Era Pump System Inc. Farmingdale, NY, USA). Each dose was given until the response of MAP reached plateau (approx. 15 min). Then, the rats were sacrificed humanely and the left kidney was weighed rapidly. The t-Student test was applied to analyze the baseline data and ANOVA for repeated measures was used for other data.

3. Results

3.1. Baseline Measurement. In baseline measurements, before infusion of BK or BK + A779, the groups were not significantly different in terms of MAP, RPP, RBF, and RBF per gram kidney weight (Figure 1).

3.2. Effect of Agonist and Antagonist. MAP and RPP did not significantly alter when BK or BK + A779 was administered in both OV and OVE groups. The results also indicated that BK or BK + A779 infusion had no significant effect on RBF percentage change (%RBF, Figure 2).

3.3. Responses to Ang 1-7 Infusion. A slight increase of MAP response to Ang 1-7 infusion was observed when both A779 and BK were infused. For example, 300 ng kg^{-1} min^{-1} Ang 1-7 increased MAP from 99.8 ± 2.4 (0 ng kg^{-1} min^{-1}) to 103.7 ± 2.9 mmHg in OV group and from 99.2 ± 6 (0 ng kg^{-1} min^{-1}) to 103.8 ± 5.9 mmHg in OVE group. However, in both the OV and OVE groups, the difference of MAP alteration between the two subgroups induced by Ang 1-7 infusion was not statistically meaningful (Figure 3). As mentioned before, RPP remained constant at the basal value during Ang

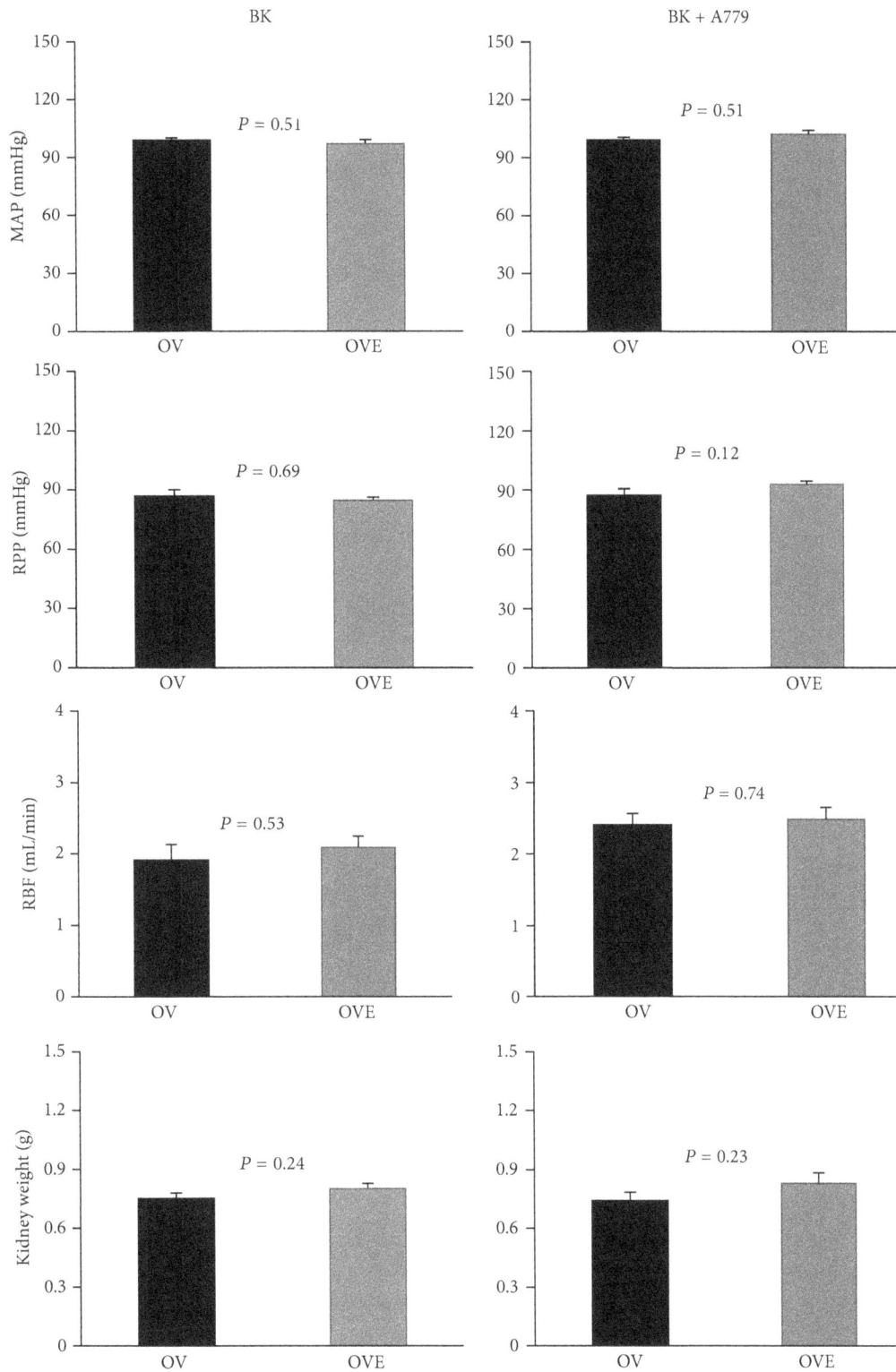

FIGURE 1: Baseline hemodynamic parameters in BK and BK + A779 groups in ovariectomized untreated and ovariectomized estradiol-treated rats. Data are presented as mean ± SEM. MAP, mean arterial pressure; RPP, renal perfusion pressure; RVR, renal vascular resistance; RBF, renal blood flow *per* gram kidney weight. There were no significant differences between the groups.

BK   BK + A779

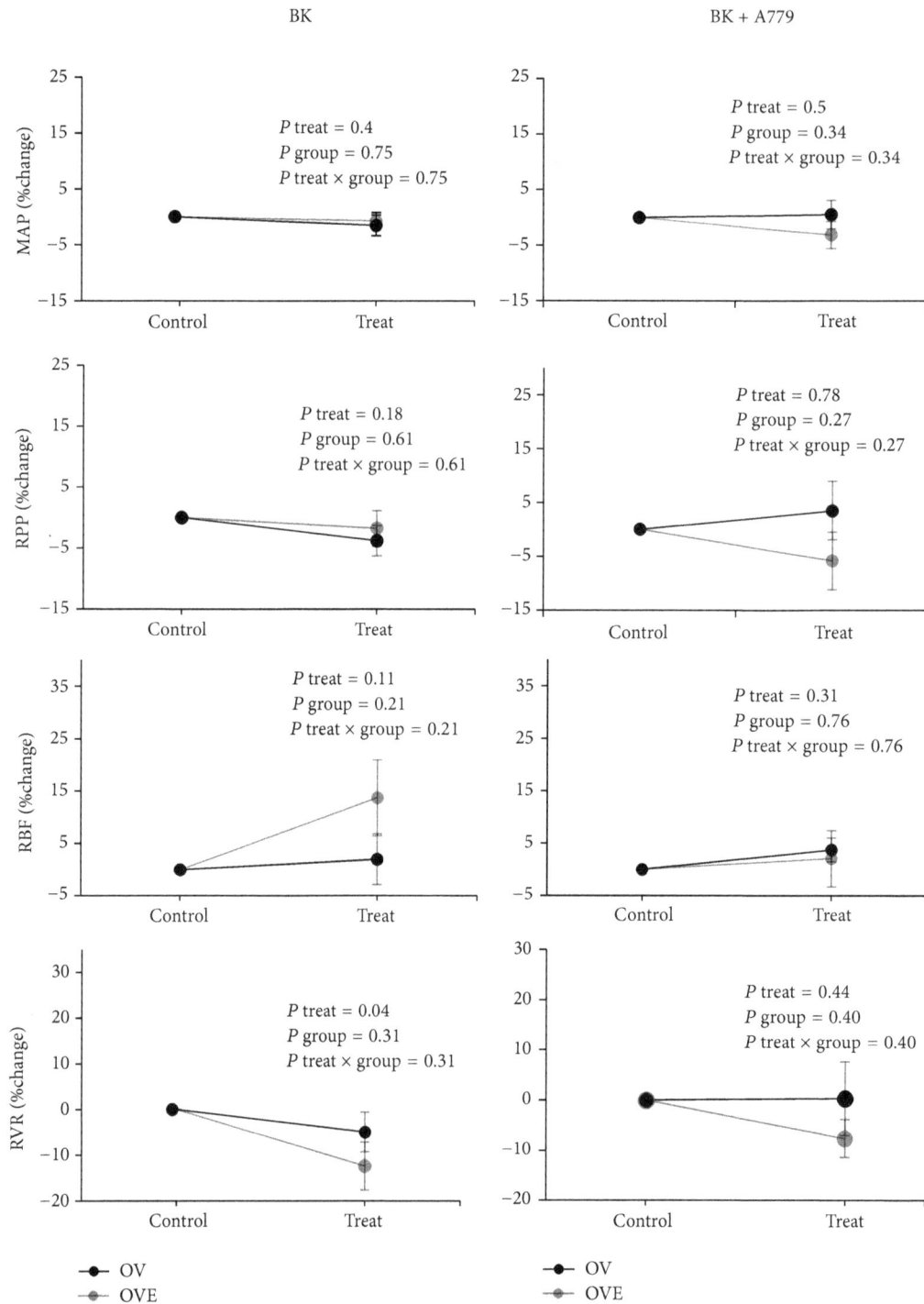

FIGURE 2: Parameters were recorded in ovariectomized and ovariectomized estradiol-treated rats before and after administration of BK or A779 + BK. Data are presented as mean ± SEM of percentage changes from the baseline. MAP, mean arterial pressure; RPP, renal perfusion pressure; RVR, renal vascular resistance; RBF, renal blood flow *per* gram kidney weight. P values were derived from repeated measures ANOVA.

1-7 infusion. Ang 1-7 infusion increased %RBF in a dose-dependent manner in all the groups (P dose < 0.001). BK alone administration increased %RBF response to Ang 1-7 in the OVE group compared with the OV group (P < 0.05).

For example, $300\,\mathrm{ng\,kg^{-1}\,min^{-1}}$ Ang 1-7 increased RBF by $6.9 \pm 1.9\%$ in OVE group versus $0.9 \pm 1.8\%$ in OV group. Interestingly, when BK plus A779 was infused, RBF response was enhanced dose-dependently in both groups with greater

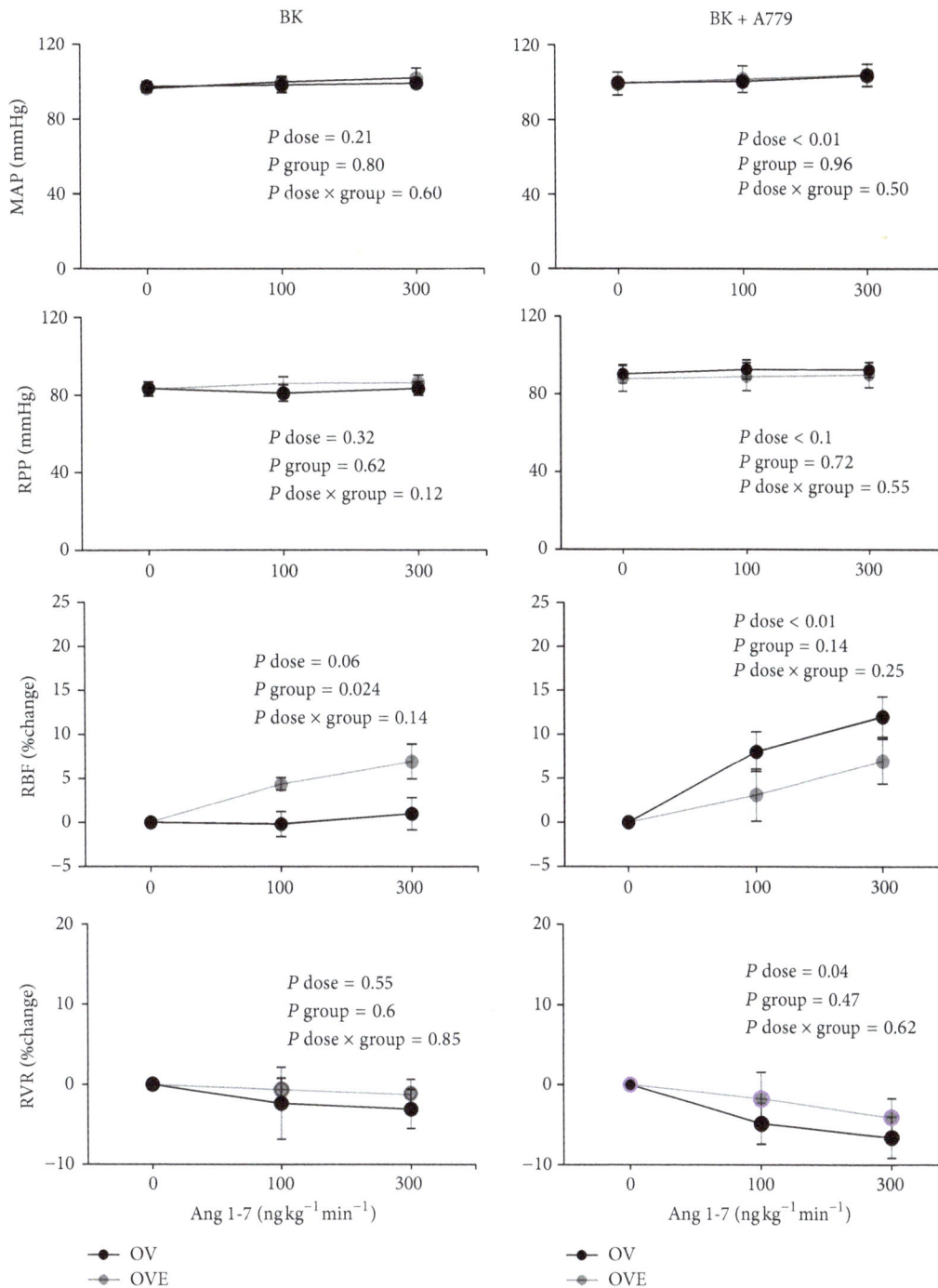

FIGURE 3: RBF, MAP, RPP, and RVR responses to Ang 1-7 were present when BK or A779 + BK was administrated. Data are shown as mean ± SEM. MAP, mean arterial pressure; RPP, renal perfusion pressure; RVR, renal vascular resistance; RBF, renal blood flow. P values were derived from repeated measures ANOVA.

response in the OV group. For example, $300 \, ng \, kg^{-1} \, min^{-1}$ Ang 1-7 increased RBF by $12 \pm 2.2\%$ in OV group versus $7 \pm 2.5\%$ in OVE group.

4. Discussion

The present study was performed to determine the effect of MasR antagonist, A779, on the RBF response to Ang 1-7 in the presence of BK in ovariectomized rats that were treated with vehicle or estradiol. Our major finding is that administration of BK promotes RBF response to Ang 1-7 in estradiol-treated rats when MasR is not blocked. However, surprisingly, when A779 was added, RBF response to Ang 1-7 increased in a dose-dependent manner in both the OV and OVE groups, while RBF response in the OV group was insignificantly greater than that in the OVE group.

Some observations show that estrogen contributes to modulate components of renal KKS and RAS, and it regulates renal hemodynamics via these two systems [6–8, 39]. B2 receptor mRNA levels were reduced by ovariectomy in the aorta and kidney, and this alteration is reformed by estrogen replacement [7]. Animal study also supports that renal kallikrein and kallikrein mRNA levels of rats are enhanced in females compared with males; and these factors were decreased by ovariectomy and estrogen treatment returns them back to normal levels [39]. Additionally, hormone replacement therapy (HRT) in postmenopausal women increases plasma concentration of BK and decreases ACE activity [40]. Estradiol enhances expression of renal ACE2 and consequently increases Ang 1-7 level [6]. Previous study showed that, in the heart of ovariectomized rats, estrogen depletion does not alter MasR expression, but estradiol therapy reduces its expression [41]. Estrogen replacement also enhances the relaxation response of Ang 1-7 in female ovariectomized rats, and this alternation is blocked by Ang 1-7 receptor antagonist, D-[Ala^7]-Ang 1-7 [42]. In the uterine arteries of sheep, estrogen stimulates the vasodilator response to BK by enhancement of NO release and NO synthase (NOS) activity [43]. Therefore, renoprotective role of estrogen may result from enhanced plasma levels of NO, BK, and Ang 1-7 and reduction in the arterial blood pressure and ACE activity. Our results are in accordance with the findings of the studies that declare that in the presence of BK estradiol enhances the RBF response to Ang 1-7.

The kidney effects of Ang 1-7 and BK are a complex pathway. Ang 1-7 regulates renal hemodynamics, glomerular filtration rate, and tubular transport [44–47]. It also modifies RBF through release of prostanoids and NO [47–50], where Ang 1-7 via MasR regulates renal function [51] in a gender dependent manner [34]. It is reported that Ang 1-7 increases blood flow in the kidney, brain, and mesentery [48]. Nematbakhsh and Safari suggested that RBF response to Ang 1-7 is different between males and females [34] possibly due to higher MasR expression in females [52]. This is while BK exerts variable effects on the renal vascular bed. Ren et al. demonstrated that BK has a vasodilator effect on efferent arterioles [53], and its effect on vascular tone is modulated by releasing vasodilator mediators such as NO and prostaglandins [24, 54, 55]. It seems that renal B2 receptor causes vasodilation. Hock et al. confirmed that the selective B2 receptor antagonist, icatibant, inhibits relaxation response to BK in renal vascular preparation [56]. In another study, it was demonstrated that des-Arg9-BK, a selective B1 receptor agonist, was involved in vasoconstriction in the kidney and this response is abolished by B1 receptor antagonist [57]. In fact, the main renal vascular response to BK in the isolated perfused kidney was vasodilation [58]. The dose of BK is also another factor contributing to different actions of BK on renal circulation. BK in high doses produces vasoconstriction in renal vessels, while at low doses it causes vasodilation [59]. Hoagland et al. observed that intravenous administration of BK induces significant increase in RBF and decrease in RVR [33]. In addition, BK increases medullary RBF but does not alter cortical RBF [55]. Our data supports that BK enhances RBF in response to Ang 1-7 in a dose-dependent manner.

It is reported that, in B2 receptor knockout mice, RBF and blood pressure do not alter compared with the control mice. However, when the two groups were subjected to high salt diet, RBF decreased in B2 receptor knockout mice [60]. Therefore, the regulatory action of endogenous BK on renal function and blood pressure is dependent on physiological and pharmacological conditions [60].

Another point is the MasR effects. An in vivo experiment showed that Ang 1-7 induces vasodilation of mesenteric vessels by facilitation of BK, while losartan, as an AT1R blocker, does not affect this mechanism. However, A779 blocks this vasodilation, suggesting that BK-potentiating activity of Ang 1-7 is not dependent on its interaction with AT1R while MasR is involved [29]. MasR deficient vessels show vascular endothelium dysfunction. Peiró et al. evaluated response to Ang 1-7 in Mas deficient vessels compared with wild type mice treated with A799 [61]. According to the results, Ang 1-7 mediated relaxation was reduced by 40% in isolated vessels of knockout MasR; and A799 diminished dilation response to Ang 1-7 [61]. Additionally, residual vascular relaxation was demonstrated in response to Ang 1-7; therefore, this peptide may act via another pathway [62]. In another study, mesenteric vessels were isolated and A779 and NO synthase (NOS) inhibitor, L-NAME, were administrated and it was shown that the vasorelaxant responses of Ang 1-7 and BK were abolished by A779 and L-NAME [63]. It is concluded that MasR has a central role in endothelial NO-mediated relaxation by Ang 1-7 and BK [63]. In the current study, not only did blockade of MasR significantly enhance RBF response to Ang 1-7, but also this RBF alternation is higher in the vehicle group than in the estradiol-treated animals. Consequently, when MasR is blocked, RBF response to Ang 1-7 may be related to another pathway. We cannot provide the exact mechanism for such observation, but one explanation is that BK potentiates vasodilatory effect of Ang 1-7 by its receptor and also other angiotensin receptors such as AT2R may be involved [64]. To summarize, RBF response to Ang 1-7 seems to be related to several factors including RAS receptors, BK, NO, and prostaglandins. All those factors integrate to control renal hemodynamics. In the absence of one factor, others help compensate and make a greater response.

5. Conclusion

Some data support the exclusive MasR mediated vasodilator response of Ang 1-7 [29, 63], while others confirm that other receptors are involved and MasR has a partial role [61, 62]. Furthermore, cooperation between BK and Ang 1-7 appears to have a critical role in the vasodilatory effect that is mediated by BK receptor. Considering the role of estrogen on RAS and KKS, we concluded that BK and estradiol increased RBF response to Ang 1-7 infusion and this action may not be related to MasR.

Conflict of Interests

The authors declare that there is no conflict of interests regarding the publication of this paper.

Acknowledgment

This study was supported by Isfahan University of Medical Sciences.

References

[1] L. Gouva and A. Tsatsoulis, "The role of estrogens in cardiovascular disease in the aftermath of clinical trials," *Hormones*, vol. 3, no. 3, pp. 171–183, 2004.

[2] M. C. Chappell, A. C. Marshall, E. M. Alzayadneh, H. A. Shaltout, and D. I. Diz, "Update on the angiotensin converting enzyme 2-angiotensin (1–7)-Mas receptor axis: fetal programing, sex differences, and intracellular pathways," *Frontiers in Endocrinology*, vol. 4, article 201, 2013.

[3] S. L. Seliger, C. Davis, and C. Stehman-Breen, "Gender and the progression of renal disease," *Current Opinion in Nephrology and Hypertension*, vol. 10, no. 2, pp. 219–225, 2001.

[4] A. K. Sampson, K. M. Moritz, E. S. Jones, R. L. Flower, R. E. Widdop, and K. M. Denton, "Enhanced angiotensin II type 2 receptor mechanisms mediate decreases in arterial pressure attributable to chronic low-dose angiotensin II in female rats," *Hypertension*, vol. 52, no. 4, pp. 666–671, 2008.

[5] I. Armando, M. Jezova, A. V. Juorio et al., "Estrogen upregulates renal angiotensin II AT2 receptors," *The American Journal of Physiology—Renal Physiology*, vol. 283, no. 5, pp. F934–F943, 2002.

[6] H. Ji, S. Menini, W. Zheng, C. Pesce, X. Wu, and K. Sandberg, "Role of angiotensin-converting enzyme 2 and angiotensin(1–7) in 17β-oestradiol regulation of renal pathology in renal wrap hypertension in rats," *Experimental Physiology*, vol. 93, no. 5, pp. 648–657, 2008.

[7] P. Madeddu, C. Emanueli, M. V. Varoni et al., "Regulation of bradykinin B_2-receptor expression by oestrogen," *British Journal of Pharmacology*, vol. 121, no. 8, pp. 1763–1769, 1997.

[8] H. Sumino, S. Ichikawa, T. Kanda et al., "Hormone replacement therapy in postmenopausal women with essential hypertension increases circulating plasma levels of bradykinin," *American Journal of Hypertension*, vol. 12, no. 10, pp. 1044–1047, 1999.

[9] C. M. Ferrario and S. N. Iyer, "Angiotensin-(1–7): a bioactive fragment of the renin-angiotensin system," *Regulatory Peptides*, vol. 78, no. 1–3, pp. 13–18, 1998.

[10] J. Joyner, L. A. A. Neves, J. P. Granger et al., "Temporal-spatial expression of ANG-(1-7) and angiotensin-converting enzyme 2 in the kidney of normal and hypertensive pregnant rats," *The American Journal of Physiology—Regulatory Integrative and Comparative Physiology*, vol. 293, no. 1, pp. R169–R177, 2007.

[11] R. A. S. Santos, A. C. Simoes e Silva, C. Maric et al., "Angiotensin-(1–7) is an endogenous ligand for the G protein-coupled receptor Mas," *Proceedings of the National Academy of Sciences of the United States of America*, vol. 100, no. 14, pp. 8258–8263, 2003.

[12] Z. Zhu, J. Zhong, S. Zhu, D. Liu, M. van der Giet, and M. Tepel, "Angiotensin-(1–7) inhibits angiotensin II-induced signal transduction," *Journal of Cardiovascular Pharmacology*, vol. 40, no. 5, pp. 693–700, 2002.

[13] M. Iwai and M. Horiuchi, "Devil and angel in the renin-angiotensin system: ACE-angiotensin II-AT1 receptor axis vs. ACE2-angiotensin-(1-7)-Mas receptor axis," *Hypertension Research*, vol. 32, no. 7, pp. 533–536, 2009.

[14] R. A. S. Santos, A. J. Ferreira, and A. C. S. e Silva, "Recent advances in the angiotensin-converting enzyme 2-angiotensin(1–7)-Mas axis," *Experimental Physiology*, vol. 93, no. 5, pp. 519–527, 2008.

[15] M. Luque, P. Martin, N. Martell, C. Fernandez, K. B. Brosnihan, and C. M. Ferrario, "Effects of captopril related to increased levels of prostacyclin and angiotensin-(1–7) in essential hypertension," *Journal of Hypertension*, vol. 14, no. 6, pp. 799–805, 1996.

[16] C. M. Ferrario, J. Jessup, P. E. Gallagher et al., "Effects of renin-angiotensin system blockade on renal angiotensin-(1–7) forming enzymes and receptors," *Kidney International*, vol. 68, no. 5, pp. 2189–2196, 2005.

[17] M. Donoghue, F. Hsieh, E. Baronas et al., "A novel angiotensin-converting enzyme-related carboxypeptidase (ACE2) converts angiotensin I to angiotensin 1–9," *Circulation Research*, vol. 87, no. 5, pp. e1–e9, 2000.

[18] M. C. Chappell, A. J. Allred, and C. M. Ferrario, "Pathways of angiotensin-(1-7) metabolism in the kidney," *Nephrology Dialysis Transplantation*, vol. 16, supplement 1, pp. 22–26, 2001.

[19] M. C. Chappell, N. T. Pirro, A. Sykes, and C. M. Ferrario, "Metabolism of angiotensin-(1-7) by angiotensin-converting enzyme," *Hypertension*, vol. 31, no. 1, pp. 362–367, 1998.

[20] H. S. Margolius, "Kallikreins and kinins: molecular characteristics and cellular and tissue responses," *Diabetes*, vol. 45, supplement 1, pp. S14–S19, 1996.

[21] K. D. Bhoola, C. D. Figueroa, and K. Worthy, "Bioregulation of kinins: kallikreins, kininogens, and kininases," *Pharmacological Reviews*, vol. 44, no. 1, pp. 1–80, 1992.

[22] D. J. Campbell, "Towards understanding the kallikrein-kinin system: insights from measurement of kinin peptides," *Brazilian Journal of Medical and Biological Research*, vol. 33, no. 6, pp. 665–677, 2000.

[23] R. L. Hébert, D. Regoli, H. Xiong, M. D. Breyer, and G. E. Plante, "Bradykinin B2 type receptor activation regulates fluid and electrolyte transport in the rabbit kidney," *Peptides*, vol. 26, no. 8, pp. 1308–1316, 2005.

[24] N.-E. Rhaleb, X.-P. Yang, and O. A. Carretero, "The Kallikrein-kinin system as a regulator of cardiovascular and renal function," *Comprehensive Physiology*, vol. 1, no. 2, pp. 971–993, 2011.

[25] J.-V. Mombouli and P. M. Vanhoutte, "Heterogeneity of endothelium-dependent vasodilator effects of angiotensin-converting enzyme inhibitors: role of bradykinin generation during ACE inhibition," *Journal of Cardiovascular Pharmacology*, vol. 20, no. 9, pp. S74–S82, 1992.

[26] E. G. Erdös, F. Tan, and R. A. Skidgel, "Angiotensin I-converting enzyme inhibitors are allosteric enhancers of kinin B1 and B2 receptor function," *Hypertension*, vol. 55, no. 2, pp. 214–220, 2010.

[27] K. B. Brosnihan, P. Li, and C. M. Ferrario, "Angiotensin-(1-7) dilates canine coronary arteries through kinins and nitric oxide," *Hypertension*, vol. 27, no. 3, pp. 523–528, 1996.

[28] A. Abbas, G. Gorelik, L. A. Carbini, and A. G. Scicli, "Angiotensin-(1-7) induces bradykinin-mediated hypotensive responses in anesthetized rats," *Hypertension*, vol. 30, no. 2, pp. 217–221, 1997.

[29] M. A. Oliveira, Z. B. Fortes, R. A. S. Santos, M. C. Kosla, and M. H. C. De Carvalho, "Synergistic effect of angiotensin-(1-7) on bradykinin arteriolar dilation in vivo," *Peptides*, vol. 20, no. 10, pp. 1195–1201, 1999.

[30] R. W. Schrier and W. Wang, "Acute renal failure and sepsis," *The New England Journal of Medicine*, vol. 351, no. 2, pp. 159–169, 2004.

[31] C. J. Lote, L. Harper, and C. O. S. Savage, "Mechanisms of acute renal failure," *British Journal of Anaesthesia*, vol. 77, no. 1, pp. 82–89, 1996.

[32] V. E. Torres, B. F. King, A. B. Chapman et al., "Magnetic resonance measurements of renal blood flow and disease progression in autosomal dominant polycystic kidney disease," *Clinical Journal of the American Society of Nephrology*, vol. 2, no. 1, pp. 112–120, 2007.

[33] K. M. Hoagland, D. A. Maddox, and D. S. Martin, "Bradykinin B2-receptors mediate the pressor and renal hemodynamic effects of intravenous bradykinin in conscious rats," *Journal of the Autonomic Nervous System*, vol. 75, no. 1, pp. 7–15, 1999.

[34] M. Nematbakhsh and T. Safari, "Role of Mas receptor in renal blood flow response to angiotensin (1–7) in male and female rats," *General Physiology and Biophysics*, vol. 33, no. 3, pp. 365–372, 2014.

[35] K. D. da Silveira, K. S. P. Bosco, L. R. L. Diniz et al., "ACE2-angiotensin-(1–7)-Mas axis in renal ischaemia/reperfusion injury in rats," *Clinical Science*, vol. 119, no. 9, pp. 385–394, 2010.

[36] S. Bachmann and P. Mundel, "Nitric oxide in the kidney: synthesis, localization, and function," *American Journal of Kidney Diseases*, vol. 24, no. 1, pp. 112–129, 1994.

[37] Z. Pezeshki, M. Nematbakhsh, S. Mazaheri et al., "Estrogen abolishes protective effect of erythropoietin against cisplatin-induced nephrotoxicity in ovariectomized rats," *ISRN Oncology*, vol. 2012, Article ID 890310, 7 pages, 2012.

[38] S. Bosnyak, E. S. Jones, A. Christopoulos, M.-I. Aguilar, W. G. Thomas, and R. E. Widdop, "Relative affinity of angiotensin peptides and novel ligands at AT1 and AT2 receptors," *Clinical Science*, vol. 121, no. 7, pp. 297–303, 2011.

[39] P. Madeddu, N. Glorioso, M. Maioli et al., "Regulation of rat renal kallikrein expression by estrogen and progesterone," *Journal of Hypertension*, vol. 9, no. 6, pp. S244–S245, 1991.

[40] A. J. Proudler, D. Crook, J. C. Stevenson, A. I. H. Ahmed, J. M. Rymer, and I. Fogelman, "Hormone replacement therapy and serum angiotensin-converting-enzyme activity in post-menopausal women," *The Lancet*, vol. 346, no. 8967, pp. 89–90, 1995.

[41] H. Wang, J. A. Jessup, Z. Zhao et al., "Characterization of the cardiac renin angiotensin system in oophorectomized and estrogen-replete mRen2. Lewis rats," *PLoS ONE*, vol. 8, no. 10, Article ID e76992, 2013.

[42] L. A. A. Neves, D. B. Averill, C. M. Ferrario, J. L. Aschner, and K. B. Brosnihan, "Vascular responses to angiotensin-(–7) during the estrous cycle," *Endocrine*, vol. 24, no. 2, pp. 161–165, 2004.

[43] J.-C. Veille, P. Li, J. C. Eisenach, A. G. Massmann, and J. P. Figueroa, "Effects of estrogen on nitric oxide biosynthesis and vasorelaxant activity in sheep uterine and renal arteries in vitro," *American Journal of Obstetrics and Gynecology*, vol. 174, no. 3, pp. 1043–1049, 1996.

[44] E. A. van der Wouden, P. Ochodnický, R. P. E. van Dokkum et al., "The role of angiotensin(1–7) in renal vasculature of the rat," *Journal of Hypertension*, vol. 24, no. 10, pp. 1971–1978, 2006.

[45] V. Vallon, N. Heyne, K. Richter, M. C. Khosla, and K. Fechter, "[7-D-ALA]-angiotensin 1–7 blocks renal actions of angiotensin 1–7 in the anesthetized rat," *Journal of Cardiovascular Pharmacology*, vol. 32, no. 1, pp. 164–167, 1998.

[46] R. K. Handa, C. M. Ferrario, and J. W. Strandhoy, "Renal actions of angiotensin-(1–7): in vivo and in vitro studies," *American Journal of Physiology*, vol. 270, no. 1, pp. F141–F147, 1996.

[47] Y. Ren, J. L. Garvin, and O. A. Carretero, "Vasodilator action of angiotensin-(1–7) on isolated rabbit afferent arterioles," *Hypertension*, vol. 39, no. 3, pp. 799–802, 2002.

[48] W. O. Sampaio, A. A. S. Nascimento, and R. A. S. Santos, "Systemic and regional hemodynamic effects of angiotensin-(1–7) in rats," *The American Journal of Physiology—Heart and Circulatory Physiology*, vol. 284, no. 6, pp. H1985–H1994, 2003.

[49] G. A. Botelho-Santos, W. O. Sampaio, T. L. Reudelhuber, M. Bader, M. J. Campagnole-Santos, and R. A. S. Dos Santos, "Expression of an angiotensin-(1–7)-producing fusion protein in rats induced marked changes in regional vascular resistance," *The American Journal of Physiology—Heart and Circulatory Physiology*, vol. 292, no. 5, pp. H2485–H2490, 2007.

[50] I. F. Benter, D. I. Diz, and C. M. Ferrario, "Cardiovascular actions of angiotensin (1–7)," *Peptides*, vol. 14, no. 4, pp. 679–684, 1993.

[51] S. V. B. Pinheiro, A. J. Ferreira, G. T. Kitten et al., "Genetic deletion of the angiotensin-(1–7) receptor Mas leads to glomerular hyperfiltration and microalbuminuria," *Kidney International*, vol. 75, no. 11, pp. 1184–1193, 2009.

[52] A. K. Sampson, K. M. Moritz, and K. M. Denton, "Postnatal ontogeny of angiotensin receptors and ACE2 in male and female rats," *Gender Medicine*, vol. 9, no. 1, pp. 21–32, 2012.

[53] Y. Ren, J. Garvin, and O. A. Carretero, "Mechanism involved in bradykinin-induced efferent arteriole dilation," *Kidney International*, vol. 62, no. 2, pp. 544–549, 2002.

[54] L. G. Navar, E. W. Inscho, D. S. A. Majid, J. D. Imig, L. M. Harrison-Bernard, and K. D. Mitchell, "Paracrine regulation of the renal microcirculation," *Physiological Reviews*, vol. 76, no. 2, pp. 425–536, 1996.

[55] B. Badzyńska and J. Sadowski, "Differential action of bradykinin on intrarenal regional perfusion in the rat: waning effect in the cortex and major impact in the medulla," *The Journal of Physiology*, vol. 587, no. 15, pp. 3943–3953, 2009.

[56] F. Hock, K. Wirth, U. Albus et al., "Hoe 140 a new potent and long acting bradykinin–antagonist: in vitro studies," *British Journal of Pharmacology*, vol. 102, no. 3, pp. 769–773, 1991.

[57] F. Gobeil, W. Neugebauer, C. Filteau et al., "Structure-activity studies of B₁ receptor-related peptides. Antagonists," *Hypertension*, vol. 28, no. 5, pp. 833–839, 1996.

[58] K. Bagaté, L. Develioglu, J.-L. Imbs, B. Michel, J.-J. Helwig, and M. Barthelmebs, "Vascular kinin B1 and B2 receptor-mediated effects in the rat isolated perfused kidney—differential regulations," *British Journal of Pharmacology*, vol. 128, no. 8, pp. 1643–1650, 1999.

[59] K. G. Hofbauer, H. Dienemann, P. Forgiarini, R. Stalder, and J. M. Wood, "Renal vascular effects of angiotensin II, arginine-vasopressin and bradykinin in rats: interactions with prostaglandins," *General Pharmacology: The Vascular System*, vol. 14, no. 1, pp. 145–147, 1983.

[60] A. F. Milia, V. Gross, R. Plehm, J. A. De Silva Jr., M. Bader, and F. C. Luft, "Normal blood pressure and renal function in mice lacking the bradykinin B2 receptor," *Hypertension*, vol. 37, no. 6, pp. 1473–1479, 2001.

[61] C. Peiró, S. Vallejo, F. Gembardt et al., "Endothelial dysfunction through genetic deletion or inhibition of the G protein-coupled receptor Mas: a new target to improve endothelial function," *Journal of Hypertension*, vol. 25, no. 12, pp. 2421–2425, 2007.

[62] D. M. R. Silva, H. R. Vianna, S. F. Cortes, M. J. Campagnole-Santos, R. A. S. Santos, and V. S. Lemos, "Evidence for a new angiotensin-(1–7) receptor subtype in the aorta of Sprague-Dawley rats," *Peptides*, vol. 28, no. 3, pp. 702–707, 2007.

[63] C. Peiró, S. Vallejo, F. Gembardt et al., "Complete blockade of the vasorelaxant effects of angiotensin-(1–7) and bradykinin in murine microvessels by antagonists of the receptor Mas," *The Journal of Physiology*, vol. 591, no. 9, pp. 2275–2285, 2013.

[64] P. E. Walters, T. A. Gaspari, and R. E. Widdop, "Angiotensin-(1–7) acts as a vasodepressor agent via angiotensin II type 2 receptors in conscious rats," *Hypertension*, vol. 45, no. 5, pp. 960–966, 2005.

24

Olive Mill Waste Extracts: Polyphenols Content, Antioxidant, and Antimicrobial Activities

Inass Leouifoudi,[1] Hicham Harnafi,[2] and Abdelmajid Zyad[1]

[1]*Laboratory of Biological Engineering, Faculty of Science and Technologies, Sultan Moulay Slimane University, 23 000 Beni-Mellal, Morocco*
[2]*Laboratory of Biochemistry, Faculty of Science, Mohamed First University, 60 000 Oujda, Morocco*

Correspondence should be addressed to Inass Leouifoudi; inass.leouifoudi@gmail.com

Academic Editor: Ismail Laher

Natural polyphenols extracts have been usually associated with great bioactive properties. In this work, we investigated *in vitro* antioxidant and antimicrobial potential of the phenolic olive mill wastewater extracts (OWWE) and the olive cake extracts (OCE). Using the Folin Ciocalteux method, OWWE contained higher total phenol content compared to OCE (8.90 ± 0.728 g/L versus 0.95 ± 0.017 mg/g). The phenolic compounds identification was carried out with a performance liquid chromatograph coupled to tandem mass spectrometry equipment (HPLC-ESI-MS). With this method, a list of polyphenols from OWWE and OCE was obtained. The antioxidant activity was measured in aqueous (DPPH) and emulsion (BCBT) systems. Using the DPPH assay, the results show that OWWE was more active than OCE and interestingly the extracts originating from mountainous areas were more active than those produced from plain areas ($EC_{50} = 12.1 \pm 5.6$ µg/mL; $EC_{50} = 157.7 \pm 34.9$ µg/mL, resp.). However, when the antioxidant activity was reversed in the BCBT, OCE produced from plain area was more potent than mountainous OCE. Testing by the gel diffusion assay, all the tested extracts have showed significant spectrum antibacterial activity against *Staphylococcus aureus*, whereas the biophenols extracts showed more limited activity against *Escherichia coli* and *Streptococcus faecalis*.

1. Introduction

In the recent years, the interest of natural antioxidants, particularly polyphenols, in relation to their therapeutic and health beneficial properties has significantly increased. Indeed, polyphenols are known for decades for their antioxidant activity [1], which was then confirmed by more recent studies [2, 3]. Mediterranean olive mill wastes are rich on these active ingredients and antioxidant activity of olive oil mill waste phenolic extracts had already been tested [4, 5]. These *in vitro* tests have usually shown an inhibitor effect of oxidation reactions and have attracted increasing attention as potential agents for preventing and treating many oxidative stress-related diseases. One of the first works, which has used olive mill waste as a potential source of natural antioxidants, was published in 1988 [6]. The current work evaluates the phenolic content of olive byproducts and its bioactivities. It may be considered as one of the rarely investigations of antioxidant activity of Moroccan olive mill wastes witch is distinguished from the most Mediterranean olive mill wastes by the nature of the bioclimatic conditions.

Furthermore, the antimicrobial activity was identified in the early twentieth century but has been rarely explored [7]. Most studies of antimicrobial activity have focused on ecological and environmental consequences [8] or on agronomic applications [9]. Antimicrobial activity of olive mill waste extracts was early recognized and linked to the biophenols content [10]. However, the antimicrobial activity of olive cake and olive wastewater phenolic extracts and pure biophenols has been rarely tested against human pathogens [11, 12].

Moreover, beyond demonstrating the antioxidant and antimicrobial activity of olive byproducts polyphenol extracts, a few studies have an interest in comparing both the antioxidant and the antimicrobial effects of phenolic OCE to OWWE extracts, much less evaluating these effects in relation to the bioclimatic collection areas, from which they are originating. Therefore, this work aims to study the *in vitro* antioxidant and antibacterial potentials of Moroccan olive mill waste extracts and the relationship with their phenolic composition.

2. Materials and Methods

2.1. Chemical Reagents. All solvents and chemicals were obtained from Sigma Chemical Co., Saint Quentin (France). Bacteria strains were originally obtained from the laboratory of Biological Engineering, Faculty of Science and Technology, Sultan Moulay Slimane University, Beni-Mellal, Morocco.

2.2. Plant Material. Moroccan *Picholine* olives variety was identified and authenticated by Pr. A. Boulli, Department of life sciences, Sultan Moulay Slimane University, and stored as a voucher specimen in the Faculty of Science and Technologies, Beni-Mellal, Morocco. Samples of olive cake (solid waste) and olive wastewaters (liquid waste) were collected in mills from two areas of Tadla-Azilal region in Morocco, plain and mountainous areas, during the winter of 2012. These samples were produced from the three-phase centrifugation oil extraction process of red-black olives maturation stage.

2.3. Phenolic Compounds Extraction

2.3.1. Olive Cake Samples. Dry olive cake samples (60 g each) were grounded, sifted, and then defatted with 500 mL of hexane in a soxhlet apparatus for four hours. Defatted olive cake samples were subjected to soxhlet extractions using ethanol solvent. Olive cake samples (60 g) were placed in extraction thimbles into the soxhlet apparatus. 500 mL of ethanol was placed in a round flask (500 mL capacity) and then the flask was connected to the soxhlet extractor for 12 h at 70°C of continuous extraction [13]. The resulting olive cake extracts (OCE) were concentrated by rotary evaporator and freeze stored at −18°C for further analysis.

2.3.2. Olive Wastewater Samples. Olive mill wastewater was defatted with hexane (1 : 1, (v/v)) and then clarified by centrifugation (4000 rpm, 15 min). Phenolic compounds in defatted and clarified olive mill wastewaters were twice extracted by the liquid-liquid extraction method using ethyl acetate (1 : 1, v/v) and 4000 rpm, 10 min centrifugation. The ethyl acetate phase was evaporated and the residue was stored at −18°C for subsequent analysis.

2.4. Total Phenolic Compounds Content (Spectrometric Measurement). The total phenolic compounds content in each extract was determined by spectrophotometry using the Folin-Ciocalteu method [31, 32] with some modifications. Briefly, 2.5 mL portion of Folin-Ciocalteu reagent 0.2 N was mixed with 0.5 mL of the sample. The reaction was kept in the dark for 5 min. Then, 2 mL of a sodium carbonate solution (75 g/L) was added to the mixture and the reaction was kept in the dark for 1 h. the absorbance was measured at 760 nm

and 765 nm for OCE and OWWE, respectively. Results were expressed as gallic acid equivalents (GAE).

2.5. HPLC/ESI-MS Analysis. High-performance liquid chromatography-mass spectrometry analysis was performed at 279 nm and 30°C using a RP C18 column (150 × 4.6) × 5 μm with a Thermo Fisher apparatus equipped with a Surveyor quaternary pump coupled at a PDA detector (diode array detector: 200–600 nm) and an LCQ Advantage (ESI) ion trap mass spectrometer (Thermo Finnigan, San Jose, CA). The injected volume was 20 μL. The mobile phase (0.5 mL/min) consisted of solvent A: TFA 0.05% in water and solvent B: TFA 0.05% in ACN. A Six-step gradient was applied, for a total run time of 76 min, as follows: starting from 80% solvent A and 20% solvent B increasing to 30% solvent B over 30 min, then isocratic elution for 10 min, increased to 30% solvent B over 10 min, to 40% over 30 min, and to 20% solvent B over 2 min, and finally isocratic elution for 4 min. ESI ionization conditions were spray voltage 4 KV, capillary 350°C, 14 V. Pure nitrogen was the sheath gas and pure helium was the collusion gas. The full scan mass data m/z was obtained in positive mode and ranged from 100 to 2000 Da.

2.6. Antioxidant Activity

2.6.1. Free Radical Scavenging Activity Measurement (DPPH Method) [26]. The DPPH (2,2-diphenyl-1-picrylhydrazyl) assay was carried out in a 96-well microtiter plate. The samples and positive control, Vitamin C, were diluted with methanol to prepare sample concentrations equivalent to 200, 100, 50, 25, 12.5, 6.25, and 3.125 μg of dried sample/mL solutions. 150 μL of 0.004% DPPH solution was pipetted into each well of 96-well plate followed by 8 μL of the sample solutions. The plates were incubated at 37°C for 30 min and the absorbance was measured at 540 nm, using ELISA microtiter plate reader. The experiment was performed in triplicate and % scavenging activity was calculated using the following equation:

$$\% \text{ Scavenging} = \left(A_o - \frac{A_s}{A_o} \right) * 100, \tag{1}$$

where A_o is the absorbance of the control and A_s is the absorbance of the sample at 540 nm.

2.6.2. Antioxidant Activity Measurement Using β-Carotene Bleaching Test (BCBT) [33]. In this assay, linoleic acid (2 mg) was added to Tween 40 (200 mg) and β-carotene solution (2 mg in 1 mL chloroform) in a round bottom flask. The chloroform was evaporated completely by heating at 37°C under vacuum for 10 min. Aerated water (100 mL) was added in portions with vigorous shaking. 2 mL of this reaction was transferred to test tubes and 0,5 mL of the tested samples prepared at different concentrations (10 μg/mL, 25 μg/mL, 50 μg/mL, 100 μg/mL, and 200 μg/mL) was added. Absorbance at 490 nm of the control (linoleic acid ID ß-carotene) was measured immediately and time was assigned as T_0. The absorbance was remeasured after 24 h incubation at room temperature (T_{24}). Values are presented as means ± SD of three parallel measurements.

The percentage inhibition of ß-carotene bleaching was calculated using the following formula:

$$\% \text{ Inhibition} = \left[\frac{(A_{24} - C_{24})}{(C_0 - C_{24})} \right] * 100, \qquad (2)$$

where A_{24} is the absorbance of the test extract at T_{24}, C_{24} is absorbance of the control at T_{24}, and C_0 is the absorbance of the control at T_0.

2.7. Antimicrobial Activity [34]. Antimicrobial activity was tested against three microorganisms: *Staphylococcus aureus* and *Streptococcus faecalis*, both Gram-positive bacteria, and *Escherichia coli* as Gram-negative bacteria. Bacteria were cultured in a Mueller Hinton agar medium for 12 h at 37°C. The disc diffusion method was used to determine the antimicrobial activities of OCE and OWWE diluted in DMSO so as to test concentrations of 1.5, 3, and 6 mg/disc for OCE and 1, 2, and 4 mg/disc for OWWE. Agar plates (4 mL/plate) were prepared, allowed to set, and surface dried at 25°C for 15 min. Bacterial cultures were incubated at 37°C for 24 h in order to have a microbial suspension having turbidity nearest 10^5–10^6 CFU/mL. 100 μL of the inoculum (3×10^6 CFU/mL) was spread plated on nutrient agar plates. Blank sensitivity discs, 6 mm, were allowed to warm to room temperature for 1 h and then impregnated with 25 μL of each extract or controls and then left to dry in a sterile Petri dish for 90 min. Negative controls for standards and extracts were 25%, 50%, and 100% DMSO. Positive controls were amoxicillin discs (25 μg), chloramphenicol (30 μg), and ceftriaxone (30 μg). The plates were then incubated for 24 h at 37°C. The diameter of the inhibition zone was measured in mm (including disc) with calipers; three replicates were performed and the assays were duplicated.

3. Results

3.1. Phenolic Compounds Content. The characterization of the biophenols content of OWWE and OCE is provided in Table 1. OWWE has the higher amounts of total phenols compared to OCE, as measured by Folin Ciocalteu assay. The OWWE phenolic content was about 10 times more than OCE phenolic content (Table 1). The levels of mountainous biophenols extracts were interestingly higher than plain biophenols extracts. This difference in total phenolic content can be explained by the impact of geographic and climatic conditions on the determination of polyphenols content in plants [23, 35].

3.2. Phenolic Compounds Identification. HPLC provided separation of individual biophenols in the OCE and OWWE as illustrated in Figures 1 and 2, respectively, for detection at 279 nm, where both qualitative and quantitative differences between mountainous and plain areas are observed. Identification of biophenols was performed by comparing retention times of standards in HPLC-ESI and confirmed

TABLE 1: Total phenolic content in OCE and OWWE.

Area	Total phenolic content	
	OCE (mg GAE*/g)	OWWE (g GAE/L)
Mountain	0.950 ± 0.017^a	8.90 ± 0.728^c
Plain	0.551 ± 0.027^b	5.17 ± 0.057^d

Values are means of duplicate analysis and expressed as gallic acid equivalent. Different letters mean significant differences ± standard deviation ($P < 0.05$) (Student's test).
*GAE: gallic acid equivalent.

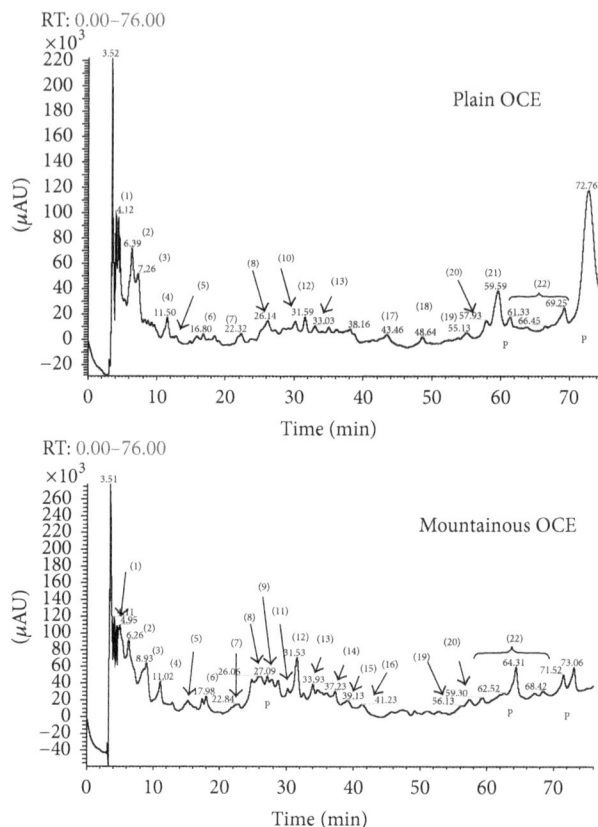

FIGURE 1: HPLC chromatograms of the phenolic profile of OCE. Peaks identities: (1) hydroxytyrosol glucoside, (2) hydroxytyrosol, (3) tyrosol, (4) vanillic acid, (5) sinapic acid, (6) syringic acid, (7) caffeic acid, (8) elenolic acid, (9) oleuropein aglycone, (10) verbascoside, (11) rutin, (12) luteolin, (13) quercetin, (14) luteolin-7-rutinoside, (15) luteolin-7-glucoside, (16) apigenin, (17) methoxyluteolin, (18) naringenin (19) ligstroside aglycon, (20) ligstroside, (21) oleuropein, (22) secoiridoids derivatives and (P) polymeric substances.

by relevant molecular mass data from LC–MS. The major individual biophenols identified in the OCE and OWWE were particularly characterized at five classes, namely, simple phenols, phenolic acids, derivatives secoiridoids, flavonoids, and lignans (Tables 2 and 3). Furthermore, the phenolic composition seems to be related to the impact of bioclimatic conditions.

As the main aim of this study was to screen olive mill waste extracts for biological activities, a detailed characterization of individual compounds was not attempted and

RT: 0.00–76.00 SM: 7B

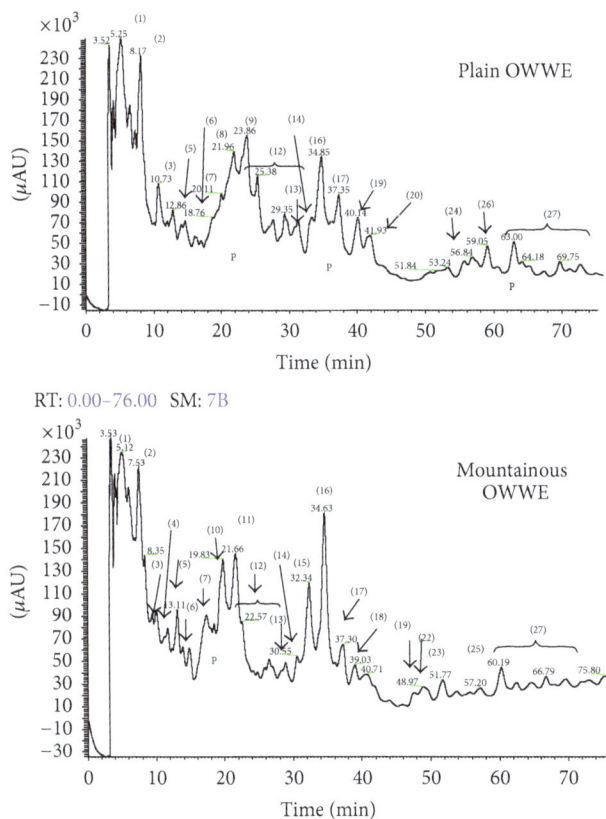

FIGURE 2: HPLC chromatogram of the phenolic profile of OWWE. Peaks identities: (1) hydroxytyrosol glucoside, (2) hydroxytyrosol, (3) tyrosol, (4) vanillic acid (5) sinapic acid, (6) syringic acid, (7) caffeic acid, (8) p-coumaric acid, (9) dihydroxymandelic acid, (10) vanillin, (11) 3,4,5 trimethoxybenzoic acid, (12) secoiridoids derivatives, (13) verbascoside, (14) rutin, (15) luteolin-7-rutinoside, (16) luteolin-7-glucoside, (17) luteolin, (18) apigenin, (19) nüzhenide, (20) quercetin, (21) apigenin-7-rutinoside, (22) apigenin-7-glucoside, (23) oleuropein, (24) oleuropein aglycon (25) ligstroside, (26) ligstroside aglycon, (27) secoiridoids derivatives and (P) polymeric substances.

only the major peaks appearing at 279 nm were identified to assist in understanding the relation between the chemical composition and the observed bioactivities.

3.3. Antioxidant Activity

3.3.1. DPPH Assay.

Both OCE and OWWE showed concentration-dependent DPPH radical scavenging activity with a high correlation at concentrations less than 200 μg/mL (OWWE-Plain; $R^2 = 0.869$, OWWE-Mountain $R^2 = 0.952$, OCE-Plain; $R^2 = 0.722$, OCE- Mountain; $R^2 = 0.883$, Vitamin C; $R^2 = 0.998$) (Figure 3). EC$_{50}$ is inversely proportional to antioxidant activity and hence OWWE was more active than OCE in trapping DPPH radicals (Table 4).

Antiradical activity EC$_{50}$ (μg/mL) was defined as the concentration of extracts necessary to decrease the initial DPPH radical concentration by 50%. Values are means standard deviation (SD) of three measurements ($P < 0.05\%$).

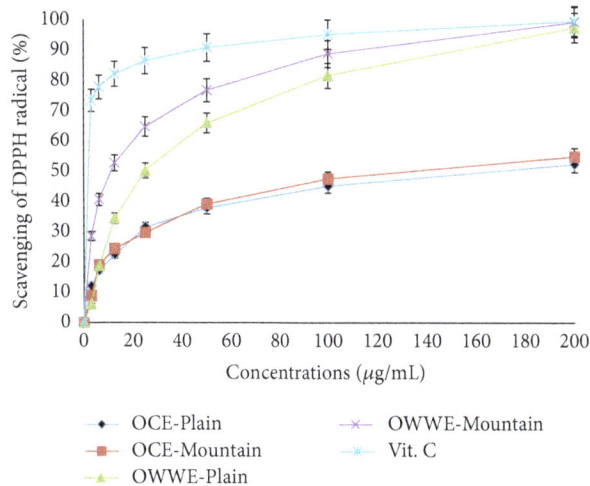

FIGURE 3: Kinetics of DPPH radical scavenging activity of OCE and OWWE.

The difference in activity decreased gradually upon increasing the dose; at EC$_{50}$, OWWE was 13 times more active than OCE in comparison to the mountainous area extracts (EC$_{50}$ = 12.1 ± 5.6; EC$_{50}$ = 157.7 ± 34.9 μg/mL, resp.) while it was only 5 times more active for plain area extracts (EC$_{50}$ = 30.7 ± 4.4; EC$_{50}$ = 168.0 ± 48 μg/mL) (Table 4). This result may be attributed to the highest concentrations of antioxidant phenolic compounds and the nature of the individual phenolic compounds present in the OCE and OWWE extracts. However, for the positive control, EC$_{50}$ value was 3.2 ± 0.6 μg/mL.

3.3.2. BCBT Assay.

Both OCE and OWWE protected linoleic acid and hence minimize decolorization of ß-carotene in the BCBT test (Figure 4). OWWE, particularly that originating from mountainous area, showed the higher capacity for oxidation's inhibition with an EC$_{50}$ = 81.3 ± 1.2 μg/mL compared to that originating from plain area (EC$_{50}$ = 131.8 ± 10.3 μg/mL). However, OCE have shown a lower antioxidant activity, and conversely of the results of the DPPH assay, mountainous extracts have shown a very low antioxidant activity in the BCBT test (less than 50% of oxidation's inhibition for the highest concentration: 200 μg/mL) compared to the plain extract (EC$_{50}$ = 139.1 ± 4.56 μg/mL).

3.4. Antimicrobial Activity.

No antimicrobial activity was observed for the negative control (DMSO) at the tested concentration, while positive controls were active against the studied bacteria except amoxicillin (25 μg) which did not show any antibacterial activity against *Escherichia coli* and *Staphylococcus aureus* [36, 37] (Table 5).

Excepting OWWE mountainous extract (5 mg), no significant antibacterial activity of the tested extracts was observed against *Escherichia coli* and *Streptococcus faecalis*. However, *Staphylococcus aureus* was sensitive to the major tested extracts in a dose-dependent manner. At lower concentrations, the extracts showed various antibacterial effects, but at 5 mg/disc all the samples were active against this

TABLE 2: Major phenolic compounds identified in OCE.

Compounds	$[M-H]^+$ $(m/z)^a$	Main fragments ESI-MS	Area P	M	References[b]
Phenolic alcohols					
Tyrosol	139		ID	ID	[5, 14–19]
Hydroxytyrosol	155		ID	ID	[5, 14–16, 20–22]
Phenolic acids					
Vanillic acid	169		ID	ID	[15, 17, 19, 22–24]
Caffeic acid	181		ID	NI	[4, 5, 13, 14, 16, 19, 23]
Sinapic acid	225		ID	ID	[22, 23]
Dihydroxymandelic acid	185		ID	ID	[15]
Vanillin	153		ID	ID	[5, 16, 23, 24]
Secoiridoids and derivatives					
Oleuropein	541	227/225, 303/301	ID	ID	[4, 5, 14, 15, 17, 24, 25]
3,4-DHPEA-EA[b]	379		ID	ID	[5, 16, 17, 19, 20]
3,4-DHPEA-EDA[b]	321		ID	NI	[5, 17]
Oleuropein derivatives	369	225/223, 141/139	NI	ID	[5, 17]
Elenolic acid (p-HPEA-EDA)	243	225/223, 197/195, 179/177	ID	ID	[5, 15–17, 19, 22]
Ligstroside	525	395/393	ID	ID	[5, 14, 15, 23]
p-DHPA-EA[b]	363		NI	ID	[5, 16, 17, 19, 20]
Ligstroside derivatives	337	217/215, 155/153	ID	ID	[5, 20, 24]
Ligstroside derivatives	293		ID	NI	[20]
Ligstroside derivatives	395	259/257	ID	ID	[20]
Hydroxytyrosol glucoside	317	137/135	ID	NI	[5, 15, 16]
Oleoside	391		ID	NI	[14, 15, 23, 26]
Verbascoside	365		ID	NI	[14, 15, 23, 24]
Flavonoids					
Apigenin	271		NI	ID	[5, 14, 16, 19, 22, 23]
Luteolin	287	153/151	ID	ID	[5, 14, 15, 20, 22, 24]
Luteolin-7-glucoside	449	287/285	NI	ID	[5, 14–16, 19, 23, 24]
Nüzhenide	685		NI	ID	[19]
Quercetin	303		ID	ID	[14, 22, 23]

[a]Masse/charge, in the positive mode.
ID: Identified; NI: not identified.
P: plain/M: mountain.
[b]3,4-DHPEA-EA: oleuropein aglycon, p-DHPA-EA: ligstroside aglycon, 3,4-DHPEA-EDA: oleuropein aglycon isomer in aldehyde form, and 3,4-DHPEA-AC: hydroxytyrosol acetate.

strain with similar inhibition zones to those of the positive controls (chloramphenicol 14.2 ± 0.5 mm; ceftriaxone: 15.6 ± 0.4 mm). *Streptococcus faecalis* and *Escherichia coli* seem to be resistant to even high concentrations. No significant differences in activity were observed between OCE and OWWE phenolic extracts whatever their geographical origin (plain or mountain).

4. Discussion

4.1. Phenolic Composition Extracts. The difference of OCE and OWWE phenolic composition may be attributed to several parameters. It can be according to the olive variety, climate conditions, cultivation practices, the olive storage time, and the olive oil extraction process [22, 29]. Olive mill waste samples were chosen, as the purpose of this study was not to assess differences due to olive variety and olive oil

extraction process. Indeed, the total content of phenolic compounds in our extracts appears to be interestingly correlated with the bioclimatic origin and climate conditions (Table 1) but varietal differences cannot be ignored. In this context, other studies have been clearly demonstrated the impact of geographical and climatic conditions on the determination of polyphenols content in plants [23, 28, 35]. Moreover, olive mill waste's composition was studied in various recent studies [17, 35]. It was characterized by its complexity and it was found being rich in hydroxytyrosol and secoiridoids derivatives [3, 14, 28]. HPLC with detection by ESI-MS provides valuable information on phenolic composition. The individual biophenols identified in the OCE and OWWE were classified at five classes, namely, simple phenols, phenolic acids, derivatives secoiridoids, flavonoids, and lignans (Tables 2 and 3). These results were consistent with those found by Suárez et al. [19] and Ramos et al. [17]. Qualitative

TABLE 3: Major phenolic compounds identified in OWWE.

Compounds	$[M-H]^-$ $(m/z)^a$	Main fragments ESI-MS^b	Areas P	M	References
Phenolic alcohols					
Tyrosol	137		ID	ID	[3, 14, 27, 28]
Hydroxytyrosol	153		ID	ID	[3, 18, 27–29]
Phenolic acids					
Vanillic acid	167		NI	ID	[18, 24]
Sinapic acid	223		ID	NI	[22, 23]
Syringic acid	197		ID	ID	[3, 22, 23, 30]
Caffeoylquinic acid	353	191	ID	NI	[24]
3,4,5 Trimethoxybenzoic acid	211		NI	ID	[30]
Vanillin	151		NI	ID	[23, 24, 27]
Secoiridoids and derivatives					
3,4-DHPEA-EDA^b	319	227, 183	ID	NI	[28]
ME 3,4 DHPEA-EA^b	409		ID	NI	[5]
Oleuropein derivatives	365	214, 307	NI	ID	[5]
Ligstroside	523	335, 259	NI	ID	[20, 23]
p-DHPA-EA^b	361		ID	NI	[28]
Ligstroside derivatives	337	155	ID	NI	[20]
Ligstroside derivatives	393	257, 137	ID	NI	[20]
Elenolic acid	241		NI	ID	[15]
3,4-DHPEA-AC^b	195		ID	NI	[15]
Hydroxytyrosol glucoside	315	150	ID	ID	[17]
Oleoside	389	209	ID	NI	[17]
Verbascoside	623	526, 277	ID	ID	[14, 18, 24, 28]
Flavonoids					
Apigenin-7-rutinoside	577		NI	ID	[22, 23]
Apigenin-7-glucoside	477		NI	ID	[22, 23]
Luteolin	285		ID	ID	[20, 22, 23, 28]
Luteolin-7-glucoside	447		ID	ID	[18, 23, 24, 28]
Luteolin-7-rutinoside	593		NI	ID	[22–24]
Nüzhenide	685		ID	NI	[22, 23]
Rutin	609		ID	ID	[18, 23, 24]
Lignans					
1 Acetoxypinoresinol	415		ID	ID	[22]
Pinoresinol	357		NI	ID	[22]

^{a}Masse/charge, in the negative mode.
ID: identified; NI: not identified.
P: plain/M: mountain.
^{b}3,4-DHPEA-EA: oleuropein aglycon, p-DHPA-EA: ligstroside aglycon, 3,4-DHPEA-EDA: oleuropein aglycon isomer in aldehyde form, ME 3,4 DHPEA-EA: oleuropein aglycon in methyl form, and 3,4-DHPEA-AC: hydroxytyrosol acetate.

TABLE 4: Scavenging effects (EC$_{50}$ μg/mL) of OCE and OWWE on DPPH free radicals.

	OCE Plain area	Mountainous area	OWWE Plain area	Mountainous area	Vitamin C
EC$_{50}$ (μg/mL)	168.0 ± 48	157.7 ± 34.9	32.7 ± 4.5	12.1 ± 5.6	3.2 ± 0.6

Antiradical activity EC$_{50}$ (μg/mL) was defined as the concentration of extracts necessary to decrease the initial DPPH radical concentration by 50%. Values are means standard deviation (SD) of three measurements ($P < 0.05\%$).

TABLE 5: Antimicrobial activity of OCE and OWWE.

Test substance (dose/disc)	Inhibition zone (mm) Bacteria		
	Escherichia coli	*Staphylococcus aureus*	*Streptococcus faecalis*
OCE			
Plain extract (1.25 mg)	0	13,2 ± 0,4	0
Plain extract (2.50 mg)	0	14,6 ± 0,1	0
Plain extract (5 mg)	11,65 ± 0,75	15,7 ± 0,7	11,1 ± 0,1
Mountainous extract (1.25 mg)	0	0	0
Mountainous extract (2.50 mg)	0	12,7 ± 0,7	0
Mountainous extract (5 mg)	12,65 ± 0,65	15 ± 0,8	0
OWWE			
Plain extract (1.25 mg)	0	0	0
Plain extract (2.50 mg)	0	12,7 ± 0,3	0
Plain extract (5 mg)	0	14,55 ± 0,35	0
Mountainous extract (1.25 mg)	0	0	0
Mountainous extract (2.50 mg)	0	0	0
Mountainous extract (5 mg)	11,3 ± 0,3	15,85 ± 0,55	15 ± 0,2
Amoxicillin (25 µg)	0	0	15,45 ± 0,45
Chloramphenicol (30 µg)	28,75 ± 0,55	14,2 ± 0,5	22,3 ± 0,5
Ceftriaxone (30 µg)	19,05 ± 0,45	15,6 ± 0,4	25,8 ± 0,2

Diameter of zone of inhibition (mm) including diameter of 6 mm disc. Results quoted as the average of three readings ± standard deviation. 0 mm indicates no visible zone of inhibition.

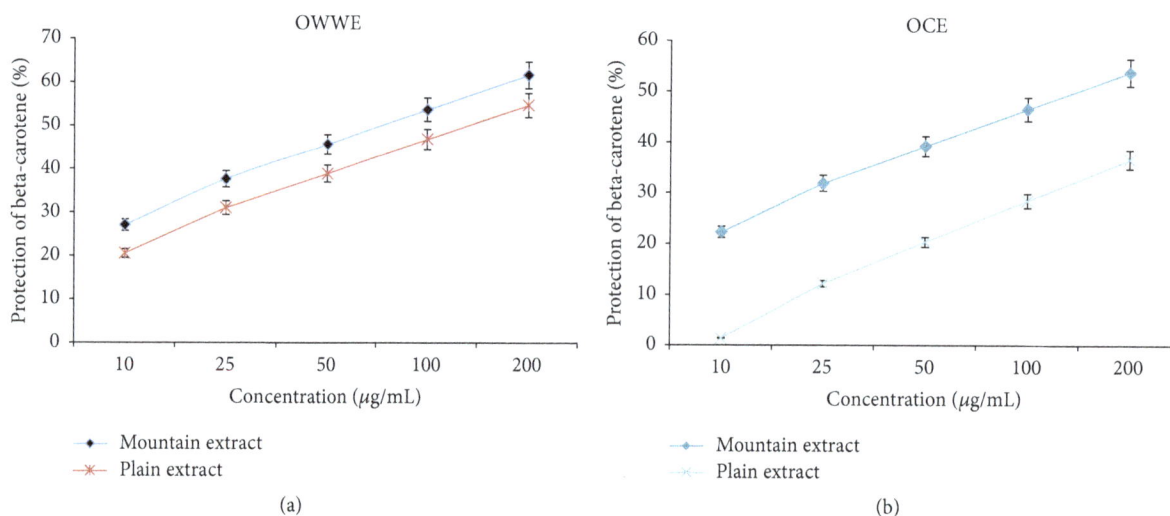

FIGURE 4: Dose-response curve of antioxidant activity of OCE and OWWE in BCBT.

and quantitative differences are obvious between the profiles of OWWE and OCE (Figures 1 and 2). OWWE had the higher total phenol content consistent with its greater abundance of individual phenols with the exception of oleuropein, ligstroside, and verbascoside, which were higher in OCE. Our results show that hydroxytyrosol is the major compound identified in Moroccan olive cake and olive wastewater phenolic extracts. It has been identified and characterized in the olive cake and olive mill wastewater and had been demonstrated as a major antioxidant agent [5, 17]. Tyrosol was also detected in both extracts at an important level. This phenol

was particularly characterized by its important antioxidant effect [14]. The reduced levels of oleuropein, ligstroside, and verbascoside can be attributed to hydrolysis of hydroxytyrosol, tyrosol, and hydroxytyrosol glucoside. Oleuropein and verbascoside have been identified in various studies for their important antioxidant and antimicrobial potential [4, 17]. The amount of flavonoids recovered from OWWE was notably larger than OCE. Moreover, apigenin-7-glucoside and apigenin-7-rutinoside, which could not be detected in OCE, were identified in OWWE chromatograms (Figure 2). Other secoiridoids derivatives were detected as well as those of OCE and OWWE with an observed abundance in OWWE especially those from mountainous areas. The most answered were 3,4-DHPEA-EA, 3,4-DHPEA-EDA, and hydroxytyrosol glucoside [4, 5, 19]. The elenolic acid, the main fragment of the oleuropein degradation, was mostly found in OCE. It can be considered as an important antimicrobial and antiviral agent [22].

4.2. Antioxidant Activity. The determination of the antioxidant activity of plant extracts requires a multidimensional evaluation of antioxidant activities combined with special tests. Thus, the free radical scavenging DPPH and the bleaching test BCBT were chosen for this study. The results differ depending on the test used. This can be explained by the sensitivity of each test to the analyzed extracts. With the DPPH method, both extracts tested have been active for trapping free radicals DPPH according to the phenolic extract dose (Figure 3). The EC_{50} values, inversely proportional to the antiradical scavenging DPPH showed that OWWE was more active than OCE and interestingly, the mountainous phenolic extract were more active than the plain phenolic extracts (Table 4). The results confirmed the existence of a good correlation between the antioxidant potential and the total polyphenol content [17, 38]. OCE and OWWE showed a linear correlation coefficient: $R^2 = 0.954$ and $R^2 = 0.977$, respectively, indicating that 95% and 97% of the antioxidant capacity were due to the contribution of the phenolic compounds and they represent the dominant antioxidants in these extracts [5, 39]. In contrast to the DPPH assay, OCE mountainous extract was more efficient to protect elenolic acid than OCE plain extract in BCBT assay, which can be attributed to the high specificity of the BCBT assay for lipophilic compounds. This suggests the more hydrophobic nature of antioxidants present in OCE originating from plain area compared to those originating from mountainous area. This result could be attributed to the hydrolysis of some compounds present in olive mill waste extracts such as verbascoside [14]. Interestingly, hydroxytyrosol glucoside and caffeic acid, the major constituent compounds of verbascoside, were detected at significant level in OCE plain extract with reduced level of verbascoside concentration. The observed antioxidant activity can also be related to the chemical composition of the evaluated extracts, which were rich in hydroxytyrosol, secoiridoids and derivatives, phenolic acids, and flavonoids. With reference to the phenolic compounds chemical structures, hydroxytyrosol, which usually proved high radical scavenging activity, has a 3,4 dihydroxyl structure bonded to an aromatic ring. This gives it a greater activity compared to tyrosol, for example, which has a similar structure, but with only one hydroxyl group bound to an aromatic ring [17]. These data suggest the importance of the hydroxylation of the aromatic ring of the compounds compared to the phenolic compounds with a single hydroxyl group. The extracts with the highest levels of secoiridoids and derivatives mainly oleuropein, verbascoside, hydroxytyrosol glucoside, and oleuropein aglycon showed also a significant antiradical potential [5, 14]. Furthermore, Fki, et al. [40] measured the antiradical activity of phenolic acids and have demonstrated a high antioxidant activity of caffeic acid. However, the compounds with one hydroxyl group such as p-coumaric acid and syringic acid have showed low antioxidant activity. Moreover, flavonoids, especially luteolin, luteolin-7-glucoside, quercetin, and rutin, were identified among the major phenolic compounds of the olive mill waste. Their characteristic structure with three aromatic rings gives them an important antioxidant activity specifically due to the presence of 3 to 5 hydroxyl groups [5]. However, further purification and fractionation are required to identify the potent antioxidant from the individual active compounds of these naturel extracts.

4.3. Antimicrobial Activity. In comparison to the antibiotic antibacterial activity, none of the extracts exhibit a significant activity against *Escherichia coli* and *Streptococcus faecalis* except OWWE mountainous extract at higher concentration (5 mg/mL) against *Streptococcus faecalis* (Table 5). In contrast, *Staphylococcus aureus* was susceptible to the major tested phenolic extracts. Most plant extracts show activity against Gram-positive bacteria but activity against Gram-negative bacteria is a critical measure of success [14]. Yangui et al. [41] demonstrated that hydroxytyrosol, tyrosol, and luteolin showed a good antimicrobial activity against Gram-positive bacteria. Indeed, Figures 1 and 2 showed that hydroxytyrosol and luteolin were among the major constituents of both extracts with a higher content in mountainous OWWE. This was consistent with the significant antibacterial activity of OWWE against *Staphylococcus aureus* and *Streptococcus faecalis* at higher concentration. Other studies showed that flavonoids in particular quercetin [42] and luteolin [43] could be considered as important antibacterial compounds especially against Gram-positive bacteria. Moreover, various antimicrobial activities were mainly attributed to phenolic acid especially caffeic acid, vanillic acid, p-coumaric acid, and 4-hydroxybenzoic acid [12, 44], verbascoside [45], and oleuropein and hydroxytyrosol [14]. Furthermore, no antibacterial activity was observed against *Escherichia coli*. This bacterial strain seems to be very resistant to both of olive mill waste extracts. The different activities against Gram-negative and Gram-positive bacteria may be rationalized by considering differences in cell wall composition. Gram-negative bacteria have a lipopolysaccharide component in their outer membrane that makes them more resistant to antibacterial compounds. OMW biophenols are essentially hydrophilic; the more lipophilic constituents are partitioned into the olive oil during processing. Furthermore, no correlation has been observed between antimicrobial activity and the polyphenol content ($R^2 = 0.00$). Similar results were obtained by Pérez et al. [46] in the evaluation of antibacterial activity of olive mill wastewater extracts. Confirming these data, there is no standard method evaluation criteria for the detection of antimicrobial activity in plant extracts [47]. Differences in bacterial strains, growth media and the inoculum size, make comparison of antimicrobial data of plant extracts from different sources very difficult. Other similar works suggested differences in used methods and the relative purity of the extract used in the tests [48]. Nevertheless, some studies showed no selective antimicrobial activity against both Gram-positive and Gram-negative bacteria [49].

5. Conclusion

In addition to the extraction and identification of OMW biophenols, OCE and OWWE phenolic extracts in the present study gave promising results in antioxidant and antibacterial activities. It was demonstrated that OWWE, especially those from mountainous areas, were rich on biophenols compounds and more active than those of OCE in the inhibition of the oxidation reactions. This activity has been suggested to be related to the phenolic content amount and to the nature of the phenolic composition extracts. Thus, it was concluded that OWWE was the most promising antioxidant source to contribute to further potential biological properties in the biomedical domains especially as natural anticancer agents. Indeed, studies in cells cancer molecular biology of these extracts will be considered in our further research works. Furthermore, the studied extracts were effective in inhibiting the growth of *Staphylococcus aureus* indicating that such extracts may present an antimicrobial activity against Gram-positive bacteria.

Conflict of Interests

The authors do not have any conflict of interests regarding the content of the present work.

Acknowledgments

The authors thank the CNRST, Rabat, Morocco, for HPLC-MS analysis and gratefully acknowledge the assistance of Dr. Abdessalam Jaafari, Laboratory of Biological Engineering, Sultan Moulay Slimane University. The authors also wish to thank Professor Jamal Koubali, Department of English at the Sultan Moulay Slimane University, for reading the paper and improving the English.

References

[1] D. Harman, "Aging: a theory based on free radical and radiation chemistry," *Journal of Gerontology*, vol. 11, no. 3, pp. 298–300, 1956.

[2] A. Djeridane, M. Yousfi, B. Nadjemi, D. Boutassouna, P. Stocker, and N. Vidal, "Antioxidant activity of some Algerian medicinal plants extracts containing phenolic compounds," *Food Chemistry*, vol. 97, no. 4, pp. 654–660, 2006.

[3] L. Bertin, F. Ferri, A. Scoma, L. Marchetti, and F. Fava, "Recovery of high added value natural polyphenols from actual olive mill wastewater through solid phase extraction," *Chemical Engineering Journal*, vol. 171, no. 3, pp. 1287–1293, 2011.

[4] H. K. Obied, D. R. Bedgood, P. D. Prenzler, and K. Robards, "Effect of processing conditions, prestorage treatment, and storage conditions on the phenol content and antioxidant

activity of olive mill waste," *Journal of Agricultural and Food Chemistry*, vol. 56, no. 11, pp. 3925–3932, 2008.

[5] M. Suárez, M.-P. Romero, T. Ramo, A. Macià, and M.-J. Motilva, "Methods for preparing phenolic extracts from olive cake for potential application as food antioxidants," *Journal of Agricultural and Food Chemistry*, vol. 57, no. 4, pp. 1463–1472, 2009.

[6] F. Z. Sheabar and I. Neeman, "Separation and concentration of natural antioxidants from the rape of olives," *Journal of the American Oil Chemists' Society*, vol. 65, no. 6, pp. 990–993, 1988.

[7] K. P. Link, H. Angell, and J. Walker, "The isolation of protocatechic acid from pigmented onion scales and its significance in relation to disease resistance in onions," *The Journal of Biological Chemistry*, vol. 81, no. 2, pp. 369–375, 1929.

[8] E. Moreno, J. Quevedo-Sarmiento, and A. Ramos-Cormenzana, "Antibacterial activity of wastewaters from olive oil mills," *Encyclopedia of Environmental Control Technology*, vol. 4, pp. 731–757, 1989.

[9] R. Capasso, A. Evidente, L. Schivo, G. Orru, M. A. Marcialis, and G. Cristinzio, "Antibacterial polyphenols from olive oil mill waste waters," *Journal of Applied Bacteriology*, vol. 79, no. 4, pp. 393–398, 1995.

[10] M. Niaounakis and C. P. Halvadakis, "Olive-mill waste management," Literature Review and Patent Survey, Typothito-George Dardanos Publications, Athens, Greece, 2004.

[11] G. Bisignano, A. Tomaino, R. Lo Cascio, G. Crisafi, N. Uccella, and A. Saija, "On the *in vitro* antimicrobial activity of oleuropein and hydroxytyrosol," *Journal of Pharmacy and Pharmacology*, vol. 51, no. 8, pp. 971–974, 1999.

[12] N. H. Aziz, S. E. Farag, L. A. A. Mousa, and M. A. Abo-Zaid, "Comparative antibacterial and antifungal effects of some phenolic compounds," *Microbios*, vol. 93, no. 374, pp. 43–54, 1998.

[13] M. H. Alu'datt, I. Alli, K. Ereifej, M. Alhamad, A. R. Al-Tawaha, and T. Rababah, "Optimisation, characterisation and quantification of phenolic compounds in olive cake," *Food Chemistry*, vol. 123, no. 1, pp. 117–122, 2010.

[14] H. K. Obied, D. R. Bedgood Jr., P. D. Prenzler, and K. Robards, "Bioscreening of Australian olive mill waste extracts: biophenol content, antioxidant, antimicrobial and molluscicidal activities," *Food and Chemical Toxicology*, vol. 45, no. 7, pp. 1238–1248, 2007.

[15] E. Aranda, I. García-Romera, J. A. Ocampo et al., "Chemical characterization and effects on *Lepidium sativum* of the native and bioremediated components of dry olive mill residue," *Chemosphere*, vol. 69, no. 2, pp. 229–239, 2007.

[16] A. Serra, L. Rubió, X. Borràs, A. Macià, M.-P. Romero, and M.-J. Motilva, "Distribution of olive oil phenolic compounds in rat tissues after administration of a phenolic extract from olive cake," *Molecular Nutrition & Food Research*, vol. 56, no. 3, pp. 486–496, 2012.

[17] P. Ramos, S. A. O. Santos, Â. R. Guerra et al., "Valorization of olive mill residues: antioxidant and breast cancer antiproliferative activities of hydroxytyrosol-rich extracts derived from olive oil by-products," *Industrial Crops and Products*, vol. 46, pp. 359–368, 2013.

[18] C. Romero, M. Brenes, P. García, and A. Garrido, "Hydroxytyrosol 4-β-D-glucoside, an important phenolic compound in olive fruits and derived products," *Journal of Agricultural and Food Chemistry*, vol. 50, no. 13, pp. 3835–3839, 2002.

[19] M. Suárez, M.-P. Romero, and M.-J. Motilva, "Development of a phenol-enriched olive oil with phenolic compounds from olive cake," *Journal of Agricultural and Food Chemistry*, vol. 58, no. 19, pp. 10396–10403, 2010.

[20] K. De La Torre-Carbot, O. Jauregui, E. Gimeno, A. I. Castellote, R. M. Lamuela-Raventós, and M. C. López-Sabater, "Characterization and quantification of phenolic compounds in olive oils by solid-phase extraction, HPLC-DAD, and HPLC-MS/MS," *Journal of Agricultural and Food Chemistry*, vol. 53, no. 11, pp. 4331–4340, 2005.

[21] M. N. Alhamad, T. M. Rababah, M. Al-u'datt et al., "The physicochemical properties, total phenolic, antioxidant activities, and phenolic profile of fermented olive cake," *Arabian Journal of Chemistry*, 2012.

[22] H. K. Obied, M. S. Allen, D. R. Bedgood, P. D. Prenzler, K. Robards, and R. Stockmann, "Bioactivity and analysis of biophenols recovered from olive mill waste," *Journal of Agricultural and Food Chemistry*, vol. 53, no. 4, pp. 823–837, 2005.

[23] S. Dermeche, M. Nadour, C. Larroche, F. Moulti-Mati, and P. Michaud, "Olive mill wastes: biochemical characterizations and valorization strategies," *Process Biochemistry*, vol. 48, no. 10, pp. 1532–1552, 2013.

[24] S. M. Cardoso, S. Guyot, N. Marnet, J. A. Lopes-da-Silva, C. M. G. C. Renard, and M. A. Coimbra, "Characterisation of phenolic extracts from olive pulp and olive pomace by electrospray mass spectrometry," *Journal of the Science of Food and Agriculture*, vol. 85, no. 1, pp. 21–32, 2005.

[25] B. Amro, T. Aburjai, and S. Al-Khalil, "Antioxidative and radical scavenging effects of olive cake extract," *Fitoterapia*, vol. 73, no. 6, pp. 456–461, 2002.

[26] K. S. Kim, S. Lee, Y. S. Lee et al., "Anti-oxidant activities of the extracts from the herbs of *Artemisia apiacea*," *Journal of Ethnopharmacology*, vol. 85, no. 1, pp. 69–72, 2003.

[27] L. Lesage-Meessen, D. Navarro, S. Maunier et al., "Simple phenolic content in olive oil residues as a function of extraction systems," *Food Chemistry*, vol. 75, no. 4, pp. 501–507, 2001.

[28] E. De Marco, M. Savarese, A. Paduano, and R. Sacchi, "Characterization and fractionation of phenolic compounds extracted from olive oil mill wastewaters," *Food Chemistry*, vol. 104, no. 2, pp. 858–867, 2007.

[29] N. Allouche, I. Fki, and S. Sayadi, "Toward a high yield recovery of antioxidants and purified hydroxytyrosol from olive mill wastewaters," *Journal of Agricultural and Food Chemistry*, vol. 52, no. 2, pp. 267–273, 2004.

[30] M. J. B. Juárez, A. Zafra-Gómez, B. Luzón-Toro et al., "Gas chromatographic-mass spectrometric study of the degradation of phenolic compounds in wastewater olive oil by *Azotobacter chroococcum*," *Bioresource Technology*, vol. 99, no. 7, pp. 2392–2398, 2008.

[31] V. L. Singleton and J. A. Rossi Jr., "Colorimetry of total phenolics with phosphomolybdic-phosphotungstic acid reagents," *American Journal of Enology and Viticulture*, vol. 16, no. 3, pp. 144–158, 1965.

[32] A. Scalbert, B. Monties, and G. Janin, "Tannins in wood: comparison of different estimation methods," *Journal of Agricultural and Food Chemistry*, vol. 37, no. 5, pp. 1324–1329, 1989.

[33] N. Kartal, M. Sokmen, B. Tepe, D. Daferera, M. Polissiou, and A. Sokmen, "Investigation of the antioxidant properties of *Ferula orientalis* L. using a suitable extraction procedure," *Food Chemistry*, vol. 100, no. 2, pp. 584–589, 2007.

[34] O. Y. Celiktas, E. E. H. Kocabas, E. Bedir, F. V. Sukan, T. Ozek, and K. H. C. Baser, "Antimicrobial activities of methanol extracts and essential oils of *Rosmarinus officinalis*, depending on location and seasonal variations," *Food Chemistry*, vol. 100, no. 2, pp. 553–559, 2007.

[35] I. Leouifoudi, A. Zyad, A. Amechrouq, M. A. Oukerrou, H. A. Mouse, and M. Mbarki, "Identification and characterisation of phenolic compounds extracted from Moroccan olive mill wastewater," *Food Science and Technology*, vol. 34, no. 2, pp. 249–257, 2014.

[36] M. S. Rafiq, M. I. Rafiq, T. Khan, M. Rafiq, and M. M. Khan, "Effectiveness of simple control measures on methicillin resistant *Staphylococcus aureus* infection status and characteristics with susceptibility patterns in a teaching hospital in Peshawar," *Journal of the Pakistan Medicine Association*, vol. 65, no. 9, pp. 915–920, 2015.

[37] V. da Costa Andrade, B. del Busso Zampieri, E. R. Ballesteros, A. B. Pinto, and A. J. Fernandes Cardoso de Oliveira, "Densities and antimicrobial resistance of *Escherichia coli* isolated from marine waters and beach sands," *Environmental Monitoring and Assessment*, vol. 187, no. 6, article 342, 2015.

[38] A. C. P. Do Prado, H. S. Da Silva, S. M. Da Silveira et al., "Effect of the extraction process on the phenolic compounds profile and the antioxidant and antimicrobial activity of extracts of pecan nut [*Carya illinoinensis* (Wangenh) C. Koch] shell," *Industrial Crops and Products*, vol. 52, pp. 552–561, 2014.

[39] S. Athamena, I. Chalghem, A. Kassah-Laouar, S. Laroui, and S. Khebri, "Activité antioxydante et antimicrobienne d'extraits de Cumain Cyminum L.," *Lebanese Science Journal*, vol. 11, no. 1, pp. 69–81, 2010.

[40] I. Fki, M. Bouaziz, Z. Sahnoun, and S. Sayadi, "Hypocholesterolemic effects of phenolic-rich extracts of *Chemlali* olive cultivar in rats fed a cholesterol-rich diet," *Bioorganic and Medicinal Chemistry*, vol. 13, no. 18, pp. 5362–5370, 2005.

[41] T. Yangui, S. Sayadi, A. Gargoubi, and A. Dhouib, "Fungicidal effect of hydroxytyrosol-rich preparations from olive mill wastewater against *Verticillium dahliae*," *Crop Protection*, vol. 29, no. 10, pp. 1208–1213, 2010.

[42] B. Shan, Y.-Z. Cai, J. D. Brooks, and H. Corke, "The *in vitro* antibacterial activity of dietary spice and medicinal herb extracts," *International Journal of Food Microbiology*, vol. 117, no. 1, pp. 112–119, 2007.

[43] T. Askun, G. Tumen, F. Satil, and M. Ates, "*In vitro* activity of methanol extracts of plants used as spices against *Mycobacterium tuberculosis* and other bacteria," *Food Chemistry*, vol. 116, no. 1, pp. 289–294, 2009.

[44] C. Soler-Rivas, J. C. Espín, and H. J. Wichers, "Oleuropein and related compounds," *Journal of the Science of Food and Agriculture*, vol. 80, no. 7, pp. 1013–1023, 2000.

[45] N. Didry, V. Seidel, L. Dubreuil, F. Tillequin, and F. Bailleul, "Isolation and antibacterial activity of phenylpropanoid derivatives from *Ballota nigra*," *Journal of Ethnopharmacology*, vol. 67, no. 2, pp. 197–202, 1999.

[46] J. Pérez, T. Dela Rubia, J. Moreno, and J. Martínez, "Phenolic content and antibacterial activity of olive oil waste waters," *Environmental Toxicology and Chemistry*, vol. 11, no. 4, pp. 489–495, 1992.

[47] F. Hadacek and H. Greger, "Testing of antifungal natural products: methodologies, comparability of results and assay choice," *Phytochemical Analysis*, vol. 11, no. 3, pp. 137–147, 2000.

[48] E. A. Hayouni, M. Abedrabba, M. Bouix, and M. Hamdi, "The effects of solvents and extraction method on the phenolic contents and biological activities *in vitro* of Tunisian *Quercus coccifera* L. and *Juniperus phoenicea* L. fruit extracts," *Food Chemistry*, vol. 105, no. 3, pp. 1126–1134, 2007.

[49] A. Guesmi and A. Boudabous, "Activité antimicrobienne de cinq huiles essentielles associées dans les produits de thalassothérapie," *Revue des Régions Arides*, no. 1, pp. 224–230, 2006.

25

Crude *Aloe vera* Gel Shows Antioxidant Propensities and Inhibits Pancreatic Lipase and Glucose Movement *In Vitro*

Urmeela Taukoorah and M. Fawzi Mahomoodally

Department of Health Sciences, Faculty of Science, University of Mauritius, 230 Réduit, Mauritius

Correspondence should be addressed to M. Fawzi Mahomoodally; f.mahomoodally@uom.ac.mu

Academic Editor: Robert Gogal

Aloe vera gel (AVG) is traditionally used in the management of diabetes, obesity, and infectious diseases. The present study aimed to investigate the inhibitory potential of AVG against α-amylase, α-glucosidase, and pancreatic lipase activity *in vitro*. Enzyme kinetic studies using Michaelis-Menten (K_m) and Lineweaver-Burk equations were used to establish the type of inhibition. The antioxidant capacity of AVG was evaluated for its ferric reducing power, 2-diphenyl-2-picrylhydrazyl hydrate scavenging ability, nitric oxide scavenging power, and xanthine oxidase inhibitory activity. The glucose entrapment ability, antimicrobial activity, and total phenolic, flavonoid, tannin, and anthocyanin content were also determined. AVG showed a significantly higher percentage inhibition (85.56 ± 0.91) of pancreatic lipase compared to Orlistat. AVG was found to increase the Michaelis-Menten constant and decreased the maximal velocity (V_{max}) of lipase, indicating mixed inhibition. AVG considerably inhibits glucose movement across dialysis tubes and was comparable to Arabic gum. AVG was ineffective against the tested microorganisms. Total phenolic and flavonoid contents were 66.06 ± 1.14 (GAE)/mg and 60.95 ± 0.97 (RE)/mg, respectively. AVG also showed interesting antioxidant properties. The biological activity observed in this study tends to validate some of the traditional claims of AVG as a functional food.

1. Introduction

Aloe vera is one of nature's most sacred therapeutic medicinal food plants. The medicinal potential of this tropical succulent has urged recurrent myths about its properties that have persisted from the fourth century BC throughout world history [1]. There are also reports that tend to show that Alexander the Great used *Aloe vera* to treat his wounded soldiers and Cleopatra used it for skin care [2]. Over the years, this exquisite plant has acquired names such as "the wand of heaven," "heaven's blessing," and "the silent healer" [3]. Native to Northern Africa, this plant has been in existence for over 2000 years [2].

Parenchymatous gel from *Aloe vera* leaves is extensively used in folk medicine, health drinks, topical creams, toiletries, and cosmetics [4]. Without any doubt, the commercialisation of *Aloe vera* is a success story. Various kinds of natural-based industries have a share in the *Aloe vera* market, most notably the cosmetic, food, beverage, and

dietary supplement industries. The major constituents of *Aloe vera* gel can be classified into five groups, namely, phenolics, saccharides, vitamins, enzymes, and low molecular weight substances [5]. *Aloe vera* gel has an assortment of pharmacological properties which encompasses antiviral, antibacterial, laxative, protection against radiation, antioxidant, anti-inflammation, anticancer, antidiabetic, antiallergic, and immunostimulation properties amongst others [5, 6].

Apart from skin disorders, *Aloe vera* gel can also be also applied on superficial or partial thickness burns to fasten healing process and reduce pain [7, 8]. It helps in soothing skin injuries affected by burning, skin irritations, cuts, and insect bites. Faster wound closure has also been demonstrated in rats treated with isolated and characterised *Aloe vera* polysaccharides [9]. *Aloe vera* further reduces inflammation by downregulating proinflammatory cytokine production in activated human macrophages and thus interfering with the cytokine overproduction during early sepsis or in chronic inflammatory or autoimmune disease, thereby ameliorating

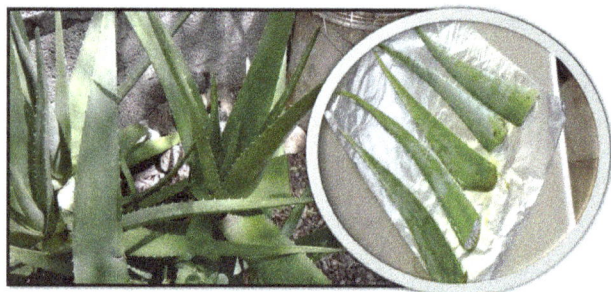

FIGURE 1: Freshly cut *Aloe vera* leaves.

the outcome and quality of life of patients [10]. *Aloe vera* polysaccharides have also been speculated to enhance immunity activity and exert antioxidant effects in oral ulcer animal models [11].

Furthermore, *Aloe vera* has shown its potential in the management of diabetes mellitus (DM). Clinical trials have shown that, in obese individuals with prediabetes or early untreated diabetes mellitus, *Aloe vera* gel complex reduced body weight, body fat mass, and insulin resistance [12]. Abo-Youssef and Messiha (2013) also proved the antidiabetic effect of *Aloe vera* leaf pulp extract *in vivo* and *in vitro* as compared to glimepiride [13–16].

Despite the availability of panoply of information on *Aloe vera*, there is insufficient scientific evidence on the efficacy of untreated or unprocessed local cultivar of Mauritian *Aloe vera* gel and its mechanism of action. Additional work is required to probe into the antidiabetic, antimicrobial, and antioxidant properties of the Mauritian *Aloe vera* gel which may help to validate its traditional claims. This endeavour will also delineate further health benefits of *A. vera* so as to encourage its use as a herbal medicine or functional food. Therefore, the main aim of this *in vitro* study was to investigate the antidiabetic, antimicrobial, and antioxidant activities of crude *Aloe vera* gel.

2. Methodology

2.1. Plant Material. Fresh *Aloe vera* leaves (Figure 1) were collected from Vacoas in October 2013. They were authenticated and an identification code (UTAV201301) was assigned to the specimen.

2.2. Preparation of Plant Material. The leaves were washed thoroughly under running tap water and then patted dry using clean filter papers. The peels were discarded while the gel was finely crushed using an electric blender. The resulting gel paste was used in all the tests.

2.3. Alpha-Amylase Inhibition Assay. The activity of α-amylase was carried out according to the method of Mao and Kinsella [17], based on the starch-iodine colour changes with minor modifications. Soluble starch solution (1%) was used as substrate. The starch solution was prepared by adding 1 g of soluble potato starch in 10 mL water and then boiled for

2 minutes. After cooling, water was added to reach a final volume of 100 mL. α-amylase solution (0.1 mL of 15 μg/mL in 0.1 M acetate buffer at pH 7.2 containing 0.0032 M sodium chloride) was added to a mixture of 3 mL of 1% soluble starch solution and 2 mL of acetate buffer (0.1 M, pH 7.2) preequilibrated at 30°C in a water bath. Substrate and α-amylase blank determinations were undertaken under the same conditions.

At zero time ($t = 0$ min) and at the end of the incubation period ($t = 60$), 0.1 mL of reaction mixture was withdrawn from each tube after mixing and transferred into 10 mL of an iodine solution (0.254 g iodine and 4.0 g potassium iodide in 1 litre). After mixing, the absorbance of the starch-iodine mixture was measured immediately at room temperature at 565 nm using a spectrophotometer. The absorbance of the starch blank was subtracted from the sample reading. One unit of amylase activity was arbitrarily defined as follows: $(A_o - A_t / A_o) * 100$, where A_o and A_t are absorbance of the iodine complex of the starch digest at zero time and after 60 minutes of hydrolysis. Specific activity of α-amylase was defined as units/mg protein/60 min. Percentage inhibition was calculated using the following equation:

$$\% \text{ inhibition} = \left[\left(A_o - A_t\right)_{\text{control}} - \frac{\left(A_o - A_t\right)_{\text{sample}}}{\left(A_o - A_t\right)_{\text{control}}} \right] \quad (1)$$

$$* \, 100.$$

2.4. Alpha-Glucosidase Inhibition Assay. Alpha-glucosidase inhibitory activity was performed following the modified method of Pistia-Brueggeman and Hollingsworth [18]. In test-tubes, a reaction mixture containing 500 μL of phosphate buffer (50 mM, pH 6.9), 100 μL of α-glucosidase (1 U/mL), and 200 μL of plant extract of varying concentrations was preincubated for 5 minutes at 37°C and then 200 μL of 1 mM PNPG (4-nitrophenyl-alpha-D-glucopyranoside) substrate was added to the mixture. After further incubation at 37°C for 30 minutes, the reaction was stopped by the addition of 500 μL of sodium carbonate (0.1 M). Enzyme, inhibitor, and substrate solutions were all prepared using the same buffer. Acarbose (5 mg/mL) was used as a positive control and water as a negative control. The yellow colour produced (due to *p*-nitrophenol formation) was quantitated by colorimetric analysis and reading the absorbance at 405 nm. Each experiment was performed in triplicate, along with appropriate blanks. The percentage inhibition was calculated using the formula

$$\% \text{ inhibition} = \left[\frac{\left(A_{\text{control}} - A_{\text{sample}}\right)}{A_{\text{control}}} \right] * 100. \quad (2)$$

2.5. Porcine Pancreatic Lipase Inhibitory Assay. The porcine pancreatic lipase inhibitory assay was adapted from Zheng et al. and Bustanji et al. [19, 20]. Briefly, 50 μL of porcine pancreatic lipase (1 mg/mL) was added to a mixture containing 100 μL extract and 50 μL tris-HCl buffer (2.5 mM, pH 7). The resulting mixture is then incubated at 37°C for 15 minutes. After the incubation period, 100 μL of PNPB is then added to the test-tube. The mixture is again incubated for 1 h at 37°C.

The absorbance is read at 405 nm. Percentage inhibition is calculated using the equation below:

$$\% \text{ inhibition} = \left[\frac{(A_{\text{control}} - A_{\text{blank}})}{A_{\text{blank}}} \right] * 100. \quad (3)$$

2.6. Enzyme Kinetics Using Michaelis-Menten and Lineweaver-Burk Equations.

The assay was adapted from Zheng et al. [19] and p-nitrophenol calibration curve was generated. The extract and porcine pancreatic lipase were mixed in a ratio of $2:1$, respectively, and preincubated for 15 minutes. After 15 minutes, 150 μL of enzyme-extract mixture was added to each well containing 50 μL buffer and 100 μL PNPB of varying concentrations (with starting concentration 25.5 mM). The plate was then put in the incubator at 37°C for 30 minutes. After the incubation period, absorbance was determined at 405 nm. A double reciprocal plot using Michaelis-Menten and Lineweaver-Burk equations was generated.

2.7. Effect of Aloe vera Gel on In Vitro Glucose Movement.

In vitro glucose diffusion studies were carried out by following the method with slight modifications described by Gallagher et al. and Edwards et al. [21, 22]. Briefly, the system consisted of a one-sided sealed dialysis tube (10 cm × 15 mm, dialysis tubing membrane, Sigma-Aldrich MW12173) into which 2 mL of 22 mM D-glucose in 0.15 M NaCl and 1 mL extract (50 g/L)/control (water) were incorporated. The other end was then sealed and the membrane was placed into a 100 mL glass beaker containing 40 mL 0.15 M NaCl and 10 mL distilled water to equilibrate the strength of internal and external medium. The beakers were placed into an orbital shaking incubator (JISICO) at 37°C at 100 rpm. The movement of the glucose into the external medium with respect to a negative control was monitored at set time intervals, that is, 0, 1, 2, 3, and 4 hrs. The absorbance was read at 500 nm. All tests were carried out in triplicate and glucose concentrations were measured using glucose oxidase kit method (GIBCO, Italy).

2.8. Antimicrobial Assay.

The antibacterial and antifungal properties of the extracts were assessed by using modified antimicrobial assay utilising microtitre plate described by Drummond and Waigh [23]. Briefly, using aseptic techniques a single colony of microbe was transferred into a 100 mL bottle of peptone water broth, capped, and placed in incubator overnight at 35°C. After 12–18 h of incubation, using aseptic preparation and the aid of a centrifuge, a clean sample of microbe was prepared. To the sterile microtitre plates, 100 μL of peptone water broth is first added to all wells, followed by 100 μL of extract or control. Then, 100 μL of microbial culture was further added. The resulting mixtures were then left to incubate for 24 h at ambient temperature. After incubation, 40 μL INT (iodonitrotetrazolium) (0.2 mg/mL) was added to all the wells and left to incubate for a further 20 minutes. The microplates were then assessed visually to determine the minimum inhibitory concentration (MIC). Controls used

for bacteria are Gentamicin, Chloramphenicol, and Streptomycin while controls used for fungi are Ampicillin and Amphotericin.

2.9. Ferric Reducing Antioxidant Power (FRAP) Assay.

The ability of the extracts to reduce iron was determined according to the modified method of Benzie and Strain [24] where Trolox was used as standard. Plant extracts of varying concentrations were mixed with 2850 μL FRAP solution (25 mL acetate buffer (300 mM, pH 3.6), 2.5 mL 2-4-6 tripyridyl-s-triazine (10 mM in 40 mM hydrochloric) (TPTZ; Sigma-Aldrich, Sydney, Australia), and 2.5 mL hydrated ferric chloride solution (20 mM) previously equilibrated for 30 minutes in the dark at 37°C). The reaction was allowed to take place for 30 minutes in the dark. The absorbance was determined at 593 nm. All determinations were done in triplicate and data obtained were expressed as mM Trolox Equivalent (TE)/mg crude extract.

2.10. Nitric Oxide Radical Scavenging Assay.

Nitric oxide (NO) was generated from sodium nitroprusside (SNP) (Sigma-Aldrich, Sydney, Australia) and was measured by the Griess Ilosvay reagent [25], using 0.1% w/v naphthylethylene-diamine-dihydrochloride (Sigma-Aldrich, Sydney, Australia) instead of 5% 1-naphthylamine. Plant extract (0.5 mL) was added to a mixture containing SNP (2 mL) and phosphate buffer saline (PBS) (0.5 mL, pH 7.4). The reaction mixture was incubated for 2.5 hrs at 25°C. Following incubation, 0.5 mL of the reaction mixture was added to 1 mL sulphanilic acid (0.33% in 20% glacial acetic acid) (Sigma-Aldrich, Sydney, Australia) and allowed to stand for 5 minutes. Naphthylethylene-diamine-dihydrochloride (1 mL of 0.1% w/v) was then added to the mixture. The resulting solution was vortexed and allowed to stand for further 30 minutes. The absorbance of the chromophores formed during the diazotization of nitrite with sulphanilamide and subsequent coupling with naphthylethylene-diamine-dichloride was read at 546 nm. Percentage inhibition was calculated as follows:

$$\% \text{ inhibition} = \left[\frac{(A_{\text{blank}} - A_{\text{sample}})}{A_{\text{blank}}} \right] * 100. \quad (4)$$

2.11. DPPH Free Radical Scavenging Assay.

The free radical scavenging activity of the different extracts was measured by using 1,1-diphenyl-2-picrylhydrazyl (DPPH) (Sigma-Aldrich, Sydney, Australia) according to the modified method of Umamaheswari and Chatterjee [26]. Plant extract (100 μL) was added to 200 μL freshly prepared DPPH solution (100 μM in methanol). The reaction mixture was incubated at 37°C for 30 minutes. After incubation, absorbance was determined at 517 nm. The percentage inhibition of DPPH was calculated using (4).

2.12. Xanthine Oxidase Inhibitory Activity.

The xanthine oxidase (Sigma-Aldrich, Germany) inhibitory activity was determined using modified method of Abdullahi et al. [27]. Samples were assayed for their in vitro xanthine oxidase inhibitory activity which was evaluated spectrophotometrically using xanthine as the substrate. The assay mixture consisted of 1 mL of the fraction, 2.9 mL phosphate buffer (pH 7.5), and 2 mL xanthine (0.15 mM) prepared in buffer. The mixture was vortexed and left to stand for 15 minutes. After 15 minutes, 0.1 mL of xanthine oxidase enzyme solution (0.1 unit/mL in phosphate buffer, pH 7.5), prepared immediately before use, was added. The mixture was then incubated at ambient temperature for 30 minutes. After the incubation period, reaction was stopped by the addition of 1 mL of 1 M hydrochloric acid. The absorbance was measured at 290 nm using a UV spectrometer. Allopurinol (100 μL/mL), a known inhibitor of XO, was used as a positive control. One unit of XO is defined as the amount of enzyme required to produce 1 mmol of uric acid/min at 25°C. XO inhibitory activity was expressed as the percentage inhibition of XO by using the following equation:

$$\% \text{ inhibition} = \left[1 - \left(\frac{B}{A}\right)\right] * 100, \quad (5)$$

where A represents the activity of the enzyme without plant extract and B is the activity of XO in the presence of plant extract.

2.13. Determination of Total Phenol, Flavonoid, and Anthocyanin Tannin Content. The total phenolic content was evaluated using the modified Folin-Ciocalteu assay described by Nickavar and Esbati [28]. The plant extract (0.50 mL) was added to a test-tube containing a tenfold diluted Folin-Ciocalteu reagent solution (2.50 mL) and sodium carbonate (2.00 mL, 7.5%). The mixture was allowed to react for 30 minutes at room temperature. The total phenolic content was then spectrophotometrically determined at 760 nm. All determinations were carried out in triplicate and results obtained were expressed as μg gallic acid equivalent (GAE)/mg crude extract.

The total flavonoid content was evaluated according to the aluminium chloride colorimetric method [29]. The plant extract (2 mL) was added to 2% aluminium chloride solution (2 mL). The mixture was allowed to react for 30 minutes at room temperature and the absorbance was read at 420 nm. All determinations were performed in triplicate and results obtained were expressed as μg rutin equivalent (RE)/mg crude extract.

The total anthocyanin content was calculated using the pH differential method [30]. Briefly, 1 mL of plant extract was transferred into 10 mL volumetric flask and the volume was adjusted with buffer pH 1.0 and pH 4.5. Mixtures were allowed to equilibrate for 15 minutes. Absorbance of each dilution was spectrophotometrically determined at 510 and 700 nm. Absorbance of diluted samples was evaluated using the following equation:

$$A = \left(A_{510} - A_{700}\right)_{\text{pH1.0}} - \left(A_{510} - A_{700}\right)_{\text{pH4.5}}. \quad (6)$$

TABLE 1: Percentage inhibition of AVG against key enzymes.

Sample	Percentage inhibition		
	α-amylase	α-glucosidase	Pancreatic lipase
Acarbose	96.64 ± 0.10	62.70 ± 0.15	70.58 ± 0.50
Aloe vera	-4.88 ± 0.09	-0.81 ± 0.33	$85.56 \pm 0.91^{*}$

$^{*}p < 0.05$ compared to the control (Acarbose), one-way ANOVA.

The monomeric anthocyanin pigment concentration in the original sample was calculated according to the following equation:

$$\text{Anthocyanin content (mg/mL)}$$
$$= A * \text{MW} * \text{DF} * \frac{1000}{(\varepsilon * 1)}, \quad (7)$$

where MW is the molecular weight of cyanidin-3-glucoside (484.5), DF the dilution factor, and ε the molar extinction coefficient (26,900).

Quantitative estimation of tannin, as catechin equivalent, was evaluated using the vanillin-HCl method with slight modifications. Extract (1 mL) was added in 5 mL of reagent mix containing 4% vanillin (in methanol) and 8% concentrated hydrochloric acid (in methanol). The resulting reaction mixture was vortexed and kept in the dark for 20 minutes. The absorbance was then determined at 500 nm using a spectrophotometer, using catechin (400 μg/mL) as standard.

2.14. Statistical Analysis. All data were expressed as means $\pm$ SD for 3 experiments. Statistical analyses were performed using statistical software, namely, SPSS version 21.0 for Windows 7 and Excel software (Microsoft 2010).

3. Results

3.1. Inhibitory Activity of Aloe vera Gel on Key Enzymes. Data obtained from the α-amylase inhibition assay (Table 1) indicated no enzyme inhibitory activity for the *Aloe vera* extract when compared to the positive control (Acarbose, 400 μg/mL) which had percentage of inhibition (96.64 $\pm$ 0.09%). Results from α-glucosidase inhibition assay showed no enzyme inhibitory activity for the *Aloe vera* extract when compared to the positive control (Acarbose, 5 mg/mL). *Aloe vera* gel exhibits a significantly higher ($p < 0.05$) percentage inhibition of 85.56$\pm$0.91% than the positive control (Orlistat, 0.48 mM) against pancreatic lipase.

3.2. Enzyme Kinetic Studies. *Aloe vera* was further assessed through kinetic studies to determine the type of inhibition on pancreatic lipase (Figure 2). The Lineweaver-Burk plot was generated using the calibration curve of nitrophenol, mentioned in Section 2. The double reciprocal Lineweaver-Burk plots showed a decrease in maximal velocity (V_{max}) and an increase in Michaelis-Menten constant (K_m), thereby suggesting mixed inhibition. V_{max} decreases from (4.25 $\times$ 10^{-5}) mM min^{-1} to (1.83 $\times$ 10^{-5}) mM min^{-1} while K_m increases from 0.99 to 10.66.

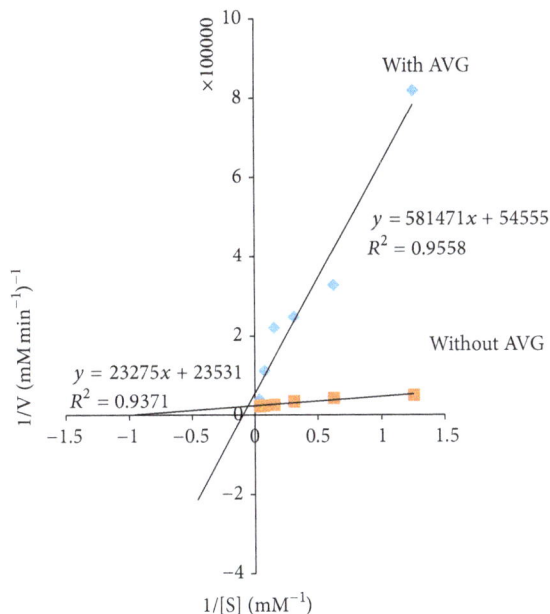

FIGURE 2: The Lineweaver-Burk plots in the presence and absence of *Aloe vera* gel.

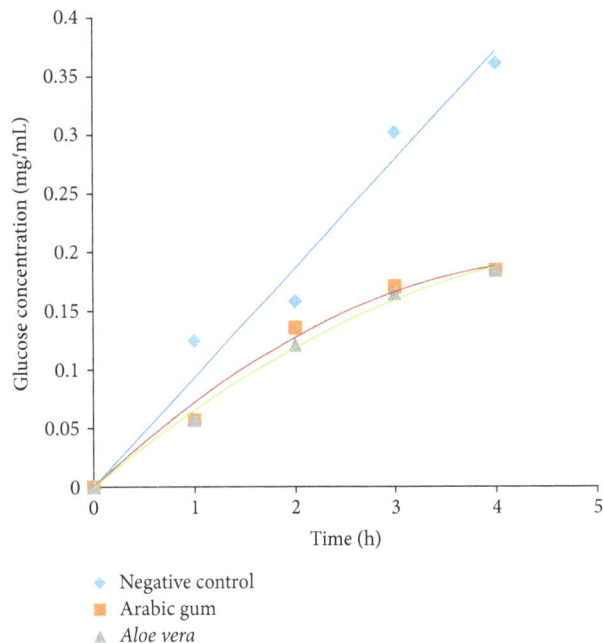

FIGURE 3: Glucose movement *in vitro*.

3.3. Effect of Aloe vera Gel on Glucose Movement In Vitro. Figure 3 shows that *Aloe vera* mimics the action of Arabic gum (positive control) and thus retards glucose movement considerably. No significant difference ($p > 0.05$) was observed between the positive control and *Aloe vera* gel. The glucose content in dialysate and GDRI are depicted in Tables 2 and 3, respectively.

3.4. Antimicrobial Screening. *Aloe vera* gel did not inhibit the growth of any of the microbes tested (Table 4). However, when compared to the blank, the results showed a less intensive red colour for *Staphylococcus aureus*, *Escherichia coli*, and *Pseudomonas aeruginosa*. This tends to suggest that *Aloe vera* (though it did not inhibit bacterial growth) showed reduced growth. The controls used against bacteria are Streptomycin, Chloramphenicol, and Ciprofloxacin while the one used against fungi is Amphotericin.

3.5. Antioxidant Activities of Aloe vera Gel. In FRAP assay, the antioxidant activity was determined by generating the standard curve in the range of 0–400 μM and the results were expressed as mM Trolox Equivalent (TE)/mg crude extract ($y = 0.0022x$, $R^2 = 0.996$). *Aloe vera* gel showed a value of 72.42 ± 0.95 mM Trolox Equivalent (TE). Table 5 shows the percentage inhibition of *Aloe vera* in the different assays. *Aloe vera* gel exhibits significantly lower percentage inhibition against DPPH and NO$^\bullet$ free radicals than the corresponding control ($p < 0.05$). It also inhibits xanthine oxidase at a significantly lower percentage than the control ($p < 0.05$).

3.6. Phytochemical Screening. Total phenolic content is reported as gallic acid equivalents by reference to standard curve ($y = 0.0099x$ and $R^2 = 0.9879$) and was found

to be 66.1 ± 1.14 mg GAE/g of extract. The total flavonoid content was 60.9 ± 0.97 μg rutin equivalent (RE)/mL crude extract, respectively, by reference to standard curve ($y = 0.0092x + 0.4896$ and $R^2 = 0.883$). *Aloe vera* also showed a total tannin content of 21.1 ± 1.9 μg catechin equivalent by reference to standard curve ($y = 0.0003x$ and $R^2 = 0.9903$). No anthocyanin was found. The results are summarised in Table 6.

4. Discussion

In the present study, unprocessed *Aloe vera* gel was assessed in terms of its ability to inhibit key carbohydrate hydrolysing enzymes. No significant inhibition was found explaining that the antidiabetic property of *Aloe vera* gel may not be due to enzyme inhibition. This contradicts the findings of Abu Soud et al., where dried *Aloe vera* crude extract showed significant (more than 80%) α-amylase inhibitory activity [31–33]. These disparities can be explained based on the fact that different extraction method was used. Another study reported moderate α-amylase inhibitory activity with low percentage inhibition by *Aloe vera* extracts [33]. However, the previous study has used soxhlet apparatus where dried plant parts were finely crushed, powdered, and extracted with methanol [34]. Methanol and ethanol are more efficient than water in cell walls and seeds degradation which have nonpolar character and cause active ingredients to be released from cells [35]. The decrease in activity of aqueous extract can also be ascribed to the enzyme polyphenol oxidase, which degrades polyphenols in water extracts but is inactive in methanol and ethanol [35]. Additionally, ethanol was found to penetrate the cellular membrane more easily to extract the intracellular ingredients from the plant material [35].

Table 2: Glucose content in dialysate.

Sample	Glucose content in dialysate (mg/mL)				One-way ANOVA ($t = 4$)	
	1 hour	2 hours	3 hours	4 hours	F	p value
Arabic gum	0.057 ± 0.005	0.136 ± 0.003	0.171 ± 0.003	0.185 ± 0.001	1088.047	>0.05
Aloe vera	0.057 ± 0.005	0.124 ± 0.003	0.165 ± 0.005	0.185 ± 0.005		

Table 3: Glucose diffusion retardation index.

Sample	Glucose diffusion retardation index			
	1 hour	2 hours	3 hours	4 hours
Arabic gum	9954	9914	9943	9949
Aloe vera	9954	9923	9945	9949

Dialysis tubing technique is a simple model to evaluate the potential of soluble dietary fibres to retard the diffusion and movement of glucose in the intestinal tract [36, 37]. There are experimental evidences suggesting that the retardation of the nutrient flow into the external medium is an indication of the modulating effect of fibre on glucose absorption in the intestine [36]. Hence, this assay may help to evaluate the hypoglycaemic effect of a particular extract. The effects of plant extracts on glucose movement *in vitro* have gained much attention due to the fact that in recent years national and international diabetes associations have emphasised the need to increase fibre intake which interacts with food nutrients reducing absorption, especially postprandial glucose after carbohydrate-rich meals [38].

In the present study, *Aloe vera* gel proved to be an efficient agent to retard glucose movement across the dialysis tubing. It followed almost the same trend as Arabic gum, used as a control. As reported by Ahmed et al., the retardation in glucose diffusion might be attributed to the physical obstruction towards glucose molecules or the entrapment of glucose molecules within the fibre network [39]. Hence, it can be deduced that the viscous and mucilaginous nature of *Aloe vera* gel entrapped the glucose molecules preventing them from moving into the external solution. The results thus support the use of *Aloe vera* gel to maintain blood glucose level in diabetic patients. The diabetic activity could also be attributed to reduced intestinal absorption of postprandial glucose, in order to prevent high peaks of glucose in the blood. Most of the studies carried out on the antidiabetic properties of *Aloe vera* used homogenised or processed *Aloe vera* extract. To our best knowledge, no information concerning effect of *Aloe vera* gel (in its natural form) on antidiabetic activities has been published. Abo-Youssef and Messiha [13] reported the antidiabetic role of *Aloe vera* and explained that this could be due to the potent antioxidant potential of *Aloe vera*. Another study used aqueous extract of *Aloe vera* (100 g *Aloe vera* boiled with 200 mL distilled water and then cooled) which was fed to diabetic rats which in turn resulted in lowered blood glucose level [40].

A varying range of lipases, responsible for the catalysis of hydrolysis of ester bonds in triacylglycerols, are produced by the human body [41]. Some pharmacological obesity treatments, for example, Orlistat, function through specific, irreversible inhibition of gastrointestinal lipases, of which pancreatic lipase is the most biologically active and important one in healthy humans [41]. Serious adverse effects are commonly reported for Orlistat, including steatorrhoea, bloating, oily spotting, faecal urgency, and faecal incontinence that can affect up to 40% of patients [41]. Hence, a product which inhibits pancreatic lipase and lowers/eliminates the adverse effects of present treatment would be of substantial benefit to patients.

The present study attempted to probe into the hypolipidemic effect of *Aloe vera* gel through the inhibition of pancreatic lipase. The results showed that *Aloe vera* gel exhibited a significantly higher percentage of inhibition than the positive control Orlistat. Furthermore, kinetics parameters were evaluated from the double reciprocal plot for *Aloe vera* gel. The results showed an increase in the Michaelis constant (K_m) and a decrease in maximal velocity (V_{max}) of the reaction, suggesting a mixed inhibition of pancreatic lipase. This is a major type of inhibition that occurs when the inhibitor is capable of binding to both the free-enzyme and the enzyme-substrate complex. Generally, when the inhibitor binds favourably to the free-enzyme, mixed inhibition leads to an increase in K_m value while if it binds preferentially to the enzyme-substrate complex, K_m value is decreased. Both cases are accompanied by a decrease in V_{max}. In the present study, an increase in K_m and a decrease in V_{max} were observed suggesting that *Aloe vera* gel has a greater affinity for the free-enzyme that is pancreatic lipase. This offers the advantage of not being affected by higher concentrations of substrate compared to Orlistat which acts as a competitive inhibitor [42]. Our result tends to support a study conducted by Kim et al. [43] which showed that the administration of processed *Aloe vera* gel lowered triacylglyceride levels in liver. Additionally, the plasma and histological examinations of periepididymal fat pad showed that processed *Aloe vera* gel reduced the average size of adipocytes. Choi et al. [12] showed reduced body weight, body fat mass, and insulin resistance in obese individuals treated with *Aloe vera*. Choudhary et al. also proved the efficacy of *Aloe vera* by showing significant reduction in blood glucose, lipid profile, and blood pressure of the diabetic patients [44]. According to the present study's results, it can be deduced that *Aloe vera* gel inhibits porcine pancreatic lipase and thus deserves to be further explored as a weight lowering agent to combat obesity.

The present study also aimed to investigate the antimicrobial attributes of *Aloe vera* gel. The extract was tested against 5 common microorganisms. Results clearly demonstrate that *Aloe vera* gel, in its natural form, does not inhibit microbial growth. This tends to contradict results obtained by Khaing, where he demonstrated that *Aloe vera* inhibited numerous human pathogens except *Candida albicans* [45]. The present

TABLE 4: Antimicrobial activity of *Aloe vera*.

Antimicrobial strains	MIC (mg/mL)				
	Aloe vera	Streptomycin	Chloramphenicol	Ciprofloxacin	Amphotericin
Staphylococcus aureus	—	0.002	0.004	No growth	—
Escherichia coli	—	0.016	0.002	No growth	—
Pseudomonas aeruginosa	—	0.008	0.063	No growth	—
Candida albicans	—	—	—	—	0.063
Candida tropicalis	—	—	—	—	0.063

TABLE 5: Antioxidant activity of *Aloe vera*.

Assays	Percentage inhibition		One-way ANOVA	
	Aloe vera	Control	F	p value
DPPH free radical scavenging assay	17.11 ± 1.30	81.78 ± 0.24^a	7153.206	<0.05
NO$^\bullet$ scavenging assay	34.88 ± 0.52	87.25 ± 0.74^b	9935.925	<0.05
Xanthine oxidase inhibitory assay	73.85 ± 2.02	85.94 ± 0.11^c	106.801	<0.05

[a]Ascorbic acid (400 μg/mL), [b]ascorbic acid (2 mg/mL), and [c]allopurinol (100 μg/mL).

TABLE 6: Phytochemical content of *A. vera*.

Assays	Aloe vera
Total phenolic content	66.06 ± 1.14^a
Total flavonoid content	60.95 ± 0.97^b
Total tannin content	21.11 ± 1.92^c
Total anthocyanin content	ND

[a]μg gallic acid equivalent (GAE)/mg, [b]μg rutin equivalent (RE)/mg, and [c]μg catechin equivalent; ND: not detected.

results also contradicted the results obtained by Nejatzadeh-Barandozi [46], where *Aloe vera* suppressed the growth of *Staphylococcus aureus*, *Escherichia coli*, and *Pseudomonas aeruginosa* amongst others. The disparity can be explained by the use of ethanol extract which contains more bioactive components than the unprocessed *Aloe vera* gel. Hence, it can be deduced from preliminary data gathered in the present study that unprocessed *Aloe vera* gel is not an effective antimicrobial agent.

Reactive oxygen species (ROS) have potent oxidative effects on cellular constituents which can in turn impair cellular functions [47]. Therefore, they are associated with pathogenesis of insulin resistance via the inhibition of insulin signals and dysregulation of adipocytokines/adipokines which play an important role in the progression of diabetes, hypertension, atherosclerosis, and even cancer [48]. Scavenging of free radicals is believed to be a valuable measure to prevent or treat diseases like diabetes mellitus [49].

For the determination of antioxidant properties of *Aloe vera* gel, different antioxidant assays like DPPH, NO, FRAP, and xanthine oxidase inhibitory assay were performed. *Aloe vera* gel showed low DPPH and NO$^\bullet$ scavenging abilities in the current study. Though significantly lower than the positive control, it is evident that the extract did show some proton-donating ability and could serve as free radical inhibitor or scavenger, acting possibly as antioxidants. The results however contradict the findings of Khaing [45].

The latter proved that *Aloe vera* had strong DPPH scavenging ability. The difference can be explained by the fact that 95% ethanol *Aloe vera* extract was used which has a higher percentage yield of bioactive ingredients. Yet, here also, the antioxidant activity was not as high as the positive controls. Another study compared the antioxidant activity of *Aloe vera* extracted in different solvents and obtained highest DPPH inhibition in methanol extract of *Aloe vera* [34]. The results also displayed xanthine oxidase inhibition. Xanthine oxidase is a form of xanthine oxidoreductase, a type of enzyme that generates ROS. These enzymes catalyze the oxidation of hypoxanthine to xanthine and can further convert the oxidation of xanthine to uric acid. *Aloe vera* gel also showed significant ferric reducing antioxidant power which adds up to its antioxidant properties. However, a study showed that *Aloe vera* extracts obtained from supercritical carbon dioxide extraction and ethanol showed stronger antioxidant activities than BHT and α-tocopherol [50].

Over the past 10 years, there has been a growing interest in the potential of polyphenols among researchers and food manufacturers mainly because of their antioxidant properties, their abundance in our diet, and their role in the prevention of various diseases associated with oxidative stress such as cancer, cardiovascular disease, and neurodegeneration [46]. Polyphenols are reputed for their antioxidant activities and these compounds are multifunctional and can act as reducing agents, hydrogen-donating antioxidants, and singlet oxygen quenchers. The current study showed that *Aloe vera* gel possesses significant amount of phenols and flavonoids which contribute to the antioxidant activities but contain little tannins and no anthocyanins. This support the findings of Patel et al. [51] which reported that the *Aloe vera* extract contained significant amount of phenol, flavonoids, berberine, and gallic acid through HPLC techniques. However, the crude *Aloe vera* extract used in the experiments was from a commercial source.

Therefore, the present *in vitro* study has provided sound scientific footing to enhance assurance on the traditional remedy of *Aloe vera*, which may be efficient as a preventive agent in the pathogenesis of some diseases. It is anticipated that data amassed in the present study will open new avenues for the development of potential drugs that can be used to treat and/or manage DM, obesity, and related complications.

Conflict of Interests

The authors declare that they have no competing interests.

Authors' Contribution

M. Fawzi Mahomoodally and Urmeela Taukoorah designed the study and contributed to the preparation of the paper. Both authors read and approved the final paper.

References

[1] F. Mahomoodally, "Let food be thy medicine: exotic fruits and vegetables as therapeutic components for obesity and other metabolic syndromes," in *Novel Plant Bioresources: Applications in Food, Medicine and Cosmetics*, A. Gurib-Fakim, Ed., pp. 350–351, Wiley-Blackwell, 1st edition, 2014.

[2] B. O. Akinyele and A. C. Odiyi, "Comparative study of vegetative morphology and the existing taxonomic status of *Aloe vera* L.," *Journal of Plant Sciences*, vol. 2, no. 5, pp. 558–563, 2007.

[3] V. K. Gupta and S. Malhotra, "Pharmacological attribute of *Aloe vera*: revalidation through experimental and clinical studies," *Ayu*, vol. 33, no. 2, pp. 193–196, 2012.

[4] D. Vijayalakshmi, R. Dhandapani, S. Jayaveni, P. S. Jithendra, C. Rose, and A. B. Mandal, "*In vitro* anti inflammatory activity of *Aloe vera* by down regulation of MMP-9 in peripheral blood mononuclear cells," *Journal of Ethnopharmacology*, vol. 141, no. 1, pp. 542–546, 2012.

[5] A. Ray, S. D. Gupta, and S. Ghosh, "Evaluation of anti-oxidative activity and UV absorption potential of the extracts of *Aloe vera* L. gel from different growth periods of plants," *Industrial Crops and Products*, vol. 49, pp. 712–719, 2013.

[6] E. R. Rodríguez, J. D. Martín, and C. D. Romero, "*Aloe vera* as a functional ingredient in foods," *Critical Reviews in Food Science and Nutrition*, vol. 50, no. 4, pp. 305–326, 2010.

[7] S. K. Gediya, R. B. Mistry, U. K. Patel, M. Blessy, and H. N. Jain, "Herbal plants: used as a cosmetics," *Journal of Natural Products and Plant Resources*, vol. 1, no. 1, pp. 24–32, 2011.

[8] M. N. Shahzad and N. Ahmed, "Effectiveness of *Aloe vera* gel compared with 1% silver sulphadiazine cream as burn wound dressing in second degree burns," *Journal of the Pakistan Medical Association*, vol. 63, no. 2, pp. 225–230, 2013.

[9] A. Oryan, A. Mohammadalipour, A. Moshiri, and M. R. Tabandeh, "Topical application of *Aloe vera* accelerated wound healing, modeling, and remodeling: an experimental study with significant clinical value," *Annals of Plastic Surgery*, 2014.

[10] M. M. Budai, A. Varga, S. Milesz, J. Tozsér, and S. Benko, "*Aloe vera* downregulates LPS-induced inflammatory cytokine production and expression of NLRP3 inflammasome in human macrophages," *Molecular Immunology*, vol. 56, no. 4, pp. 471–479, 2013.

[11] Z. Yu, C. Jin, M. Xin, and H. JianMin, "Effect of *Aloe vera* polysaccharides on immunity and antioxidant activities in oral ulcer animal models," *Carbohydrate Polymers*, vol. 75, no. 2, pp. 307–311, 2009.

[12] H.-C. Choi, S.-J. Kim, K.-Y. Son, B.-J. Oh, and B.-L. Cho, "Metabolic effects of aloe vera gel complex in obese prediabetes and early non-treated diabetic patients: Randomized controlled trial," *Nutrition*, vol. 29, no. 9, pp. 1110–1114, 2013.

[13] A. M. H. Abo-Youssef and B. A. Messiha, "Beneficial effects of *Aloe vera* in treatment of diabetes: comparative *in vivo* and *in vitro* studies," *Bulletin of Faculty of Pharmacy, Cairo University*, vol. 51, no. 1, pp. 7–11, 2013.

[14] H. A. El-Shemy, M. A. M. Aboul-Soud, A. A. Nassr-Allah, K. M. Aboul-Enein, A. Kabash, and A. Yagi, "Antitumor properties and modulation of antioxidant enzymes' activity by *Aloe vera* leaf active principles isolated via supercritical carbon dioxide extraction," *Current Medicinal Chemistry*, vol. 17, no. 2, pp. 129–138, 2010.

[15] Republic of Mauritius, *National Diabetes Management System to be Introduced Shortly, Says Health Minister*, 2015, http://www.govmu.org/English/News/Pages/National-Diabetes-Management-System-to-be-Introduced-Shortly,-says-Health-Minister-.aspx.

[16] M. I. Issack, V. N. Pursem, T. M. S. Barkham, L.-C. Ng, M. Inoue, and S. S. Manraj, "Reemergence of dengue in mauritius," *Emerging Infectious Diseases*, vol. 16, no. 4, p. 716, 2010.

[17] W. W. Mao and J. E. Kinsella, "Amylase activity in banana fruit: properties and changes in activity with ripening," *Journal of Food Science*, vol. 46, no. 5, pp. 1400–1403, 1981.

[18] G. Pistia-Brueggeman and R. I. Hollingsworth, "A preparation and screening strategy for glycosidase inhibitors," *Tetrahedron*, vol. 57, no. 42, pp. 8773–8778, 2001.

[19] C.-D. Zheng, Y.-Q. Duan, J.-M. Gao, and Z.-G. Ruan, "Screening for Anti-lipase Properties of 37 Traditional Chinese Medicinal Herbs," *Journal of the Chinese Medical Association*, vol. 73, no. 6, pp. 319–324, 2010.

[20] Y. Bustanji, A. Issa, M. Mohammad et al., "Inhibition of hormone sensitive lipase and pancreatic lipase by *Rosmarinus officinalis* extract and selected phenolic constituents," *Journal of Medicinal Plants Research*, vol. 4, no. 21, pp. 2235–2242, 2010.

[21] A. M. Gallagher, P. R. Flatt, G. Duffy, and Y. H. A. Abdel-Wahab, "The effects of traditional antidiabetic plants on *in vitro* glucose diffusion," *Nutrition Research*, vol. 23, no. 3, pp. 413–424, 2003.

[22] C. A. Edwards, N. A. Blackburn, L. Craigen et al., "Viscosity of food gums determined in vitro related to their hypoglycemic actions," *The American Journal of Clinical Nutrition*, vol. 46, no. 1, pp. 72–77, 1987.

[23] A. J. Drummond and R. D. Waigh, "The development of microbiological methods for phytochemical screening," *Recent Research Developments in Phytochemistry*, vol. 4, pp. 143–152, 2000.

[24] I. F. F. Benzie and J. J. Strain, "The ferric reducing ability of plasma (FRAP) as a measure of 'antioxidant power': the FRAP assay," *Analytical Biochemistry*, vol. 239, no. 1, pp. 70–76, 1996.

[25] P. Mandal, T. K. Misra, and M. Ghosal, "Free-radical scavenging activity and phytochemical analysis in the leaf and stem of *Drymaria diandra* Blume," *International Journal of Integrative Biology*, vol. 7, no. 2, pp. 80–84, 2009.

[26] M. Umamaheswari and T. Chatterjee, "*In vitro* antioxidant activities of the fractions of *Coccinia grandis* L. leaf extract," *African Journal of Traditional, Complementary and Alternative Medicines*, vol. 5, no. 1, pp. 61–73, 2008.

[27] A. Abdullahi, R. Hamzah, A. Jigam et al., "Inhibitory activity of xanthine oxidase by fractions *Crateva adansonii*," *Journal of Acute Disease*, vol. 1, no. 2, pp. 126–129, 2012.

[28] B. Nickavar and N. Esbati, "Evaluation of the antioxidant capacity and phenolic content of three *Thymus* species," *Journal of Acupuncture and Meridian Studies*, vol. 5, no. 3, pp. 119–125, 2012.

[29] O. U. Amaeze, G. A. Ayoola, M. O. Sofidiya, A. A. Adepoju-Bello, A. O. Adegoke, and H. A. B. Coker, "Evaluation of antioxidant activity of *Tetracarpidium conophorum* (Müll. Arg) Hutch & Dalziel leaves," *Oxidative Medicine and Cellular Longevity*, vol. 2011, Article ID 976701, 7 pages, 2011.

[30] J. Sutharut and J. Sudarat, "Total anthocyanin content and antioxidant activity of germinated colored rice," *International Food Research Journal*, vol. 19, no. 1, pp. 215–221, 2012.

[31] P. Kumar, M. Mehta, S. Satija, and M. Garg, "Enzymatic *in vitro* anti-diabetic activity of few traditional Indian medicinal plants," *Journal of Biological Sciences*, vol. 13, no. 6, pp. 540–544, 2013.

[32] S. Pulipaka, S. R. Challa, and R. B. Pingili, "Comparative antidiabetic activity of methanolic extract of *Operculina turpethum* stem and root against healthy and streptozotocin induced diabetic rats," *International Current Pharmaceutical Journal*, vol. 1, no. 9, pp. 272–278, 2012.

[33] R. S. Abu Soud, I. I. Hamdan, and F. U. Afifi, "Alpha amylase inhibitory activity of some plant extracts with hypoglycemic activity," *Scientia Pharmaceutica*, vol. 72, no. 1, pp. 25–33, 2004.

[34] V. Saritha, K. R. Anilakumar, and F. Khanum, "Antioxidant and antibacterial activity of *Aloe vera* gel extracts," *International Journal of Pharmaceutical and Biological Archive*, vol. 1, no. 4, pp. 376–384, 2010.

[35] P. Tiwari, B. Kumar, M. Kaur, G. Kaur, and H. Kaur, "Phytochemical screening and extraction: a review," *Internationale Pharmaceutica Sciencia*, vol. 1, no. 1, pp. 98–106, 2011.

[36] D. Qujeq and A. Babazadeh, "The entrapment ability of aqueous and ethanolic extract of *Teucrium polium*: glucose diffusion into the external solution," *International Journal of Molecular and Cellular Medicine*, vol. 2, no. 2, pp. 93–96, 2013.

[37] C. M. Picot, A. H. Subratty, and F. M. Mahomoodally, "Inhibitory potential of five traditionally used native antidiabetic medicinal plants on alpha-amylase, alpha-glucosidase, glucose entrapment and amylolysis kinetics in-vitro," *Advances in Pharmacological Sciences*, vol. 2014, Article ID 739834, 7 pages, 2014.

[38] M. O. Weickert and A. F. H. Pfeiffer, "Metabolic effects of dietary fiber consumption and prevention of diabetes," *Journal of Nutrition*, vol. 138, no. 3, pp. 439–462, 2008.

[39] F. Ahmed, N. S. Siddaraju, and A. Urooj, "*In vitro* hypoglycemic effects of *Gymnema sylvestre*, *Tinospora cordifolia*, *Eugenia jambolana* and *Aegle marmelos*," *Journal of Natural Pharmaceuticals*, vol. 2, no. 2, pp. 52–55, 2011.

[40] S. A. J. Saif-Ur-Rehman, S. Hassan, I. Ahmed, and M. Naim, "Study on Antidiabetic effect of *Aloe vera* extract on alloxan induced diabetic rats," *Libyan Agriculture Research Center Journal International*, vol. 2, no. 1, pp. 29–32, 2011.

[41] B. S. Drew, A. F. Dixon, and J. B. Dixon, "Obesity management: update on orlistat," *Vascular Health and Risk Management*, vol. 3, no. 6, pp. 817–821, 2007.

[42] V. Ghadyale, S. Takalikar, V. Haldavnekar, and A. Arvindekar, "Effective control of postprandial glucose level through inhibition of intestinal alpha glucosidase by *Cymbopogon martinii* (Roxb.)," *Evidence-Based Complementary and Alternative Medicine*, vol. 2012, Article ID 372909, 6 pages, 2012.

[43] K. Kim, H. Kim, J. Kwon et al., "Hypoglycemic and hypolipidemic effects of processed *Aloe vera* gel in a mouse model of non-insulin-dependent diabetes mellitus," *Phytomedicine*, vol. 16, no. 9, pp. 856–863, 2009.

[44] M. Choudhary, A. Kochhar, and J. Sangha, "Hypoglycemic and hypolipidemic effect of *Aloe vera* L. in non-insulin dependent diabetics," *Journal of Food Science and Technology*, vol. 51, no. 1, pp. 90–96, 2014.

[45] T. A. Khaing, "Evaluation of the antifungal and antioxidant activities of the leaf extract of *Aloe vera* (*Aloe barbadensis* Miller)," *World Academy of Science, Engineering and Technology*, vol. 75, pp. 610–612, 2011.

[46] F. Nejatzadeh-Barandozi, "Antibacterial activities and antioxidant capacity of *Aloe vera*," *Organic and Medicinal Chemistry Letters*, vol. 3, no. 1, p. 5, 2013.

[47] M. Carocho and I. C. F. R. Ferreira, "A review on antioxidants, prooxidants and related controversy: natural and synthetic compounds, screening and analysis methodologies and future perspectives," *Food and Chemical Toxicology*, vol. 51, no. 1, pp. 15–25, 2013.

[48] M. Matsuda and I. Shimomura, "Increased oxidative stress in obesity: implications for metabolic syndrome, diabetes, hypertension, dyslipidemia, atherosclerosis, and cancer," *Obesity Research and Clinical Practice*, vol. 7, no. 5, pp. e330–e341, 2013.

[49] L. Fu, B.-T. Xu, R.-Y. Gan et al., "Total phenolic contents and antioxidant capacities of herbal and tea infusions," *International Journal of Molecular Sciences*, vol. 12, no. 4, pp. 2112–2124, 2011.

[50] Q. Hu, Y. Hu, and J. Xu, "Free radical-scavenging activity of *Aloe vera* (*Aloe barbadensis* Miller) extracts by supercritical carbon dioxide extraction," *Food Chemistry*, vol. 91, no. 1, pp. 85–90, 2005.

[51] D. K. Patel, K. Patel, B. Duraiswamy, and S. P. Dhanabal, "Phytochemical analysis and standardization of *Strychnos nux-vomica* extract through HPTLC techniques," *Asian Pacific Journal of Tropical Disease*, vol. 2, no. 1, pp. S56–S60, 2012.

26

Potential Effects of Silymarin and Its Flavonolignan Components in Patients with β-Thalassemia Major: A Comprehensive Review in 2015

Hadi Darvishi Khezri,[1] Ebrahim Salehifar,[2] Mehrnoush Kosaryan,[1] Aily Aliasgharian,[1] Hossein Jalali,[1] and Arash Hadian Amree[1]

[1]*Thalassemia Research Center, Mazandaran University of Medical Sciences, Sari, Iran*
[2]*Faculty of Pharmacy, Thalassemia Research Center, Mazandaran University of Medical Sciences, Sari 48175-861, Iran*

Correspondence should be addressed to Ebrahim Salehifar; Esalehifar@mazums.ac.ir

Academic Editor: Mahmoud S. Ahmed

Major β-thalassemia (β-TM) is one of the most common inherited hemolytic types of anemia which is caused as a result of absent or reduced synthesis of β-globin chains of hemoglobin. This defect results in red blood cells lysis and chronic anemia that can be treated by multiple blood transfusions and iron chelation therapy. Without iron chelation therapy, iron overload will cause lots of complications in patients. Antioxidant components play an important role in the treatment of the disease. Silymarin is an antioxidant flavonoid isolated from *Silybum marianum* plant. In the present study, we reviewed clinical and experimental studies investigating the use of silymarin prior to September 1, 2015, using PubMed, ISI Web of Knowledge, Science Direct, Scopus, Ovid, and Cochrane Library databases and we evaluated the potential effects of silymarin on controlling the complications induced by iron overload in patients with β-TM. Based on the results of the present study, we can conclude that silymarin may be useful as an adjuvant for improving multiple organ dysfunctions.

1. Introduction

β-Thalassemia (β-TM) is a chronic hereditary disease with a high prevalence in the Mediterranean region, Middle East, Indian subcontinent, and South East Asia. So far, around 230 different mutations have been reported on β-globin gene worldwide [1, 2]. The ineffective red blood cell (RBC) synthesis in these patients due to unbalanced hemoglobin chains production cause increased RBCs turnover and anemia that can be ameliorated by blood transfusions [3]. Although recurrent blood transfusion could be an effective treatment and reduces disease-specific morbidity and mortality, it is a comprehensive source of iron overload that can have several side effects [4, 5]. Despite iron chelation therapy, chronic transfusion therapy often leads to massive iron overload in liver, heart, brain, and endocrine organs and subsequent organ dysfunction that ultimately results in death [3, 6, 7]. Iron overload may also occur in patients who do not receive multiple blood transfusions due to the absorption from the gut [8]. Oxidative stress, inflammation, hepatic involvements, osteoporosis, and cardiac and renal insufficiency are major causes of iron overload related morbidity in patients with β-TM [9].

In the past decade, the protective activities of various herbal flavonoids have been investigated. *Silybum marianum* (St. Mary's thistle, milk thistle; Asteraceae/Flavonolignan) was widely used in traditional European medicine for 2000 years especially for the treatment of the liver, spleen, and gallbladder disorders [10]. The seeds are the active part of the plant and the main flavonoid of them is called silymarin which consists of a mixture of four flavonolignans (70–80%): silibinin (silybin) (50%), silychristin (20%), silydianin (10%), and isosilybin (5%) [11]. Silybin is the most important biologically active component of silymarin complex [12].

In the present study, we investigated the protective properties of silymarin and its constituents in β-TM patients to

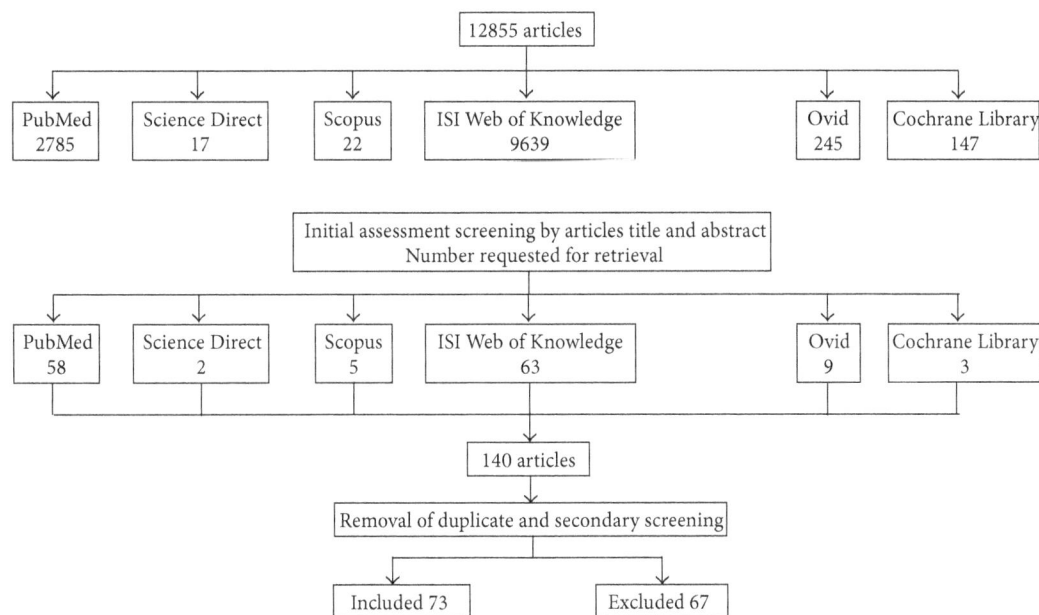

FIGURE 1: Literature search and retrieval flowchart.

consider the clinical applications of this herbal extract for protection against iron-induced organs damage.

2. Methods

We searched the English literature in PubMed, ISI Web of Knowledge, Science Direct, Scopus, Ovid, and Cochrane Library databases to find studies published from January 2000 to September 2015. The titles of the searches were appropriate MESH headings including "Milk thistle", "silymarin", "silybum", "silibinin", "silybin", "silydianin", "silychristin", "herbs", "medicinal plant", "natural product", "herbal medicine", "plant medicine", "phytomedicine", and "thalassemia". Moreover, in addition to the electronic searches, manual searches of reference lists used in all of the retrieved review articles and primary studies were carried out to identify other studies that were not found in the electronic searches. The literature was searched by two authors independently. The inclusion criteria of the papers were as follows: (1) the studies on antioxidant effects, iron chelating, liver protective, anti-inflammatory, immunomodulatory, and antiosteoporotic activities, and cardiac and renal protective effects that were conducted on animals and humans; (2) plant extracts or compounds isolated from plant. The exclusion criteria consisted of (1) the studies that were about an herbal formula and (2) the articles that were not written in English or translated to English. Two researchers independently read the full texts and extracted the following contents: publication data; study design; sample size; patient characteristics; treatment protocol; and outcome measures.

The search strategy generated 12855 titles and abstracts. After initial screening and evaluation, 12715 articles were rejected and 140 articles were founded to be potentially eligible for the review. These articles were retrieved for full text review. Removing duplicates and using secondary screening resulted in 73 articles to be included for the review (Figure 1).

3. Results

3.1. Antioxidant Effects. Iron toxicity in β-TM is the main cause of oxidative stress. Oxidative stress, associated with the formation of reactive oxygen species (ROS), plays an important role in the development of inflammation, decreased level of plasma antioxidants, depletion of erythrocyte glutathione (GSH), increased lipid peroxidation of RBC membranes, and immunosuppression in these patients [13, 14]. Several studies have shown that silymarin modulates imbalance between cell survival and apoptosis through interference with the expressions of the cell cycle regulators and proteins involved in apoptosis [15]. Silymarin protects cells from ROS damages by increasing endogenous antioxidant enzymes such as glutathione peroxidase (GPx) and superoxide dismutase (SOD). Moreover, it also inhibits the activation of NF-κB [16, 17].

Alidoost et al. surveyed intracellular GSH and proliferative response of peripheral blood mononuclear cells (PBMC) before and after 72-hour incubation of PBMC with various concentrations of silymarin (0, 5, 10, or 20 μg/mL) in 28 patients with β-TM and 28 healthy age-matched individuals [14]. Results of that study showed a significant restoration of GSH and its normalization in β-TM cells following treatment with silymarin. GSH is a primary intracellular antioxidant and plays an essential role in several functions in T cells [14]. Considerably, low levels of GSH and depressed proliferative response of PBMC in β-TM may be responsible for the cell mediated immune abnormalities in iron overload conditions [14]. These data indicate the benefit of using silymarin to normalize immune dysfunction via antioxidant and immunostimulatory activities in β-thalassemia major.

Moreover, Jeong et al. found that silibinin can successfully prompt apoptosis and as a result it leads to human glioma tumor cells death through calpain-dependent mechanism involving protein kinase C (PKC), ROS, and apoptosis-inducing factor (AIF) nuclear translocation [18].

3.2. Iron Chelation Effects. For the first time, Borsari et al. introduced silybin as a new iron-chelating agent [19] and since then the in vitro studies have showed that silybin has a high affinity for Fe (III) at acidic pH and makes an iron-silybin complex [12, 20]. Consequently, some clinical trials have reported that silymarin and silybin may act as iron-chelating agents in patients with β-TM [11, 21, 22]. These studies argued that treatment with silymarin and silybin leads to reduction in the body iron stores and decrease of serum ferritin level.

Navidi-Shishaone et al. investigated the effect of desferrioxamine (DFO) and silymarin combination therapy against kidney and heart iron deposition in an iron overload rat model. The iron overload condition was performed by iron dextran (100 mg/kg/day) every other day. Administration of iron dextran was stopped after 2 weeks and the animals were treated daily with combination of silymarin (200 mg/kg/day, intraperitoneally) and DFO (50 mg/kg/day, intraperitoneally). The results displayed that although coadministration of silymarin and DFO may be potentially considered as an iron chelator, combination of these two agents does not reduce the intensity of iron deposition in the kidney, liver, and heart [23]. In a clinical trial by Gharagozloo et al., 59 patients with β-TM were randomized into two groups. First group received silymarin plus DFO while DFO with placebo was administered for the second group for 3 months (Table 1 shown). Findings of the mentioned study indicated that the combination therapy was well tolerated and more effective than DFO alone in reducing serum ferritin level. However, no significant differences were detected between silymarin and placebo groups in serum ferritin level after 1.5 and 3 months of treatment. In that study, it was also argued that the observed slight changes in ferritin level between two groups probably may be because of small sample size. That was the first report showing the beneficial effects of silymarin in β-TM patients [11]. In another study, patients were treated with the combination of DFO and silymarin (420 mg/day) or DFO plus placebo (49//versus 48//) for 9 months. Serum iron and total iron binding capacity (TIBC) levels were significantly reduced after silymarin therapy. Moreover, serum ferritin levels strongly decreased in silymarin group in comparison to placebo group (Table 1). That shows potential effectiveness of silymarin alone as an iron-chelating agent in reducing body iron load in β-TM [21]. Balouchi et al. stated that although 69.23% of patients have a little drop in the serum ferritin level in combination therapy group (DFO plus 420 mg/day silymarin), reduction of serum ferritin level was not significant after 6 months (Table 1 shown). Besides, they mentioned that silymarin has iron chelator effects and the little sample size was the reason why the nonsignificant decrease in serum ferritin level was observed [24]. Recently, Hagag et al. investigated therapeutic effects of silymarin plus deferiprone (DFP) in 80 β-TM patients with > 1000 ng/mL serum ferritin level

[22]. They indicated that, after treatment, the serum ferritin and iron levels were dramatically decreased. In addition, higher TIBC was also observed after combination therapy (Table 1). These findings are supported by results of their previous study with deferasirox (DFX) and silymarin combination therapy [25]. Moreover, after combination therapy, serum iron level was significantly decreased from 248.85 ± 38.2 to 137.4 ± 31.1 ng/dL ($P = 0.001$). Based on the results of these two studies, it can be concluded that the iron chelator effects of silymarin are related to its ability of Fe (III) binding. Similarly, Bares et al. evaluated that administration of oral silybin for 12 weeks decreases body iron stores in patients with chronic hepatitis C [26]. It seems that silymarin could potentially have an iron-chelating effect via strong antioxidant activity and reducing nonhaem iron [20]. More studies are required to clarify the role of silymarin in the decrease of iron overload in clinical condition.

3.3. Hepatic Protection. Iron overload can affect various tissues including liver in patients with β-TM. Liver injury and chronic hepatitis (B and C) are serious medical problems in the transfusion dependent β-TM patients. The high incidence of hepatitis C was observed in β-TM patients after a screening during a fourteen-year study (at two 7-year intervals; 1996–2002 and 2003–2009). Of the 395 patients, 109 (27.5%) were anti-HCV positive, and 21 (19.2%) out of these 109 cases were exposed after 1996. The incidence rate of HCV was 4.2/1000 person-years during that time. The incidence rates of HCV in the first and second seven-year periods were 6.2/1000 and 1.3/1000 person-years, respectively [27].

Silymarin has been extensively used as a hepatoprotective agent in Asia and Europe [18]. Although it has been widely used in the treatment of liver disease, few clinical trials have been conducted about its effects on patients. In animal models, silymarin was shown to protect the patients against liver injury induced by toxins [28]. Based on findings of cellular morphological changes in rat using light microscope, the protective roles of silymarin plus DFO on iron overload-induced hepatotoxicity were introduced by Najafzadeh et al. [29]. The mentioned study showed antihepatotoxic effects of silymarin, improvement of liver function, and decrease of total protein and total albumin in animal models. Studies of silymarin at high concentrations in the HCV replicon system also show an effect on HCV core and NS5A gene expression [30, 31]. In these studies, an anticarcinogenic role of silymarin was argued to be the main mechanism of its actions [10]. The results of these studies demonstrate that silymarin has antiviral and hepatoprotective effects and it may be useful in the treatment of β-TM patients with hepatitis as a complementary approach.

3.4. Immunomodulatory and Anti-Inflammatory Effects. There are several immune abnormalities in transfusions dependent β-TM patients such as increased number and enhanced activities of suppressor T-cells (CD8), reduced proliferative capacity of helper T-cells (CD4), and decreased CD4/CD8 ratios [32–34]. Moreover, iron overload in β-TM patients reduces the proliferative activities of T cells [35, 36]. Iron overload and continuous immune stimulation are the

TABLE 1: Summary of carried-out randomized clinical trials of silymarin in patients with β-TM.

| Study author (reference) | Methods | | | | | Ferritin (ng/mL) | | | | P value between groups |
| | Groups | | Silymarin dose | Study design | Period of study (week) | Intervention group | | Control group | | |
	Intervention (N)	Control (N)				Baseline	End	Baseline	End	
Gharagozloo et al., 2009 [11]	DFO plus silymarin ($n = 29$)	DFO plus placebo ($n = 30$)	40 mg/kg/day	Parallel	12	4285.4 ± 2181.3	3548.3 ± 2012.8	3772.7 ± 1806.6	3727.8 ± 2025.0	NS
Moayedi et al., 2013 [21]	DFO plus silymarin ($n = 49$)	DFO plus placebo ($n = 48$)	40 mg/kg/day	Parallel	36	3028.8 ± 2002.6	1972.2 ± 1250.6	1780.19 ± 1089.5	2213.8 ± 1375.1	0.01
Gharagozloo et al., 2013 [3]	silymarin ($n = 5$)	DFO plus silymarin ($n = 25$)	40 mg/kg/day	Parallel	12	NM	NM	NM	NM	—
Balouchi et al., 2014 [24]	DFO plus silymarin ($n = 13$)	DFO plus placebo ($n = 9$)	40 mg/kg/day	Parallel	24	2292.20 ± 1382.26	1935.70 ± 1649.35	1701.56 ± 773.51	1794.67 ± 870.65	NS
Hagag et al., 2013 [25]	DFX plus silymarin ($n = 20$)	DFX plus placebo ($n = 20$)	40 mg/kg/day	Parallel	24	$3253.7 + 707.1$	$1067.2 + 297.9$	$3049.2 + 527.7$	$1795.3 + 551.6$	0.001
Hagag et al., 2015 [22]	DFP plus silymarin ($n = 40$)	DFP plus placebo ($n = 40$)	40 mg/kg/day	Parallel	36	$1901 + 563.38$	$989.5 + 178.57$	$1885.2 + 510.54$	$1260 + 212.26$	<0.001

NS: nonsignificant.
NM: nonmeasured.

key causes of suppressed cell mediated immunity in these patients [36, 37].

Immunomodulatory and anti-inflammatory effects of silibinin have been shown in some studies. Silibinin inhibits tumor necrosis factor alpha (TNF-α) production [38, 39]. Silibinin suppresses the growth of HMC-1 cells and it also decreases expression of proinflammatory cytokines through inhibition of NF-κB signaling pathway in HMC-1 human mast cells (such as TNF-α, IL-6, and IL-8) [40]. An in vitro study showed that silymarin has anti-inflammatory and immunomodulatory effects through inhibition of NF-κB [41, 42]. Wilasrusmee et al. reported that in vitro treatment of PBMC with silymarin leads to restoration of the thiol status and increases T cell proliferation and activation, and it enhances interferon gamma (IFNγ), interleukin- (IL-) 4, and IL-10 secretions via stimulating of the lymphocytes in a dose dependent pattern [43]. So, they recommended the silymarin as a possible effective immunomodulatory herbal medication in the management of β-TM patients because of its antioxidant, cytoprotective, and iron-chelating activities [3].

Gharagozloo et al., in a 12-week randomized clinical trial, examined the immunomodulatory effects of silymarin. Twenty-five patients received DFO (40 mg/kg/day) and 420 mg of silymarin daily as a combination therapy while five cases took only silymarin. The serum levels of neopterin and TNF-α were dramatically diminished in two groups. Neopterin is created by monocytes and macrophages upon stimulation with IFN-γ. Measurement of neopterin blood concentrations provides important information about the triggering of cellular immune activation in humans under the control of T helper cells type 1. This analysis allows researchers to evaluate the extent of oxidative stress stimulated by the immune system [3]. Moreover, increased production of IFN γ and IL-4 was observed in activated T cells following silymarin therapy in both groups. Based on these results, Gharagozloo et al. concluded that silymarin may stimulate cell-mediated immune response via a direct effect on cytokine-producing mononuclear cells in β-TM. Besides, there were no evidences of lymphocyte subsets percentage, concentration of serum immunoglobulins, complement levels, and T cell proliferation between intervention groups [3].

Researchers proposed that probable iron-chelating and antioxidant activities of silymarin can be considered as an important mechanism of its immune-stimulatory effect. They also stated that silymarin has strong dose dependent immunomodulatory effects. Interestingly, it shows an immune-stimulatory activity at low doses (40/mg/kg/day) and immunosuppressive effects at high doses [3, 44]. Schümann et al. indicated that silymarin suppresses T cell-dependent liver injury and inhibits intrahepatic expression of TNF-α, IFN-γ, IL-4, IL-2, and inducible nitric oxide synthase (iNOS) in in vitro condition [45]. It has been shown that silymarin strongly disturbs the activation of NF-κB and mTOR in activated T lymphocytes with inhibition of IL-2 and IFN-γ production and cell proliferation [46, 47].

A clinical study investigated the immunomodulatory effect of silymarin (420 mg/day) by measuring the serum levels of TGF-β, IL-10, IL-17, and IL-23 in patients with β-TM in comparison to healthy controls. The results showed a significant higher concentration of TGF-β and IL-23 in the patient group than the controls. Among cytokines, only a significant reduction in serum IL-10 levels was found due to silymarin administration. In patients treated with silymarin, a fall in serum TGF-β (38%), IL-10 (84.6%), IL-17 (61.5%), and IL-23 (61.5%) levels was noted. This data propose that the immune abnormality, inflammation, and immunosuppression caused by iron overload in β-TM patients could be modulated by silymarin [24]. These results suggest that silymarin and its compounds could ameliorate immune abnormalities and inflammation in β-TM patients.

3.5. Osteoprotective Effects. Osteoporosis is a common bone-related metabolic disease characterized by low bone density and increased bone fragility and fractures [48]. Patients with β-TM are susceptible to osteopenia and osteoporosis. The mechanism of osteoporosis in these patients is multifactorial. Iron deposition in endocrine organs following multiple transfusion leads to impaired growth hormone secretion, hypothyroidism, hypoparathyroidism, lack of gonadal steroids, and vitamin D deficiency which contribute to the defect in achieving an acceptable bone density [49]. Recently, estrogenic and osteoprotective effects of silymarin were studied in animal models. Some studies found that silibinin has a potential to increase osteoblastogenesis and inhibit osteoclast formation by attenuating the downstream signaling cascades associated with receptor activator of NF-κB ligand or TNF-α in murine preosteoblastic cell. In addition, silibinin might act as bone morphogenetic protein (BMP) modulator, osteoprotective, and inhibitor of osteoclastic bone resorption. BMPs are a group of growth factors known as cytokines and metabologens that induce the development of bone and cartilage. BMPs are now considered to constitute a group of pivotal morphogenetic signals and orchestrating tissue architecture throughout the body [50, 51]. Silymarin therapy may also heighten collagen secretion, osteocalcin transcription, and BMP expression [52]. Seidlová-Wuttke et al. demonstrated that silymarin is a selective estrogen receptor modulator (SERM) on the ERβ-subtype of the estrogen receptor and it can be considered as pure ERβ-specific ligands [53]. ERα and ERβ are the classical estrogen receptors that engage in the regulation of many complex physiological processes in humans. Modulation of these receptors is now considered for the treatment and prevention of osteoporosis [54]. Although several studies have established the various roles of silymarin in both in vitro and in vivo models, the effect of silymarin and its flavonolignan components as an osteoprotective agent in clinical practice is required to be investigated.

3.6. Cardiac Protective Effects. Cardiac complications such as cardiomyopathy and heart failure secondary to iron overload are still the main cause of mortality in β-TM [55]. It has been shown that around 70% of deaths are related to this complication [56]. Recently, some randomized clinical trials were carried out on these patients regarding cardiac protective property of silymarin [11, 19, 21]. It seems that decrease of oxidative stress markers such as ROS inside the heart cells is caused by strong antioxidant properties of silymarin and their cytoprotective and anti-inflammatory effects could be responsible for cardioprotective effects [57, 58]. Moreover, silymarin protects cardiac myocytes via decrease of lactate dehydrogenase (LDH) and malondialdehyde (MDA) [59]. However, the cardiac protective effects of silymarin are not clear in clinical researches.

3.7. Renal Protective Effects. Renal dysfunction as result of tissue iron deposition is one of the main problems in patients with β-TM [60]. Currently, a few researches showed that silymarin can protect kidney against induced iron toxicity in β-TM and diabetics patients and also after chemotherapy in cancer patients [61–65]. Silymarin significantly can reduce kidney iron deposition in rat model and it has nephroprotective properties in acute iron overload animal models. Fallahzadeh et al. stated that silymarin can be considered as a new addition to the antidiabetic nephropathy armamentarium [66]. In this clinical trial, urinary albumin-creatinine ratio (UACR), urinary levels of TNF-α, and urinary and serum levels of MDA were significantly reduced in the intervention group. Silymarin could improve diabetic nephropathy at 140 mg doses 3 times a day for 3 months in type 2 diabetes patients with macroalbuminuria. For better understanding of the renal protective effects of silymarin, more studies are recommended to carry out, especially, evaluation of administration of silymarin in combination with standard iron chelation.

4. Conclusion

According to the current review, it seems that silymarin plus standard iron chelation may have a better result to protect organ induced iron overload. Silymarin which is a safe and well-tolerated adjuvant is introduced as a drug without adverse effects in many clinical studies. We recommend that more well-designed randomized clinical trials are required considering silymarin pharmacokinetic behavior in order to generate strong evidence about improvement of iron overload complications among patients with β-TM.

Conflict of Interests

None of the authors have any conflict of interests to disclose.

References

[1] N. Achoubi, M. Asghar, K. N. Saraswathy, and B. Murry, "Prevalence of β-thalassemia and hemoglobin e in two migrant populations of Manipur, North East India," *Genetic Testing and Molecular Biomarkers*, vol. 16, no. 10, pp. 1195–1200, 2012.

[2] M. Kosaryan, K. Vahidshahi, H. Karami, M. A. Forootan, and M. Ahangari, "Survival of thalassemic patients referred to the Boo Ali Sina teaching hospital, Sari, Iran," *Hemoglobin*, vol. 31, no. 4, pp. 453–462, 2007.

[3] M. Gharagozloo, M. Karimi, and Z. Amirghofran, "Immunomodulatory effects of silymarin in patients with β-thalassemia major," *International Immunopharmacology*, vol. 16, no. 2, pp. 243–247, 2013.

[4] J.-A. Ribeil, J.-B. Arlet, M. Dussiot, I. Cruz Moura, G. Courtois, and O. Hermine, "Ineffective erythropoiesis in β-thalassemia,"

[5] C. Sengsuk, O. Tangvarasittichai, P. Chantanaskulwong et al., "Association of iron overload with oxidative stress, hepatic damage and dyslipidemia in transfusion-dependent β-thalassemia/HbE patients," *Indian Journal of Clinical Biochemistry*, vol. 29, no. 3, pp. 298–305, 2014.

[6] N. E. Piloni, V. Fermandez, L. A. Videla, and S. Puntarulo, "Acute iron overload and oxidative stress in brain," *Toxicology*, vol. 314, no. 1, pp. 174–182, 2013.

[7] E. Vichinsky, E. Butensky, E. Fung et al., "Comparison of organ dysfunction in transfused patients with SCD or β thalassemia," *American Journal of Hematology*, vol. 80, no. 1, pp. 70–74, 2005.

[8] T. E. D. J. dos Santos, G. F. de Sousa, M. C. Barbosa, and R. P. Gonçalves, "The role of iron overload on oxidative stress in sickle cell anemia," *Biomarkers in Medicine*, vol. 6, no. 6, pp. 813–819, 2012.

[9] M. Y. Abdalla, M. Fawzi, S. R. Al-Maloul, N. El-Banna, R. F. Tayyem, and I. M. Ahmad, "Increased oxidative stress and iron overload in Jordanian β-thalassemic children," *Hemoglobin*, vol. 35, no. 1, pp. 67–79, 2011.

[10] E. Shaker, H. Mahmoud, and S. Mnaa, "Silymarin, the antioxidant component and Silybum marianum extracts prevent liver damage," *Food and Chemical Toxicology*, vol. 48, no. 3, pp. 803–806, 2010.

[11] M. Gharagozloo, B. Moayedi, M. Zakerinia et al., "Combined therapy of silymarin and desferrioxamine in patients with β-thalassemia major: a randomized double-blind clinical trial," *Fundamental & Clinical Pharmacology*, vol. 23, no. 3, pp. 359–365, 2009.

[12] M. Gharagozloo, Z. Khoshdel, and Z. Amirghofran, "The effect of an iron (III) chelator, silybin, on the proliferation and cell cycle of Jurkat cells: a comparison with desferrioxamine," *European Journal of Pharmacology*, vol. 589, no. 1–3, pp. 1–7, 2008.

[13] A. Svobodová, D. Walterová, and J. Psotová, "Influence of silymarin and its flavonolignans on H_2O_2-induced oxidative stress in human keratinocytes and mouse fibroblasts," *Burns*, vol. 32, no. 8, pp. 973–979, 2006.

[14] F. Alidoost, M. Gharagozloo, B. Bagherpour et al., "Effects of silymarin on the proliferation and glutathione levels of peripheral blood mononuclear cells from β-thalassemia major patients," *International Immunopharmacology*, vol. 6, no. 8, pp. 1305–1310, 2006.

[15] K. Ramasamy and R. Agarwal, "Multitargeted therapy of cancer by silymarin," *Cancer Letters*, vol. 269, no. 2, pp. 352–362, 2008.

[16] M. C. Comelli, U. Mengs, C. Schneider, and M. Prosdocimi, "Toward the definition of the mechanism of action of silymarin: activities related to cellular protection from toxic damage induced by chemotherapy," *Integrative Cancer Therapies*, vol. 6, no. 2, pp. 120–129, 2007.

[17] A. J. Hanje, B. Fortune, M. Song, D. Hill, and C. McClain, "The use of selected nutrition supplements and complementary and alternative medicine in liver disease," *Nutrition in Clinical Practice*, vol. 21, no. 3, pp. 255–272, 2006.

[18] J. C. Jeong, W. Y. Shin, T. H. Kim et al., "Silibinin induces apoptosis via calpain-dependent AIF nuclear translocation in U87MG human glioma cell death," *Journal of Experimental and Clinical Cancer Research*, vol. 30, article 44, 2011.

[19] M. Borsari, C. Gabbi, F. Ghelfi et al., "Silybin, a new iron-chelating agent," *Journal of Inorganic Biochemistry*, vol. 85, no. 2-3, pp. 123–129, 2001.

The Scientific World Journal, vol. 2013, Article ID 394295, 11 pages, 2013.

[20] C. Hutchinson, A. Bomford, and C. A. Geissler, "The iron-chelating potential of silybin in patients with hereditary haemochromatosis," *European Journal of Clinical Nutrition*, vol. 64, no. 10, pp. 1239–1241, 2010.

[21] B. Moayedi, M. Gharagozloo, N. Esmaeil, M. R. Maracy, H. Hoorfar, and M. Jalaeikar, "A randomized double-blind, placebo-controlled study of therapeutic effects of silymarin in β-thalassemia major patients receiving desferrioxamine," *European Journal of Haematology*, vol. 90, no. 3, pp. 202–209, 2013.

[22] A. Hagag, M. Elfaragy, S. Elrifaey, and A. Abd El-Lateef, "Therapeutic value of combined therapy with Deferiprone and Silymarin as iron chelators in Egyptian Children with Beta Thalassemia major," *Infectious Disorders—Drug Targets*, vol. 15, no. 3, pp. 189–195, 2015.

[23] M. Navidi-Shishaone, S. Mohhebi, M. Nematbakhsh et al., "Co-administration of silymarin and deferoxamine against kidney, liver and heart iron deposition in male iron overload rat model," *International Journal of Preventive Medicine*, vol. 5, no. 1, pp. 110–116, 2014.

[24] S. Balouchi, M. Gharagozloo, N. Esmaeil, M. Mirmoghtadaei, and B. Moayedi, "Serum levels of TGFβ, IL-10, IL-17, and IL-23 cytokines in β-thalassemia major patients: the impact of silymarin therapy," *Immunopharmacology and Immunotoxicology*, vol. 36, no. 4, pp. 271–274, 2014.

[25] A. A. Hagag, M. S. Elfrargy, R. A. Gazar, and A. E. A. El-Lateef, "Therapeutic value of combined therapy with deferasirox and silymarin on iron overload in children with beta thalassemia," *Mediterranean Journal of Hematology and Infectious Diseases*, vol. 5, no. 1, pp. 1–7, 2013.

[26] J. M. Bares, J. Berger, J. E. Nelson et al., "Silybin treatment is associated with reduction in serum ferritin in patients with chronic hepatitis C," *Journal of Clinical Gastroenterology*, vol. 42, no. 8, pp. 937–944, 2008.

[27] A. Azarkeivan, M. N. Toosi, M. Maghsudlu, S. A. Kafiabad, B. Hajibeigi, and M. Hadizadeh, "The incidence of hepatitis C in patients with thalassemia after screening in blood transfusion centers: a fourteen-year study," *Transfusion*, vol. 52, no. 8, pp. 1814–1818, 2012.

[28] R. P. Singh and R. Agarwal, "Flavonoid antioxidant silymarin and skin cancer," *Antioxidants and Redox Signaling*, vol. 4, no. 4, pp. 655–663, 2002.

[29] H. Najafzadeh, M. R. Jalali, H. Morovvati, and F. Taravati, "Comparison of the prophylactic effect of silymarin and deferoxamine on iron overload-induced hepatotoxicity in rat," *Journal of Medical Toxicology*, vol. 6, no. 1, pp. 22–26, 2010.

[30] M. W. Fried, V. J. Navarro, N. Afdhal et al., "Effect of silymarin (milk thistle) on liver disease in patients with chronic hepatitis C unsuccessfully treated with interferon therapy: a randomized controlled trial," *The Journal of the American Medical Association*, vol. 308, no. 3, pp. 274–282, 2012.

[31] V. Bonifaz, Y. Shan, R. W. Lambrecht, S. E. Donohue, D. Moschenross, and H. L. Bonkovsky, "Effects of silymarin on hepatitis C virus and haem oxygenase-1 gene expression in human hepatoma cells," *Liver International*, vol. 29, no. 3, pp. 366–373, 2009.

[32] E. M. Walker Jr. and S. M. Walker, "Effects of iron overload on the immune system," *Annals of Clinical & Laboratory Science*, vol. 30, no. 4, pp. 354–365, 2000.

[33] G. Weiss, "Iron and immunity: a double-edged sword," *European Journal of Clinical Investigation*, vol. 32, supplement 1, pp. 70–78, 2002.

[34] D. Farmakis, A. Giakoumis, A. Aessopos, and E. Polymeropoulos, "Pathogenetic aspects of immune deficiency associated with ß thalassemia," *Medical Science Review*, vol. 9, no. 1, pp. RA19–RA22, 2003.

[35] S. Cunningham-Rundles, P. J. Giardina, R. W. Grady, C. Califano, P. McKenzie, and M. De Sousa, "Effect of transfusional iron overload on immune response," *Journal of Infectious Diseases*, vol. 182, supplement 1, pp. S115–S121, 2000.

[36] Ü. Ezer, F. Gülderen, V. K. Çulha, N. Akgül, and Ö. Gürbüz, "Immunological status of Thalassemia syndrome," *Pediatric Hematology and Oncology*, vol. 19, no. 1, pp. 51–58, 2002.

[37] M. Gharagozloo, M. Karimi, and Z. Amirghofran, "Double-faced cell-mediated immunity in β-thalassemia major: stimulated phenotype versus suppressed activity," *Annals of Hematology*, vol. 88, no. 1, pp. 21–27, 2009.

[38] L. Al-Anati, E. Essid, R. Reinehr, and E. Petzinger, "Silibinin protects OTA-mediated TNF-α release from perfused rat livers and isolated rat Kupffer cells," *Molecular Nutrition & Food Research*, vol. 53, no. 4, pp. 460–466, 2009.

[39] J. C. Peraçoli, M. V. C. Rudge, and M. T. S. Peraçoli, "Tumor necrosis factor-alpha in gestation and puerperium of women with gestational hypertension and pre-eclampsia," *American Journal of Reproductive Immunology*, vol. 57, no. 3, pp. 177–185, 2007.

[40] B.-R. Kim, H.-S. Seo, J.-M. Ku et al., "Silibinin inhibits the production of pro-inflammatory cytokines through inhibition of NF-κB signaling pathway in HMC-1 human mast cells," *Inflammation Research*, vol. 62, no. 11, pp. 941–950, 2013.

[41] C. Morishima, M. C. Shuhart, C. C. Wang et al., "Silymarin inhibits in vitro T-cell proliferation and cytokine production in hepatitis C virus infection," *Gastroenterology*, vol. 138, no. 2, pp. 671.e2–681.e2, 2010.

[42] S. J. Polyak, C. Morishima, V. Lohmann et al., "Identification of hepatoprotective flavonolignans from silymarin," *Proceedings of the National Academy of Sciences of the United States of America*, vol. 107, no. 13, pp. 5995–5999, 2010.

[43] C. Wilasrusmee, S. Kittur, G. Shah et al., "Immunostimulatory effect of *Silybum Marianum* (milk thistle) extract," *Medical Science Monitor*, vol. 8, no. 11, pp. BR439–BR443, 2002.

[44] M. Gharagozloo and Z. Amirghofran, "Effects of silymarin on the spontaneous proliferation and cell cycle of human peripheral blood leukemia T cells," *Journal of Cancer Research and Clinical Oncology*, vol. 133, no. 8, pp. 525–532, 2007.

[45] J. Schümann, J. Prockl, A. K. Kiemer, A. M. Vollmar, R. Bang, and G. Tiegs, "Silibinin protects mice from T cell-dependent liver injury," *Journal of Hepatology*, vol. 39, no. 3, pp. 333–340, 2003.

[46] M. Gharagozloo, E. Velardi, S. Bruscoli et al., "Silymarin suppress CD4$^+$ T cell activation and proliferation: effects on NF-κB activity and IL-2 production," *Pharmacological Research*, vol. 61, no. 5, pp. 405–409, 2010.

[47] M. Gharagozloo, E. N. Javid, A. Rezaei, and K. Mousavizadeh, "Silymarin inhibits cell cycle progression and mTOR activity in activated human T cells: therapeutic implications for autoimmune diseases," *Basic & Clinical Pharmacology & Toxicology*, vol. 112, no. 4, pp. 251–256, 2013.

[48] J.-L. Kim, Y.-H. Kim, M.-K. Kang, J.-H. Gong, S.-J. Han, and Y.-H. Kang, "Antiosteoclastic activity of milk thistle extract after ovariectomy to suppress estrogen deficiency-induced osteoporosis," *BioMed Research International*, vol. 2013, Article ID 919374, 11 pages, 2013.

[49] N. Valizadeh, F. Farrokhi, V. Alinejad, S. S. Mardani, S. Hejazi, and M. Noroozi, "Bone density in transfusion dependent thalassemia patients in Urmia, Iran," *Iranian Journal of Pediatric Hematology and Oncology*, vol. 4, no. 2, pp. 68–71, 2014.

[50] C. V. Kavitha, G. Deep, S. C. Gangar, A. K. Jain, C. Agarwal, and R. Agarwal, "Silibinin inhibits prostate cancer cells-and RANKL-induced osteoclastogenesis by targeting NFATc1, NF-κB, and AP-1 activation in RAW264.7 cells," *Molecular Carcinogenesis*, vol. 53, no. 3, pp. 169–180, 2014.

[51] X. Ying, L. Sun, X. Chen et al., "Silibinin promotes osteoblast differentiation of human bone marrow stromal cells via bone morphogenetic protein signaling," *European Journal of Pharmacology*, vol. 721, no. 1–3, pp. 225–230, 2013.

[52] J.-L. Kim, S.-H. Park, D. Jeong, J.-S. Nam, and Y.-H. Kang, "Osteogenic activity of silymarin through enhancement of alkaline phosphatase and osteocalcin in osteoblasts and tibia-fractured mice," *Experimental Biology and Medicine*, vol. 237, no. 4, pp. 417–428, 2012.

[53] D. Seidlová-Wuttke, T. Becker, V. Christoffel, H. Jarry, and W. Wuttke, "Silymarin is a selective estrogen receptor β (ERβ) agonist and has estrogenic effects in the metaphysis of the femur but no or antiestrogenic effects in the uterus of ovariectomized (ovx) rats," *The Journal of Steroid Biochemistry and Molecular Biology*, vol. 86, no. 2, pp. 179–188, 2003.

[54] I. Paterni, C. Granchi, J. A. Katzenellenbogen, and F. Minutolo, "Estrogen receptors alpha (ERα) and beta (ERβ): subtype-selective ligands and clinical potential," *Steroids*, vol. 90, pp. 13–29, 2014.

[55] M. A. Tanner, R. Galanello, C. Dessi et al., "A randomized, placebo-controlled, double-blind trial of the effect of combined therapy with deferoxamine and deferiprone on myocardial iron in thalassemia major using cardiovascular magnetic resonance," *Circulation*, vol. 115, no. 14, pp. 1876–1884, 2007.

[56] C. Borgna-Pignatti, M. D. Cappellini, P. De Stefano et al., "Cardiac morbidity and mortality in deferoxamine- or deferiprone-treated patients with thalassemia major," *Blood*, vol. 107, no. 9, pp. 3733–3737, 2006.

[57] A. Zholobenko and M. Modriansky, "Silymarin and its constituents in cardiac preconditioning," *Fitoterapia*, vol. 97, pp. 122–132, 2014.

[58] B. A.-S. Moayedi Esfahani, N. Reisi, and M. Mirmoghtadaei, "Evaluating the safety and efficacy of silymarin in β-thalassemia patients: a review," *Hemoglobin*, vol. 39, no. 2, pp. 75–80, 2015.

[59] B. Zhou, L.-J. Wu, N.-H. Li et al., "Silibinin protects against isoproterenol-induced rat cardiac myocyte injury through mitochondrial pathway after up-regulation of SIRT1," *Journal of Pharmacological Sciences*, vol. 102, no. 4, pp. 387–395, 2006.

[60] M. Economou, N. Printza, A. Teli et al., "Renal dysfunction in patients with beta-thalassemia major receiving iron chelation therapy either with deferoxamine and deferiprone or with deferasirox," *Acta Haematologica*, vol. 123, no. 3, pp. 148–152, 2010.

[61] A. Baradaran, "Comment on: the protective role of silymarin and deferoxamine against iron dextran-induced renal iron deposition in male rats," *International Journal of Preventive Medicine*, vol. 4, no. 6, pp. 734–735, 2013.

[62] M. Nematbakhsh, Z. Pezeshki, B.-A. Moaeidi et al., "Protective role of silymarin and deferoxamine against iron dextran-induced renal iron deposition in male rats," *International Journal of Preventive Medicine*, vol. 4, no. 3, pp. 286–292, 2013.

[63] C. Ninsontia, K. Pongjit, C. Chaotham, and P. Chanvorachote, "Silymarin selectively protects human renal cells from cisplatin-induced cell death," *Pharmaceutical Biology*, vol. 49, no. 10, pp. 1082–1090, 2011.

[64] G. Kaur, M. Athar, and M. S. Alam, "Dietary supplementation of silymarin protects against chemically induced nephrotoxicity, inflammation and renal tumor promotion response," *Investigational New Drugs*, vol. 28, no. 5, pp. 703–713, 2010.

[65] N. Sheela, M. A. Jose, D. Sathyamurthy, and B. N. Kumar, "Effect of silymarin on streptozotocin-nicotinamide-induced type 2 diabetic nephropathy in rats," *Iranian Journal of Kidney Diseases*, vol. 7, no. 2, pp. 117–123, 2013.

[66] M. K. Fallahzadeh, B. Dormanesh, M. M. Sagheb et al., "Effect of addition of silymarin to renin-angiotensin system inhibitors on proteinuria in type 2 diabetic patients with overt nephropathy: a randomized, double-blind, placebo-controlled trial," *American Journal of Kidney Diseases*, vol. 60, no. 6, pp. 896–903, 2012.

27

Validated HPTLC Method for Quantification of Luteolin and Apigenin in *Premna mucronata* Roxb., Verbenaceae

Nayan G. Patel,[1] Kalpana G. Patel,[2] Kirti V. Patel,[3] and Tejal R. Gandhi[4]

[1]*Department of Pharmacology and Toxicology, Faculty of Pharmacy, Dharmsinh Desai University, College Road, Nadiad, Gujarat 387001, India*

[2]*Department of Quality Assurance, Anand Pharmacy College, Shri Ram Krishna Seva Mandal Campus, Near Town Hall, Anand, Gujarat 388001, India*

[3]*Department of Pharmacology, Pharmacy Department, The MS University of Baroda, Vadodara, Gujarat 390002, India*

[4]*Department of Pharmacology, Anand Pharmacy College, Shri Ram Krishna Seva Mandal Campus, Near Town Hall, Anand, Gujarat 388001, India*

Correspondence should be addressed to Nayan G. Patel; nayan_pharma87@yahoo.in

Academic Editor: Mohammad A. Rashid

A simple, rapid, and precise high-performance thin-layer chromatographic method was developed for quantitative estimation of luteolin and apigenin in *Premna mucronata* Roxb., family Verbenaceae. Separation was performed on silica gel 60 F_{254} HPTLC plates using toluene : ethyl acetate : formic acid (6 : 4 : 0.3) as mobile phase for elution of markers from extract. The determination was carried out in fluorescence mode using densitometric absorbance-reflection mode at 366 nm for both luteolin and apigenin. The methanolic extract of *Premna mucronata* was found to contain 10.2 mg/g % luteolin and 0.165 mg/g % of apigenin. The method was validated in terms of linearity, LOD and LOQ, accuracy, precision, and specificity. The calibration curve was found to be linear between 200 and 1000 ng/band for luteolin and 50 and 250 ng/band for apigenin. For luteolin and apigenin, the limit of detection was found to be 42.6 ng/band and 7.97 ng/band while the limit of quantitation was found to be 129.08 ng/band and 24.155 ng/band, respectively. This developed validated method is capable of quantifying and resolving luteolin and apigenin and can be applicable for routine analysis of extract and plant as a whole.

1. Introduction

Quality control of medicinal plants is highly essential to ensure authenticity, stability, and consistency. Safety and efficacy studies along with the standardization of bioactive extract on the basis of active principle or major compound(s) as a quality assurance parameter shall open up unlimited possibilities for herbal medicine in pharmacotherapeutics [1–3]. Standardization can be carried out by obtaining a chemical fingerprint/profile in terms of one or more marker compounds (chemical or biomarker). Use of chromatography for standardization of plant products was introduced by the WHO and is accepted as a strategy for identification and evaluation of the quality of plant medicines [4–6]. HPTLC is becoming a routine analytical technique because of its advantages of low operating cost, high sample throughput, simplicity and speed, the need for minimum sample cleanup, reproducibility, accuracy, and reliability [7–10].

Premna mucronata, family Verbenaceae, commonly known as Arni is a large shrub or small tree of about 20 to 25 feet's height found in Northern India, the Gangetic plains, Uttar Pradesh, Bihar, and Bengal province of India. Besides, it is also found in hill area from Kumaon to Bhutan up to the height of 5000 feet from sea level [11]. The plant possesses antioxidant and hypocholesterolemics activities and is also known for improving digestion, acts as a blood purifier, cardiac stimulant, and expectorant, and is also useful in skin disorders [11–13]. It has been reported that the plant *Premna mucronata* contains flavonoids, luteolin, apigenin, clerodendrin, hispidulin, and pectolinarigenin. The plant also contains clerodin, clerosterol, D-mannitol, palmitic acid, ceryl alcohol, and cerotic acid. Within the complex mixture of phytoconstituents in this plant, luteolin and apigenin can be used as analytical markers for determination of its quality. Preliminary studies performed at our laboratory have established the efficacy of the plant *Premna mucronata* in cardioprotection against experimentally induced myocardial infarction in rats by isoprenaline and coronary artery ligation method [14–18]. Literature survey also has revealed that the flavonoid glycosides possess antioxidant properties and strong scavenging properties for superoxide radicals [19–22]. Moreover, luteolin, a flavonoid, is also capable of protecting the myocardium against IR injury, partly mediated through downregulation of NO production and its own antioxidant properties [16]. Hence, further work was focused on identification and quantification of flavonoids, luteolin and apigenin, in *Premna mucronata*. However, to the best of our knowledge, there is no report on thin-layer chromatographic method for quantitative analysis of luteolin and apigenin in methanolic extract prepared from whole plant *Premna mucronata*. Here, we have developed HPTLC method for quantitative estimation of luteolin and apigenin. The developed method was also validated in terms of system suitability, specificity, linearity, LOD, and LOQ according to ICH guidelines [23].

2. Materials and Methods

2.1. Equipment. Linomat 5 applicator (CAMAG, Switzerland), twin trough chamber (20 × 10 cm; CAMAG, Switzerland), TLC scanner IV (CAMAG, Switzerland), winCATS version 1.4.6 software (CAMAG, Switzerland), microsyringe (Linomat syringe 659.0014, Hamilton-Bonaduz Schweiz, CAMAG, Switzerland), UV chamber (CAMAG, Switzerland), and precoated silica gel 60 F_{254} aluminium plates (20 × 10 cm, 100 μm thickness; Merck, Darmstadt, Germany) were used in the study.

2.2. Reference Compounds and Chemicals. Reference standard luteolin (L9283-10MG), apigenin (A3145-5MG), and NP reagent (2-aminoethyl diphenylborinate) (D9754-1G) were obtained from Sigma Aldrich Ltd. Analytical grade solvents were obtained from SD Fine Chemicals. Precoated silica gel 60 F_{254} HPTLC aluminium plates (10 × 10 cm, 0.2 mm thick) were obtained from E. Merck Ltd. (Mumbai, India).

2.3. Plant. Premna mucronata was obtained from commercial supplier of Anand. The plant was identified and authenticated by Dr. Geetha K A, Directorate of Medicinal and Aromatic Plants Research, Boriavi, Anand, Gujarat, India.

2.4. Preparation of Standard Luteolin Solution. A stock solution of luteolin was prepared by dissolving 5 mg of accurately weighed luteolin in methanol and making up the volume to 10 mL with methanol. Working solution of luteolin (200 μg/mL) was prepared by appropriate dilutions of the stock solution with methanol.

2.5. Preparation of Standard Apigenin Solution. A stock solution of apigenin was prepared by dissolving 5 mg of accurately weighed apigenin in methanol and making up the volume to 10 mL with methanol. The stock solution was further diluted with methanol to give a standard solution of apigenin (50 μg/mL).

2.6. Chromatographic Conditions. Chromatographic conditions are as follows:

> Stationary phase: precoated silica gel 60 F_{254} HPTLC aluminium plates (10 × 10 cm, 0.2 mm thick).
>
> Mobile phase: toluene : ethyl acetate : formic acid (6 : 4 : 0.3).
>
> Saturation time: 15 minutes.
>
> Wavelength: 366 nm.
>
> Lamp: mercury.

The HPTLC analysis was performed in an air conditioned room maintained at 22°C and 55% humidity using precoated silica gel 60 F_{254} aluminium backed plates (10 × 10 cm, 0.2 mm layer thickness, 5-6 μm particle size; Merck, Darmstadt, Germany). 6 μL and 5 μL of the standard solutions of luteolin and apigenin were spotted using a Linomat 5 autosampler fitted with a 100 μm Hamilton syringe (CAMAG, Muttenz, Switzerland) and operated with settings of a band length of 8 mm; distance between bands of 5 mm; distance from the plate edge of 10 mm; and distance from the bottom of the plate of 10 mm. The plates were developed to a distance of 80 mm using toluene : ethyl acetate : formic acid (6 : 4 : 0.3, v/v) mobile phase in CAMAG twin trough chamber presaturated with mobile phase. The developed plates were air dried and scanned with a CAMAG TLC Scanner 4 equipped with winCATS planar chromatography manager (version 1.4.6) software that was used for densitometry measurements, spectra recording, and data processing. The absorption/remission measurement mode was used at a scan speed of 20 mm/s. Zones of luteolin and apigenin were scanned from 200 to 400 nm to record their absorption and fluorescence spectra, respectively. Densitogram was recorded in fluorescence mode for both luteolin and apigenin.

2.7. Calibration Curve for Standard Luteolin. The standard solution of luteolin (200 to 1000 ng/band) was applied in triplicate on HPTLC plate. The plate was developed and scanned as per the chromatographic conditions mentioned above. The peak areas were recorded. Calibration curve of luteolin was prepared by plotting peak area versus concentration of luteolin applied.

2.8. Calibration Curve for Standard Apigenin. The standard solution of apigenin (50 to 250 ng/band) was applied in triplicate on HPTLC plate. The plate was developed and scanned as per the chromatographic conditions mentioned above. The peak areas were recorded. Calibration curve of apigenin was prepared by plotting peak area versus concentration of apigenin applied.

2.9. Preparation of Methanolic Extract of Premna mucronata (MEPM). Accurately weighed 10 gm of powdered drug of whole plant was extracted for 15 min with methanol (4 × 25 mL) under reflux on water bath at 100°C. The methanolic extract was filtered through Whatman number 1 filter paper. The filtrates were combined, concentrated, and transferred to a 50 mL volumetric flask, and the volume was made up to 50 mL with methanol.

2.10. HPTLC Analysis of Plant Extract. Samples of methanolic extract of *Premna mucronata* were filtered through 0.45 μm filter, and HPTLC was performed under the conditions optimized for the reference compound. The plates after development were dried in air and photographed at 254 nm. The plates were then derivatized by spraying with NP-PEG reagent followed by photographing the plates in visible and fluorescence mode and scanned at 366 nm for both luteolin and apigenin. The amount of luteolin and apigenin in plant extract was quantified using calibration curve plotted with luteolin and apigenin.

2.11. Validation of the Method. The method was validated according to International Conference on Harmonization guidelines.

Linearity was studied by applying different aliquots of standard stock solution in the ranges 200 to 1000 ng/band for luteolin and 50 to 250 ng/band for apigenin. The calibration curves were developed by plotting peak area versus concentrations. The areas of peaks were treated by least square linear regression analysis. The limit of detection (LOD) and limit of quantification (LOQ) were determined using the following equations:

$$
\begin{aligned}
\text{LOD} &= \frac{3.3 \times \text{Standard Deviation of the } y\text{-intercept}}{\text{Slope of the calibration curve}}, \\
\text{LOQ} &= \frac{10 \times \text{Standard Deviation of the } y\text{-intercept}}{\text{Slope of the calibration curve}}.
\end{aligned}
\tag{1}
$$

The intermediate precision of the method was studied by analyzing aliquots of standard in triplicate at 3 concentration levels for luteolin and apigenin on the same day for intraday precision. The study was also repeated on different days with freshly prepared samples in order to determine interday precision. The results were expressed as relative standard deviation (RSD). The specificity of the method was ascertained by determining the peak purity of the component by overlaying the fluorescence spectra of luteolin and apigenin in the sample extract with the spectra of reference standard luteolin and apigenin at the start, middle, and end positions of the bands. The accuracy of the method was determined by recovery studies at 3 levels in triplicate. For recovery studies, known amount of standard was added.

2.12. Statistical Analysis. The statistical analysis was performed using Microsoft Excel 2007.

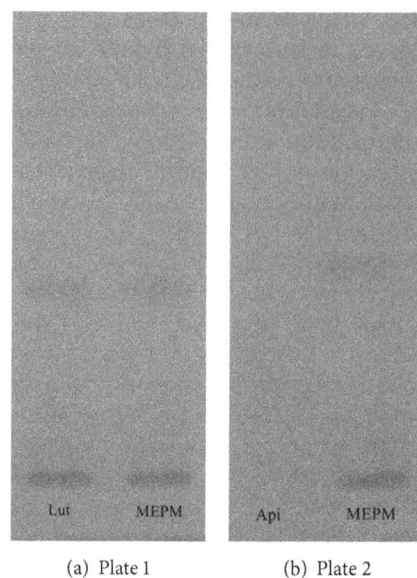

(a) Plate 1   (b) Plate 2

FIGURE 1: ((a) and (b)) Visible mode after spray with NP-PEG reagent, Lut: luteolin standard, Api: apigenin standard, and MEPM: methanolic extract of *Premna mucronata*.

3. Results and Discussion

Different proportions of toluene and ethyl acetate were tried as the mobile phase on silica gel HPTLC plates and a ratio of (6 : 4 v/v) gave good resolution. Well resolved symmetric band for luteolin and apigenin in extract was obtained under the optimized conditions using precoated HPTLC plates with 0.2 mm thickness, 5-6 mm particle size, and the mobile phase toluene : ethyl acetate : formic acid (6 : 4 : 0.3). Luteolin and apigenin on derivatization with NP-PEG reagent (natural products polyethylene glycol reagent) appeared orange in visible mode (Figures 1(a) and 1(b)) and gave bright yellow and parrot green fluorescence in fluorescence mode (Figures 2(a) and 2(b)) [24]. Standard luteolin (R_f 0.45) and standard apigenin (R_f 0.49) showed single peak in HPTLC chromatogram (Figures 3 and 4). Calibration curve of luteolin and apigenin was prepared by plotting concentration of luteolin versus area of the peak and concentration of apigenin versus area of the peak, respectively (Figures 5 and 6).

3.1. Determination of Marker in Extract. The methanolic extract of *Premna mucronata* was found to contain 10.2 mg/g % luteolin and 0.165 mg/g % of apigenin. Furthermore, the methanolic extract of *Premna mucronata* shows peak in the chromatogram at same R_f value as luteolin (0.45) standard and apigenin (0.49) standard (Figure 7).

3.2. Linearity. Luteolin and apigenin showed good correlation coefficient of 0.9942 and 0.9917, respectively, when peak area of the resolved band was plotted against concentration, thus exhibiting good linearity between concentration and peak area. Table 1 summarizes Beer's law limit, linear regression equation, and correlation coefficient for the method.

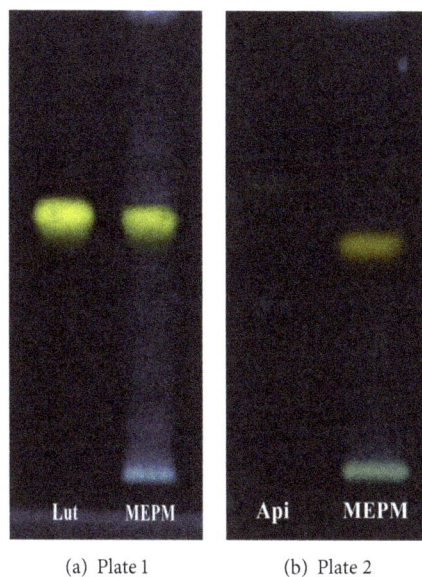

(a) Plate 1   (b) Plate 2

FIGURE 2: ((a) and (b)) Fluorescence mode after spray with NP-PEG reagent, Lut: luteolin standard, Api: apigenin standard, and MEPM: methanolic extract of *Premna mucronata*.

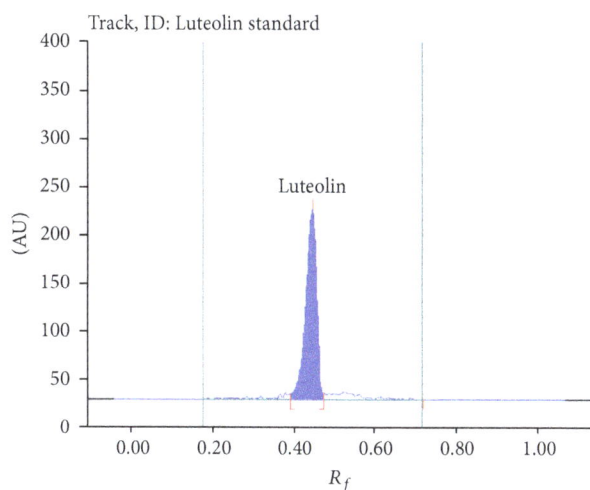

FIGURE 3: Chromatogram of luteolin standard.

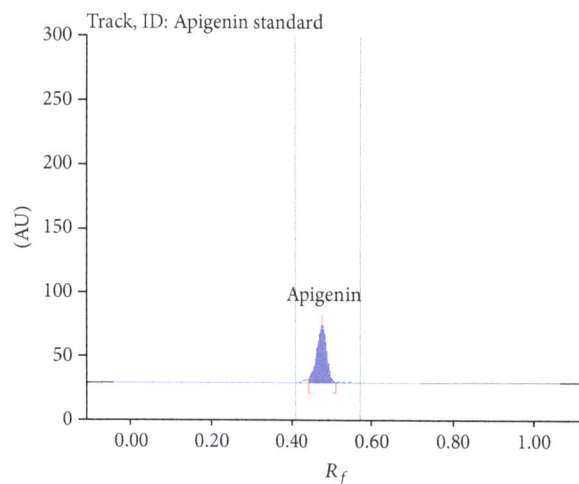

FIGURE 4: Chromatogram of apigenin standard.

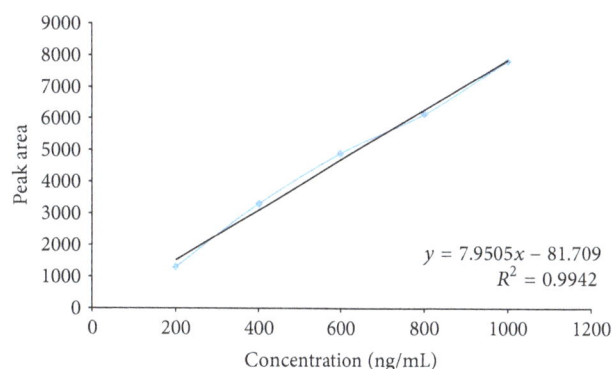

$$y = 7.9505x - 81.709$$
$$R^2 = 0.9942$$

FIGURE 5: Calibration curve of luteolin standard.

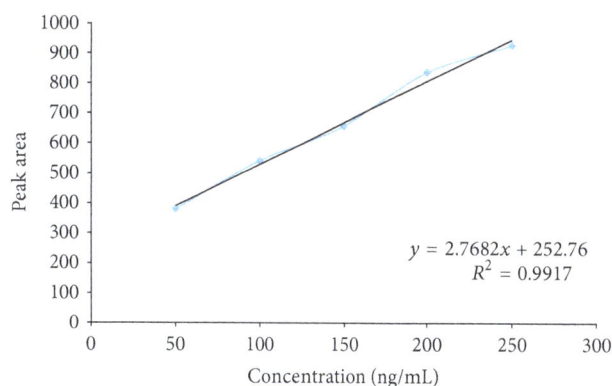

$$y = 2.7682x + 252.76$$
$$R^2 = 0.9917$$

FIGURE 6: Calibration curve of apigenin standard.

3.3. Precision. The proposed method was found to be precise as indicated by intermediate precision studies expressed as percent RSD (relative standard deviation) for intraday and interday variations as shown in Tables 2 and 3.

3.4. Accuracy. The proposed method when used for quantitation of marker after spiking with standard afforded recovery of luteolin and apigenin in the range of 96.67%–102.92% and 97.72%–99.29%, respectively, at three concentration levels as shown in Tables 4 and 5.

3.5. Limit of Detection and Limit of Quantification. For luteolin and apigenin, the limit of detection was found to be 42.6 ng/band and 7.97 ng/band while the limit of quantitation

was found to be 129.08 ng/band and 24.155 ng/band, respectively.

3.6. Specificity. The identity of the bands in the sample extracts was confirmed by comparing R_f, absorption spectra, and fluorescence spectra and by overlaying with those of their respective standard using CAMAG TLC Scanner 4.

TABLE 1: Method validation parameters for estimation of luteolin and apigenin.

Parameters	Luteolin	Apigenin
Wavelength, nm	366	366
Linearity range, ng/band	200–1000	50–250
Regression equation	$y = 7.950x - 81.70$	$2.768x + 252.7$
Correlation coefficient	0.9942	0.9917
Limit of detection, ng/band	42.6	7.97
Limit of quantification, ng/band	129.08	24.155
Specificity	Specific	Specific

TABLE 2: Intermediate precision studies for luteolin.

Concentration (ng/band)	Concentration[a] (ng/band)	Intraday[b] (% RSD)	Concentration[a] (ng/band)	Interday[b] (% RSD)
400	402.3	1.08	403.69	1.32
600	604.3	0.57	606.71	0.65
800	798.8	0.38	799.20	0.43

[a]Mean of three determinations; [b]% RSD—relative standard deviation.

TABLE 3: Intermediate precision studies for apigenin.

Concentration (ng/band)	Concentration[a] (ng/band)	Intraday[b] (% RSD)	Concentration[a] (ng/band)	Interday[b] (% RSD)
100	101.43	0.67	101.3	0.60
150	150.3	0.43	150.3	0.41
200	201.1	0.27	201.15	0.18

[a]Mean of three determinations; [b]% RSD—relative standard deviation.

TABLE 4: Recovery studies of luteolin.

Amount of luteolin in sample (ng)	Amount of standard luteolin added (ng)	Total amount of luteolin taken (ng)	Total amount of luteolin found (ng)	Percent of recovery[a] (%)
454.89	200	654.89	633.13	96.67 ± 1.20
454.89	400	854.89	842.58	98.56 ± 0.69
454.89	600	1054.89	1085.66	102.92 ± 0.85

[a]Mean of three determinations ± % relative standard deviation.

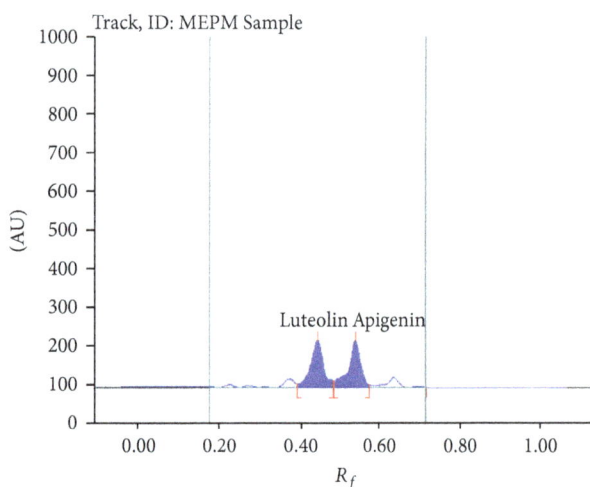

FIGURE 7: Chromatogram of methanolic extract of *Premna mucronata* Roxb. showing presence of luteolin (R_f 0.45) and apigenin (R_f 0.5).

There were no interfering spots by the plant constituents at R_f values of the marker. The absorption spectra of standard marker luteolin (R_f 0.45) and apigenin (R_f 0.49) and the corresponding spot present in extract matched exactly, indicating no interference by the other plant constituents (Figures 8 and 9). The purity of the bands due to luteolin and apigenin in the sample extract was confirmed by overlaying the absorption and fluorescence spectra recorded at start, middle, and end position of the band in the sample tracks, respectively (Figures 10 and 11).

4. Conclusion

The proposed HPTLC method was found to be rapid, simple, and accurate for quantitative estimation of luteolin and apigenin. The recovery of luteolin and apigenin from whole part of *Premna mucronata* was found to be 96.67%–102.92% and 97.72%–99.29%, respectively, revealing accuracy of the developed method and hence can be applicable for routine

TABLE 5: Recovery studies of apigenin.

Amount of apigenin in sample (ng)	Amount of standard apigenin added (ng)	Total amount of apigenin taken (ng)	Total amount of apigenin found (ng)	Percent of recovery[a] (%)
131.57	100	231.57	229.91	99.29 ± 1.22
131.57	200	331.57	328.23	98.99 ± 1.21
131.57	300	431.57	421.77	97.72 ± 0.82

[a]Mean of three determinations ± % relative standard deviation.

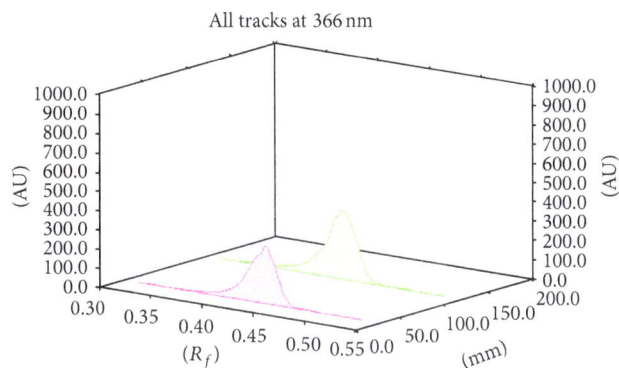

FIGURE 8: TLC densitograms for comparison of methanol extract of *Premna mucronata* Roxb. with reference standard, luteolin at 366 nm. Standard luteolin (shows peak at R_f 0.45), methanol extract (shows peak at R_f 0.45).

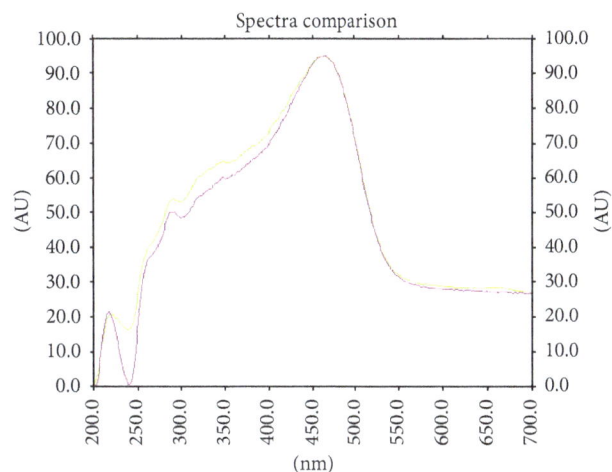

FIGURE 10: Overlain UV spectra at 254 nm for peak purity of luteolin.

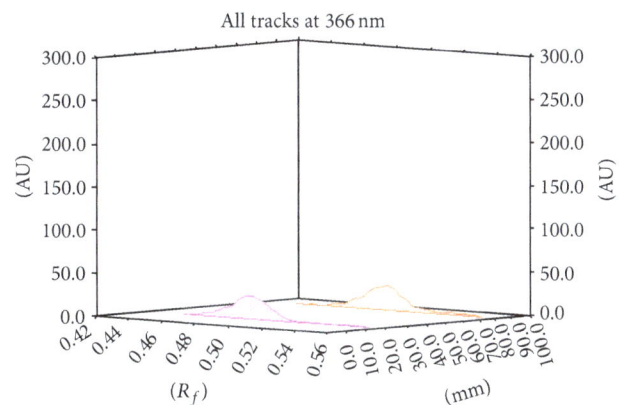

FIGURE 9: TLC densitograms for comparison of methanol extract of *Premna mucronata* Roxb. with reference standard, apigenin at 366 nm. Standard apigenin (shows peak at R_f 0.49), methanol extract (shows peak at R_f 0.49).

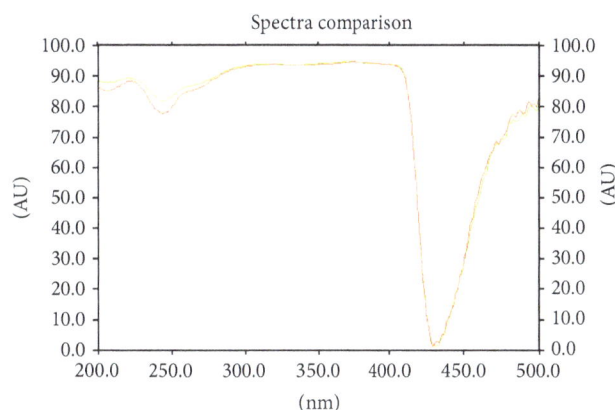

FIGURE 11: Overlain fluorescence spectra at 366 nm for peak purity of apigenin.

analysis of extract and plant as a whole. Moreover, HPTLC profile by co-TLC can be used for fingerprinting thereby providing assurance of standardization and quality. And HPTLC has various advantages of low operating cost, high sample throughput, simplicity, and the need for minimum sample clean-up. In future, as the plant shows good cardio-protective activity, dosage form of the same can be formulated where fingerprinting and quantification of both the chemical markers will be used.

Conflict of Interests

The authors declare that there is no conflict of interests regarding the publication of this paper.

References

[1] V. P. Kamboj, "Herbal medicine," *Current Science*, vol. 78, no. 1, pp. 35–39, 2000.

[2] A. R. Bilia, "*Ginkgo biloba* L.," *Fitoterapia*, vol. 73, no. 3, pp. 276–279, 2002.

[3] P. J. Houghton, "Establishing identification criteria for botanicals," *Drug Information Journal*, vol. 32, no. 2, pp. 461–469, 1998.

[4] N. R. Farnsworth, O. Akerele, A. S. Bingel, D. D. Soejarto, and Z. Guo, "Medicinal plants in therapy," *Bulletin of the World Health Organization*, vol. 63, no. 6, pp. 965–981, 1985.

[5] World Health Organization, "Quality control methods for medicinal plant material," WHO/PHARM 92.559, World Health Organization, Geneva, Switzerland, 1992.

[6] J. G. Brun, "The use of natural products in modern medicine [phytotherapy]," *Acta Pharmaceutica Nordica*, vol. 1, no. 3, pp. 117–130, 1989.

[7] P. Xie, S. Chen, Y.-Z. Liang, X. Wang, R. Tian, and R. Upton, "Chromatographic fingerprint analysis-a rational approach for quality assessment of traditional Chinese herbal medicine," *Journal of Chromatography A*, vol. 1112, no. 1-2, pp. 171–180, 2006.

[8] K. Dhalwal, V. M. Shinde, K. R. Mahadik, and A. G. Namdeo, "Rapid densitometric method for simultaneous analysis of umbelliferone, psoralen, and eugenol in herbal raw materials using HPTLC," *Journal of Separation Science*, vol. 30, no. 13, pp. 2053–2058, 2007.

[9] M. Bagul, H. Srinivasa, H. Padh, and M. Rajani, "A rapid densitometric method for simultaneous quantification of gallic acid and ellagic acid in herbal raw materials using HPTLC," *Journal of Separation Science*, vol. 28, no. 6, pp. 581–584, 2005.

[10] M. N. Ravishankara, N. Shrivastava, H. Padh, and M. Rajani, "HPTLC method for the estimation of alkaloids of *Cinchona officinalis* stem bark and its marketed formulations," *Planta Medica*, vol. 67, no. 3, pp. 294–296, 2001.

[11] Agnimanth, http://www.ayurvedaconsultants.com/.

[12] D. Thirumalai, M. Paridhavi, and M. Gowtham, "A phytochemical review on premna species," *International Journal of Research in Phytochemistry and Pharmacology*, vol. 1, no. 4, pp. 196–200, 2011.

[13] Premna mucronata, http://www.holistic-herbalist.com/agnimantha.html.

[14] P. S. M. Prince, S. Suman, P. T. Devika, and M. Vaithianathan, "Cardioprotective effect of 'Marutham' a polyherbal formulation on isoproterenol induced myocardial infarction in Wistar rats," *Fitoterapia*, vol. 79, no. 6, pp. 433–438, 2008.

[15] J. Wang, H. Bo, X. Meng, Y. Wu, Y. Bao, and Y. Li, "A simple and fast experimental model of myocardial infarction in the mouse," *Texas Heart Institute Journal*, vol. 33, no. 3, pp. 290–293, 2006.

[16] P.-H. Liao, L.-M. Hung, Y.-H. Chen et al., "Cardioprotective effects of luteolin during ischemia-reperfusion injury in rats," *Circulation Journal*, vol. 75, no. 2, pp. 443–450, 2011.

[17] N. G. Patel, K. V. Patel, T. R. Gandhi, K. G. Patel, and H. B. Gevariya, "Evaluation of the cardioprotective effect of *Premna mucronata* Roxb. (Verbenaceae) in the experimental model of myocardial ischemia-reperfusion injury," *International Journal of Modern Pharmaceutical Research*, vol. 1, no. 1, pp. 1–20, 2012.

[18] N. G. Patel, K. G. Patel, K. V. Patel, and T. R. Gandhi, "Myocardial salvaging effect of *Premna mucronata* Roxb. (Verbenaceae) on isoproterenol induced myocardial necrosis in rats," *Der Pharmacia Lettre*, vol. 7, no. 7, pp. 137–147, 2015.

[19] N. Cotelle, J.-L. Bernier, J.-P. Catteau, J. Pommery, J.-C. Wallet, and E. M. Gaydou, "Antioxidant properties of hydroxyflavones," *Free Radical Biology and Medicine*, vol. 20, no. 1, pp. 35–43, 1996.

[20] Q. Cai, R. O. Rahn, and R. Zhang, "Dietary flavonoids, quercetin, luteolin and genistein, reduce oxidative DNA damage and lipid peroxidation and quench free radicals," *Cancer Letters*, vol. 119, no. 1, pp. 99–107, 1997.

[21] M. Nagao, N. Morita, T. Yahagi et al., "Mutagenicities of 61 flavonoids and 11 related compounds," *Environmental Mutagenesis*, vol. 3, no. 4, pp. 401–419, 1981.

[22] M. Noroozi, W. J. Angerson, and M. E. J. Lean, "Effects of flavonoids and vitamin C on oxidative DNA damage to human lymphocytes," *American Journal of Clinical Nutrition*, vol. 67, no. 6, pp. 1210–1218, 1998.

[23] International Conference on Harmonization, Validation of Analytical Procedures: Text and Methodology ICH-Q2 (R1), Geneva, Switzerland, 2005, http://private.ich.org/LOB/media/MEDIA417.pdf.

[24] H. Wagner and S. Bladt, *Plant Drug Analysis: A Thin Layer Chromatography Atlas*, Springer, Berlin, Germany, 2nd edition, 1996.

28

Development of an Experimental Model of Diabetes Co-Existing with Metabolic Syndrome in Rats

Rajesh Kumar Suman,[1] **Ipseeta Ray Mohanty,**[1] **Manjusha K. Borde,**[1]
Ujwala Maheshwari,[2] **and Y. A. Deshmukh**[1]

[1]*Department of Pharmacology, MGM Medical College, Kamothe, Navi Mumbai 410209, India*
[2]*Department of Pathology, MGM Medical College, Kamothe, Navi Mumbai 410209, India*

Correspondence should be addressed to Rajesh Kumar Suman; rajesh_suman1986@hotmail.com

Academic Editor: Thérèse Di Paolo-Chênevert

Background. The incidence of metabolic syndrome co-existing with diabetes mellitus is on the rise globally. *Objective.* The present study was designed to develop a unique animal model that will mimic the pathological features seen in individuals with diabetes and metabolic syndrome, suitable for pharmacological screening of drugs. *Materials and Methods.* A combination of High-Fat Diet (HFD) and low dose of streptozotocin (STZ) at 30, 35, and 40 mg/kg was used to induce metabolic syndrome in the setting of diabetes mellitus in Wistar rats. *Results.* The 40 mg/kg STZ produced sustained hyperglycemia and the dose was thus selected for the study to induce diabetes mellitus. Various components of metabolic syndrome such as dyslipidemia {(increased triglyceride, total cholesterol, LDL cholesterol, and decreased HDL cholesterol)}, diabetes mellitus (blood glucose, HbA1c, serum insulin, and C-peptide), and hypertension {systolic blood pressure} were mimicked in the developed model of metabolic syndrome co-existing with diabetes mellitus. In addition to significant cardiac injury, atherogenic index, inflammation (hs-CRP), decline in hepatic and renal function were observed in the HF-DC group when compared to NC group rats. The histopathological assessment confirmed presence of edema, necrosis, and inflammation in heart, pancreas, liver, and kidney of HF-DC group as compared to NC. *Conclusion.* The present study has developed a unique rodent model of metabolic syndrome, with diabetes as an essential component.

1. Introduction

Metabolic syndrome encompasses cluster of risk factors for cardiovascular disease which includes abdominal obesity, dyslipidemia, hypertension, and hyperglycemia [1]. The incidence of metabolic syndrome is on the rise globally [2]. World Health Organization (WHO), International Diabetes Federation (IDF), and National Cholesterol of Adult Treatment Panel III (NCEPATPIII) have laid down specific criteria for metabolic syndrome. Later, these organizations jointly developed a new definition of metabolic syndrome known as "harmonized criteria" which included central obesity, raised blood pressure, elevated triglyceride levels, low high-density lipoprotein (HDL), and raised glucose levels [1]. Metabolic syndrome increases the risk of developing type II diabetes by impeding the critical regulatory influence of insulin on glucose, lipid, and protein metabolism. Patients developing type II diabetes have often gone through a state of obesity associated with reduced insulin sensitivity along with an activated beta cell compensatory mechanism, such as excess basal insulin secretion and hyperinsulinemia, as a part of their metabolic profile [3–5]. Thus, metabolic syndrome and diabetes mellitus are interrelated metabolic disorders which may co-exist on several occasions.

Diabetes mellitus co-existing with metabolic syndrome has become a common predicament in society due to change in lifestyle and dietary habits. The number of diabetics with metabolic syndrome is substantial and the prevalence is increasing throughout the world [6, 7]. Efforts should be directed to treating both the diseases together as a whole rather than independently by finding better treatments and novel prevention strategies for type II diabetes co-existing with metabolic syndrome. In order to do so appropriate characterized and clinically relevant experimental models are considered as essential tools for testing new agents, understanding the molecular basis, pathogenesis, and mechanism of actions of these therapeutic agents. Thus to control these diseases, it is of paramount importance to establish such unique animal models that closely mimic the changes subsequent to development of diabetes and metabolic syndrome in humans. These viable animal models should address all the aspects of this human disease, developing all major signs of diabetes as well as metabolic syndrome, especially obesity, dyslipidemia, hypertension, and possibly fatty liver disease and kidney dysfunction.

The streptozotocin and the Alloxan models of chemically induced diabetes are commonly used to screen antidiabetic drugs [8, 9]. However, these methods cause marked destruction of the pancreatic mass and may therefore mimic changes closer to type I diabetes rather than type II diabetes mellitus. Recently, it has been reported that rats fed with High-Fat Diet and combination of streptozotocin developed type II diabetes more closely to humans. High-Fat Diet will cause insulin resistance in peripheral tissues due to lipotoxicity; meanwhile, low dose of streptozotocin will induce mild defect in insulin secretion [10]. Combination of High-Fat Diet with low dose streptozotocin model has therefore successfully mimicked natural progress of diabetes development as well as metabolic features in human type II diabetes [11–13]. Similarly, for the study of metabolic syndrome, several investigators have used carbohydrate (fructose, sucrose) and fat-rich dietary components in rodents. Combinations of carbohydrate and fat-rich dietary components have been used in rodents to mimic these signs and symptoms of human metabolic syndrome. However there are no chronic animal models where diabetes and metabolic syndrome co-exist which may be useful to screen therapeutic agents beneficial in such conditions.

The present study was designed to develop a unique animal model that will mimic the pathological features seen in a large pool of individuals with long term diabetes and metabolic syndrome, suitable for pharmacological screening of drugs beneficial in this condition. Such a model should replicate the components of metabolic syndrome such as hyperlipidemia, hypertension, and obesity along with type II diabetes mellitus.

2. Materials and Methods

2.1. Experimental Animal. Adult male Wistar rats, 10 to 12 weeks old, weighing 150 to 200 gm, were used in the study. The rats were housed in the Central Animal Facility of our own MGM Medical College, Navi Mumbai, India. They were maintained under standard laboratory conditions in the animal house. The study protocol was approved by the Institutional Animal Ethics Committee and conforms to the Committee for the Purpose of Control and Supervision of Experiments on Animals and Indian National Science Academy and Guidelines for the Use and Care of Experimental Animals in Research. Rats were kept in polyacrylic cages (38 × 23 × 15 cm) with not more than four animals per cage, housed in an air-conditioned room, and kept under natural light-dark cycles. The animals were allowed free access to standard diet or High-Fat Diet as the case may be and water *ad* libitum.

2.2. Preparation of High-Fat Diet. The High-Fat Diet (HFD) was prepared indigenously in our laboratory by using normal pellet diet, raw cholesterol, and mixture of vanaspati ghee and coconut oil (2 : 1). Normal rat pellet diet was powdered by grinding and mixed with 2.5% cholesterol and mixture of vanaspati ghee and coconut oil (5%). The mixture was made into pellet form and put into freezer to solidify. In addition 2% raw cholesterol powder was mixed in coconut oil and administered to the rats by oral route (3 mL/kg).

2.2.1. Standardization of Streptozotocin Dose for Induction of Diabetes Mellitus. The HFD along with 2% liquid cholesterol (3 mL/kg) was orally fed to rats for 3 weeks to induce metabolic syndrome. A pilot study was carried out with different doses of STZ (30, 35, and 40 mg/kg) in order to select the appropriate dose of STZ for induction of diabetes. Based on the pilot study results, it was found that 40 mg/kg STZ produced diabetes in experimental rats. Therefore, a single STZ injection (40 mg/kg body wt, i.p., dissolved in 0.01 M citrate buffer, pH 4.5) was standardized to induce diabetes mellitus. Serum glucose estimations (blood sugar >200 mg/dL) were undertaken periodically (days 0, 3, and 7) from the tail vein to confirm the production of diabetes mellitus.

2.2.2. Experimental Model of Diabetes with Metabolic Syndrome. After 3 weeks of dietary manipulation, rats were injected intraperitoneally with STZ (40 mg/kg). The body weight and biochemical parameters (blood glucose, total cholesterol) were estimated 7 days after the vehicle or STZ injection; that is, on 4 weeks of dietary manipulation in rats. The rats with blood glucose (>200 mg/dL), total cholesterol (>110 mg/dL), triglyceride (>150 mg/dL), change in body weight (8% of initial weight), systolic blood pressure (>130 mm Hg), and reduced HDL levels (<35 mg/dL) confirmed presence of metabolic syndrome with diabetes. Thereafter the rats were either fed normal diet or HFD as per the protocol for 10 weeks. Blood samples were collected from the retroorbital plexus under light anesthesia at 0, 4, 7, and 10 weeks for estimation of biochemical parameters. At the ends of experimental period, rats were sacrificed for histopathological evaluation of injury to the heart, aorta, pancreas, liver, and kidney.

2.3. Experimental Groups

2.3.1. Group 1: Normal Control (NC). In Normal Control group, rats were administered distilled water orally using a feeding cannula for study period of 10 weeks. At the end of 3 weeks, 0.01 M citrate buffer, pH 4.5, was injected intraperitoneally to mimic the STZ injections.

2.3.2. Group 2: High Fat Diabetic Control (HF-DC). The HFD were fed to rats for 10 weeks to produce metabolic syndrome.

Table 1: Time course of changes in anthropometric parameters in the experimental group.

SN	Variable	Baseline		4 weeks		7 weeks		10 weeks	
		NC	HF-DC	NC	HF-DC	NC	HF-DC	NC	HF-DC
1	Body weight	157.63 ± 7.11	161.14 ± 5.11	188.87 ± 6.22	$235.14 \pm 4.59^{***}$	214.12 ± 5.33	$226.42 \pm 4.68^{*}$	237.88 ± 4.99	$219.14 + 9.92$
2	AC	14.13 ± 0.49	14.28 ± 0.39	15.00 ± 0.26	$17.72 \pm 0.48^{**}$	16.31 ± 0.25	$17.00 \pm 0.40^{*}$	17.68 ± 0.70	16.58 ± 0.45
3	TC	13.06 ± 00.40	13.14 ± 0.55	13.93 ± 0.41	$16.71 \pm 0.48^{**}$	15.25 ± 0.26	$16.00 \pm 0.41^{*}$	16.62 ± 0.74	15.57 ± 0.47
4	AC/TC	1.081	1.086	1.076	1.060	1.069	1.062	1.063	1.064

NC: Normal Control group ($n = 8$); HF-DC: High Fat Diabetic Control group ($n = 7$). Values are expressed as mean $\pm$ SD. $^{*}p < 0.05$, $^{**}p < 0.01$, and $^{***}p < 0.001$, NC versus HF-DC.

At the end of 3 weeks diabetes was induced by a single STZ injection (40 mg/kg body wt, i.p., dissolved in 0.01 M citrate buffer, pH 4.5).

2.4. Evaluation Parameters

(1) *Anthropometric parameter*: body weight (gm), abdominal circumference (AC), thoracic circumference (TC), and AC/TC ratio were recorded every 4 weeks and the changes in these parameters were calculated.

(2) *Biochemical parameters (metabolic, cardiac, liver, and kidney function markers)*: the rat blood samples of all experimental groups were collected from the retroorbital plexus under light anesthesia at 0, 4, 7, and 10 weeks for estimation of blood glucose, TC, TG, and CPK-MB. In addition, after the completion of the experimental duration (10 weeks), serum was used for the determination of the parameters like lipid profile, serum insulin, C-peptide, creatinine, SGPT, and hs-CRP by autoanalyzer or ELISA kits in the Pathology (NABL accredited) or Pharmacology Laboratory.

(3) *Blood pressure recording*: the blood pressure was measured using the noninvasive tail-cuff method at the end of the experiment. Three readings were taken and average was taken as final reading for systolic blood pressure.

(4) *Histopathological studies*: at the end of the experiment (10 weeks), the animals were sacrificed. The heart, thoracic aorta, liver, kidney, and pancreas were immediately fixed in 10% buffered neutral formalin solution. The tissues were carefully embedded in molten paraffin with the help of metallic blocks, covered with flexible plastic moulds, and kept under freezing plates to allow the paraffin to solidify. Cross sections (5 μm thick) of the fixed tissues were cut. These sections were stained with hematoxyline and eosin and visualized under light microscope to study the microscopic architecture of the tissues. The investigator performing the histological evaluation was blind to biochemical results and to treatment allocation.

(5) *Immunohistochemical localization of insulin*: the pancreas was immediately fixed in 10% buffered neutral formalin solution after scarification (10 weeks). The tissues were carefully cut, 3-micrometer thick, and obtained on poly-L-lysine coated slides and transferred to three changes of xylene for 30 min, followed

by rehydrating with decreasing grades of alcohol. The Antigen Retrieval was in microwave oven, 800 watt for 10 min, 420 watt for 10 min, and 360 watt for 5 min in Citrate buffer pH 6. Immunostaining was done by Peroxidase block with 3% hydrogen peroxide in methanol for 5 min and incubated sections for 10 min. Primary Antibody Incubation was undertaken for 30 min at room temperature and thereafter incubated with superenhancer for 10 min. The tissues were incubated with poly-HRP for 30 min followed by substrate DAB. The slides were then visualized under light microscope to study the immunohistochemical localization of insulin.

3. Results

3.1. Standardization of HFD with Different Dose of Streptozotocin. Standardization of HFD and dose of STZ (30, 35, and 40) mg/kg to induce metabolic syndrome co-existing with diabetes mellitus was undertaken in the laboratory. The doses of STZ (30 and 35 mg/kg) did not produce sustained increase in blood glucose (>200 mg/dL). Hence diabetes was not produced by 30 and 35 mg/kg dose of STZ. The 40 mg/kg of STZ produced desired increase in blood glucose levels in HFD fed rats that was maintained through the study period. Hence, 40 mg/kg dose of STZ was selected for the present study.

3.1.1. Anthropometric Parameter. The HF-DC group showed significant ($p < 0.001$) increase in body weight on 4th and 7th week as compared with NC group rats. The increase in body weight of HF-DC group rats was not sustained at the end of 10th week. Similarly, the AC and TC of the HF-DC group rats also increased significantly only at 4th and 7th week as compared to the NC rats at similar time points. The AC/TC ratio of HF-DC group rats was not statistically different form NC rats. The weight difference between NC and HF-DC in baseline weight and 10th week weight is 50.91% in NC and 35.99% in HF-DC. The figure shows weight loss at 10th week in HF-DC group (Table 1, Figure 1).

3.1.2. Biochemical Parameters

(a) Metabolic Parameters. The blood glucose, total cholesterol, and triglycerides levels in the HF-DC group rats were significantly higher ($p < 0.001$) as compared to NC group

TABLE 2: Metabolic parameters in the experimental groups.

SN	Variable	NC	HF-DC
1	TG (mg/dL)	63.75 ± 11.47	$312.85 \pm 62.24^{***}$
2	HDL (mg/dL)	32.62 ± 2.56	$26.57 \pm 5.74^{**}$
3	LDL (mg/dL)	12.6 ± 2.41	$62.57 \pm 12.44^{***}$
4	HbA1c (%)	6.22 ± 0.43	$12.78 \pm 1.50^{***}$
5	Insulin (μU/mL)	6.46 ± 0.65	$2.94 \pm 1.11^{**}$
6	C-Peptide (ng/mL)	0.07 ± 0.02	0.05 ± 0.035
7	HOMA-IR	1.57 ± 0.16	2.17 ± 0.63
8	HOMA-β	66.6 ± 5.86	$5.9 \pm 1.2^{***}$
9	Atherogenic index	1.36 ± 0.20	$11.34 \pm 5.01^{***}$

NC: Normal Control group ($n = 8$); HF-DC: High Fat Diabetic Control group ($n = 7$). Values are expressed as mean $\pm$ SD. $^{**}p < 0.01$, $^{***}p < 0.001$, NC versus HF-DC.

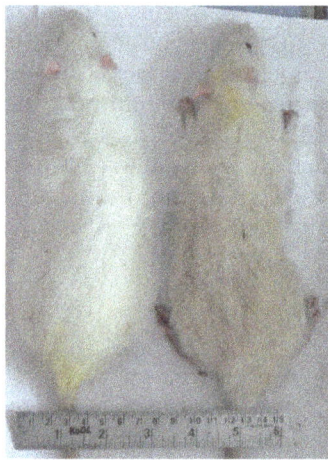

FIGURE 1: Rats of the Normal Control and High Fat Diabetic control groups at 10th weeks.

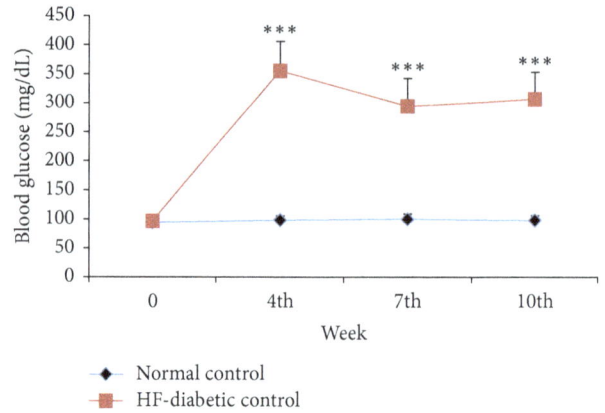

FIGURE 2: Time course changes of blood glucose level of NC ($n = 8$), HF-DC group ($n = 7$). Values are expressed as mean $\pm$ SD. $^{***}p < 0.001$, NC versus HF-DC.

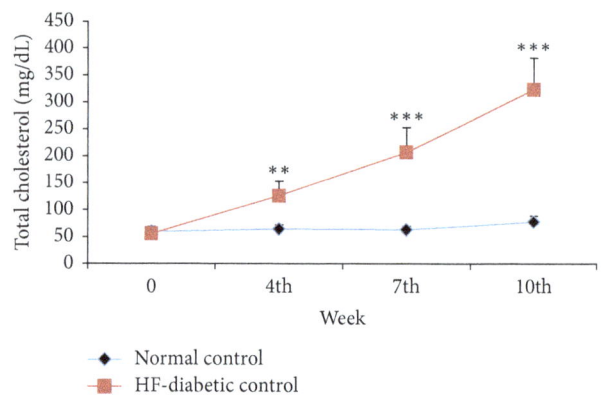

FIGURE 3: Time course changes in total cholesterol among experimental groups of NC ($n = 8$), HF-DC group ($n = 7$). Values are expressed as mean $\pm$ SD. $^{**}p < 0.01$, $^{***}p < 0.001$, NC versus HF-DC.

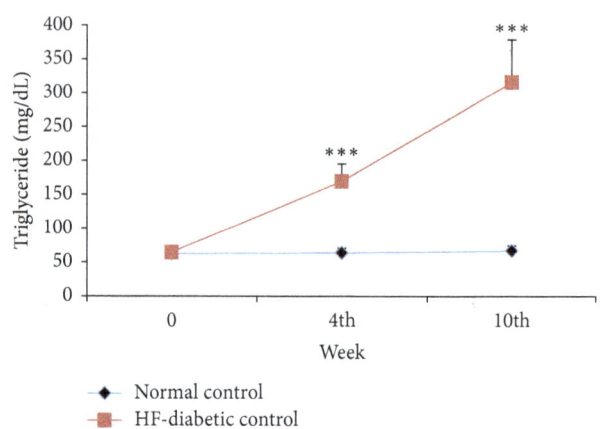

FIGURE 4: Time course changes in triglyceride of NC ($n = 8$), HF-DC group ($n = 7$). Values are expressed as mean $\pm$ SD. $^{***}p < 0.001$, NC versus HF-DC.

rats at 4th, 7th, and 10th week. Glycosylated hemoglobin, total cholesterol, low-density lipoprotein, and atherogenic index were significantly increased in HF-DC group as compared with NC group at the end of 10 weeks. HOMA-IR increased in HF-DC, while serum insulin and HOMA-β are significantly reduced in HF-DC group as compared with NC. High-density lipoprotein was significantly decreased in HF-DC as compared with NC. The C-peptide levels in HF-DC were decreased though statistically not significant as compared to NC rats (Figures 2, 3, and 4 and Table 2).

(b) *Cardiac Variables.* There was a significant ($p < 0.001$) increase in serum CPK-MB levels in HF-DC rats at 7th and 10th week as compared with NC. However, the CPK-MB levels did not rise significantly at 4th week (Figure 4). The other cardiac markers hs-CRP and systolic blood pressure were measured on 10th week of study and were found to be significantly raised ($p < 0.01$) in HF-DC group as compared with NC (Figure 5, Table 3).

(c) *Liver and Kidney Function Markers.* The HF-DC group rats showed a significant ($p < 0.01$) increase in the level of SGPT

TABLE 3: Study variables in the experimental groups.

SN	Variables	NC	HF-DC
	Cardiac variables		
1	Hs-CRP (mg/dL)	0.86 ± 0.11	$2.2 \pm 0.52^{**}$
2	Systolic blood pressure (mm Hg)	101.7 ± 1.52	$149.6 \pm 4.04^{***}$
	Liver function		
1	SGPT	62.77 ± 11.58	$98.50 \pm 10.35^{**}$
	Kidney function		
1	Creatinine	0.35 ± 0.07	$1.36 \pm 0.45^{*}$

NC: Normal Control group ($n = 8$); HF-DC: High Fat Diabetic Control group ($n = 7$). Values are expressed as mean $\pm$ SD. $^{*}p < 0.05$, $^{**}p < 0.01$, and $^{***}p < 0.001$, NC versus HF-DC.

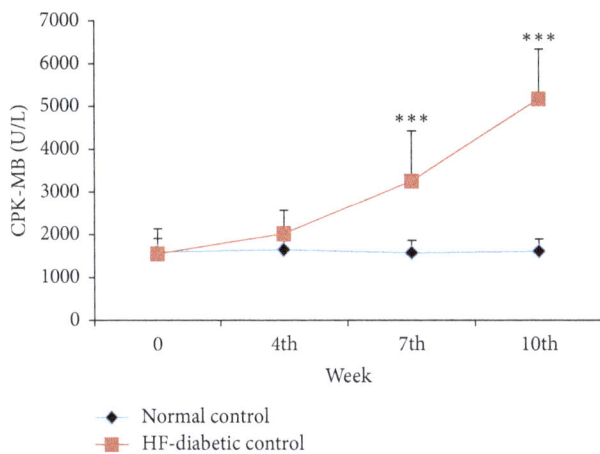

FIGURE 5: Time course changes in CPK-MB of NC ($n = 8$), HF-DC group ($n = 7$). Values are expressed as mean $\pm$ SD. $^{***}p < 0.001$, NC versus HF-DC.

(U/L) and creatinine (mg/dL) when compared to NC group rats at 10th week (Table 3).

3.1.3. Blood Pressure Recordings. The systolic blood pressure was raised significantly ($p < 0.001$) in HF-DC group as compared with NC group (Table 3).

3.1.4. Histopathological Assessment

(a) Myocardium and Aorta. Histopathological assessment of NC group rat heart revealed the noninfarcted architecture of the myocardium (Figure 6(a)). In contrast, the HF-DC group rats subjected to HFD and STZ injury (Figure 6(b)) demonstrated marked edema, confluent areas of necrosis and separation of myofibers, congested blood vessels, and mild inflammation as compared to the NC group. Figure 6(c) depicts the normal architecture seen in the NC group. In contrast, the histology of the aorta of HF-DC group rats showed atherosclerotic deposition in the vessel wall (Figure 6(d)).

(b) Histopathology of the Pancreas. The pancreas of the NC group (Figure 7(a)) rats was characterized by an organized pattern and showed normal architecture of islets of

Langerhans and the beta cells. In contrast, the HF-DC group (Figure 7(b)) of rats demonstrated damaged islets of Langerhans, atrophy of beta cells, and reduced beta cell mass as compared to NC.

(c) Histopathology of the Liver. Histological assessment of the liver of the NC group (Figure 8(a)) rats shows normal architecture of central vein, peripheral vein, and hepatocytes. In contrast, the liver cells of the HF-DC group (Figure 8(b)) showed degeneration, scattered necrotic cells, congestion in the central vein, and fat deposition as compared to NC.

(d) Histopathology of the Kidney. Histopathology of NC group (Figure 9(a)) kidney showed absence of congestion of glomerular blood vessels, tubular necrosis, and inflammation. In contrast histological assessment of the HF-DC group (Figure 9(b)) demonstrated congestion of glomerular blood vessels, tubular necrosis, inflammation, and cloudy degeneration as compared to NC group.

3.1.5. Immunohistochemistry of Pancreas for Insulin Localisation. Immunohistochemistry of NC group pancreas showed increased localization of insulin in the NC as compared to HF-DC (Figure 10(a)). The HF-DC group showed loss of beta cell mass resulting in decrease in insulin secretion (Figure 10(b)).

4. Discussion

Metabolic syndrome includes central obesity, insulin resistance, elevated blood pressure, impaired glucose tolerance, and dyslipidaemia. The number of adults with metabolic syndrome is substantial and the prevalence is increasing throughout the world. In the Indian subcontinent, 45% of males and 38% of females are diagnosed with metabolic syndrome. Majority of individuals diagnosed as metabolic syndrome are also diabetics. With the increase in proportion of such individuals with both the disease conditions co-existing, diabetes and metabolic syndrome need to be addressed not as independent diseases or separate entities but as a unique disease combination that requires urgent attention.

There are several animal models of diabetes as well as metabolic syndrome. However, there is no experimental model where both diabetes and metabolic syndrome co-exist. Hyperglycemia, hypertension, hyperlipidemia, and low grade inflammation confer combined architecture of metabolic derangements which may initiate changes in heart, pancreas, liver, and kidney. It is therefore essential to establish models to target all these risk factors for the treatment and reduction of clustering factors of diabetes with metabolic syndrome as such unique pathogenesis cannot be adequately studied in either the diabetes or metabolic syndrome animal models alone. In the search to combat these risk factors together, efforts were directed to develop a suitable animal model that would mimic all the symptoms of human metabolic syndrome as well as diabetes to screen the potential target compounds [14].

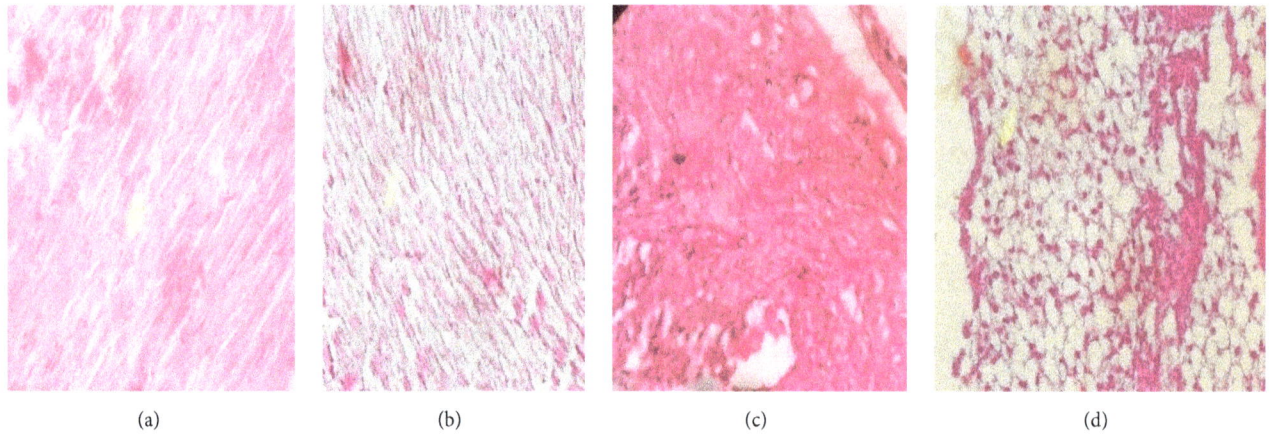

(a)   (b)   (c)   (d)

FIGURE 6: Histopathological changes of the myocardium and aorta. (a) The NC group rat heart revealed the noninfarcted architecture of the myocardium. (b) The HF-DC group rats showed myofibril damage and demonstrated marked edema, confluent areas of myonecrosis separation of myofibers, congested blood vessels, and mild inflammation. (c) NC group rat aorta showed the normal architecture. (d) Histopathology of HF-DC aorta showed fat cell deposition in vessel wall (atherosclerosis).

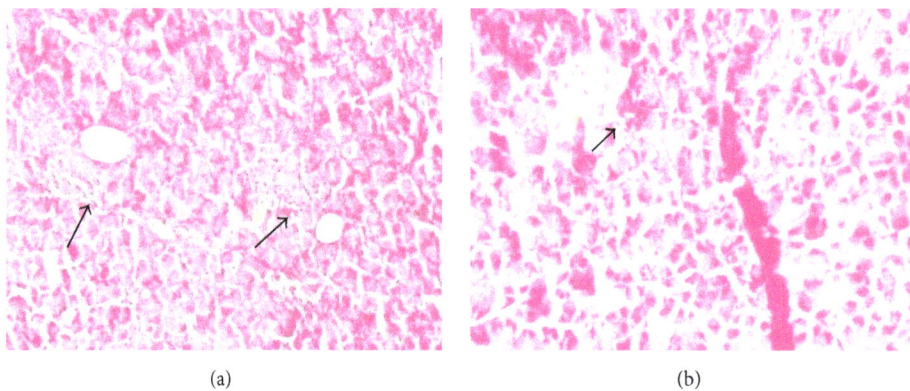

(a)   (b)

FIGURE 7: Histopathological changes of the Pancreas. (a) The NC group of rats pancreas were characterized by an organized pattern and showed normal architecture of beta cell mass. (b) The HF-DC group of rat pancreas damaged islets of Langerhans and the atrophy of beta cells showed reduced beta cell mass. The arrow showed beta cell mass.

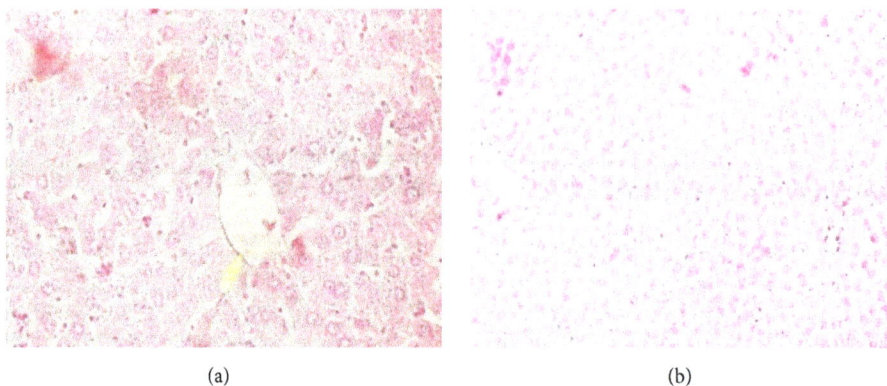

(a)   (b)

FIGURE 8: Histopathology of the liver. (a) The liver of the NC group rats shows normal architecture of central vein, peripheral vein, and hepatocytes. (b) The HF-DC group showed degeneration of hepatocyte and congestion in liver.

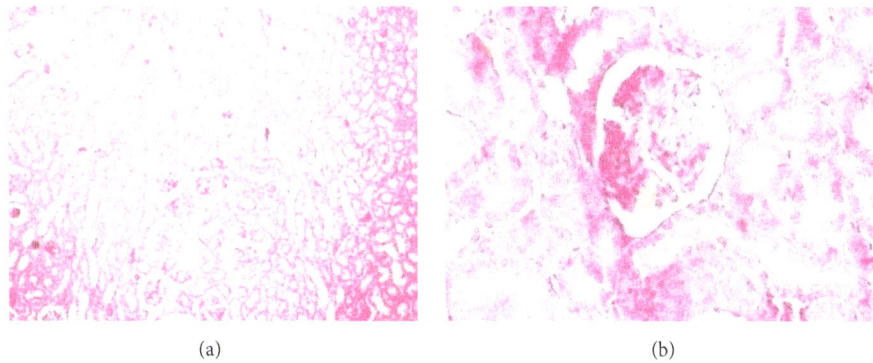

(a)   (b)

FIGURE 9: Histopathology of the kidney. (a) Histopathology of NC group kidney showed normal structure of the kidney. (b) The HF-DC group showed congestion of glomerulus, damaged tubules, inflammation, and cloudy degeneration in tubules.

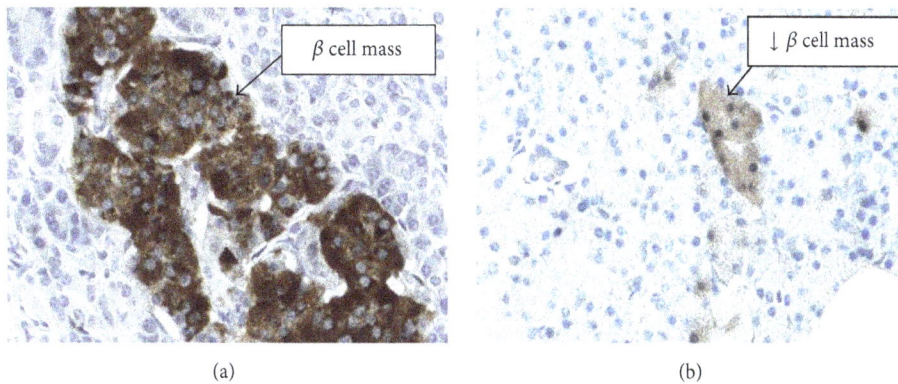

(a)   (b)

FIGURE 10: Immunohistochemical localization of insulin. (a) Immunohistochemistry of NC group pancreas showed increased localization of insulin. (b) The HF-DC group showed decreased insulin localization and hence loss of beta cell functions.

Such a unique experimental model would closely reflect the natural history and characteristic of metabolic syndrome along with human type II diabetes as well as respond to the pharmacological treatment. Further, it was kept in mind while developing the model that it should be less expensive, easily available, taking relatively short periods for development, reproducible, and displaying the various components of metabolic syndrome and diabetes mellitus. In the absence of such a unique experimental model where both the disease conditions co-exist, development of an animal model is of paramount importance and utility.

Metabolic syndrome includes central obesity, insulin resistance, elevated blood pressure, impaired glucose tolerance, and dyslipidaemia. Patients of metabolic syndrome may not have overt diabetes. However the objective of the present study was to develop an animal model which was essentially diabetic and in addition should possess the other components of metabolic syndrome such as dyslipidemia, central obesity, and hypertension.

The present study standardized different doses of STZ (30, 35, and 40 mg/kg) to be used for induction of diabetes after HFD was fed to the experimental rats. Diabetes co-existing with metabolic syndrome was successfully established with 40 mg/kg dose of STZ in the present study.

4.1. Anthropometric Parameters. Various anthropometric parameters such as body weight, thoracic circumferences (TC), abdominal circumference (AC), and their ratios (AC/TC) were evaluated in the healthy normal control (NC) and High Fat Diabetic control (HF-DC) groups. The HF-DC group showed significant ($p < 0.001$) increase in body weight on 4th and 7th week as compared with NC group rats. The increase in body weight of HF-DC group rats was not sustained till the end of 10th week. Similarly, the AC and TC of the HF-DC group rats also increased significantly only at 4th and 7th week as compared to the NC rats at similar time points. The AC/TC ratio of HF-DC group rats was not statistically different form NC rats. These anthropometric findings are in contrast to other study results in published literature. A previous study by Novelli et al. [15] (2007) showed an increase in all anthropometric parameters till the end of the study duration in rats induced with metabolic syndrome. The difference observed in the anthropometric results may be attributed to the diabetic state that is known to cause weight loss as shown by Kuate et al. [14]. Therefore this unique model of metabolic syndrome co-existing with diabetes would differ in the anthropometric results which are typically seen in various models of metabolic syndrome. Challenge with streptozotocin causes decrease in body weight which is typically seen in type II diabetes but not metabolic syndrome.

4.2. Hyperglycemia. The present study evaluated several metabolic parameters such as blood glucose, glycosylated hemoglobin (HbA1c), serum insulin, and C-Peptide. The blood glucose levels in the HF-DC group rats were significantly higher as compared to NC group rats at 4th, 7th, and 10th week. Results do not coincide with the observations made in various animal models of metabolic syndrome as overt diabetes is not an essential requirement for this syndrome. Kuate et al. [14] (2015) also demonstrated that high carbohydrate and fat diet does not induce frank diabetes in experimental rats. Results of Mansor et al. [16] (2013) and Wang et al. [17] (2011) are also in contrast to the findings of the present study as they also did not record significant hyperglycemia. The previous study by Mansor et al. [16] (2013) and Wang et al. [17] (2011) has studied the diabetes related changes 3-4 weeks subsequent to streptozotocin administration. However in the present study, long term effects of diabetes, that is, 7 weeks after streptozocin administration, were studied. It may be hypothesized that the metabolic changes of diabetes are manifested after a longer duration. Therefore the present model is more suitable to study the metabolic syndrome in the setting of diabetes.

In addition to hyperglycemia, the present study results also found poor glycemic control as indicated by increased HbA1c levels in HF-DC group as compared with NC. Kehkashan and Waseem [18] (2011) also determined HbA1c in diabetic rats and showed elevated glycosylated hemoglobin levels, similar to present study results. However hyperglycemia and glycemic control have not been established so far in an animal model of metabolic syndrome. A deficiency of insulin and a decline in pancreatic function were evidenced by a reduced level of serum insulin, C-peptide, and HOMA-β, respectively, in HF-DC group as compared to NC group rats. The HOMA-IR was raised in HF-DC group as compared with NC at the end of the study though the results were not statistically significant. The C-peptide determined by El-Sheikh [19] (2012) and Kamal et al. [20] (2011) showed reduced level in diabetic rats similar to present study. The study by Mansor et al. [16] (2013) and Wang et al. [17] (2011) estimated serum insulin levels in High-Fat Diet and STZ challenged diabetic rats. Results showed reduced level of serum insulin as seen in present study. These results do not concur with the various models of metabolic syndrome induced with High-Fat Diet. In contrast to our results, Shahraki et al. [21] (2011) demonstrated that the High-Fat Diet causes increase in the insulin levels as it causes insulin resistance. However, in the present study, administration of STZ causes reduced level of Insulin secretion because it damages the pancreas. Thus, deficiency of insulin rather than insulin resistance was the hallmark of this animal model developed to study metabolic syndrome in the setting of diabetes mellitus.

Thus, the biochemical results showed increase in blood glucose with concomitant decrease in insulin and C-peptide levels in conformity with histopathological and immuno-histochemical findings. The pancreas HF-DC group of rats

demonstrated damaged islets of Langerhans, atrophy of beta cells, and reduced beta cell mass as compared to NC. Immunohistochemical localization of insulin showed increased secretion of insulin in the NC as compared to HF-DC group. This suggests that those beta cells are functional in the NC group, secreting insulin as compared to HF-DC group. HF-DC caused beta cell dysfunction and loss of beta cell mass resulting in decreased insulin localization as seen in the slide.

4.3. Dyslipidemia. The triglycerides and cholesterol levels in the HF-DC group rats were significantly higher as compared to NC group rats at 4th, 7th, and 10th week. Dyslipidemia is a hallmark of metabolic syndrome. These results concur with studies undertaken by Kuate et al. [14] (2015), Mansor et al. [16] (2013), and Wang et al. [17] (2011). However the present model has a unique pathogenesis which is not shared with the models used by these investigators.

The present study also determined total cholesterol (TC), low-density lipoprotein (LDL), and high-density lipoprotein (HDL) at the end of the 10th week (end parameter). Abnormal lipid profile as reflected by raised LDL, TC, and reduced HDL levels was observed in the HF-DC group as compared with NC group. The previous studies by Munshi et al. [22] (2014), Kuate et al. [14] (2015), and Shahraki et al. [21] (2011) and Mamikutty et al. [23] (2014) evaluated the metabolic parameter in high carbohydrate/fat; fructose diet induced metabolic syndrome showed similar results, that is, raised level of TC, LDL and reduced level of HDL in control groups. However, these investigators have not administered STZ to induce diabetes in their study.

4.4. Cardiac Variables and Hypertension. Individuals with metabolic syndrome and diabetes have a twofold elevated risk of having a heart attack or stroke. Thus, it is critical that the cardiovascular complication of metabolic syndrome and diabetes are also replicated in the experimental models. Atherogenic index of plasma which assesses the risk of developing atherosclerosis log (TG/HDL-C) was also calculated. Universally, atherogenic index of plasma has been used by researchers as a significant predictor of atherosclerosis and as an independent cardiovascular risk factor. In the present study increase in the atherogenic index was observed in the HF-DC group as compared with NC group. Atherogenic dyslipidemia as evidenced by elevated serum triglyceride levels, increased levels of small dense low-density lipoprotein (sd LDL) particles, and decreased levels of HDL-C was observed in the HF-DC suggesting that the HF-DC rats are more prone to developing coronary artery diseases.

CPK-MB, an enzyme found primarily in the myocardium, is widely used to evaluate the existence and extent of myocyte injury [24]. When myocardial cells are damaged due to deficient oxygen supply or glucose, the integrity of cell membrane gets disturbed and it might become more porous which results in the leakage of these enzymes. The present study determined the CPK-MB levels to confirm the myocardial injury induced by High-Fat Diet and STZ in rats. The CPK-MB levels did not rise significantly at 4th week in the HF-DC group as compared to NC group. However, a significant increase in serum CPK-MB levels in HF-DC rats at 7th and 10th week as compared with NC was observed. The time course of changes in CPK-MB suggests that the deleterious cardiovascular changes are slow but progressive in nature. The study by Zhang et al. [24] (2014) showed increase in the CPK-MB levels in isoproterenol model of myocardial necrosis. However this cardiovascular marker of myocardial injury has not been studied so far in either the diabetic or diabetic with metabolic syndrome rats.

The myocardial injury induced by High-Fat Diet and STZ shown by biochemical marker was also confirmed by histopathological assessment. The present study showed that the HF-DC group rats subjected to HFD and STZ injury demonstrated marked edema, confluent areas of necrosis and separation of myofibers, congested blood vessels, and mild inflammation as compared to the NC group. The histology of the aorta of HF-DC group rats also showed atherosclerotic deposition in the vessel wall. Munshi et al. [22] (2014) also demonstrated similar fatty deposition in tunica intima of aorta and myocardial injury in hyperlipidemic rats. Similar to the present findings Renna et al. [25] (2014) also found raised hs-CRP in fructose fed hypertensive rats as compared with normal rats; similar results are shown by present study.

The other cardiac markers hs-CRP and systolic blood pressure were measured at 10th week of study and were found to be significantly raised in HF-DC group as compared with NC. Hypertension, one of the important components of metabolic syndrome, was mimicked successfully in the experimental model of diabetes and metabolic syndrome. Raised blood pressure confirmed presence of hypertension, one of the important components of metabolic syndrome in present experimental model induced by High-Fat Diet and STZ. The study by Kuate et al. [14] (2015) and Mamikutty et al. [23] (2014) also showed increase in systolic blood pressure in metabolic syndrome induced in rats by high carbohydrate and fructose diet.

Metabolic syndrome is also associated with an increased risk of nonalcoholic fatty liver disease and kidney dysfunction. The present study also confirmed a decline in hepatic and renal function as shown by biochemical findings and histopathological assessment. Hepatic cells of the HF-DC group showed degeneration, scattered necrotic cells, congestion in the central vein, and fat deposition as compared to NC. The HF-DC group rats also demonstrated congestion of glomerular blood vessels, tubular necrosis, inflammation, and cloudy degeneration as compared to NC group. Therefore, this model may also be used to study hepatic steatosis and nephropathy.

4.5. Uniqueness of the Animal Model of Metabolic Syndrome in the Setting of Diabetes Mellitus. There are no reported experimental models using High-Fat Diet and low dose streptozotocin where pathogenesis of diabetes with metabolic syndrome has been mimicked. However, recently, Kuate et al. [14] (2015) reported a model of high-carbohydrate, High-Fat Diet induced obese and type 2 diabetic rats with metabolic

syndrome features. This study aimed at evaluating the potential therapeutic action of the polyphenol-rich hydroethanolic extract (HET) of this fruit in experimentally induced obese and type 2 diabetic rats (T2DM) with characteristic metabolic syndrome (MetS). As reported by Kuate et al. [14], rats were fed high-carbohydrate, high-fat diet, for 7 weeks; subsequently STZ (30 mg/kg) was administered to produce diabetes. The test drug was further administered for 28 days. The experimental parameters were evaluated 4 weeks after induction of diabetes. However the present model is unique in the following ways. Only High-Fat Diet instead of high-carbohydrate, High-Fat Diet was used to induce metabolic syndrome. The present study has formulated a unique formulation of HFD which can be prepared indigenously in laboratory and is therefore feasible and cost effective. Dose of streptozotocin used is 40 mg/kg instead of 30 mg/kg used in the reported study. Induction of the features of metabolic syndrome and diabetes is faster. Feeding of high diets for 3 weeks results in metabolic syndrome compared to 7 weeks in the reported model. Long term changes produced by metabolic syndrome and diabetes are studied. This experimental model was monitored for 8 weeks after induction of the pathological features of metabolic syndrome and diabetes compared to 4 weeks in the reported model.

Absolute insulin deficiency (significant fall in serum insulin levels) in the HFD-diabetic control group rats as compared to normal control group rats was observed in the present model, in contrast to the model reported by Kuate et al. [14]. Deficiency of insulin levels as well as insulin resistance (increased HOMA-IR) was the hallmark of this animal model in contrast to only insulin resistance reported by Kuate et al. [14] to study the features of metabolic syndrome in the setting of diabetes mellitus. The biochemical results showed increase in blood glucose with concomitant decrease in insulin, C-peptide levels in conformity with histopathological findings. The pancreas of HF-DC group of rats demonstrated damaged islets of Langerhans, atrophy of beta cells, and reduced beta cell mass as compared to NC. It may be hypothesized that the beta cell mass was decreased in the HF-DC group rats resulting in decrease in secretion of insulin and C-peptide because of necrosis of pancreatic cell mass. Besides beta cell function (secretion of insulin), beta cell mass (intact beta cells available for insulin) has also been studied by histopathological and immunohistochemical studies. This would provide valuable information regarding the pathogenesis of the disease. Dyslipidemia resulting in alteration in the atherogenic index, subsequent deposition of fat droplets. and atherosclerosis in the thoracic aorta have also been studied to delineate the underlying mechanism of deleterious effects of altered lipid profile. The metabolic syndrome has become one of the most important diseases in this decade because of the marked increase in cardiovascular risk associated with a clustering of risk factors. Therefore studying the cardiovascular changes subsequent to diabetes as well as metabolic syndrome as undertaken in the present model has major clinical implications.

Thus, the present study has attempted to develop a unique rodent model of metabolic syndrome in the setting of diabetes mellitus. Although presently there is no perfect animal model of these comorbidities, the present study for the first time has successfully developed an experimental model with specific attributes (dyslipidemia, hypertension, and diabetes) that makes them useful for studying the mechanisms and potential therapies of metabolic syndrome in the setting of diabetes.

5. Conclusion

The present study has developed a unique rodent model of metabolic syndrome, with diabetes as an essential component. The developed model will be helpful in screening of different pharmacological compounds.

Conflict of Interests

The authors declare that there is no conflict of interests regarding the publication of this paper.

Acknowledgment

The study is funded by Indian Council of Medical Research vide grants received, no. 58/2/2014-BMS.

References

[1] K. G. M. M. Alberti, R. H. Eckel, S. M. Grundy et al., "Harmonizing the metabolic syndrome: a joint interim statement of the international diabetes federation task force on epidemiology and prevention; National Heart, Lung, and Blood Institute; American Heart Association; World Heart Federation; International Atherosclerosis Society; and International Association for the study of obesity," *Circulation*, vol. 120, no. 16, pp. 1640–1645, 2009.

[2] J. S. Torgerson, J. Hauptman, M. N. Boldrin, and L. Sjöström, "XENical in the Prevention of Diabetes in Obese Subjects (XENDOS) Study. A randomized study of orlistat as an adjunct to lifestyle changes for the prevention of type 2 diabetes in obese patients," *Diabetes Care*, vol. 27, no. 1, pp. 155–161, 2004.

[3] A. Guilherme, J. V. Virbasius, V. Puri, and M. P. Czech, "Adipocyte dysfunctions linking obesity to insulin resistance and type 2 diabetes," *Nature Reviews Molecular Cell Biology*, vol. 9, no. 5, pp. 367–377, 2008.

[4] K.-H. Yoon, J.-H. Lee, J.-W. Kim et al., "Epidemic obesity and type 2 diabetes in Asia," *The Lancet*, vol. 368, no. 9548, pp. 1681–1688, 2006.

[5] G. I. Bell and K. S. Polonsky, "Diabetes mellitus and genetically programmed defects in β-cell function," *Nature*, vol. 414, no. 6865, pp. 788–791, 2001.

[6] J. E. Shaw, R. A. Sicree, and P. Z. Zimmet, "Global estimates of the prevalence of diabetes for 2010 and 2030," *Diabetes Research and Clinical Practice*, vol. 87, no. 1, pp. 4–14, 2010.

[7] N. Unwin, D. Gan, and D. Whiting, "The IDF Diabetes Atlas: providing evidence, raising awareness and promoting action," *Diabetes Research and Clinical Practice*, vol. 87, no. 1, pp. 2–3, 2010.

[8] X.-K. Zheng, L. Zhang, W.-W. Wang, Y.-Y. Wu, Q.-B. Zhang, and W.-S. Feng, "Anti-diabetic activity and potential mechanism of total flavonoids of *Selaginella tamariscina* (Beauv.) Spring in

[9] S. Skovsø, "Modeling type 2 diabetes in rats using high fat diet and streptozotocin," *Journal of Diabetes Investigation*, vol. 5, no. 4, pp. 349–358, 2014.

[10] R. H. Unger, G. O. Clark, P. E. Scherer, and L. Orci, "Lipid homeostasis, lipotoxicity and the metabolic syndrome," *Biochimica et Biophysica Acta (BBA)—Molecular and Cell Biology of Lipids*, vol. 1801, no. 3, pp. 209–214, 2010.

[11] F. Franconi, G. Seghieri, S. Canu, E. Straface, I. Campesi, and W. Malorni, "Are the available experimental models of type 2 diabetes appropriate for a gender perspective?" *Pharmacological Research*, vol. 57, no. 1, pp. 6–18, 2008.

[12] K. Sahin, M. Onderci, M. Tuzcu et al., "Effect of chromium on carbohydrate and lipid metabolism in a rat model of type 2 diabetes mellitus: the fat-fed, streptozotocin-treated rat," *Metabolism: Clinical and Experimental*, vol. 56, no. 9, pp. 1233–1240, 2007.

[13] K. Srinivasan, B. Viswanad, L. Asrat, C. L. Kaul, and P. Ramarao, "Combination of high-fat diet-fed and low-dose streptozotocin-treated rat: a model for type 2 diabetes and pharmacological screening," *Pharmacological Research*, vol. 52, no. 4, pp. 313–320, 2005.

[14] D. Kuate, A. Pascale, N. Kengne, C. P. N. Biapa, B. G. K. Azantsa, and W. A. B. W. Muda, "Tetrapleura tetraptera spice attenuates high-carbohydrate, high-fat diet-induced obese and type 2 diabetic rats with metabolic syndrome features," *Lipids in Health and Disease*, vol. 14, article 50, 13 pages, 2015.

[15] E. L. B. Novelli, Y. S. Diniz, C. M. Galhardi et al., "Anthropometrical parameters and markers of obesity in rats," *Laboratory Animals*, vol. 41, no. 1, pp. 111–119, 2007.

[16] L. S. Mansor, E. R. Gonzalez, M. A. Cole et al., "Cardiac metabolism in a new rat model of type 2 diabetes using high-fat diet with low dose streptozotocin," *Cardiovascular Diabetology*, vol. 12, article 136, 10 pages, 2013.

[17] Y. Wang, T. Campbell, B. Perry, C. Beaurepaire, and L. Qin, "Hypoglycemic and insulin-sensitizing effects of berberine in high-fat diet- and streptozotocin-induced diabetic rats," *Metabolism: Clinical and Experimental*, vol. 60, no. 2, pp. 298–305, 2011.

[18] P. Kehkashan and A. S. Waseem, "Protective effect of butea monospora on high fat diet and streptozotocin-induced non-genetic rat model of type 2 diabetes: biochemical & histopathological evidence," *International Journal of Pharmacy and Pharmaceutical Sciences*, vol. 3, no. 3, pp. 74–81, 2011.

[19] N. M. El-Sheikh, "*Mangifera indica* leaves extract modulates serum leptin. Asymmetric dimethylarginine and endothelin-1 leaves in experimental diabetes mellitus," *Egyptian Journal of Biochemistry & Molecular Biology*, vol. 30, no. 2, pp. 229–244, 2012.

[20] A. A. Kamal, M. A. Ezzar, and A. N. Mohammad, "Effects of *panax quindue* of olium on streptozotocin induced diabetic rats: role of C-peptide. Nitric oxide & oxitadive stress," *International Journal of Clinical and Experimental Medicine*, vol. 4, no. 2, pp. 136–147, 2011.

[21] M. R. Shahraki, M. Harati, and A. R. Shahraki, "Prevention of high fructose-induced metabolic syndrome in male wistar rats by aqueous extract of *Tamarindus indica* seed," *Acta Medica Iranica*, vol. 49, no. 5, pp. 277–283, 2011.

[22] R. P. Munshi, S. G. Joshi, and B. N. Rane, "Development of an experimental diet model in rats to study hyperlipidemia and

insulin resistance, markers for coronary heart disease," *Indian Journal of Pharmacology*, vol. 46, no. 3, pp. 270–276, 2014.

[23] N. Mamikutty, Z. C. Thent, S. R. Sapri, N. N. Sahruddin, M. R. Mohd Yusof, and F. Haji Suhaimi, "The establishment of metabolic syndrome model by induction of fructose drinking water in male Wistar rats," *BioMed Research International*, vol. 2014, Article ID 263897, 8 pages, 2014.

[24] T. Zhang, S. Yang, and J. Du, "Protective effects of berberine on isoproterenol-induced acute myocardial ischemia in rats through regulating hmgb1-tlr4 axis," *Evidence-Based Complementary and Alternative Medicine*, vol. 2014, Article ID 849783, 8 pages, 2014.

[25] N. F. Renna, E. A. Diez, and R. M. Miatello, "Effects of dipeptidyl-peptidase 4 inhibitor about vascular inflammation in a metabolic syndrome model," *PLoS ONE*, vol. 9, no. 9, Article ID e106563, 2014.

Anti-Parkinson Activity of Petroleum Ether Extract of *Ficus religiosa* (L.) Leaves

Jitendra O. Bhangale and Sanjeev R. Acharya

Institute of Pharmacy, Nirma University, Ahmedabad, Gujarat 382 481, India

Correspondence should be addressed to Jitendra O. Bhangale; jitu2586@gmail.com

Academic Editor: Antonio Ferrer-Montiel

In the present study, we evaluated anti-Parkinson's activity of petroleum ether extract of *Ficus religiosa* (PEFRE) leaves in haloperidol and 6 hydroxydopamine (6-OHDA) induced experimental animal models. In this study, effects of *Ficus religiosa* (100, 200, and 400 mg/kg, p.o.) were studied using in vivo behavioral parameters like catalepsy, muscle rigidity, and locomotor activity and its effects on neurochemical parameters (MDA, CAT, SOD, and GSH) in rats. The experiment was designed by giving haloperidol to induce catalepsy and 6-OHDA to induce Parkinson's disease-like symptoms. The increased cataleptic scores (induced by haloperidol) were significantly ($p < 0.001$) found to be reduced, with the PEFRE at a dose of 200 and 400 mg/kg (p.o.). 6-OHDA significantly induced motor dysfunction (muscle rigidity and hypolocomotion). 6-OHDA administration showed significant increase in lipid peroxidation level and depleted superoxide dismutase, catalase, and reduced glutathione level. Daily administration of PEFRE (400 mg/kg) significantly improved motor performance and also significantly attenuated oxidative damage. Thus, the study proved that *Ficus religiosa* treatment significantly attenuated the motor defects and also protected the brain from oxidative stress.

1. Introduction

Parkinson's disease (PD) is caused by the gradual and selective loss of dopaminergic neurons in the substantia nigra pars compacta (SNpc) [1, 2]. PD produces bradykinesia, muscular rigidity, rest tremor, and loss of postural balance along with some secondary manifestations like dementia, sialorrhoea [3], soft speech, and difficulty in swallowing due to uncoordinated movements of mouth and throat [4]. PD occurs due to inhibition of mitochondrial complex-1 [5, 6], different mechanisms of cell damage like excitotoxicity, calcium homeostasis, inflammation, apoptosis, distressed energy metabolism, and protein aggregation [7], and interaction between genetic and environmental factors [8].

Oxidative stress interferes with dopamine metabolism leading to Parkinson's disease. This oxidative damage leads to formation of reactive oxygen species (ROS) leading to neuronal death [9, 10]. This was evidenced by reduced level of endogenous antioxidant compounds. These findings introduced the requirement of using antioxidants as a therapeutic intervention in PD in addition to other protective agents.

The current available drug treatments for PD possess various side effects. Therefore, herbal therapies should be considered as alternative/complementary medicines for therapeutic approach.

Since ancient times, plants have been an ideal source of medicine. Plants have played a noteworthy role in maintaining human health and improving the quality of life for thousands of years and have served humans as well, as valuable components of medicines, seasonings, beverages, cosmetics, and dyes. In modern times, focus on plant research has increased all over the world and a large body of evidence has been collected to demonstrate immense potential of medicinal plants used in various traditional systems. *Ficus religiosa* Linn. (Moraceae) commonly known as "Pimpala" or "Pipal" tree is a large widely deciduous tree, heart-shaped without aerial roots from the branches, with spreading branches and grey bark [11–13]. The tree is held sacred by Hindus and Buddhists. In India it is known by several vernacular names, the most commonly used ones being Asvatthah (Sanskrit), Sacred fig (Bengali), Peepal (Hindi),

Arayal (Malayalam), Ravi (Telugu), and Arasu (Tamil). Leaves contain campesterol, stigmasterol, isofucosterol, α-amyrin, lupeol, tannic acid, arginine, serine, aspartic acid, glycine, threonine, alanine, proline, tryptophan, tyrosine, methionine, valine, isoleucine, leucine, n-nonacosane, n-hentricontane, hexacosanol, and n-octacosane [14, 15]. *Ficus religiosa* has been used in traditional medicine for a wide range of ailments. Its bark, fruits, leaves, roots, latex, and seeds are medicinally used in different forms, sometimes in combination with other herbs [16]. The whole parts of the plant exhibit wide spectrum of activities such as anti-cancer, antioxidant, antidiabetic, antimicrobial, anticonvulsant, anthelmintic, antiulcer, antiasthmatic, and antiamnesic activities. Bark of the plant has been used as astringent, cooling, aphrodisiac, and antibacterial against *Staphylococcus aureus* and *Escherichia coli*, gonorrhea, diarrhea, dysentery, hemorrhoids, and gastrohelcosis, as anti-inflammatory, and for burns. The leaves of the plant have been used for hemoptysis, epistaxis, hematuria, menorrhagia, blood dysentery, and skin diseases. Leaf juice has been used for asthma, cough, sexual disorders, diarrhea, hematuria, toothache, migraine, eye troubles, gastric problems, and scabies. Fruits of the plant were used in asthma and as laxative and digestive. Seeds of the plant were used as refrigerant and laxative and latex was used in neuralgia, inflammations, and hemorrhages [17]. As *F. religiosa* has been used traditionally in the treatment of neurodegenerative disorders (including Parkinson's disease) and has also been reported to possess antioxidant activity, this plant may prove to be effective in the remedy of PD. Hence *F. religiosa* was evaluated for its anti-Parkinson's effect using neurotoxin induced Parkinson's model in rats.

2. Materials and Methods

2.1. Collection of Plant Material. Fresh leaves of *Ficus religiosa* were collected from local area of Ahmedabad district, Gujarat, India, during July–September. This plant was identified and authenticated by Dr. A. Benniamin, Scientist D, Botanical Survey of India, Pune. Voucher specimens number BSI/WC/Tech./2015/JOB-1 have been kept in Botanical Survey of India, Pune, Maharashtra, India.

2.2. Animals. Adult male Wistar rats, weighing 180–220 g, and albino mice of either sex weighing 25–30 g were used and acclimatized to laboratory condition for one week. All animals were housed in well-ventilated polypropylene cages at 12 : 12 h light/dark schedule at $25 \pm 2°C$ and 55–65% RH. The rats were fed with commercial pelleted rats chow and water *ad libitum* as a standard diet. Institutional Animal Ethics Committee approved the experimental protocol in accordance with the Committee for the Purpose of Control and Supervision of Experiments on Animals (CPCSEA).

2.3. Preparation of Leaf Extract. The leaves were collected and dried in shade and ground. Coarsely powdered plant material (1000 g) was weighed and extracted with 5 lit of solvents like petroleum ether (60–80°C), ethyl acetate, and ethanol by successive extraction in a Soxhlet apparatus for 72 h. After each extraction, the solvent was distilled off and concentrated extract was transferred to previously weighed petri dish and evaporated to dryness at room temperature (45–50°C) to obtain dried extracts. The dried extract was weighed and the percentage yield of the extracts was calculated as follows:

$$\% \text{ of extractive yield (w/w)} = \frac{\text{Weight of dried extract}}{\text{Weight of dried leaves powder}} \times 100. \tag{1}$$

The yield of petroleum ether, ethyl acetate, and ethanol extract was 18.2, 10.6, and 26.8% (w/w), respectively.

2.4. Preliminary Phytochemical Studies. Preliminary qualitative phytochemical screening was done for the presence of different group of chemicals, that is, alkaloids, flavonoids, saponins, tannins, sterols, carbohydrates, and glycosides, as described by Harborne [18].

2.4.1. Test for Tannins and Phenols. 5 mL of extract was added to 2 mL of 5% of alcoholic $FeCl_3$ solution. Blue-Black precipitate indicated the presence of tannins and phenols.

2.4.2. Test for Alkaloids. To the dry extract (10–20 mg), dilute hydrochloric acid (1-2 mL) was added, shaken well, and filtered. With filtrate, the following tests were performed.

(1) Mayer's Test. To 2-3 mL of filtrate, 2-3 drops of Mayer's reagent were added. Appearance of precipitate indicated presence of alkaloids.

(2) Wagner's Test. To 2-3 mL of filtrate, Wagner's (3–5 drops) reagent was added. Appearance of reddish-brown precipitate indicated presence of alkaloids.

(3) Hager's Test. To 2-3 mL of filtrate, 4-5 drops of Hager's reagent were added. Appearance of yellow precipitate indicated presence of alkaloids.

(4) Dragendorff's Test. To 2-3 mL of filtrate, 4-5 drops of Dragendorff's reagent were added. Appearance of orange-brown precipitate indicated presence of alkaloids.

2.4.3. Test for Saponins. About 1 g of dried powdered sample was boiled with 10 mL distilled water. Frothing persistence indicated the presence of saponins.

2.4.4. Test for Terpenoids. 5 mL of extract was mixed with 2 mL of chloroform and few drops of concentrated H_2SO_4 were carefully added to form a layer. Red ring indicated that the terpenoids are present.

2.4.5. Test for Steroids (Liebermann-Burchard Reaction). 5 mL of extract was mixed with 10 mL $CHCl_3$ and 1 mL acetic anhydride and few drops of concentrated H_2SO_4 were added. Green ring indicated the presence of steroids.

2.4.6. Test for Flavonoids (Shinoda Test). To dry extract (10–20 mg), 5 mL of ethanol (95%), 2-3 drops of hydrochloric acid, and 0.5 g magnesium turnings were added. Change of color of solution to pink indicated presence of flavonoids.

2.4.7. Test for Carbohydrates (Molisch's Test). Few drops (2-3) of α-naphthol solution in alcohol were added to 2-3 mL of solution of extract and shaken for few minutes and then 0.5 mL of conc. sulfuric acid was added from the side of test tube. The formation of violet ring at the junction of two solutions indicated presence of carbohydrates.

2.4.8. Test for Glycosides

(1) Legal's Test. To the extract, 1 mL of pyridine and 1 mL of sodium nitroprusside were added. Change in color to pink or red indicated presence of cardiac glycosides.

(2) Keller-Kiliani Test. Glacial acetic acid (3–5 drops), one drop of 5% ferric chloride, and concentrated sulfuric acid was added to the test tube containing 2 mL of solution of extract. Appearance of reddish-brown color at the junction of two layers and bluish green in the upper layer indicated presence of cardiac glycosides.

(3) Borntrager's Test. Dilute sulfuric acid was added to 2 mL of solution of extract, boiled for few minutes, and filtered. To the filtrate, 2 mL of benzene or chloroform was added and shaken well. The organic layer was separated and ammonia was added. The change in color of ammoniacal layer to pink red indicated presence of anthraquinone glycosides.

2.4.9. Test for Phlobatannins. About 2 mL of extract was boiled with 2 mL 1% HCl. Deposition of red color indicated the presence of phlobatannins.

2.4.10. Test for Amino Acid (Ninhydrin Test). 5 to 6 drops of Ninhydrin reagent were added in 5 mL of extract and heated over boiling water bath for 5 min. Purple coloration indicated the presence of amino acid.

2.4.11. Test for Proteins (Biuret Test). 5-6 drops of 5% NaOH and 5-7 drops of 1% $CuSO_4$ were added in 2 mL of extract. Violet color indicated the presence of protein.

2.5. Acute Oral Toxicity of the Extract. The mice were divided into 5 groups of 10 animals each. The mice were fasted for 6 h and had access to only water *ad libitum* before experimental study. Group I received only vehicle (distilled water). Groups II, III, IV, and V received different doses of pet. ether extract of *F. religiosa* (PEFRE), that is, 1000, 2000, 3000, and 4000 mg/kg, respectively. All the doses and vehicle were administered orally. The animals were observed for 72 h for mortality [19].

2.6. Haloperidol Induced Catalepsy. Haloperidol causes dysfunctioning of various neurotransmitters such as acetylcholine, GABA, and serotonin. Pathology of haloperidol induced catalepsy underlying increased oxidative stress. Haloperidol, an antipsychotic drug, blocks central dopamine receptor in striatum. It also produces a behavioral state in animals like mice and rats in which they fail to correct externally imposed postures (called catalepsy); thus, keeping the above fact in mind, the haloperidol induced catalepsy model was selected. The method described by Elliott and Close in 1990 [20] was followed for the anticataleptic activity. The animals were divided into five groups (n = 6). Group I served as vehicle control, Group II served as standard, Levodopa (6 mg/kg, p.o.), and Groups III–V served as test group treated with PEFRE (100, 200, and 400 mg/kg, p.o.), respectively. Standard bar test was used to measure the catalepsy. Catalepsy was induced by haloperidol (1 mg/kg, i.p.) and examined at every 30 min interval for 210 min. The duration for which the rat retains the forepaws extended and resting on the elevated bar was considered as cataleptic score. A cut-off time of 5 min was applied.

2.7. Induction of Parkinsonism by 6-OHDA. The rats were anesthetized with an intraperitoneal injection of 50 mg/kg of sodium pentobarbital and were fixed in a stereotaxic apparatus [21, 22]. A stainless steel needle (0.28 mm o.d) was inserted unilaterally into the substantia nigra with the following coordinates: anterior/posterior: −4.8 mm; medial/lateral: −2.2 mm; ventral/dorsal: −7.2 mm–3.5 mm from bregma, and injection of 6-OHDA (20 μg of 6-OHDA hydrobromide in 4 μL 0.9% saline with 0.02 μg/mL ascorbic acid) was then made over 5 min and the needle was left in place for a further 5 min. Then the skull was secured with stainless metallic screws and the wound area was covered by dental cement. Each rat was housed individually following the surgical procedure. Sham operated animals were also treated in the same manner, but they received equivalent volumes of normal saline instead of 6-OHDA.

2.8. Experimental Design. Animals were divided into six groups of 6 rats in each group. Group I served as sham operated animals and received normal saline (10 mL/kg, p.o.); Groups II to VI were induced with parkinsonism by 6-OHDA as follows: Group II served as a 6-OHDA control and received normal saline (10 mL/kg), Group III served as a L DOPA (6 mg/kg, p.o.), and Groups IV to VI served as a test drug, PEFRE (100, 200, and 400 mg/kg, p.o., resp.). The treatment of animals was started after 48 h of induction with 6-OHDA according to their respective group once a day for 55 days.

2.9. Behavioral Assessment. All behavioral assessment was performed by an observer blinded to the group. Different tests were performed at different time points after lesion.

2.9.1. Locomotor Activity. The spontaneous locomotor activity was monitored using digital actophotometer (Hicon instrument, India) equipped with infrared sensitive photocells. The apparatus was placed in a darkened, light and sound attenuated, and ventilated testing room. Each interruption of a beam on the x or y axis generated an electric impulse, which was presented on a digital counter. Each animal was observed over a period of 5 min on days 15, 20, 25, 30, 35, 40, 45, 50, and 55 following 6-OHDA administration and values were expressed as counts per 5 min [23].

2.9.2. Rotarod Activity. All animals were evaluated for grip strength by using the rotarod. The rotarod test is widely used in rodents to assess their "minimal neurological deficit" such as motor function and coordination. Each rat was given a prior training session before initialization of therapy to acclimatize them on a rotarod apparatus (EIE instrument, India). Animal was placed on the rotating rod with a diameter of 7 cm (speed 25 rpm). Each rat was subjected to three separate trials at 5 min interval on days 15, 20, 25, 30, 35, 40, 45, 50, and 55 following 6-OHDA administration and cut-off time (180 s) was maintained throughout the experiment. The average results were recorded as fall of time [24].

2.10. Dissection and Homogenization. After the treatment period, animals were scarified by decapitation under mild anesthesia. The brains were immediately removed, forebrain was dissected out, and cerebellum was discarded. Brains were put on ice and rinsed in ice-cold isotonic saline to remove blood. A 10% (w/v) tissue homogenate was prepared in 0.1 M phosphate buffer (pH 7.4). The homogenate was centrifuged at 10,000 g for 15 minutes and aliquots of supernatant obtained were used for biochemical estimation.

2.11. Biochemical Estimation

2.11.1. Malondialdehyde (MDA) Level. The amount of malondialdehyde was used as an indirect measure of lipid peroxidation and was determined by reaction with thiobarbituric acid (TBA) [25]. Briefly, 1 mL of aliquots of supernatant was placed in test tubes and added to 3 mL of TBA reagent: TBA 0.38% (w/w), 0.25 M hydrochloric acid (HCl), and trichloroacetic acid (TCA 15%). The solution was shaken and placed for 15 min, followed by cooling in an ice bath. After cooling, solution was centrifuged to 3500 g for 10 min. The upper layer was collected and assessed with a spectrophotometer at 532 nm. All determinations were made in triplicate. Results were expressed as nanomoles per mg of protein. The concentration of MDA was calculated using the formula

$$\text{Conc. of MDA} = \frac{\text{Abs}_{532} \times 100 \times V_T}{(1.56 \times 10^5) \times W_T \times V_U}, \quad (2)$$

where Abs_{532} is absorbance, V_T is total volume of mixture (4 mL), 1.56×10^5 is molar extinction coefficient, W_T is weight of dissected brain (1 g), and V_U is aliquot volume (1 mL).

2.11.2. Superoxide Dismutase (SOD) Level. SOD activity was determined according to the method described by Beyer and Fridovich in 1987 [26]. 0.1 mL of supernatant was mixed with 0.1 mL EDTA (1×10^{-4} M), 0.5 mL of carbonate buffer (pH 9.7), and 1 mL of epinephrine (1 mM). The optical density

of formed adrenochrome was read at 480 nm for 3 min on spectrophotometer. The enzyme activity was expressed in terms of U/min/mg. One unit of enzyme activity is defined as the concentration required for the inhibition of the chromogen production by 50% in one minute under the defined assay conditions.

2.11.3. Catalase (CAT) Level. The catalase activity was assessed by the method of Aebi in 1974 [27]. The assay mixture consists of 0.05 mL of supernatant of tissue homogenate (10%) and 1.95 mL of 50 mM phosphate buffer (pH 7.0) in 3 mL cuvette. 1 mL of 30 mM hydrogen peroxide (H_2O_2) was added and changes in absorbance were followed for 30 s at 240 nm at 15 s intervals. The catalase activity was calculated using the millimolar extinction coefficient of H_2O_2 (0.071 mmol cm^{-1}) and the activity was expressed as micromoles of H_2O_2 oxidized per minute per milligram protein:

CAT activity

$$= \frac{\delta\text{O.D.}}{E \times \text{Vol. of Sample (mL)} \times \text{mg of protein}}, \quad (3)$$

where $\delta\text{O.D.}$ is change in absorbance/minute; E is extinction coefficient of hydrogen peroxide (0.071 mmol cm^{-1}).

2.11.4. GSH Level (Reduced Glutathione). For the estimation of reduced glutathione, the 1 mL of tissue homogenate was precipitated with 1 mL of 10% TCA. To an aliquot of the supernatant, 4 mL of phosphate solution and 0.5 mL of 5,5′-dithiobis-(2-nitrobenzoic acid) (DTNB) reagent were added and absorbance was taken at 412 nm [28]. The values were expressed as nM of reduced glutathione per mg of protein:

$$\text{GSH level} = \frac{Y - 0.00314}{0.0314} \times \frac{D_F}{B_T \times V_U}, \quad (4)$$

where Y is Abs_{412} of tissue homogenate, D_F is dilution factor (1), B_T is brain tissue homogenate (1 mL), and V_U is aliquot volume (1 mL).

2.12. Histopathological Studies. The brains from control and experimental groups were fixed with 10% formalin and embedded in paraffin wax and cut into longitudinal section of 5 μm thickness. The sections were stained with hemotoxylin and eosin dye for histopathological observation.

2.13. Statistical Analysis. All the values were expressed as mean ± SEM. Statistical evaluation of the data was done by one-way ANOVA (between control and drug treatments) followed by Dunnett's t-test for multiple comparisons and two-way ANOVA followed by Bonferroni's multiple comparison test, with the level of significance chosen at $p < 0.001$ using Graph-Pad Prism 5 (San Diego, CA) software.

3. Results

3.1. Phytochemical Screening. Table 1 showed the phytochemical screening of the different extract of *F. religiosa*.

TABLE 1: Phytochemical investigation of *F. religiosa* Linn. leaves.

Sr. number	Name of test	Pet. ether	Ethyl acetate	Ethanol
1	Tannins and phenols	−ve	−ve	+ve
2	Alkaloids	+ve	+ve	+ve
3	Saponins	−ve	−ve	−ve
4	Terpenoids	−ve	+ve	+ve
5	Steroids	−ve	−ve	−ve
6	Flavonoids	−ve	+ve	+ve
7	Carbohydrates	−ve	−ve	−ve
8	Glycosides	−ve	−ve	+ve
9	Phlobatannins	−ve	−ve	−ve
10	Amino acid	−ve	−ve	−ve
11	Protein	−ve	−ve	−ve

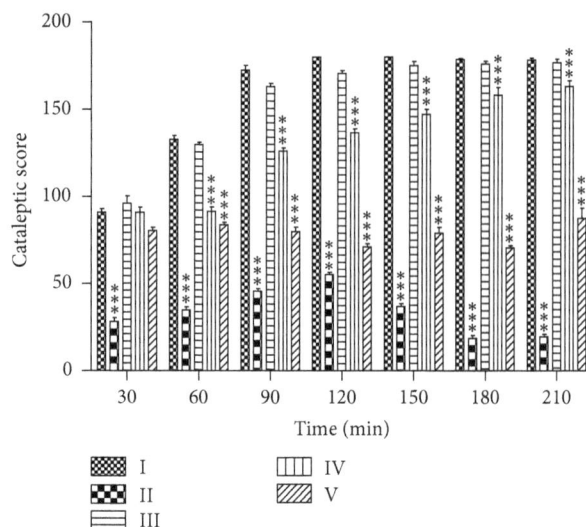

FIGURE 1: Effect of PEFRE on haloperidol induced catalepsy in rats. Group I: vehicle control group; Group II: Levodopa + haloperidol treated group; Group III: PEFRE (100 mg/kg) + haloperidol treated group; Group IV: PEFRE (200 mg/kg) + haloperidol treated group; Group V: PEFRE (400 mg/kg) + haloperidol treated group. $^{***}p < 0.001$ as compared to Vehicle treated control group.

3.2. Acute Toxicity. The PEFRE was found to be safe at all the doses used and there was no mortality found up to the dose of 4000 mg/kg of PEFRE when administered orally. Therefore, we have taken 400 mg/kg as the therapeutic dose and made variations by taking 100 mg/kg as lower dose and 400 mg/kg as higher dose.

3.3. The Effects of PEFRE on Haloperidol Induced Catalepsy. Chronic oral administration of higher doses of PEFRE (200 and 400 mg/kg) showed significant ($p < 0.001$) reduction in cataleptic score from 60 min to 210 min as compared to vehicle treated animals. Administration of PEFRE (100 mg/kg) did not show significant activity. Treatment with Levodopa (6 mg/kg) significantly ($p < 0.001$) reduced duration of catalepsy as compared to vehicle treated group (Figure 1).

3.4. The Effects of PEFRE on 6-OHDA Induced Parkinson's Disease

3.4.1. The Effects of PEFRE on 6-OHDA Induced Parkinson's Disease in the Locomotor Activity. Total locomotor activity of rats in 6-OHDA treated group was significantly ($p < 0.001$) reduced as compared to vehicle treated group. Oral administration of PEFRE of different doses (200 and 400 mg/kg) showed significant ($p < 0.001$) increase in the locomotor activity from day 20 to 55 as compared to 6-OHDA treated control animals. Administration of PEFRE (100 mg/kg) did not show significant activity. Levodopa (6 mg/kg) significantly ($p < 0.001$) increased locomotor activity (Figure 2).

3.4.2. The Effects of PEFRE on 6-OHDA Induced Parkinson's Disease in the Rotarod Performance. Treatment with 6-OHDA significantly decreased the fall of time when compared to the vehicle control animals. Chronic oral administration of PEFRE (200 and 400 mg/kg) significantly ($p < 0.001$) increased the fall of time when compared to 6-OHDA group from day 15 to day 55. Levodopa (6 mg/kg) significantly ($p < 0.001$) increased the fall of time as compared to 6-OHDA group. Administration of PEFRE (100 mg/kg) did not show significant activity (Figure 3).

3.4.3. The Effects of PEFRE on 6-OHDA Induced Parkinson's Disease in MDA, CAT, SOD, and GSH Level. Administration of 6-OHDA resulted in significant changes in biochemical parameters when compared to the vehicle control animals. The inoculation of 6-OHDA induced oxidative stress, as indicated by increased MDA level, and decreased CAT, SOD, and GSH levels when compared to vehicle control animals in brain levels. The treatment with pet. ether extract of FRE (400 mg/kg, p.o.) showed significant ($p < 0.001$) decrease in MDA level compared to OHDA rats. Similarly, daily administration of PEFRE (400 mg/kg) attenuated the increase in SOD and CAT activity with 6-OHDA treated group. Pretreatment with PEFRE (400 mg/kg) significantly ($p < 0.001$) increased GSH levels in the brain as compared to 6-OHDA treated animals, thus preventing the reduction in GSH induced by 6-OHDA (Table 2).

3.4.4. Effect of PEFRE on Histopathological Changes in the Brain of Normal and 6-OHDA Treated Animals. The histopathological study showed that neurotoxins, that is, 6-OHDA, caused marked hypertrophic changes, increased intracellular space, infiltration of neutrophils, decreased density of cells, alterations of architecture, hemorrhage, and neuronal damage and even cell death. Furthermore, many neurons were shrunken, pyknotic, and darkly stained with small nuclei (Figure 4(b)) compared with normal vehicle treated rats (Figure 4(a)). There is significant reversal of neuronal damage or neuronal alterations observed in Levodopa (6 mg/kg) treated rats (Figure 4(c)) and PEFRE treated rats at doses of 200 (Figure 4(e)) and 400 mg/kg (Figure 4(f)). Treatment with PEFRE (100 mg/kg) did not show significant recovery of neuronal damage (Figure 4(d)).

TABLE 2: Effect of PEFRE on the levels of lipid peroxidation (MDA), catalase (CAT), superoxide dismutase (SOD), and reduced glutathione (GSH) in the brain of 6-OHDA treated animals.

Group	MDA (nM/mg of protein)	CAT (μmoles of H_2O_2 used/min/mg protein)	SOD (units/mg protein)	GSH (nM/mg of protein)
Vehicle control	1.311 ± 0.09315	5.788 ± 0.046	3.185 ± 0.1852	4.371 ± 0.07576
6-OHDA control	$2.616 \pm 0.1602^{\#}$	$3.463 \pm 0.035^{\#}$	$2.06 \pm 0.1068^{\#}$	$3.985 \pm 0.020^{\#}$
Levodopa	$1.659 \pm 0.03551^{**}$	$6.525 \pm 0.20^{***}$	$9.667 \pm 0.8333^{***}$	$7.023 \pm 0.6013^{***}$
PEFRE (100)	2 ± 0.1558	3.544 ± 0.15	2.419 ± 0.8732	4.182 ± 0.01312
PEFRE (200)	1.975 ± 0.2153	4.234 ± 0.11	2.801 ± 0.5034	4.614 ± 0.1312
PEFRE (400)	$1.347 \pm 0.2501^{***}$	$6.22 \pm 0.31^{***}$	$8.833 \pm 0.8333^{***}$	$8.455 \pm 0.03936^{***}$

Values are expressed as mean ± SEM. $^{*}p < 0.05$, $^{**}p < 0.01$, and $^{***}p < 0.001$ as compared to 6-OHDA treated control group (Group II) [Groups III to VI were compared with Group II], $^{\#}p < 0.001$ as compared to vehicle treated group (Group I) [Group II was compared with Group I].

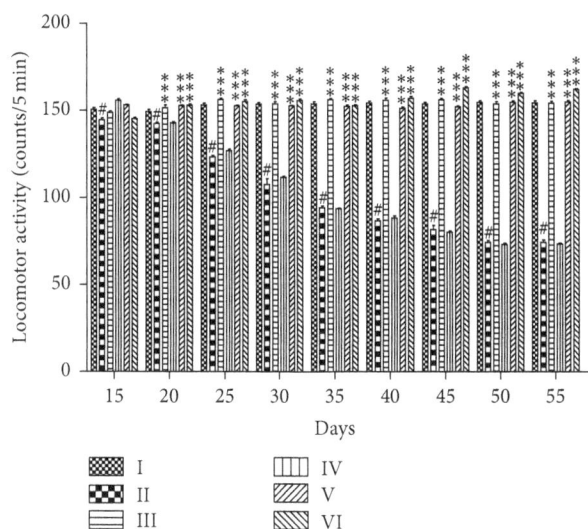

FIGURE 2: The effects of PEFRE on 6-OHDA induced Parkinson's disease in the Locomotor activity. Group I: Vehicle control group; Group II: 6-OHDA treated group; Group III: Levodopa + 6-OHDA treated group; Group IV: PEFRE (100 mg/kg) + 6-OHDA treated group; Group V: PEFRE (200 mg/kg) + 6-OHDA treated group; Group VI: PEFRE (400 mg/kg) + 6-OHDA treated group. $^{***}p < 0.001$ as compared to 6-OHDA treated negative control group (Group II). $^{\#}p < 0.001$ in 6-OHDA treated negative control group (Group II) compared to vehicle treated control group (Group I).

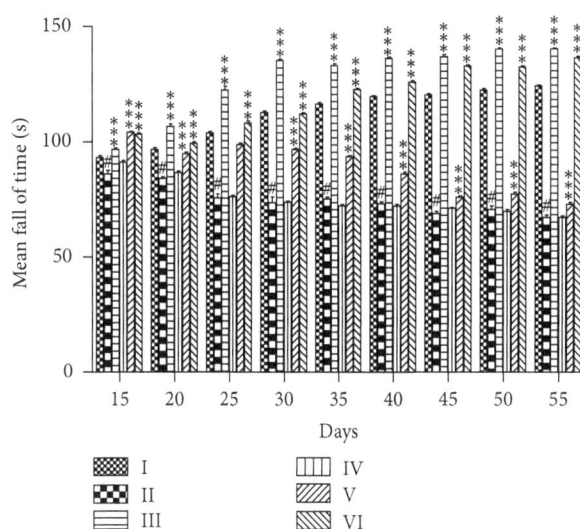

FIGURE 3: The effects of PEFRE on 6-OHDA induced Parkinson's disease in the rotarod performance. Group I: vehicle control group; Group II: 6-OHDA treated group; Group III: Levodopa + 6-OHDA treated group; Group IV: PEFRE (100 mg/kg) + 6-OHDA treated group; Group V: PEFRE (200 mg/kg) + 6-OHDA treated group; Group VI: PEFRE (400 mg/kg) + 6-OHDA treated group. $^{***}p < 0.001$ as compared to 6-OHDA treated negative control group (Group II). $^{\#}p < 0.001$ 6-OHDA treated negative control group (Group II) compared to vehicle treated control group (Group I).

4. Discussion

Parkinson's disease is a chronic neurodegenerative disorder characterized by loss of dopamine neurons of the SNpc. The pathogenesis of PD includes oxidative stress, protein accumulation like a-synuclein, mitochondrial dysfunction, apoptosis, and neuronal excitotoxicity. Among all, oxidative stress is a crucial pathological mechanism for PD. SNpc is more vulnerable to reactive oxygen species as it contains more amount of dopamine.

In the present study, we evaluated the effect of pet. ether extract of *F. religiosa* in neurotoxins (haloperidol and 6-OHDA) induced Parkinson disease in experimental animals.

Haloperidol induced catalepsy is a widely accepted animal model of PD. Haloperidol (nonselective D_2 dopamine

antagonists) provides a pharmacological model of parkinsonism by interfering with the storage of catecholamine's intracellularly, resulting in dopamine depletion in nerve endings. In the present study, haloperidol (1 mg/kg, i.p.) induced significant catalepsy in rats as evidenced by a significant increase in the time spent on the block as compared to vehicle treated animals. Treatment with *F. religiosa* significantly reduced the catalepsy in haloperidol treated rats in dose dependent manner. The PEFRE at doses of 200 and 400 mg/kg showed protective effect against haloperidol induced catalepsy indicated that this plant has an ability to protect dopaminergic neurotransmission in striatum.

There are well-known pharmacological PD models in mammalian systems including the classical and highly selective neurotoxin 6-hydroxydopamine (6-OHDA), as well as 1-methyl-4-phenyl-1,2,3,6-tetrahydropyridine (MPTP) and its

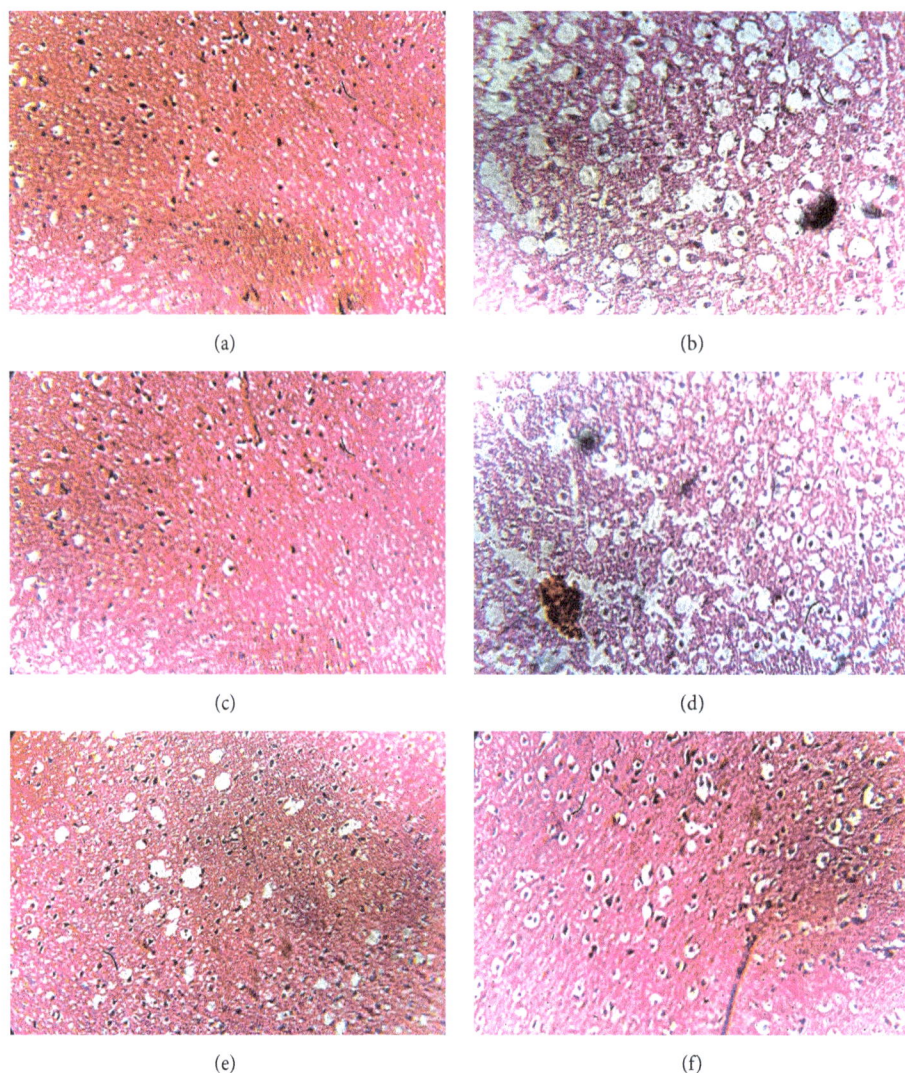

FIGURE 4: Effect of PEFRE on histopathological changes in the brain of normal and 6-OHDA treated animals (H&E staining; original magnification, 40x). (a) Normal control showing normal brain architecture. (b) Rats treated with 6-OHDA showing degeneration of neurons. (c) Rats treated with 6-OHDA and Levodopa (6 mg/kg) showing minimal changes in neuronal cell integrity and architecture. (d) Rats treated with 6-OHDA and PEFRE (100 mg/kg) showing mild decrease in neurons and cellular hypertrophy. (e) PEFRE (200 mg/kg) and (f) PEFRE (400 mg/kg) treated rats showing minimal changes in neuronal cell populations.

metabolite, MPP+ (1-methyl-4-phenylpyridinium ion). These toxins cause decreased ATP production, increased ROS production, and increased apoptosis of DAergic cells [29].

The efficacy of $F. religiosa$ in 6-OHDA induced PD has not been well established. In the present study, 6-OHDA administration to rats caused a significant decrease in locomotor activity and muscle activity. Lack of motor coordination and maintenance of normal limb posture has been reported in PD condition. The evaluated data suggested damage to the dopaminergic neurons and progression of Parkinson's disease like behavioral abnormalities in rats exposed to 6-OHDA. Pretreatment of rats with PEFRE at the doses of 200 and 400 mg/kg exhibited significant increase in locomotor activity and increase in muscle activity and thus could be proved with possible action on CNS.

Oxidative stress generated as a result of mitochondrial dysfunction particularly mitochondrial complex-1 impairment plays an important role in the pathogenesis of PD. The oxidative stress was measured through determination of levels of malondialdehyde, catalase, superoxide dismutase, and reduced glutathione in the brain tissue.

6-OHDA generates an increase in the production of hydrogen peroxide and free radicals [30, 31]. These reactive oxygen species are generated through the nonenzymatic breakdown of 6-OHDA or direct inhibition of complex-I and complex-IV of the mitochondrial electron transport chain [31–33]. The resulting ROS production from 6-OHDA breakdown leads to lipid peroxidation, protein denaturation, and increases in glutathione, which are found in PD patients [34].

Lipid peroxidation, a sensitive marker of oxidative stress, was estimated by measuring the levels of thiobarbituric acid. Lipid peroxidation occurs due to attack by radicals on double bond of unsaturated fatty acid and arachidonic acid which generate lipid peroxyl radicals and that initiate a chain reaction of further attacks on other unsaturated fatty acid. As we know, lipid peroxidation is the process of oxidative degradation of polyunsaturated fatty acids and its occurrence in biological membranes causes impaired membrane function, impaired structural integrity [35], decreased fluidity, and inactivation of number of membrane bound enzymes. Increased levels of the lipid peroxidation product have been found in the substantia nigra of PD patient. In the present investigation, similar results were observed in the brain homogenate of 6-OHDA treated control animals.

Catalase is an antioxidant which helps in neutralizing the toxic effects of hydrogen peroxide. Hydrogen peroxide is converted by the catalase enzyme to form water and nonreactive oxygen species, thus preventing the accumulation of precursor to free radical biosynthesis. Oxidative stress results in decrease in catalase level. 6-OHDA inoculation in rats induced oxidative stress, as indicated by a decrease in the catalase levels.

Superoxide dismutase (known as SOD) is an enzyme which acts as a catalyst in the process of dismutation of superoxide into nonreactive oxygen species and hydrogen peroxide. It is therefore a critical antioxidant defense which is present in nearly all cells which are exposed to oxygen [36, 37]. Superoxide dismutase helps in neutralizing the toxic effects of free radicals [38, 39]. 6-OHDA treated control group showed a decrease in the level of SOD in the brain of animals, thus indicative of production of oxidative stress.

GSH, potent enzymes, are an important factor in etiology of PD [40]. The depletion of reduced glutathione in the substantia nigra in Parkinson's disease could be the result of neuronal loss. As a matter of fact, the positive correlation has been found to exist between the extent of neuronal loss and depletion of glutathione [41]. A decrease in the availability of reduced glutathione would impair the capacity of neurons to detoxify hydrogen peroxide and increase the risk of free radical formation and lipid peroxidation. A reduction in GSH levels was evident in 6-OHDA treated control animals.

Thus, the 6-OHDA per se group showed a significant increase in the levels of thiobarbituric acid (which is an indication of extent of lipid peroxidation) and decrease in the levels of SOD and GSH in the brain as compared to the vehicle treated control animals. All these indicate an increase in the oxidative stress in the brain of animals treated with 6-OHDA. Pretreatment with higher dose of petroleum ether extract of $F.$ $religiosa$ (400 mg/kg) resulted in a decrease in MDA level and increase in the levels of SOD, catalase, and GSH, indicating its antioxidant effect in the brain of 6-OHDA treated animals.

Histopathological findings showed that pet. ether extract of $Ficus religiosa$ treated animals had decreased infiltration of neutrophils, reduced intracellular space, increased density of cells, and regained normal architecture and moderate necrosis in striatum region of brain.

5. Conclusion

In view of the above facts, we are concluding that petroleum ether extract of $Ficus religiosa$ plant showed to be an antioxidant and showed a promising effect in animals with Parkinson's disease. And we appreciate further detailed molecular studies with this drug in anti-Parkinson's pharmacology and toxicology and also characterization of active constituents responsible for neuroprotective effect.

Conflict of Interests

The authors declare that there is no conflict of interests regarding the publication of this paper.

References

[1] M. F. Beal, "Mitochondrial dysfunction in neurodegenerative diseases," *Biochimica et Biophysica Acta (BBA)—Bioenergetics*, vol. 1366, no. 1-2, pp. 211–223, 1998.

[2] P. Jenner and C. W. Olanow, "The pathogenesis of cell death in Parkinson's disease," *Neurology*, vol. 66, no. 10, supplement 4, pp. S24–S36, 2006.

[3] A. E. Lang and A. M. Lozano, "Parkinson's disease: second of two parts," *The New England Journal of Medicine*, vol. 339, no. 16, pp. 1130–1143, 1998.

[4] L. Scott, "Identifying poor symptom control in Parkinson's disease," *Nursing Times*, vol. 102, no. 12, pp. 30–32, 2006.

[5] Y. Mizuno, S. Ohta, M. Tanaka et al., "Deficiencies in complex-I subunits of the respiratory chain in Parkinson's disease," *Biochemical and Biophysical Research Communications*, vol. 163, no. 3, pp. 1450–1455, 1989.

[6] W. J. Schmidt and M. Alam, "Controversies on new animal models of Parkinson's disease pro and con: the rotenone model of Parkinson's Disease (PD)," *Journal of Neural Transmission*, vol. 70, pp. 273–276, 2006.

[7] T. J. Collier and C. E. Sortwell, "Therapeutic potential of nerve growth factors in Parkinson's disease," *Drugs and Aging*, vol. 14, no. 4, pp. 261–287, 1999.

[8] T. B. Sherer, R. Betarbet, and J. T. Greenamyre, "Environment, mitochondria, and Parkinson's disease," *Neuroscientist*, vol. 8, no. 3, pp. 192–197, 2002.

[9] L. Chen, Y. Ding, B. Cagniard et al., "Unregulated cytosolic dopamine causes neurodegeneration associated with oxidative stress in mice," *The Journal of Neuroscience*, vol. 28, no. 2, pp. 425–433, 2008.

[10] F. Zoccarato, P. Toscano, and A. Alexandre, "Dopamine-derived dopaminochrome promotes H_2O_2 release at mitochondria complex-1," *Journal of Biological Chemistry*, vol. 280, no. 16, pp. 15587–15594, 2005.

[11] A. Ghani, *Medicinal Plants of Bangladesh with Chemical Constituents and Uses*, Asiatic Society of Bangladesh, Dhaka, Bangladesh, 1998.

[12] D. Singh and R. K. Goel, "Anticonvulsant effect of *Ficus religiosa*: role of serotonergic pathways," *Journal of Ethnopharmacology*, vol. 123, no. 2, pp. 330–334, 2009.

[13] P. V. Prasad, P. K. Subhaktha, A. Narayana, and M. M. Rao, "Medico-historical study of 'aśvattha' (sacred fig tree)," *Bulletin of the Indian Institute of History of Medicine (Hyderabad)*, vol. 36, no. 1, pp. 1–20, 2006.

[14] S. K. Panda, N. C. Panda, and B. K. Sahue, "Phytochemistry and pharmacological properties of *Ficus religiosa*: an overview," *Indian Veterinary Journal*, vol. 60, pp. 660–664, 1976.

[15] R. S. Verma and K. S. Bhatia, "Chromatographic study of amino acids of the leaf protein concentrates of *Ficus religiosa* Linn and *Mimusops elengi* Linn," *Indian Journal of Pharmacy Practice*, vol. 23, pp. 231–232, 1986.

[16] O. A. Aiyegoro and A. I. Okoh, "Use of bioactive plant products in combination with standard antibiotics: implications in antimicrobial chemotherapy," *Journal of Medicinal Plants Research*, vol. 3, no. 13, pp. 1147–1152, 2009.

[17] P. K. Warrier, *Indian Medicinal Plants—A Compendium of 500 Species*, vol. 3, Orient Longman, Chennai, India, 1996.

[18] J. B. Harborne, *Phytochemical Methods*, Chapman and Hall, London, UK, 3rd edition, 1998.

[19] V. Ravichandran, B. Suresh, M. N. Sathishkumar, K. Elango, and R. Srinivasan, "Antifertility activity of hydroalcoholic extract of *Ailanthus excelsa* (Roxb): an ethnomedicines used by tribals of Nilgiris region in Tamilnadu," *Journal of Ethnopharmacology*, vol. 112, no. 1, pp. 189–191, 2007.

[20] P. J. Elliott and S. P. Close, "Neuroleptic-induced catalepsy as a model of Parkinson's disease I. Effect of dopaminergic agents," *Journal of Neural Transmission. Parkinson's Disease and Dementia Section*, vol. 2, no. 2, pp. 79–89, 1990.

[21] R. Deumens, A. Blokland, and J. Prickaerts, "Modeling Parkinson's disease in rats: an evaluation of 6-OHDA lesions of the nigrostriatal pathway," *Experimental Neurology*, vol. 175, no. 2, pp. 303–317, 2002.

[22] S. Wang, L.-F. Hu, Y. Yang, J.-H. Ding, and G. Hu, "Studies of ATP-sensitive potassium channels on 6-hydroxydopamine and haloperidol rat models of Parkinson's disease: implications for treating Parkinson's disease?" *Neuropharmacology*, vol. 48, no. 7, pp. 984–992, 2005.

[23] D. S. Reddy and S. K. Kulkarni, "Possible role of nitric oxide in the nootropic and antiamnesic effects of neurosteroids on aging- and dizocilpine-induced learning impairment," *Brain Research*, vol. 799, no. 2, pp. 215–229, 1998.

[24] S. RajaSankar, T. Manivasagam, V. Sankar et al., "*Withania somnifera* root extract improves catecholamines and physiological abnormalities seen in a Parkinson's disease model mouse," *Journal of Ethnopharmacology*, vol. 125, no. 3, pp. 369–373, 2009.

[25] H. Ohkawa, N. Ohishi, and K. Yagi, "Assay for lipid peroxides in animal tissues by thiobarbituric acid reaction," *Analytical Biochemistry*, vol. 95, no. 2, pp. 351–358, 1979.

[26] W. F. Beyer Jr. and I. Fridovich, "Assaying for superoxide dismutase activity: some large consequences of minor changes in conditions," *Analytical Biochemistry*, vol. 161, no. 2, pp. 559–566, 1987.

[27] H. Aebi, "Catalase in vitro," in *Methods in Enzymology*, vol. 105, pp. 121–126, Academic Press, New York, NY, USA, 1984.

[28] S. K. Srivastava and E. Beutler, "Accurate measurement of oxidized glutathione content of human, rabbit, and rat red blood cells and tissues," *Analytical Biochemistry*, vol. 25, pp. 70–76, 1968.

[29] F. Blandini and M.-T. Armentero, "Animal models of Parkinson's disease," *FEBS Journal*, vol. 279, no. 7, pp. 1156–1166, 2012.

[30] G. Cohen and R. E. Heikkila, "The generation of hydrogen peroxide, superoxide radical, and hydroxyl radical by 6-hydroxydopamine, dialuric acid, and related cytotoxic agents," *The Journal of Biological Chemistry*, vol. 249, no. 8, pp. 2447–2452, 1974.

[31] D. G. Graham, S. M. Tiffany, W. R. Bell Jr., and W. F. Gutknecht, "Autoxidation versus covalent binding of quinones as the mechanism of toxicity of dopamine, 6-hydroxydopamine, and related compounds toward C1300 neuroblastoma cells in vitro," *Molecular Pharmacology*, vol. 14, no. 4, pp. 644–653, 1978.

[32] Y. Y. Glinka and M. B. H. Youdim, "Inhibition of mitochondrial complexes I and IV by 6-hydroxydopamine," *European Journal of Pharmacology*, vol. 292, no. 3-4, pp. 329–332, 1995.

[33] Y. Glinka, M. Gassen, and M. B. H. Youdim, "Mechanism of 6-hydroxydopamine neurotoxicity," *Journal of Neural Transmission, Supplement*, no. 50, pp. 55–66, 1997.

[34] P. Jenner and C. W. Olanow, "Understanding cell death in Parkinson's disease," *Annals of Neurology*, vol. 44, no. 3, pp. S72–S84, 1998.

[35] B. Halliwell and J. M. C. Gutteridge, "Oxygen radicals and the nervous system," *Trends in Neurosciences*, vol. 8, pp. 22–26, 1985.

[36] L. S. Monk, K. V. Fagerstedt, and R. M. Crawford, "Oxygen toxicity and superoxide dismutase as an antioxidant in physiological stress," *Physiologia Plantarum*, vol. 76, no. 3, pp. 456–459, 1989.

[37] C. Bowler, M. Van Montagu, and D. Inzé, "Superoxide dismutase and stress tolerance," *Annual Review of Plant Physiology and Plant Molecular Biology*, vol. 43, no. 1, pp. 83–116, 1992.

[38] J. G. Scandalios, "Response of plant antioxidant defense genes to environmental stress," *Advances in Genetics*, vol. 28, pp. 1–41, 1990.

[39] E. B. Gralla and D. J. Kosman, "Molecular genetics of superoxide dismutases in yeasts and related fungi," *Advances in Genetics*, vol. 30, pp. 251–319, 1992.

[40] P. Jenner, "Oxidative mechanisms in nigral cell death in Parkinson's disease," *Movement Disorders*, vol. 13, no. 1, pp. 24–34, 1998.

[41] P. Riederer, E. Sofic, W.-D. Rausch et al., "Transition metals, ferritin, glutathione, and ascorbic acid in Parkinsonian brains," *Journal of Neurochemistry*, vol. 52, no. 2, pp. 515–520, 1989.

Permissions

List of Contributors

Waleed Barakat
Department of Pharmacology, Faculty of Pharmacy, Zagazig University, Zagazig 44519, Egypt
Department of Pharmacology, Faculty of Pharmacy, Tabuk University, Tabuk 71491, Saudi Arabia

Shimaa M. Elshazly and Amr A. A. Mahmoud
Department of Pharmacology, Faculty of Pharmacy, Zagazig University, Zagazig 44519, Egypt

Mona Fouad Mahmoud, Sara Zakaria and Ahmed Fahmy
Department of Pharmacology and Toxicology, Faculty of Pharmacy, University of Zagazig, Zagazig 44519, Egypt

Sarah Mousavi
Department of Clinical Pharmacy and Pharmacy Practice, Faculty of Pharmacy and Pharmaceutical Sciences, Isfahan University of Medical Sciences, Isfahan, Iran

Mandana Moradi
Faculty of Pharmacy, Zabol University of Medical Sciences, Zabol, Iran

Tina Khorshidahmad and Maryam Motamedi
Faculty of Pharmacy, Tehran University of Medical Sciences, Tehran, Iran

Md. Khalilur Rahman
Department of Pharmacology, Dongguk University, Gyeongju 780-714, Republic of Korea

Md. Ashraf Uddin Chowdhury and Mohammed Taufiqual Islam
Department of Systems Immunology, Kangwon National University, Chuncheon 200-701, Republic of Korea

Md. Anisuzzaman Chowdhury
Department of Pharmacy, Chosun University, Gwangju 61452, Republic of Korea

Muhammad Erfan Uddin
Department of Pharmacy, International Islamic University Chittagong, Chittagong 4203, Bangladesh

Chandra Datta Sumi
Department of Systems Biotechnology, Chung-Ang University, Anseong 456-756, Republic of Korea

Gregory Smutzer and Roni K. Devassy
Department of Biology, Temple University, 1900 N. 12th Street, Philadelphia, PA 19122, USA

Venkata Saibabu, Zeeshan Fatima and Saif Hameed
Amity Institute of Biotechnology, Amity University Haryana, Gurgaon, Manesar 122413, India

Luqman Ahmad Khan
Department of Biosciences, Jamia Millia Islamia, NewDelhi 110025, India

Ambika Srivastava, Pooja Singh and Rajesh Kumar
Department of Chemistry, Centre of Advanced Study, Faculty of Science, Banaras Hindu University, Varanasi 221005, India

Debasree Deb
Department of Pharmacology, Melaka Manipal Medical College, Manipal University, Manipal Campus, Manipal 576104, India

K. L. Bairy and Veena Nayak
Department of Pharmacology, Kasturba Medical College, Manipal University, Manipal 576104, India

Mohandas Rao
Department of Anatomy, Melaka Manipal Medical College, Manipal University, Manipal Campus, Manipal 576104, India

Bayu Lestari
Biomedical Sciences, Medical Faculty, Brawijaya University, Malang 65145, Indonesia
Department of Pharmacology, Medical Faculty, Brawijaya University, Malang 65145, Indonesia

Nur Permatasari
Department of Pharmacology, Medical Faculty, Brawijaya University, Malang 65145, Indonesia

Mohammad Saifur Rohman
Department of Cardiology and Vascular Medicine, Medical Faculty, Brawijaya University, Saiful Anwar General Hospital, Malang 65145, Indonesia

Sara M. Robledo, Karen Ligardo, Jéssica Henao, Natalia Arbeláez, Andrés Montoya and Iván D. Vélez
1PECET, Medical Research Institute, School of Medicine, University of Antioquia (UdeA), Calle 70, No. 52-21, A.A. 1226, Medellín, Colombia

Wilson Cardona, Juan M. Pérez and Jairo Sáez
Chemistry of Colombian Plants, Institute of Chemistry, Exact and Natural Sciences School, University of Antioquia (UdeA), Calle 70, No. 52-21, A.A. 1226, Medellín, Colombia

Fernando Alzate
Botanical Studies, Institute of Biology, Exact and Natural Sciences School, University of Antioquia (UdeA), Calle 70, No. 52-21, A.A. 1226, Medellín, Colombia

Victor Arango
Pharmacy School, University of Antioquia (UdeA), Calle 70, No. 52-21, A.A. 1226, Medellín, Colombia

Alis Guillén and Kevin Eduardo Rivas
Molecular Genetics Group, University of Antioquia, Calle 70, No. 52-21, A.A. 1226, Medell´ın, Colombia

Sergio Granados
Department of Physiology and Biochemistry, School of Medicine, University of Antioquia, Calle 70, No. 52-21, A.A. 1226, Medellín, Colombia

Omar Estrada
Laboratory of Cellular Physiology, Center of Biophysic and Biochemistry, IVIC, Carretera Panamericana km 11, Altos de Pipe, Caracas, Venezuela

Luis Fernando Echeverri
Group of Organic Natural Product Chemistry, Faculty of Natural and Exact Sciences, University of Antioquia, Calle 70, No. 52-21, A.A. 1226, Medell´ın, Colombia

Norman Balcázar
Molecular Genetics Group, University of Antioquia, Calle 70, No. 52-21, A.A. 1226, Medellín, Colombia
Department of Physiology and Biochemistry, School of Medicine, University of Antioquia, Calle 70, No. 52-21, A.A. 1226, Medellín, Colombia

Somayeh Moradi and Farahnaz Jazaeri
Department of Pharmacology, School of Medicine, Tehran University of Medical Sciences, Tehran, Iran

Vahid Nikoui
Razi Institute for Drug Research, Iran University of Medical Sciences, Tehran, Iran
Department of Pharmacology, Faculty of Medicine, Iran University of Medical Sciences, Tehran, Iran

Muhammad Imran Khan
Department of Pharmacology, School of Medicine, International Campus, Tehran University of Medical Sciences, Tehran, Iran

Shayan Amiri and Azam Bakhtiarian
Department of Pharmacology, School of Medicine, Tehran University of Medical Sciences, Tehran, Iran
Experimental Medicine Research Center, Tehran University of Medical Sciences, Tehran, Iran

Desak Gede Budi Krisnamurti
Department of Medical Pharmacy, Faculty of Medicine, University of Indonesia, Jakarta 10430, Indonesia

Melva Louisa
Department of Pharmacology and Therapeutics, Faculty of Medicine, University of Indonesia, Jakarta 10430, Indonesia

Erlia Anggraeni
Master Program in Biomedicine, Faculty of Medicine, University of Indonesia, Jakarta 10430, Indonesia

Septelia Inawati Wanandi
Department of Biochemistry and Molecular Biology, Faculty of Medicine, University of Indonesia, Jakarta 10430, Indonesia

Ermita I. Ibrahim Ilyas, Busjra M. Nur, Sonny P. Laksono and Anton Bahtiar
Department of Physiology, Faculty of Medicine, University of Indonesia, Jakarta 10430, Indonesia

Ari Estuningtyas, Caecilia Vitasyana and Frans D. Suyatna
Department of Pharmacology and Therapeutics, Faculty of Medicine, University of Indonesia, Jakarta 10430, Indonesia

Dede Kusmana
National Cardiovascular Center, Harapan Kita Hospital and Department of Cardiology and Vascular Medicine, University of Indonesia, Jakarta 10430, Indonesia

Muhammad Kamil Tadjudin
Department of Medical Biology, Faculty of Medicine, University of Indonesia, Jakarta 10430, Indonesia

Hans-Joachim Freisleben
Medical Research Unit, Faculty of Medicine, University of Indonesia, Jakarta 10430, Indonesia

Amir R. Afshari
Pharmacological Research Center of Medicinal Plants, School of Medicine, Mashhad University of Medical Sciences, Mashhad 917794-8564, Iran

Hamid R. Sadeghnia
Pharmacological Research Center of Medicinal Plants, School of Medicine, Mashhad University of Medical Sciences, Mashhad 917794-8564, Iran
Neurocognitive Research Center, School of Medicine, Mashhad University of Medical Sciences, Mashhad 917794-8564, Iran

Hamid Mollazadeh
Neurocognitive Research Center, School of Medicine, Mashhad University of Medical Sciences, Mashhad 917794-8564, Iran

Gaurav Gupta
Department of Life Science, School of Pharmacy, International Medical University, Bukit Jalil, Kuala Lumpur 57000, Malaysia
School of Medicine and Public Health, University of Newcastle, Newcastle, NSW 2308, Australia

Tay Jia Jia, Lim Yee Woon, Dinesh Kumar Chellappan and Mayuren Candasamy
Department of Life Science, School of Pharmacy, International Medical University, Bukit Jalil, Kuala Lumpur 57000, Malaysia

Kamal Dua
School of Biomedical Science, University of Newcastle, Newcastle, NSW 2308, Australia

Mohamed Naguib Zakaria
Department of Pharmacology and Toxicology, Faculty of Pharmacy, Zagazig University, Zagazig 44519, Egypt

HanyM. El-Bassossy
Department of Pharmacology and Toxicology, Faculty of Pharmacy, Zagazig University, Zagazig 44519, Egypt

Waleed Barakat
Department of Pharmacology and Toxicology, Faculty of Pharmacy, Zagazig University, Zagazig 44519, Egypt
Department of Pharmacology, Faculty of Pharmacy, University of Tabuk, Tabuk 71491, Saudi Arabia

Gokhan Zengin, Abdurrahman Aktumsek and Ramazan Ceylan
Department of Biology, Science Faculty, Selçuk University Campus, 42250 Konya, Turkey

Gokalp Ozmen Guler
Department of Biological Education, Ahmet Keles□ğlu Education Faculty, Necmettin Erbakan University, 42090 Konya, Turkey

Carene Marie Nancy Picot and M. Fawzi Mahomoodally
Department of Health Sciences, Faculty of Science, University of Mauritius, 230 Réduit, Mauritius

Tahereh Safari
Department of Physiology, Zahedan University of Medical Sciences, Isfahan, Iran

Mehdi Nematbakhsh
Water & Electrolytes Research Center, Isfahan University of Medical Sciences, Isfahan, Iran
Department of Physiology, Isfahan University of Medical Sciences, Isfahan, Iran
Isfahan MN Institute of Basic & Applied Sciences Research, Isfahan, Iran

Roger G. Evans and KateM. Denton
Department of Physiology, Monash University, Clayton, VIC, Australia

Syed Suhail Andrabi and Suhel Parvez
Department of Medical Elementology and Toxicology, Jamia Hamdard (Hamdard University), New Delhi 110062, India

Heena Tabassum
Department of Medical Elementology and Toxicology, Jamia Hamdard (Hamdard University), New Delhi 110062, India
Department of Biochemistry, Jamia Hamdard (Hamdard University), New Delhi 110062, India

Fatemeh Forouzanfar
Neurocognitive Research Center, School of Medicine, Mashhad University of Medical Sciences, Mashhad 917794-8564, Iran

Shaghayegh Torabi
Pharmacological Research Center of Medicinal Plants, School of Medicine, Mashhad University of Medical Sciences, Mashhad 917794-8564, Iran

Vahid R. Askari
Department of Pharmacology, School of Medicine, Mashhad University of Medical Sciences, Mashhad 917794-8564, Iran

Elham Asadpour
Anesthesiology and Critical Care Research Center, Shiraz University of Medical Sciences, Shiraz, Iran

Hamid R. Sadeghnia
Neurocognitive Research Center, School of Medicine, Mashhad University of Medical Sciences, Mashhad 917794-8564, Iran
Pharmacological Research Center of Medicinal Plants, School of Medicine, Mashhad University of Medical Sciences, Mashhad 917794-8564, Iran
Department of Pharmacology, School of Medicine, Mashhad University of Medical Sciences, Mashhad 917794-8564, Iran

Manish Kumar and Siva Hemalatha
Pharmacognosy Research Laboratory, Department of Pharmaceutics, Indian Institute of Technology (Banaras Hindu University), Varanasi 221005, India

Satyendra K. Prasad
Pharmacognosy Research Laboratory, Department of Pharmaceutics, Indian Institute of Technology (Banaras Hindu University), Varanasi 221005, India
Department of Pharmaceutical Sciences, R. T. M. Nagpur University, Nagpur 440033, India

Aghdas Dehghani and Shadan Saberi
Water & Electrolytes Research Center, Isfahan University of Medical Sciences, Isfahan 81745, Iran
Department of Physiology, Isfahan University of Medical Sciences, Isfahan 81745, Iran

Mehdi Nematbakhsh
Water & Electrolytes Research Center, Isfahan University of Medical Sciences, Isfahan 81745, Iran
Department of Physiology, Isfahan University of Medical Sciences, Isfahan 81745, Iran
IsfahanMN Institute of Basic & Applied Sciences Research, Isfahan 81546, Iran

Inass Leouifoudi and Abdelmajid Zyad
Laboratory of Biological Engineering, Faculty of Science and Technologies, Sultan Moulay Slimane University, 23 000 Beni-Mellal, Morocco

Hicham Harnafi
Laboratory of Biochemistry, Faculty of Science, Mohamed First University, 60 000 Oujda, Morocco

Urmeela Taukoorah and M. Fawzi Mahomoodally
Department of Health Sciences, Faculty of Science, University of Mauritius, 230 Réduit, Mauritius

Hadi Darvishi Khezri, Mehrnoush Kosaryan, Aily Aliasgharian, Hossein Jalali and Arash Hadian Amree
Thalassemia Research Center, Mazandaran University of Medical Sciences, Sari, Iran

Ebrahim Salehifar
Faculty of Pharmacy, Thalassemia Research Center, Mazandaran University of Medical Sciences, Sari 48175-861, Iran

Nayan G. Patel
Department of Pharmacology and Toxicology, Faculty of Pharmacy, Dharmsinh Desai University, College Road, Nadiad, Gujarat 387001, India

Kalpana G. Patel
Department of Quality Assurance, Anand Pharmacy College, Shri Ram Krishna Seva Mandal Campus, Near Town Hall, Anand, Gujarat 388001, India

Kirti V. Patel
Department of Pharmacology, Pharmacy Department, The MS University of Baroda, Vadodara, Gujarat 390002, India

Tejal R. Gandhi
Department of Pharmacology, Anand Pharmacy College, Shri Ram Krishna Seva Mandal Campus, Near Town Hall, Anand, Gujarat 388001, India

Rajesh Kumar Suman, Ipseeta Ray Mohanty, Manjusha K. Borde and Y. A. Deshmukh
Department of Pharmacology, MGM Medical College, Kamothe, Navi Mumbai 410209, India

Ujwala Maheshwari
Department of Pathology, MGM Medical College, Kamothe, Navi Mumbai 410209, India

Jitendra O. Bhangale and Sanjeev R. Acharya
Institute of Pharmacy, Nirma University, Ahmedabad, Gujarat 382 481, India

www.ingramcontent.com/pod-product-compliance
Lightning Source LLC
Chambersburg PA
CBHW080459200326
41458CB00012B/4026